PIERO VENEZIA

PASQUALE LACASELLA - ALESSIO CASUCCI - ALESSANDRO IELASI

Esthetics and function in complete denture prosthesis

DIGITAL PERSPECTIVES

Forewords by Gaetano Calesini and Mauro Fradeani

edra

Original title

Piero Venezia, Pasquale Lacasella, Alessio Casucci, Alessandro Ielasi
Estetica e funzione in protesi totale. Prospettive digitali*

ISBN 978-88-214-5025-9

* The Authors would like to thank Dr. **Francesca Izzi,** Dentist, for her precious help in revising the texts.

Book Publishing Manager: Costanza Smeraldi

Paper, Printing and Binding Manager: Paolo Ficicchia

Translation: Axis Italia, Milano, Italy

Copyediting: ALTER EDOM s.r.l., Noventa Padovana (PD), Italy

ISBN: 978-88-214-5027-3
eISBN: 978-88-214-5028-0

Edra S.p.A.
Via G. Spadolini, 7
20141 Milan
Ph. 02 881841
www.edizioniedra.it

Printed by "Starprint" S.r.l., January 2022

(*) Edra S.p.A. belongs to the LSWR GROUP

PIERO VENEZIA

Graduated summa cum laude in Dentistry at the University of Bari in 1989.
Specialisation in Esthetic prosthetics at the University of Siena in 2003.
Specialisation in Prosthetics at the University of Bari, where he also carried out teaching activities.

Lecturer in post-graduate specialisation master courses at the Universities of Siena, Genoa, Naples, Bari, Foggia, Catania and Rome.
Adjunt Professor in Prosthetic Dentistry.
Contract Professor for teaching Prosthetics at the Degree Course in Dentistry of the University of Catania.

Active member of the Italian Academy of Prosthetic Dentistry (Accademia Italiana di Odontoiatria Protesica, AIOP).
Active member of the International Academy for Digital Dental Medicine (IADDM).

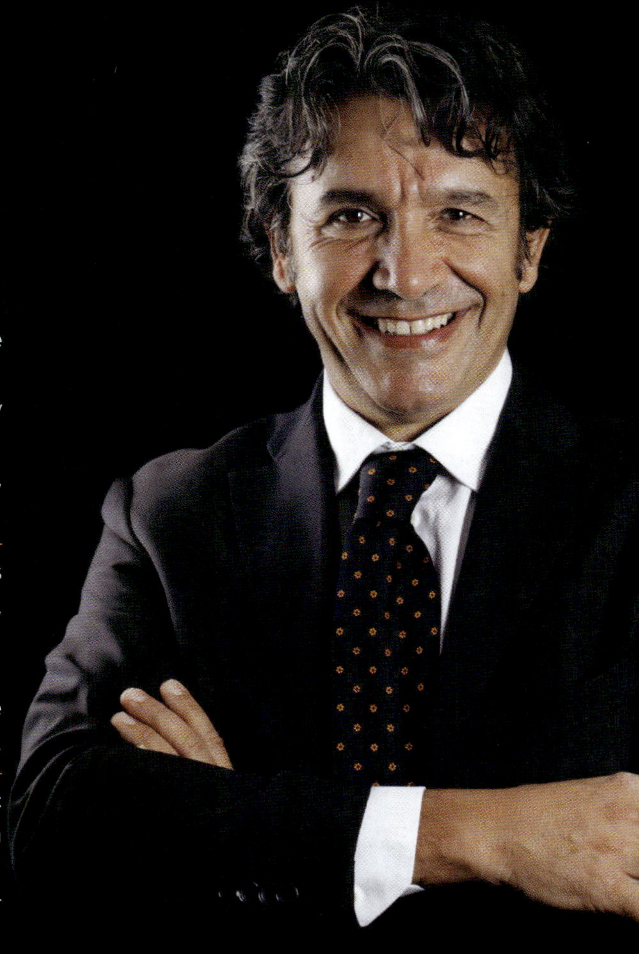

CO-AUTHORS

Pasquale Lacasella

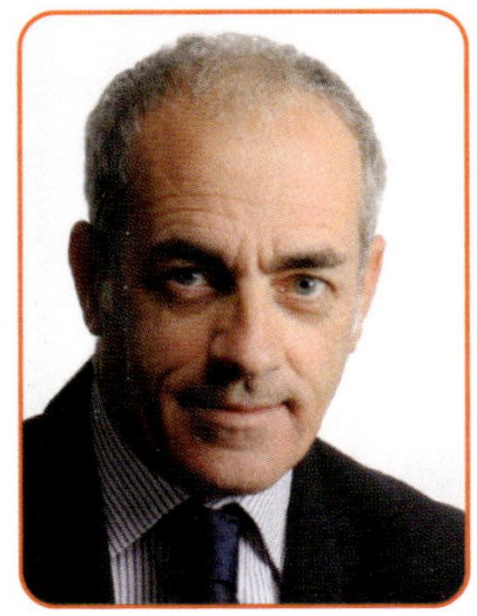

Dental technician graduated at the IPSIA Santarella school of Bari in 1985.
Specialised in complete prostheses.

Member of the Italian Academy of Prosthetic Dentistry (Accademia Italiana di Odontoiatria Protesica, AIOP).
Cultural manager of the National Association of Owners of Dental Technician Laboratory (ANTLO) Apulia.
Member of the Digital Dentistry Society (DDS).
Member of ITI (International Team for Implantology).

Author of articles concerning complete prostheses published on nationally and internationally distributed journals.

He deals with pre-implant design aimed at complex rehabilitations.
Co-owner of the Apulia Dental Lab snc laboratory in Bari.

Alessio Casucci

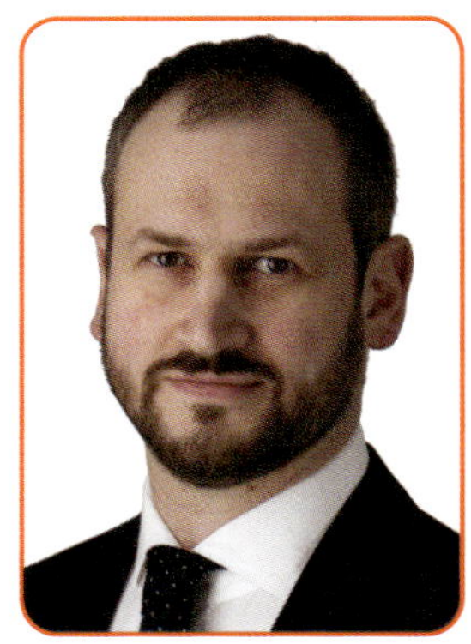

Graduated summa cum laude in Dentistry at the University of Siena.
Masters Degree in Periodontology and Master of Science in Dental Biomaterials at the University of Siena, where he also obtained an international PhD in Dental Biomaterials and their Clinical Applications.

Member of IADR (International Association for Dental Research), ICP (International College of Prosthodontics).
Lecturer on complete and implant-supported prostheses. Author of a number of publications in nationally and internationally distributed journals.

He carries out his clinical activity with a special focus on the issues concerning the rehabilitation of the edentulous patient in Montepulciano (Siena).

Alessandro Ielasi

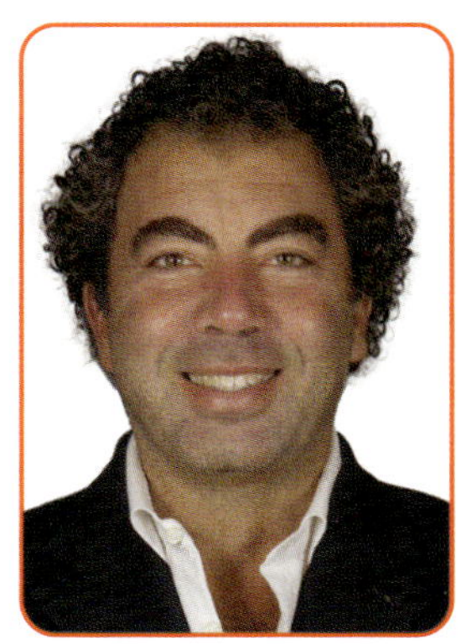

Dental technician graduated from the Fermi School of Perugia. He has attended the Zollo Laboratory since 1996 to further increase his knowledge of Complete prostheses.

Both in 2014 and 2015, he was awarded the 1st Polcan prize at the International Congress of the Italian Academy of Prosthetic Dentistry (Accademia Italiana di Odontoiatria Protesica, AIOP) for a case presented with Dr. Alessio Casucci.

Active Member of the Italian Academy of Prosthetic Dentistry (Accademia Italiana di Odontoiatria Protesica, AIOP). He carries out his work in Ischia (Naples).

CONTRIBUTORS

Salvatore D'amato
Associate Professor in Maxillofacial Surgery,
"Luigi Vanvitelli" University of Campania
Active member of the Italian Academy of Esthetic Dentistry (IAED)

Raffaele Cavalcanti
Contract professor in Periodontology,
University of Catania
Active Member of SIdP
Fellow ITI (International Team for Implantology)

Eliseo Sammarco
Member of AIC and AIOP
Practitioner in Manduria (TA)

Vincenzo Santomauro
Fellow ITI (International Team for Implantology)
Practitioner in Battipaglia (SA)

ACKNOWLEDGEMENTS

To my family, for their encouragement and support over the years. To my father Emilio who has supported and encouraged my choices and my mother Enza who, together with Elisabetta, has always stood by me, even at the most difficult times.
To Emilia, Federica and Gaia who have always borne my absences with patience and understanding.

This book could not have been published if I had not had Pasquale Lacasella by my side in the last twenty years – a friend, a truly great dental technician and a great human being: he deserves all my gratitude.

I have learned a lot from my mentors (Gaetano Calesini and Mauro Fradeani) and so much also from my dental technician friends with whom I had the good fortune to work (Lino Cipriani, Francesco Grieco, Dino Gallo, Francesco De Giovanni, Giuliano Vitale, Vincenzo L'afflitto, Aldo Grammatica, Michele Signorile and Domenico Cascione).

Special thanks to my long-time assistants who have helped me so much and have put up with me: Nunzia Carofiglio, Marika Ladisa, Stella Parrucci, Antonella Dinardo.

Finally, I'd like to thank all the friends who have collaborated in different yet essential ways to writing this book: Raffaele Cavalcanti (with whom, together with Nicola Cavalvanti, I share the duties and rewards of our office in Bari), Salvatore D'Amato, Vincenzo Santomauro and Eliseo Sammarco.
Special thanks to Paola Sammaritano of Edra, my guardian angel, who with thoroughness, timeliness and gentleness guided me in writing the book, and to my friend Massimo Gagliani who strongly believed in the fact that this beautiful idea could eventually turn into reality.

Piero Venezia

FOREWORD

When Piero Venezia asked me to write the introduction to this book, written with the participation of Dr. Casucci and of Master dental Technicians Lacasella and Ielasi I was happy to accept for several reasons.
Dr. Venezia was one of my brightest students in the nineties. We have been close friends since then and I am always happy to see his conference lectures. What is more, he plays a leading role in the family of active members of the Italian Academy of Prosthetic Dentistry, of which I am also honoured to be a member.
As professionals and mentors, we cannot teach our successors only what we know technically. The techniques are linked to our times and having been born in different eras from those of our successors, many of our favourite techniques are set to die out with us.
However, there are two values that we have a moral obligation to pass on as inheritance to those who follow: strict basic knowledge that will form the roots of their human and professional future and the wings of creativity that will allow them to evolve. In 1967, I was starting my first year as a student at the "George Eastman" school for dental technicians of Rome, a truly exclusive place, with only one course per year. There were fewer than twenty students in my course.
I still have a clear memory of three key points from the opening lesson given by Prof. Profili, an enlightened dental technician who in addition to being the principal of the school was a removable prosthesis enthusiast.
The first was a broad overview on the future of materials in dental technology. These were the years when some dental technicians had begun pioneering the use of dental ceramics in Italy but, unlike all the others, he predicted that the future would see the prevalence of polymers with much better performance than dental ceramics. Personally, I am also convinced that, in the long term, polymers will prevail over dental ceramics.
The second topic of his lectio magistralis concerned the pride of being a dental technician and choosing to only team up with good clinicians, establishing a close relationship "between equals" while respecting each other's skills, a concept that I found again a few decades later as an integral part of the Articles of Association of the Italian Academy of Prosthetic Dentistry.

He prophesied that within a few decades it would become much, much more difficult to find a good professional in the field of dental technology than in the clinical sector. He was right also on that point.

The third point concerned the recommendation not to snub the complete prosthesis since it was not the poor relative of the fixed prosthesis but, on the contrary, it was its "noble mother". Later, in the early eighties, I had the good fortune of witnessing the opening lesson of the post-graduate course on prosthetics at the University of Southern California.

The lesson was held by Alex Koper, the then director of the *advanced prosthodontic education programme* at USC.

Prof. Koper was an experienced clinician and a passionate teacher of complete removable prosthetics. During that memorable morning he retraced the history of the complete prosthesis and provided an impressive number of bibliographical references starting from the early years of the twentieth century.

Back then there were no PDFs and I spent Saturdays and Sundays in the USC library, taking photocopies of the articles cited by Koper. I remember I paid a significant extra fee on the return flight to Italy for the approximately 35 kg of photocopies I had collected during those 3 weeks in Los Angeles. It was an excellent investment! I had obtained material that I studied for a whole year... and above all, the basis of my future skills. In preparing this presentation I realised how much the times have changed but, at the same time, how little the processes of professional growth and development have changed.

None of my teachers would have ever envisioned the development of digital technology, programs and materials that we have today. Yet, while adopting the rules and concepts developed generations earlier by their teachers, they used contemporary materials and technologies of their professional generation.

That is the reality: the concepts and rules remain stable or undergo extremely slow evolutions. The materials and techniques change at an ever more mind-boggling rate.

In the last four decades, finding useful information for professional education has become much easier and more affordable due to the proliferation of congresses organised by scientific societies, magazines, books, webinars and pay per view.

In this context, an interesting fact is confirmed: professional primacy in dentistry is no longer the prerogative of the United States and reading the book "Esthetics and function in complete prostheses. Digital outlook" confirms the opinion, by now very widespread, that Italian dentistry is now the new international landmark.

In the text you will find the sound concepts underlying the prosthetic art, the most recent techniques and protocols, the concepts of the latest generation of materials, the

most up-to-date bibliography and the corresponding iconographic documentation of a standardised, top-level clinical practice.
I recommend this book to all prosthetic enthusiasts, clinical and dental technique professionals, teachers and their students as it reminds us, once again, that "there is only one mother"... and in the prosthetic field, her name is... complete prosthesis.
Enjoy the read.

Rome, 20 May 2021
Gaetano Calesini

FOREWORD

The complete prosthesis is a therapeutic option still adopted by a very large number of patients, for the most various reasons.
Back in the day, this was an immediate solution to the problems of widespread edentulism, yet over the years its substantial role among the various rehabilitation options has been confirmed, also thanks to the boost given by the development and application of CAD-CAM technology, and to the development of materials and techniques with increasingly better performance. It shares the diagnostic and clinical stages with any other type of prosthetic rehabilitation, with the complication that, often, any dental reference for making the restorations is practically lost in the patient to be rehabilitated.
Its fabrication cannot neglect a careful analysis of the patient, the esthetic-functional aspects and their expressive dynamics. Special attention should also be paid to the psychological aspects and social reflections involved by edentulism.
In the age of computerised dentistry, the complete prosthesis therefore requires implementing a precise method to achieve an accurate design and development of an item that reflects high standards.
I met Dr. Piero Venezia in the early nineties, when as a young practitioner he had decided to attend one of my courses to broaden his knowledge of fixed prostheses, with a special focus on esthetics. We then had the opportunity to meet again on many other occasions after that, also within the Italian Academy of Prosthetic Dentistry.
With this work, Piero proves that there are still multiple reasons to deal with complete prostheses, even today. He traces a clear path, from the approach to the patient to the detailed explanation of the method to the eventual fabrication of a prosthetic item which, thanks to an accurate flow of information, will allow the technician to create a tangible result that fully meets the esthetic-functional needs of the patient. All that by making use of the most advanced digital systems, as well as the most traditional analogue methods.
This work by Dr. Venezia is accurate and well laid-out, and certainly set to enrich the current dentistry literature.

Mauro Fradeani

TABLE OF CONTENTS

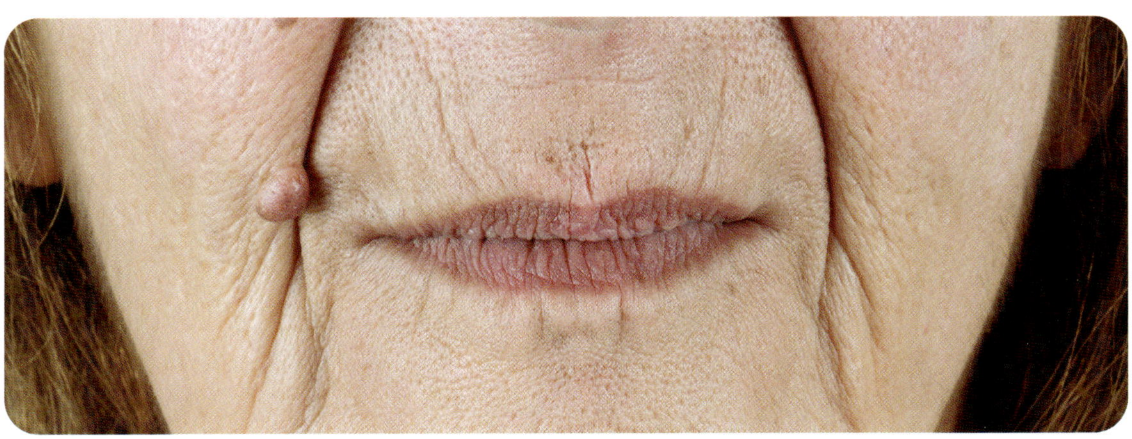

2 Biomimetic approach to complete prostheses

P. Venezia

3 New diagnostic instruments: the digital edentulous patient

P. Venezia, V. Santomauro

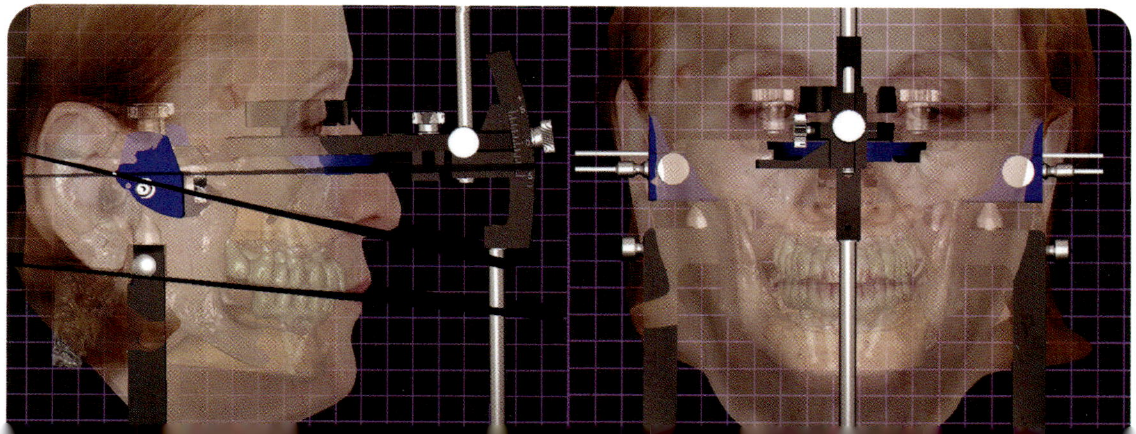

4 The complete prosthesis with analogue protocol

A. Casucci, A. Ielasi

5 Digital Denture: CAD/CAM protocols in complete prostheses

P. Venezia, P. Lacasella

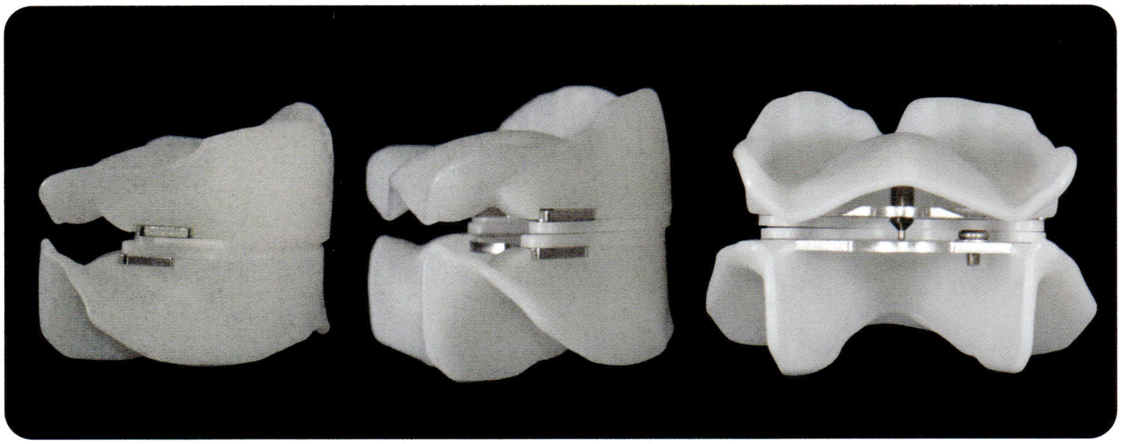

P. VENEZIA

The modern complete prosthesis

«In the development of dentistry, it has been observed that the most innovative clinical procedures are often based on a new interpretation and application of old concepts, rather than on new theories. This is even more true with regards to the complete prosthesis.»
(Sidney I. Silverman, 1956)

Prosthetic dentistry is the branch of dentistry that deals with the diagnosis, treatment plan, rehabilitation and maintenance of the oral function, comfort, appearance and health of patients, assessing their clinical situation associated to the partial or total loss of teeth and/or maxillofacial supporting structures.

The end objective, in prosthetics, is therefore to "artificially replace part of human anatomy, restoring form, function and esthetics [1].

The prosthetist must have the psycho-physical rehabilitation of the patient as the objective of their therapy and, to achieve this result, they will have to design and make, with the essential collaboration of all the other members of the dental team, a "mimetic" restoration, which integrates in the patient's mouth and especially in their face **(Figure 1)** (see Chapter 2).

Every prosthetic therapy requires, in the diagnostic stage, an adequate examination of the patient's dental occlusion and masticatory function [2].

In most prosthetic therapies, the static reference position of the occlusion between the antagonist arches ("position of maximum intercuspidation") and the dynamic occlusal relationships must not be altered during the treatment (**conformative approach**) **(Figure 2)**. Specific clinical conditions may make it necessary, in order to achieve the objectives of the therapy, to modify the occlusal relationships, static as well as dynamic (**reorganised approach**) **(Figures 3** and **4)** [3-6].

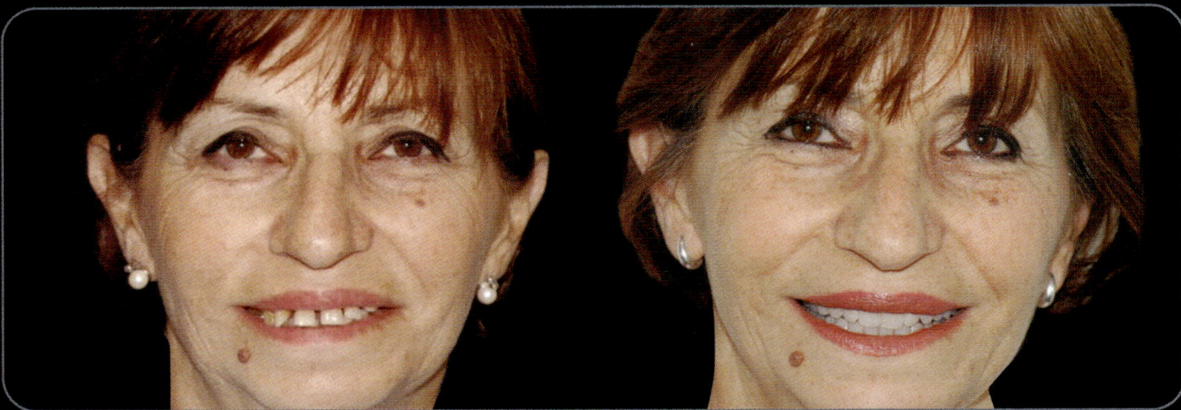

Figure 1 • Esthetic integration of a rehabilitation with removable complete prostheses.

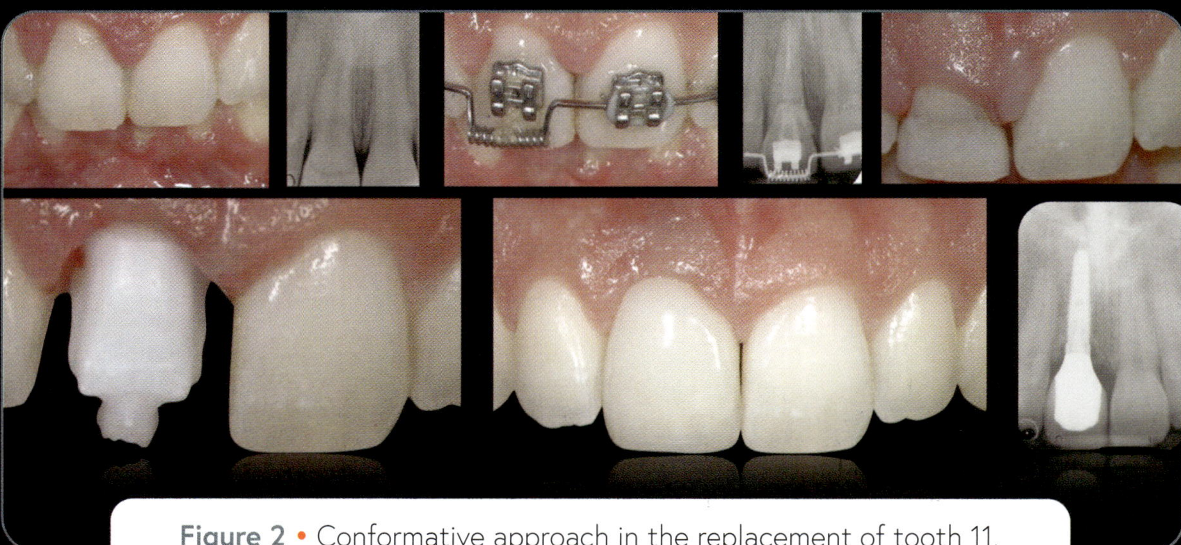

Figure 2 • Conformative approach in the replacement of tooth 11. (Orthodontics: Dr. Emilia Casiello. Surgery: Dr. Raffaele Cavalcanti.)

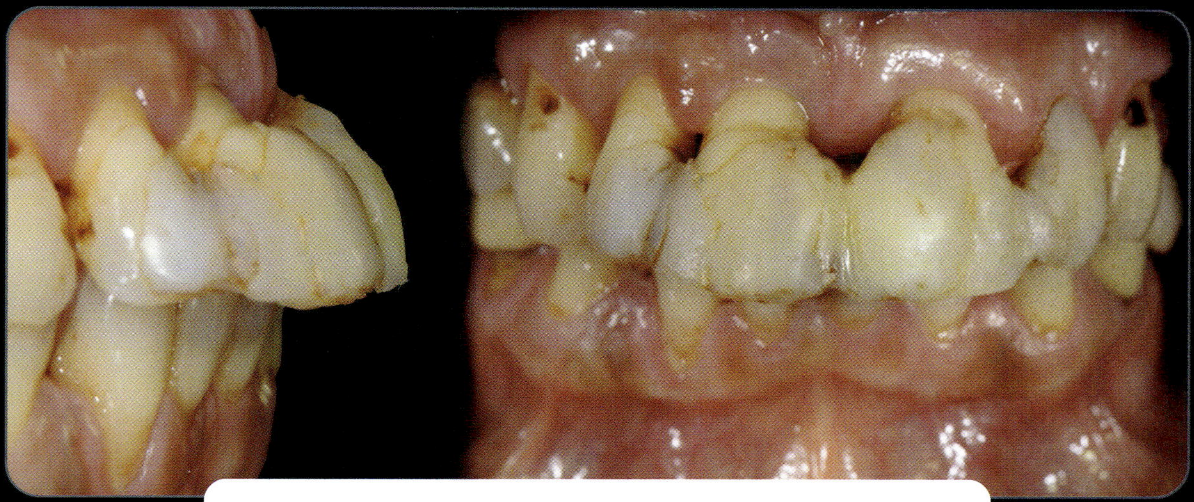

Figure 3 • Reorganised approach: initial situation.

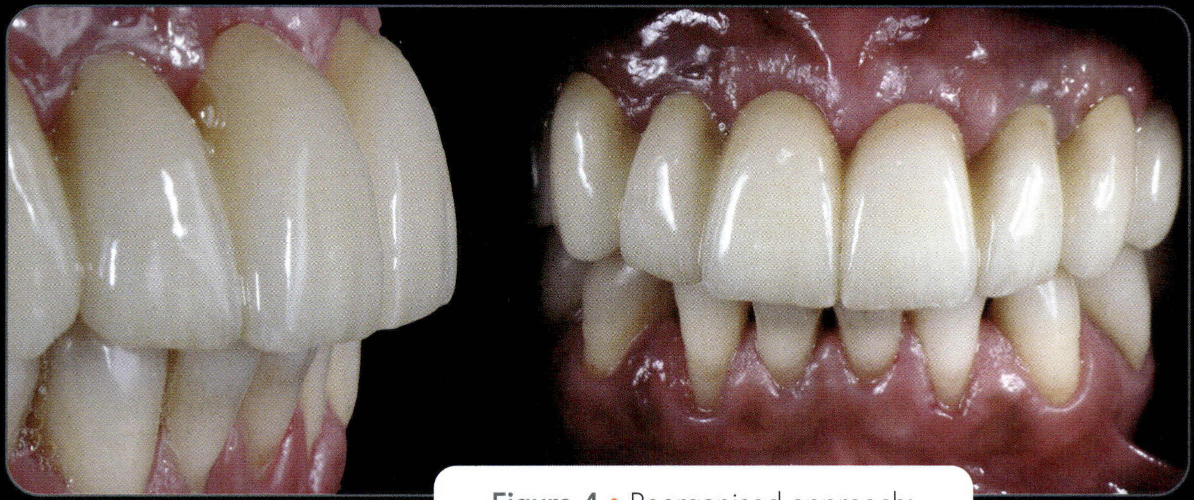

Figure 4 • Reorganised approach: final prosthetic rehabilitation.

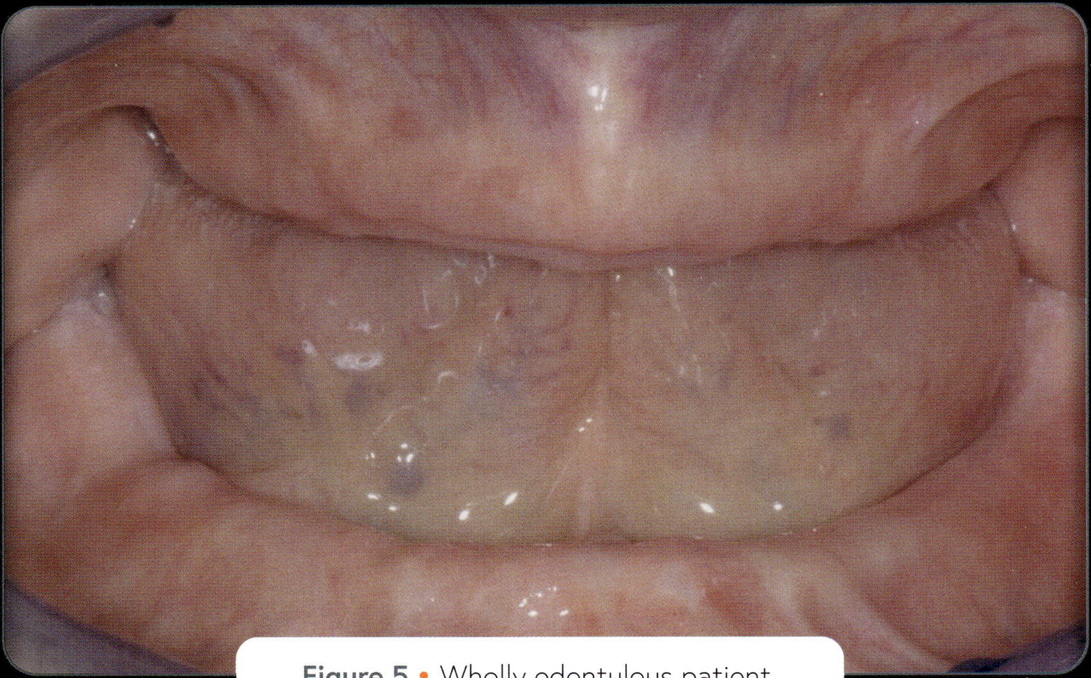

Figure 5 • Wholly edentulous patient.

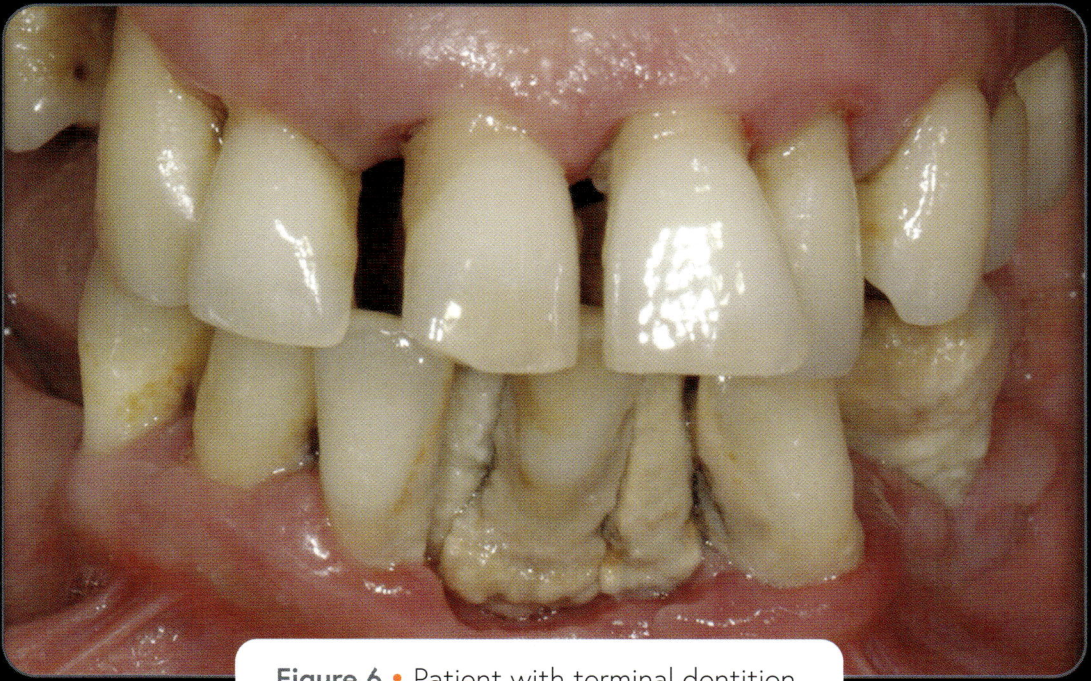

Figure 6 • Patient with terminal dentition.

As a general criterion, a conformative approach is adopted in cases where the existing relationships allow the planned prosthetic therapy to be carried out; the residual dentition can be used as reference for the construction of the static and dynamic aspects of the new prosthetic restoration in the presence of occlusal relationships deemed to be physiological.

A reorganised approach is adopted in cases where the existing relationships do not allow the planned prosthetic therapy to be carried out and when the residual dentition cannot be used as reference for the static and dynamic aspects of the prosthetic restoration.

The reorganised approach is essential when the patient to be treated is totally edentulous or in terminal dentition (**Figures 5** and **6**) [7,8]. In these cases, the diagnostic role of the complete prosthesis must not be underestimated. The rehabilitation of this complex category of patients must include four steps:

1. assessment of the relationships between prosthesis and anatomic structures;
2. obtaining the prosthetic coordinates;
3. testing the prosthetic design with temporary prostheses;
4. transfer of information from provisional prostheses to the final ones using the cross setting technique.

Compliance with the protocols described in the following chapters will achieve the objectives of prosthetic rehabilitation: function, esthetics and phonetics (**Figure 7**).

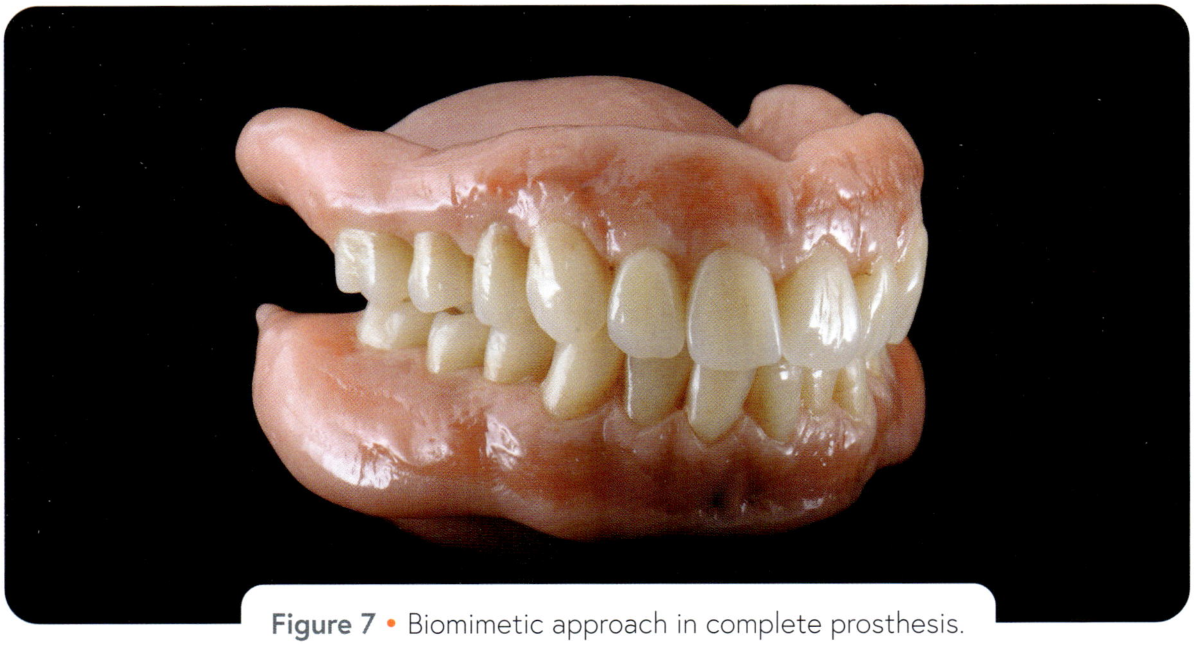

Figure 7 • Biomimetic approach in complete prosthesis.

Companies in the dental sector have greatly helped prosthetists and dental technicians in the biomimetic management of complex cases: the materials and technologies that have been placed on the market enable a completely new approach to complete prosthesis.

Artificial teeth can be produced in conventional materials (polymethyl-methacrylate) or they can be made up of several layers of materials (PMMA, composites) to increase their polishability, resistance and esthetic performance **(Figure 8)**.

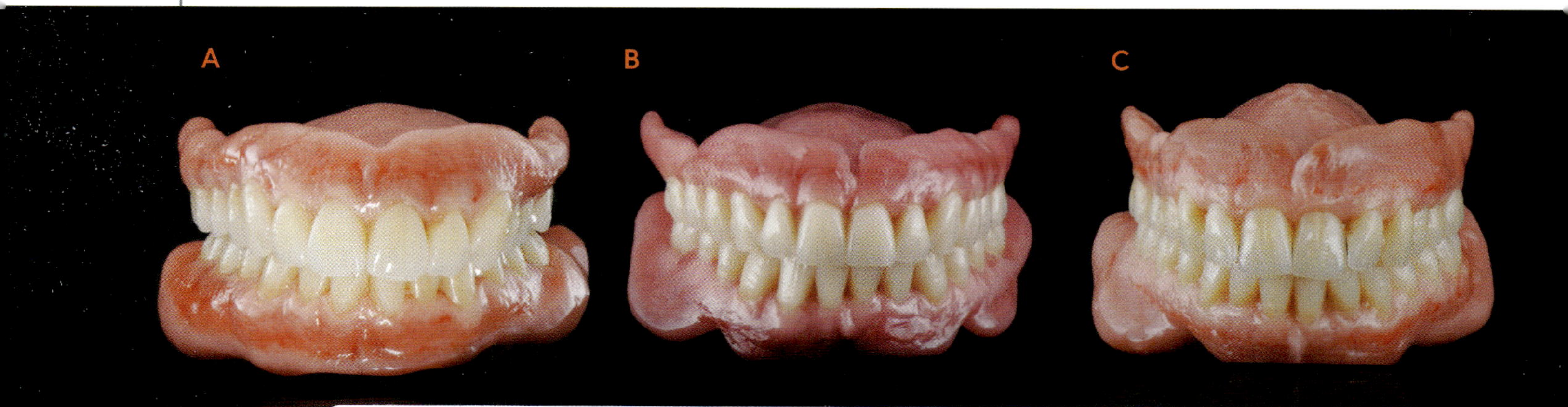

Figure 8 • Use of artificial teeth in PMMA (polymethyl-methacrylate) (**A**), in PMMA with composite surface layer (**B**), in lithium disilicate (**C**).

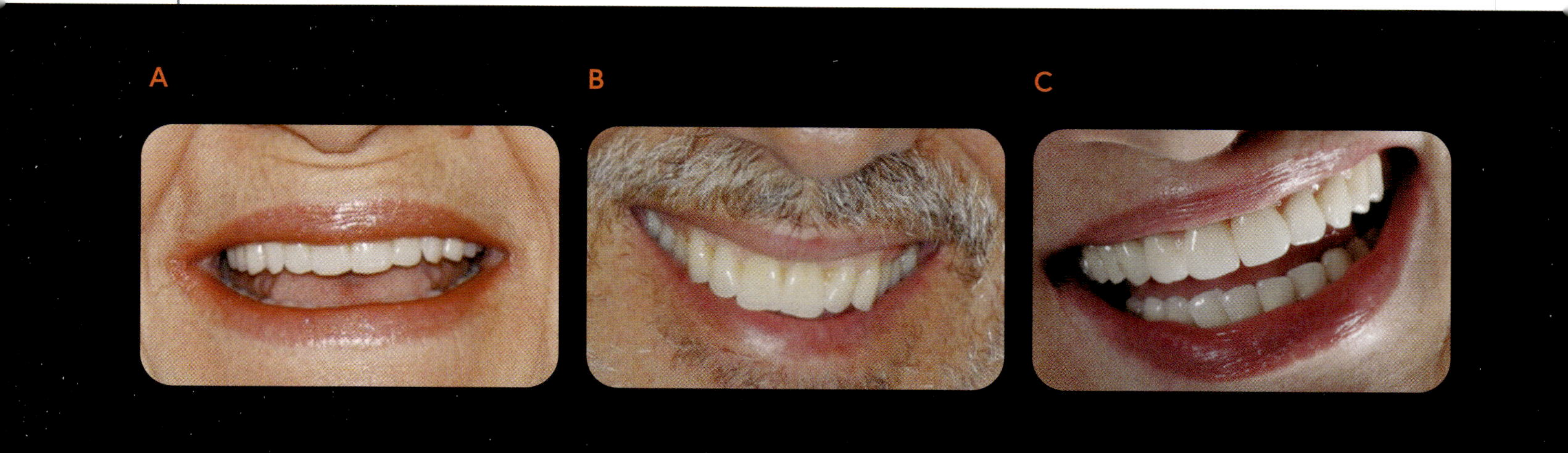

Figure 9 • Different shapes of artificial teeth: soft (**A**), medium (**B**), bold (**C**).

Ceramic teeth can also be supplied by companies or produced in the laboratory to customise the final prosthetic appearance (see Fig. 8).

Today, artificial teeth can have different volumes as well as different shapes: the teeth in production can have soft, medium or bold shapes **(Figure 9)**.

The current workflows in complete prosthesis are particularly interesting: analogue options are increasingly complemented by those involving the production of prostheses with CAD/CAM technologies as well as in the laboratory **(Figure 10)** [9,10].

The evolution is leading to the production of prostheses thanks to the acquisition of intraoral scans of the anatomical structures and the production of prostheses with 3D printers **(Figures 11** and **12)** [11].

Also, thanks to the new technologies, the complete prosthesis is again very current and rapidly evolving.

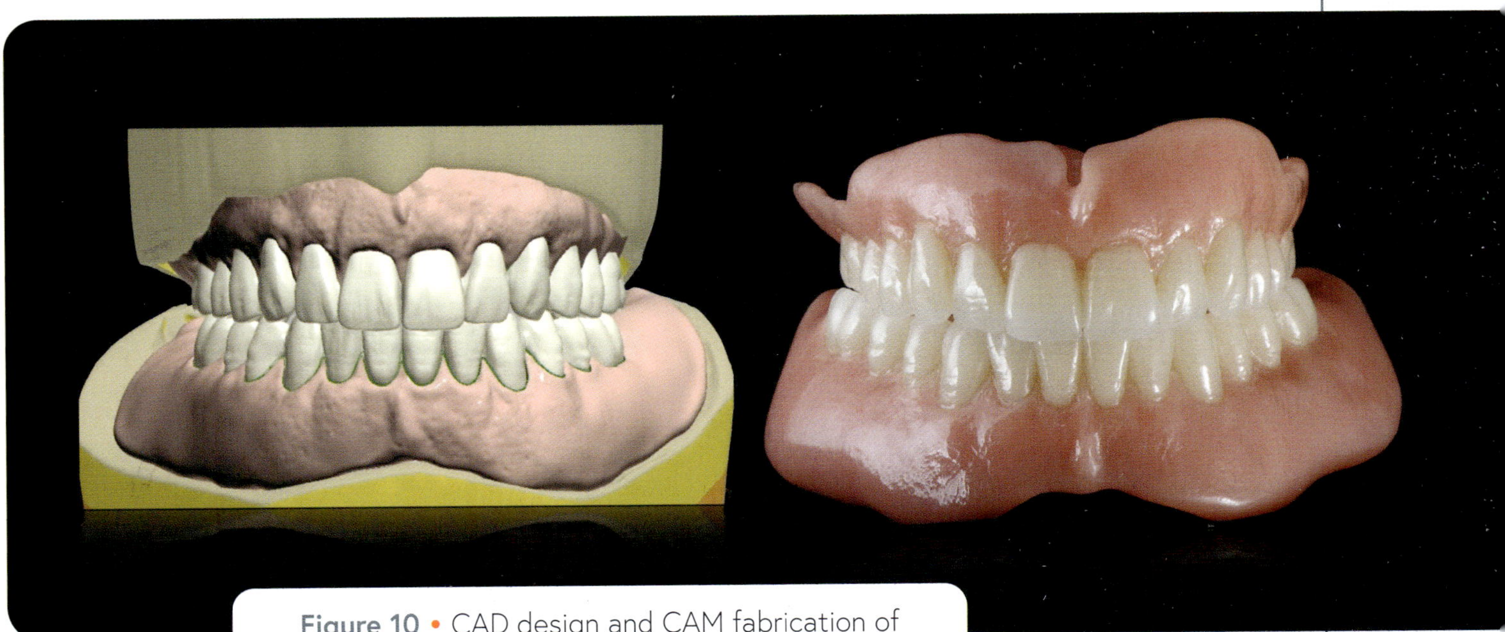

Figure 10 • CAD design and CAM fabrication of rehabilitation with removable prostheses.

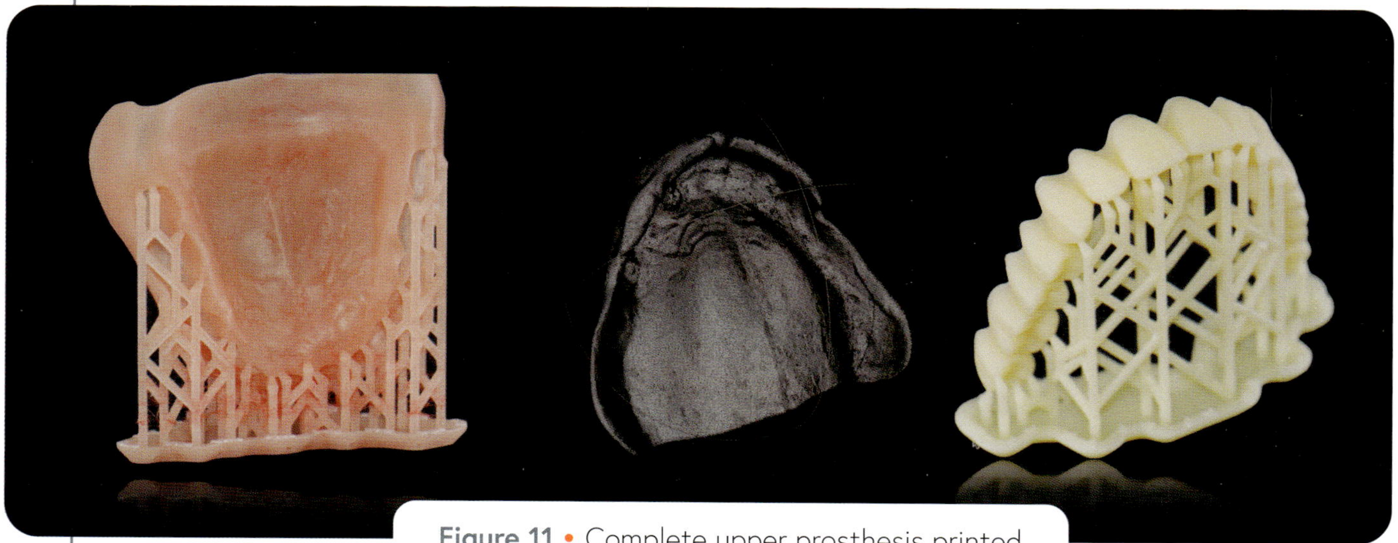

Figure 11 • Complete upper prosthesis printed with 3D printer.

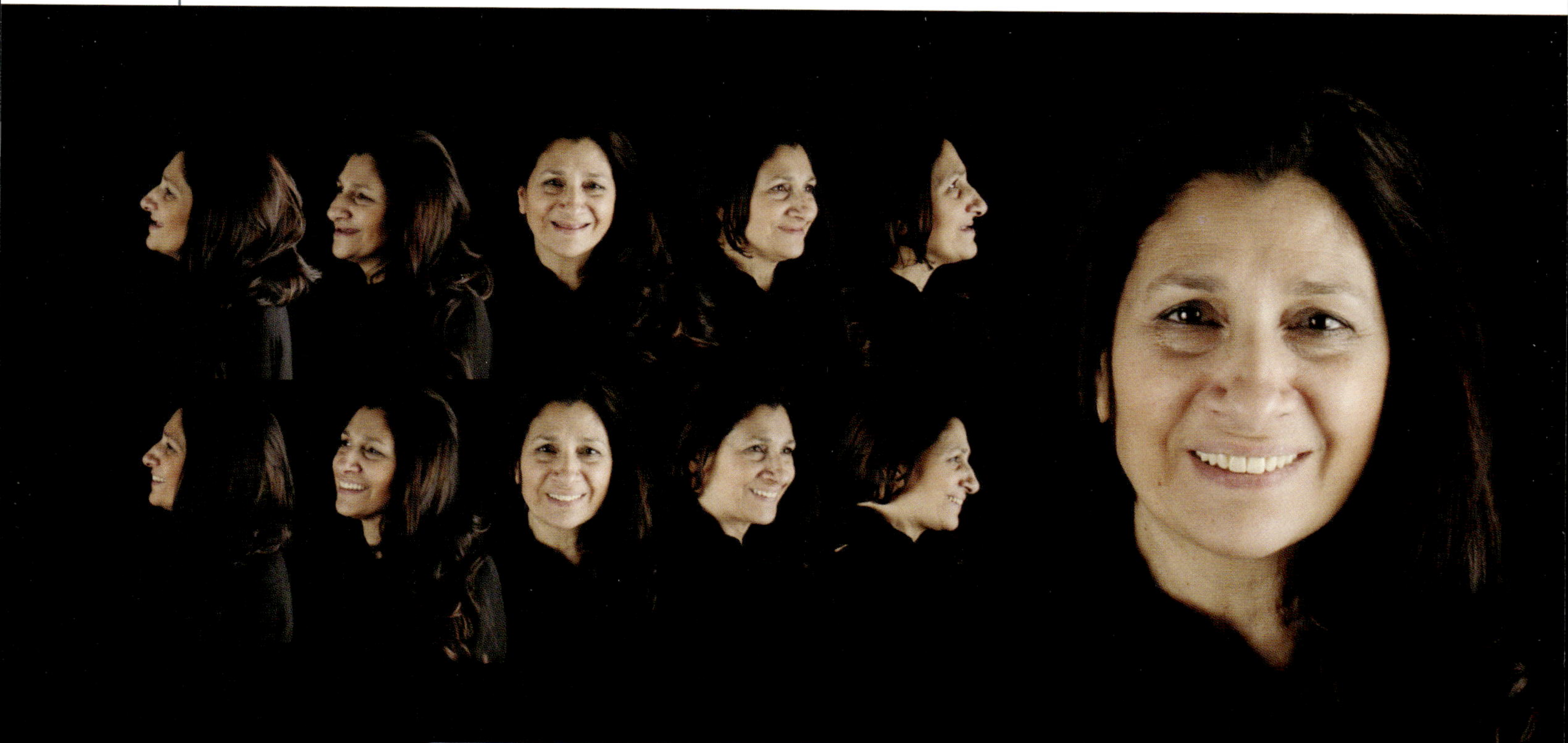

Figure 12 • Temporary rehabilitation of the upper arch carried out with prosthesis printed with a 3D printer.

References

1. The Glossary of Prosthodontic Terms: 9th ed. *J Prosthet Dent*. 2017, 117(5S).
2. Ministero della salute. *Raccomandazioni cliniche in odontoiatria*. 2014.
3. Kantor ME et al. Centric-relation recording techniques — A comparative investigation. *J Prosthet Dent*. 1972;28(6):593-600.
4. Silverman SI. Denture prosthesis and the functional anatomy of the maxillofacial structures. *J Prosthet Dent*. 1956;6(3):305-31.
5. Pound E. Esthetic dentures and their phonetic values. *J Prosthet Dent*. 1951;1(1):98-111.
6. Pound E. Let /S/ be your guide. *J Prosthet Dent*. 1977;38(5):482-9.
7. Landa JS. The free-way space and its significance in the rehabilitation of the masticatory apparatus. *J Prosthet Dent*. 1952;2(6):756-79.
8. Ceruti P et al. Simplified edentulous treatment: A multicenter randomized controlled trial to evaluate the timing and clinical outcomes of the technique. *J Prosthet Dent*. 2017;118(4):462-7.
9. Venezia P, Torsello F, Santomauro V, et al. Full digital workflow for the treatment of an edentulous patient with guided surgery, immediate loading and 3D-printed hybrid prosthesis: The BARI Technique 2.0. A case report. *Int J Environ Res Public Health*. 2019;16(24):5160.
10. Srinivasan M et al. CAD-CAM milled dentures: The Geneva protocols for digital dentures. *J Prosthet Dent*. 2020;123(1):27-37.
11. Takeda Y et al. A 3D printing replication technique for fabricating digital dentures. *J Prosthet Dent*. 2020;124(3):251-6.

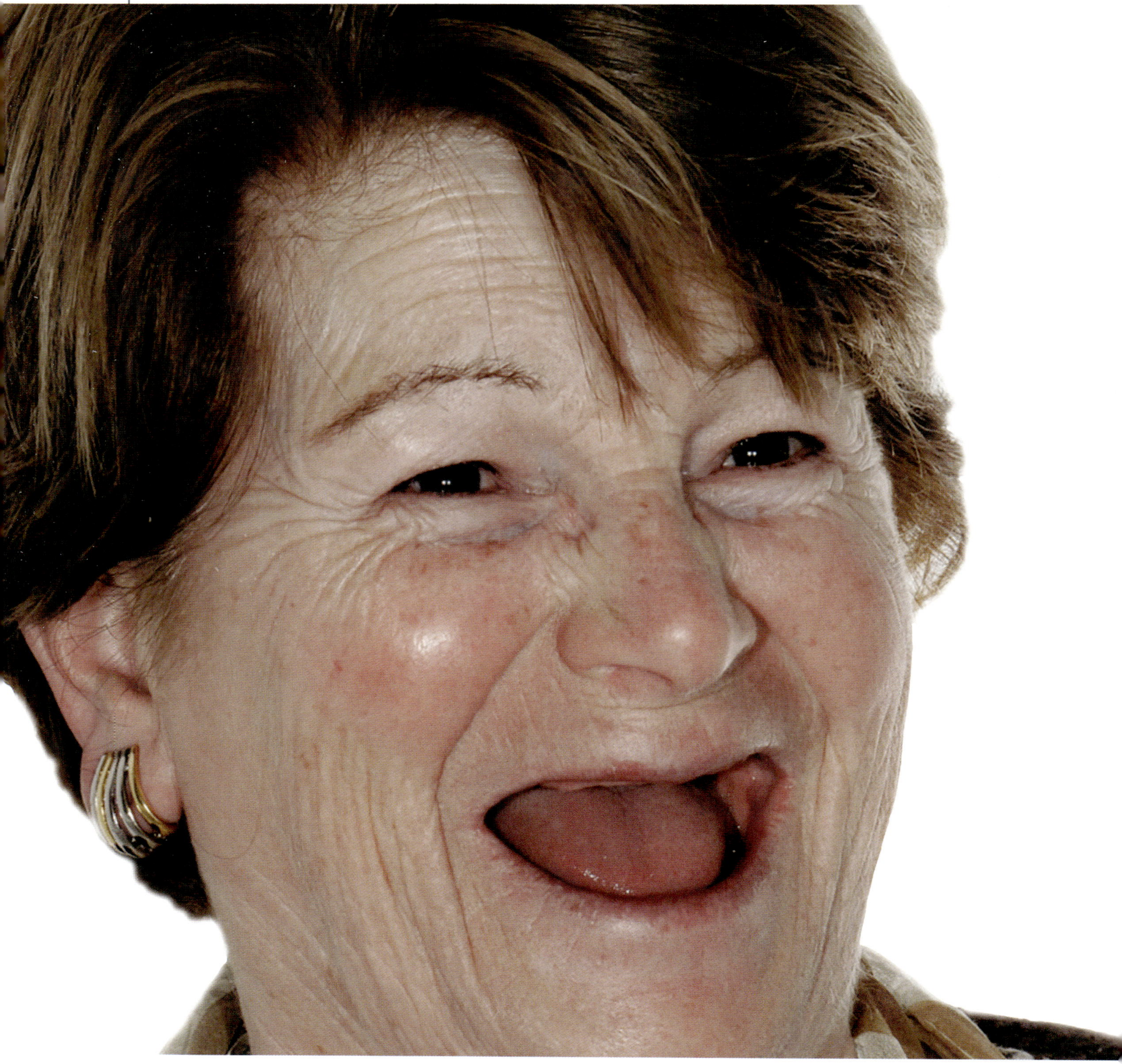

CHAPTER 1

A. CASUCCI

The edentulous patient

Definition

The World Health Organisation (WHO) defines health as "a state of complete physical, mental and social well-being" and not merely the absence of disease or infirmity [1].

This modern approach naturally also applies to the sphere of oral health, in particular to edentulism, a condition featuring the lack of teeth to varying degrees. Edentulism can be **partial**, which indicates the loss of one or more teeth, and **total**, which refers to the total lack of teeth.

These conditions can involve a significant level of disability due to impairment of chewing, phonetics and esthetics, the latter in particular when the loss of teeth affects the anterior regions. In this picture, there are consequences on social relationships, with significant psychological effects for the patient.

Epidemiology

According to Winkler, in 1977 [2], approximately 50% of the 22.6 million US citizens aged 65 or older were edentulous. Fortunately, over the past few decades, the prevalence of oral diseases has undergone significant decreases globally.

In industrialised countries, in particular, it has been documented that caries disease has already decreased in the youth population since the 1990s. As a consequence, today, an ever growing number of adults preserves their natural teeth for longer and they are at least able to maintain functional dentition **(Figure 1.1)**.

Despite this decrease in the loss of natural teeth, today it is estimated that edentulism is present in about 10.9% of the general population and in about half of the population over 65 [3].

Although there has been a general trend towards a decrease in the state of edentulism in the last decade, the WHO goal of people in their eighties having at least 20 teeth has not yet been achieved [4,5]. Furthermore, the effect of the progressive increase in the average life span of the population must also be considered, which might balance the decrease in edentulous rates, making this condition substantially constant even in the coming years in the most industrialised countries.

However, it should be underlined that, limited to European countries, with the exception of Scandinavian ones, epidemiological data concerning the prevalence and incidence of edentulism and loss of teeth are still lacking.

As regards Italy, according to the data reported by the Italian National Institute of Statistics (ISTAT) in a study made in 2013 and published later in 2015 [6], the prevalence of edentulism in the population had improved compared to the past **(Table 1.1)**. In fact, while in 2005 only 37.8% of people over 14 years of age preserved their natural teeth

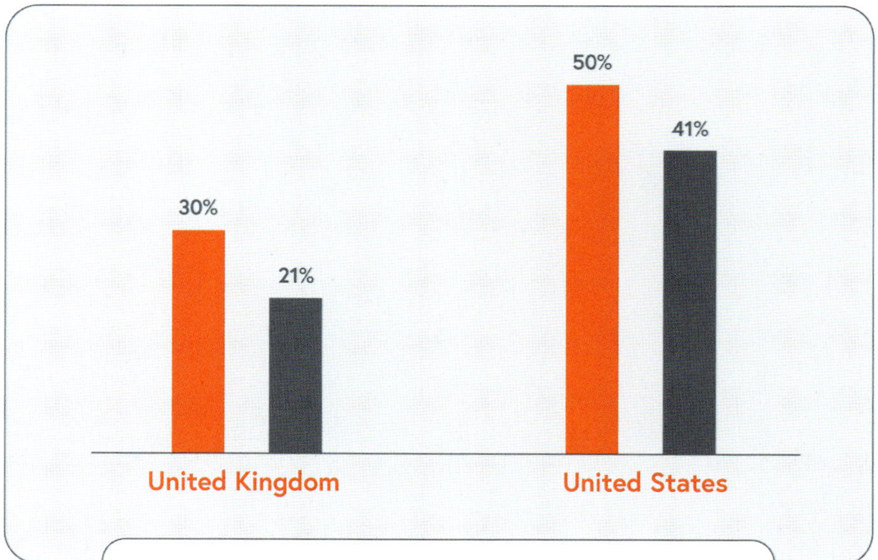

Figure 1.1 • The prevalence of edentulism above 65 years of age compared in the periods 1977-1978 and 1985-1988.

Table 1.1 Data collected in 2005 and in 2013 on prevalence or absence of natural teeth in various age groups

			NO NATURAL TOOTH (EDENTULISM)					
Years	28 natural teeth %		Total %		of which no tooth replaced %		of which with completely replaced teeth %	
14-44	64.7	70.3	0.3	0.2	–	–	0.2	0.1
45-54	30.1	32.9	3.1	2.2	0.1	0.1	2.9	1.9
55-64	17.4	18.8	10.5	9.8	0.4	0.4	9.9	8.9
65-74	8.7	10.2	28.4	25.1	0.9	0.9	27.2	22.9
over 75	3.7	4.5	53.6	50.4	4.1	4.1	49	44.1
Total	39.9	41	10.9	11	0.6	0.6	10.2	9.8
Standardised total	37.8	41.4	12	10.8	0.8	0.8	11.1	9.6

From: ISTAT. Access to dental care and dental health in Italy. ISTAT; 2015.

and complete edentulism was 12%, in 2013, 41.4% of people retained their natural teeth, and the percentage of completely edentulous people fell to 10.8%. Furthermore, the loss of teeth was more frequent in women than in men, with an estimate of 12.5% and 9.2% respectively [6].

The ISTAT figures also show that the presence of teeth or edentulism in the population changes by age group. In 2013, it was found that up to the age of 44, 70.3% of patients had all natural teeth, and then drastically decreased to 32.9% between 45-54 years old, to 10.2% in patients aged between 65 and 74, down to 4.5% in over 75s. These figures show an improvement of approximately 10% compared to those recorded in 2005.

The prevalence of edentulism follows a reverse pattern: it is present in 0.2% of patients up to the age of 44, in 2.2% of patients aged 45 to 54, in 25.1% of patients aged 65 to 74 and 50.4% in patients over 75 [6].

The loss of teeth affects the patient's general state of health and will have repercussions on chewing efficiency with consequences on the choice of foods and the digestive process. Indeed, patients who suffer the loss of many teeth often also have impaired nutritional levels, because, due to functional limitations, they prefer to consume soft or liquid foods, low in fibre and rich in fats and sugars. This is often compounded by muscle laxity that is secondary to the lack of masticatory stimuli [7].

The reasons just explained and others concerning esthetics, phonetics and muscle tone mean the clinician and patient must restore balance and oral health. It is estimated that the more teeth have been lost without being replaced, the more the complication in chewing increases: the prevalence reaches as much as 82% for patients with fewer than seven teeth in the oral cavity and without prostheses.

It is proven that at least 20 teeth in complete occlusion are required for masticatory stability [8,9]. Consequently, it is reasonable to think that the replacement of teeth, especially if posterior, is of vital importance in order not to worsen the general health of an elderly patient.

The cultural background also has a significant impact in the prevalence of edentulism. A lack of teeth was found in 2.6% of people with a degree or diploma, against 29.4% of people with elementary school leaving certificate or without any school qualifications [3,9] **(Figure 1.2)**.

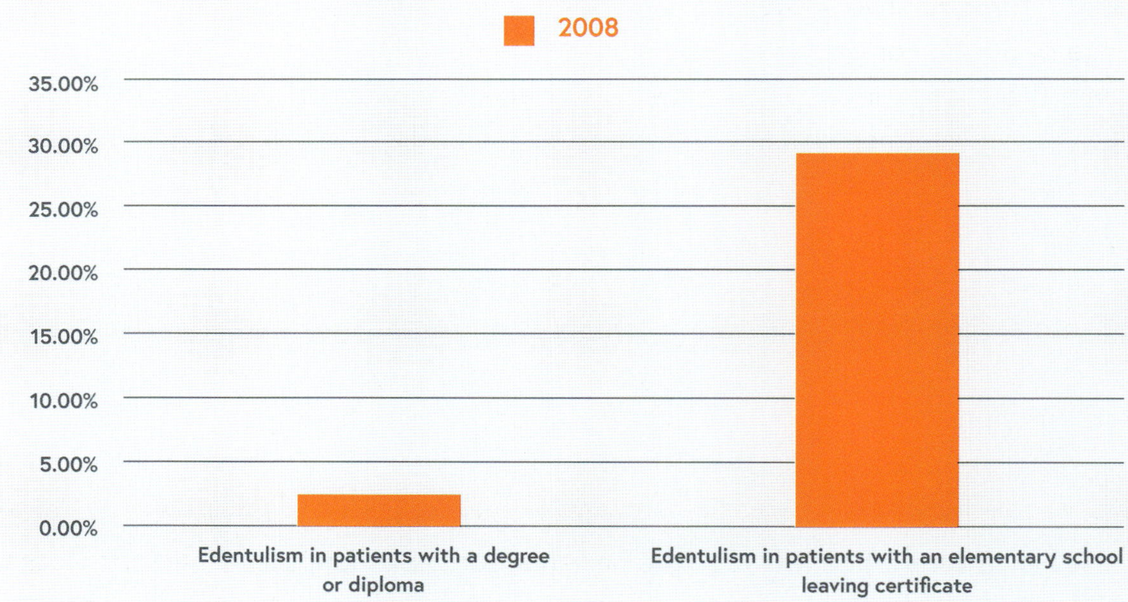

Figure 1.2 • The graph shows how the social and cultural background affects oral health: a lack of teeth is found in 2.6% of people with a degree or diploma compared to 29.4% of people with a primary school leaving certificate or without any qualifications.
(From: ISTAT. Condizioni di salute e ricorso ai servizi sanitari. ISTAT; 2008.)

In addition, a study limited to the Milan area reported that 49.6% of the elderly people hospitalised and/or living in retirement homes had to deal with edentulism, compared to 28.3% of patients residing at home [10].

Causes and risk factors

A large number of variables is associated with the loss of teeth in adulthood, although there is no unanimous acceptance of the greater importance of dental pathologies compared to socio-economic factors, which are considered as risk factors instead [11].

The main reasons why a patient loses a tooth in adulthood are: dental caries (50% incidence), periodontal disease (35% incidence) and issues caused by previous dental treatments.

The prevalence of caries is maximum among the young and the percentages decrease in old age. Periodontal disease, however, is a characteristic pathology of adulthood, in fact it shows an inverse trend compared to caries and increases significantly from the age of 34-44. For example, research by the Agostino Gemelli University Hospital in Rome (Italy) took into consideration 120 patients aged between 21 and 91 years to carry out a treatment plan. A total of 554 teeth were extracted, 289 of which for caries, 198 for periodontal disease, 38 for endodontic reasons, 16 to make prosthetics easier and 13 for failure of previous treatments [12-15].

With regard to risk factors, lifestyles, habits, genetics and systemic disease are taken into account. Neglecting oral hygiene, alcohol intake and smoking are certainly modifiable risk factors. It is estimated that the prevalence of various forms of edentulism in non-smokers is about half that of nicotine-dependent patients. Other risk factors associated with dental avulsion are diabetes, cardiovascular disease, stress, neoplastic diseases, obesity and neurological disorders [9,13].

There is also a correlation between the patients' socio-economic level and edentulism. A 2007 study conducted by Tramini et al. [16] on 321 elderly patients of a long-term care hospital in Montpellier (France) correlated partial or total edentulism of the same study subjects with conditions such as general health, behavioural attitudes, socio-economic background and above all a wide range of systemic pathologies.

In particular, the factors related to total edentulism that emerged were: older than 87 (OR = 9.4), presence of nephropathy (OR = 6.8) and inadequate oral hygiene (OR = 0.1).

A similar 1998 study by Hamasha et al. [17], highlighted how the number of missing teeth and the likelihood of being totally edentulous are significantly higher in people who have a history of atherosclerotic vascular disease, heart failure, ischemic heart disease and joint disease. There are also diseases whose correlation with tooth loss is well-established.

The patient with insulin-dependent diabetes not compensated with medicines and with concomitant periodontal disease has worsened bone resorption and therefore loss of support.

Pathologies that suppress the immune system such as, for example, HIV, neoplasms, neutropenias, leukocyte adhesion deficiency syndrome (LAD) and collagenopathies have a definite influence in the edentulous stage, like mental deficits are generally associated with poor oral hygiene, and therefore, in turn, raise the risk of caries as well as periodontal disease. Finally, therapeutic and pharmacological treatments that can promote tooth loss are cervico-facial irradiation, xerostomising medications and immunosuppressants [18].

Clinical and psycho-social implications

The loss of some or all teeth brings about anatomical changes of the stomatognathic system: at intraoral level, the edentulous condition leads to a decrease in the height and thickness of the alveolar bone. Tallgren [19] has shown that bone loss in edentulous patients is four times higher at the level of the mandible than of the maxilla. Furthermore, a highly resorbed residual ridge causes a significant decrease in the adherent gingiva, an actual "buffer surface" for the masticatory loads of any complete or partial prosthesis fabricated for that edentulous saddle. Similarly, in the maxillary region, the alveolar bone is replaced by fibrous tissue, whose presence is also a negative prognostic factor for the stability of the upper prosthesis.

Many studies corroborate the idea that edentulism causes problems in the temporomandibular joint. In the case of partial edentulism, it is hypothesised that the lack of posterior teeth leads to muscle and joint overload, with higher frequency in women than in men. However, the studies analysed to date do not confirm this hypothesis [20,21].

Edentulism in general causes physical, psychological and esthetic discomfort to the patient. If the lack of teeth is not made up for, there is a loss of vertical dimension (VD) and a protrusion of the lip and chin. This causes prognathism of the lower jaw emulating a skeletal class III (**Figure 1.3**). This esthetic discomfort damages the patient's psychological sphere [8].

There are unanimous views in the literature regarding the fact that the masticatory performance of edentulous subjects is lower than that of dentate subjects. Wayler and Chauncey [22] observed that subjects with full prostheses had greater difficulty in chewing hard foods than dentate subjects.

Österberg et al. [23] confirmed these data, noting that on average the masticatory performance of individuals with some degree of edentulism was about one sixth compared to those achieved in dentate subjects. The weak point of these studies was considering control groups formed by young dentate subjects. As a matter of fact, the masticatory ability might decrease with age regardless of the number of teeth in one's mouth.

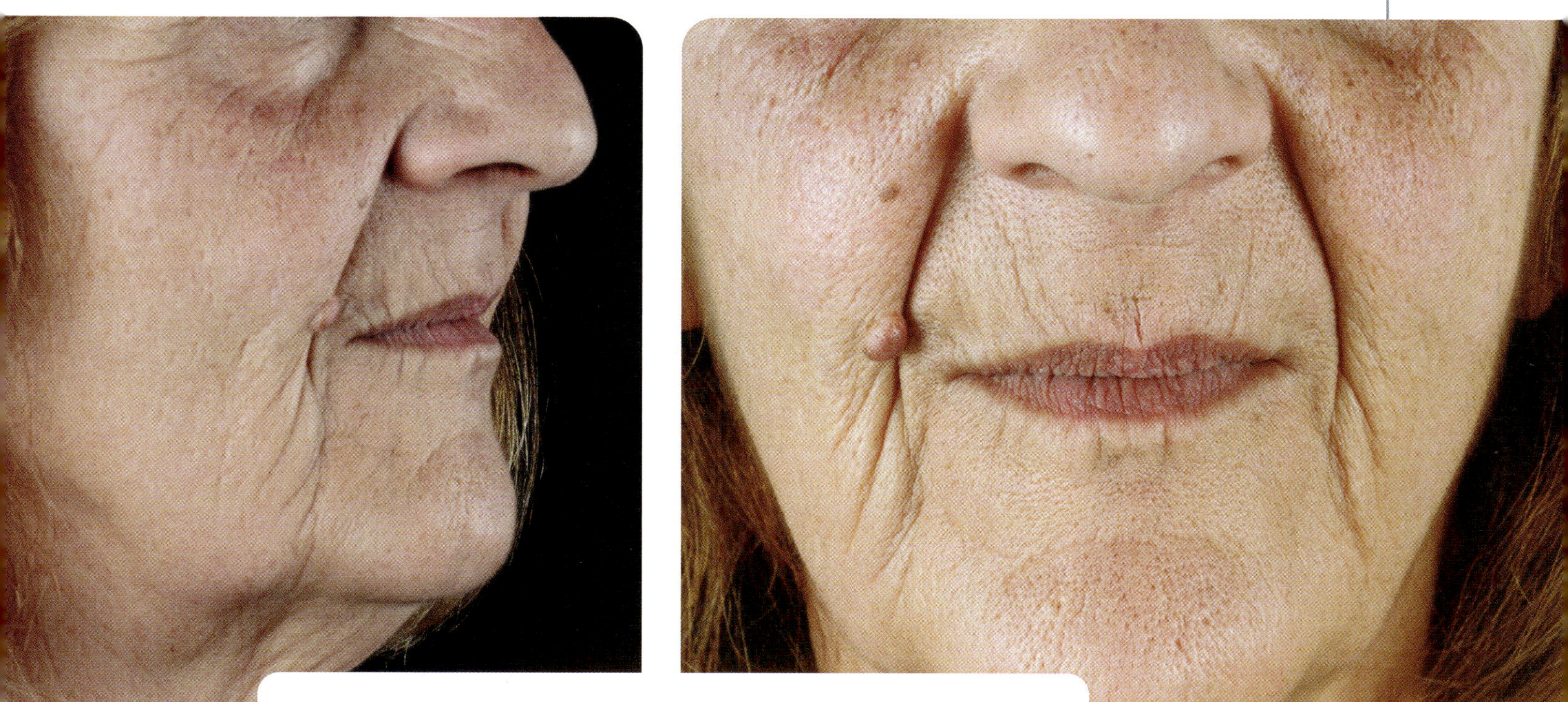

Figure 1.3 • Prognathic appearance of an edentulous patient. One may note the loss of muscle tone and lip support.

Other studies, on the other hand, have evaluated the masticatory force of fully edentulous subjects who had removable complete prostheses [24-26]. When comparing the values obtained with those of dentate individuals, all the authors observed that the masticatory force of the study subjects stood at mean force values of 20% compared to that of the control groups [7,27,28].

This might partly explain why subjects who have complete prostheses have greater difficulty in chewing harder food, especially when the lower prosthesis is unstable.

In fact, it has been reported that the masticatory efficacy increases by improving the stability level of the prostheses through the use of implants or, simply, by using adhesives for the mobile one. Furthermore, by increasing the mechanical stability of the reconstruction, the patient is better able to manage food. The muscles of the tongue and perioral structures are not engaged in the stabilisation function of the prosthesis, thereby managing to perform better the function of moving the food bolus to the surfaces of the occlusal tables [27,29,30].

Some studies [31,32] underlined that people with full or partial removable prostheses have a diet low in raw vegetables and fruit and rich in fats and carbohydrates instead. That's the reason why the goal of treating edentulous patients, by improving the functionality of the prosthesis, should also be to have a positive change in diet, but unfortunately this phenomenon hardly ever emerges. In actual fact, the literature has clearly highlighted how a new rehabilitation, even with implants, may lead to an increase in the comfort of patients and their level of satisfaction, however the change to a new prosthesis is not associated with changes in diet [8,33,34].

The absence of changes in the general diet after prosthetic therapy affects the selection of food, which, like any complex human behaviour, is influenced by the most diverse factors, even very distant from prosthetic factors, such as habits, one's identity, awareness of a healthy diet, education, traditions or social and cultural aspects; logistical aspects such as institutionalisation and economic factors may also have an impact. As a matter of fact, the perception of the masticatory ability can explain about 4% of the variation towards higher intake of fruit or vegetables [35,36]. This aspect is confirmed by the fact that in the studies carried out, the participants' diet was independent from the dental condition [37,38].

To be able to ensure a diet richer in fibre and vegetables, it is not enough to offer patients more stable rehabilitation, but it is essential to provide in-depth information on proper eating habits and that this is repeated often in order to motivate them to make general improvements towards a balanced diet [39,40]. It might be helpful to assess the quality of the patients' diet in the pre-treatment stage, so as to also consider the related factors as the goal of prosthetic therapy jointly with the esthetic-functional aspects.

With regard to the **psycho-social sphere**, the self-perception of the edentulous patient has a negative effect. These subjects will be more likely to avoid social events due to their disadvantaged chewing, phonetics and esthetics. Various studies confirm the correlation between edentulism and depression [41-43].

Edentulous patients or patients with incompatible prostheses score higher, with regard to the level of depressive anxiety, on the Global Severity Index (GSI) and on the Positive Symptom Distress Index (PSDI), general indices that are able to highlight the intensity or depth of a patient's psychological distress. Furthermore, depression often causes the subject to engage in behaviours that are harmful to their health such as, for example, smoking, drinking alcohol, following a diet full of sugars and fats, having poor hygiene or not doing any physical activity [41,44-46]

Bone resorption in the edentulous patient

Some scientific studies have confirmed the processes that the periodontium undergoes following an extraction or loss of a tooth [47,48].

Bone is considered a dynamic organ as it is subjected to a remodelling process by cells such as osteoblasts and osteoclasts.

When the balance of this mechanism fails, one is subject to pathologies such as osteopetrosis and osteoporosis, that is when bone density is higher or lower due to incorrect function of the osteoblasts or osteoclasts. Osteoclastic activity is considered to start decreasing two months after extraction, while osteoblastic activity continues being sustained [48-50].

The alveolar process is formed by bone tissue that is dependent on dental structure because it only exists if there is a tooth [47]. Following the loss of a tooth, the stimulus induced by the periodontal ligament ceases and the bone structure is subject to resorption. In actual fact, when a tooth is lost, the fibres of the desmodontium that join the dental cement to the alveolar process are interrupted.

The mode and extent of bone resorption depend on many factors such as the position (anterior or posterior), the type of bone (mandibular or maxillary), the existing bone walls (lingual or vestibular) and the patient's starting morphology, that is, whether they have a thin or thick bone wall [48].

The concept of mandibular and maxillary atrophy as a result of total edentulism is set out with a classification described by Cawood and Howell in 1988 [51]. In 1987, on the other hand, Mish and Judy focus on the concept of partial edentulism and the following year on bone density, according to the bone's microscopic structure [52].

At extraoral level, anatomical changes of the face are observed following tooth loss. Indeed, the natural teeth and the supporting bone that surrounds them support the muscles of the face lower third. In this sense, the condition of the edentulism causes considerable changes to the esthetics of the face [7,8].

Tallgren [19] analysed a series of teleradiographs in latero-lateral projection, on which cephalometric analyses of wholly edentulous subjects were made, with those of wholly edentulous patients in the upper arch and completely dentate in the lower arch. A 7-year follow-up showed how the study group (wholly edentulous) had greater average loss of facial height compared to the control group, therefore indicating the greater benefit of maintaining natural teeth in the lower arch.

The same study showed that the loss of teeth and alveolar bone also resulted in marked changes in the profile of the facial soft tissues, especially in the first year of follow-up after tooth extraction. Indeed, it is estimated that 50% of alveolar reduction takes place in the first year post-extraction [48].

Elderly patient

The latest data collected by ISTAT in 2013 on the phenomenon of edentulism report that it mainly concerns elderly people who, more than younger people, also suffer from other general chronic conditions that often cause functional limitations and disability.

Also in 2013, in Italy, there were more than 2.5 million over 65s with severe functional limitations, equal to 20%. The elderly population with mild limitations, severe chronic diseases or permanent disabilities was approximately 5.5 million, 43.4% of the overall elderly population.

People with functional limitations, disabilities or serious chronic conditions often have lower social involvement, with impaired mobility, for example, in using public transport.

The elderly may have varying degrees of dependence and medical complications and may live in different housing conditions: from their own home to the possibility of being in specialised care facilities [6].

In this context, for older patients, even access to dental care can be complicated, as is ensuring maintenance procedures, with the effect of increasing the risk of caries and the consequent failure of complex restorations. In these cases, therapeutic approaches that opt for easy solutions in terms of hygienic maintenance and that prevent the progression of caries or periodontal problems should be preferred, with the aim of reducing short and long-term risks. The demographic trend of ageing clearly indicates that there will ever more elderly people, with a higher number of teeth and implants often involved in increasingly complex restorations than the solutions applied to patients of previous generations. Preparing and adapting their clinical approach for the management of this type of patient as well is surely one of the challenges that tomorrow's dentists will have to face. As well as reducing their independence, the presence of chronic pathologies in elderly patients certainly means they must be treated with polypharmacological therapies. **Table 1.2** sets out the main interactions of systemic treatments for chronic pathologies with oral issues. In the early stages of taking the patient's history it is absolutely crucial to assess the therapies they are undergoing. Two of the many conditions that most often must be considered when taking the medical history of the elderly patient are examined here: diabetes and the intake of antiresorptive drugs.

For a more comprehensive framing of the medical history, the reader should refer to texts on geriatric pathology [53,54].

Diabetes and oral health

Diabetes mellitus type 2 (DMT2) is also referred to as non-insulin-dependent diabetes. It is a chronic metabolic disorder characterised by a lack of insulin production or its incorrect action. Insulin resistance causes insulin-sensitive organs to secrete more glucose and to decrease its absorption.

Glucose homeostasis is therefore interrupted with a dysfunction of the pancreatic β-cells. Insulin resistance and dysfunction of the islets of Langerhans are pathognomonic signs of the disease. DMT2 is considered a heterogeneous polygenic pathology as there are about 400 genetic variables as risk factors. It is one of the most widespread diseases in the 21st century. In 2010, DMT2 caused 3.96 million deaths, equal to 6.8% of global mortality [46,55].

Table 1.2 Overview of oral sequelae due to the intake of medications for systemic diseases

MEDICATION CATEGORY	ACTIVE PRINCIPLE	ORAL PATHOLOGIES
Anesthetic (local)	Benzocaine, procaine HCl, lidocaine	Taste alteration
	Procainamide	Lupus-like reactions
	Quinidine	Lichenoid reactions of the mucosa
Anti-arthritics, antipyretics, anti-inflammatory drugs	Allopurinol, auranofin, colchicine, dexamethasone, hydrocortisone, levamisole, D-penicillamine, phenylbutazone, salicylates, 5-thiopiridoxine	Taste alteration
	Gold salts	Taste alteration, lichenoid reactions, oral pigmentation, vesiculo-ulcerative stomatitis
Antibiotics and antiseptics	All	Oral candidiasis
	Erythromycin	Hypersensitivity reactions, vesiculo-ulcerative stomatitis
	Penicillin	Hypersensitivity reactions, erythema multiforme, vesiculo-ulcerative stomatitis
	Chloramphenicol, ciprofloxacin + clindamycin, dapsone, isoniazid, sulfonamides	Erythema multiforme, melanosis
	Tetracyclines	Melanosis
	Minocycline	Dark pigmentation of the teeth and tongue
	Chlorhexidine	Burning sensation of the oral cavity, irritation of the mucous membranes
	Ampicillin, cefamandole, ethambutol HCl, griseofulvin, lincomycin, metronidazole, niridazole, sulfasalazine, tetracyclines	Taste alteration
Anticancer drugs	All	Oral candidiasis, oral hemorrhage, recurrent oral viral infections, aphthous stomatitis, vesiculo-ulcerative stomatitis
Anticoagulants	All	Hemorrhage
Anticonvulsant drugs	Carbamazepine	Erythema multiforme, taste alteration
	Phenytoin	Erythema multiforme, gingival swelling, taste alteration
Antidiarrhoeal drugs	Bismuth	Brown pigmentation of the tongue
Antihistamines	All	Salivary disorders
	Chlorphenamine maleate	Taste alteration

Table 1.2 Continued

MEDICATION CATEGORY	ACTIVE PRINCIPLE	ORAL PATHOLOGIES
Antihypertensives	All	Salivary disorders
	Calcium antagonists	Swollen gingiva
	ACE-inhibitors	Vesiculo-ulcerative stomatitis, pemphigus vulgaris
	Chloramphenicol	Vesiculo-ulcerative stomatitis
	Hydralazine	Lupus-like reactions, erythema multiforme
	Methyldopa	Lupus-like reactions, lichenoid reaction of the mucosa
	Thiazide diuretics	Lichenoid reaction of the mucosa
	Minoxidil, verapamil	Erythema multiforme
	Acetazolamide, amiloride, captopril, diazoxide, diltiazem, enalapril, ethacrynic acid, nifedipine	Taste alteration
Antilipidemics	Cholestyramine, clofibrate	Taste alteration
Antimycotics	Griseofulvin	Erythema multiforme, brown pigmentation of the tongue
	Amphotericin B	Taste alteration
Antioxidants	Octyl gallate	Allergic ulcers
Antiparkinsons	All	Salivary dysfunctions
Antireflux agents	All	Salivary dysfunctions
	Cimetidine	Erythema multiforme
Antithyroid agents	Carbimazole, methimazole, methylthiouracil, propylthiouracil, thiouracil	Taste alteration
Anxiolytics	Benzodiazepines	Salivary dysfunctions
Chelating agents	Penicillamine	Ulcer and pemphigus vulgaris
Cortiscosteroids	All	Oral candidiasis, recurrent oral viral infections, vesiculo-ulcerative stomatitis
Hypoglycaemics	Sulfonylurea	Erythema multiforme
	Glipizide, phenformin and derivatives	Taste alteration
Immunosuppressants, antiproliferatives	Azathioprine, bleomycin, carmustine, doxorubicin, 5-fluorouracil, methotrexate, vincristine sulphate	Taste alteration
	Cyclosporine	Gingival swelling

Continues

Table 1.2 Continued

MEDICATION CATEGORY	ACTIVE PRINCIPLE	ORAL PATHOLOGIES
Muscle relaxants	All	Salivary dysfunctions
	Baclofen, chlorzoxazone	Taste alteration
Painkillers	Acetylsalicylic acid	Hemorrhage, erythema multiforme
	NSAIDs	Hemorrhage
	Barbiturates, codeine	Erythema multiforme
Psychiatric drugs	All	Salivary dysfunctions
	Glutethimide, meprobamate	Erythema multiforme
	Phenothiazines	Oral pigmentation, tardive dyskinesia
	Lithium carbonate	Erythema multiforme, taste alteration
	Trifluoperazine HCl	Taste alteration
Sympathomimetics	Amphetamine, amrinone	Taste alteration
Vasodilators	Bamifylline HCl, dipyridamole, nitroglycerin patches, oxyfedrine	Taste alteration
	Levodopa	Taste alteration
Others	Etidronate, germinal monoacetate, idoxuridine, iron-sorbitol, vitamin D	Taste alteration

According to the International Diabetes Federation (IDF) [56] in 2015 the disease was diagnosed in about 415 million adults and it is estimated that in 2040 about 642 million will be suffering from it. Also in 2015, ISTAT indicated that 5.4% of Italians suffer from diabetes and the predisposing factors for the onset of this condition are genetics, obesity, sedentary lifestyle, smoking, excessive alcohol consumption, arterial hypertension and HDL blood levels below normal (≤35 mg/dL) in combination or alternatively with high triglyceride values (≥250 mg/dL) [6,45,55].

Diabetic patients are more prone to dyslipidemia which in turn increases cardiovascular risk. Other complications are retinopathy, which causes blindness, cerebrovascular pathologies, nephropathy, found in 20-40% of cases, lower limb gangrene and skin ulcers. DMT2 is a preventable disease in some cases with a correct lifestyle. However, once the disease is extant, the likelihood of complications can still be reduced by following a correct diet and practising physical activity. Therefore, the prevention and management of the disease in progress are essential to prevent or even delay the first manifestation and maintain a glycaemic index below the normal reference values [45].

In addition to the systemic and general signs mentioned above, DMT2 has a very specific expression in the oral cavity: dry mouth sensation or burning mouth syndrome (BMS), dehydration of the perioral mucosa, diabetic ketoacidosis breathing, increased volume of the gums, fungal infections such as candida, stomatitis, xerostomia, ulcers, periodontal erosions and abscesses and periodontitis.

Hyperglycaemia and hypertriglyceridemia increase the inflammatory response of the immune system, resulting in a greater extension and faster progression of periodontal disease.

Research from the University of Helsinki has shown that diabetic patients are more likely to develop lesions of the oral mucosa and tongue and parasympathetic and peripheral autonomic neuropathies. Furthermore, the latter neuronal dysfunction is considered a risk factor for temporomandibular disorders. Periodontitis is the sixth most common complication for diabetic patients. Despite that, well-controlled diabetic patients have a lower risk of developing the disease than uncontrolled patients [18,55,57,58].

In these subjects, healing takes longer than normal, the mucosa is no longer resilient and osteoclastic activity is increased. The combination of these characteristics causes instability of the complete prosthesis, as it cannot precisely fit the underlying mucosa. This entails difficulties for the clinician when it comes to rehabilitation of the oral cavity in a diabetic patient [59,60].

Resorptive agents and osteonecrosis

Antiresorptive agents are used as the therapy of choice to prevent and treat osteoporosis, osteopenia, multiple myeloma, Paget's disease of the bone, osteogenesis imperfecta and tumour conditions in association with radiotherapy. The most commonly used antiresorptives are bisphosphonates, also called diphosphonates. They are therefore used for those diseases that involve bone density and the route of administration is orally or intravenously [61,62].

In 2011, Coleman [63] and Gnant [64] underlined how antiresorptive agents may alter or even postpone the onset of tumour masses. The most insidious adverse effect in patients undergoing treatment with biphosphonates is biphospohonate related osteonecrosis of the jaw (BRONJ). The same clinical picture may occur in therapies with antiangiogenic and chemotherapeutic agents [62].

The physiopathology of these agents is the inhibition of the differentiation and function of osteoclastic cells which will therefore undergo apoptosis. This mechanism results in a decrease in bone remodelling and angiogenesis. It should therefore be specified that the cause of necrosis is not the extraction of a tooth per se, but the reason for the treatment: caries, periodontal and periapical problems. Indeed, some studies have found *Actinomyces* bacterial species in combination with fungi and viruses, to underline how the inflammatory component or infection are required for the onset of necrosis [65,66].

Bisphosphonates have a half-life of months-years, that is to say that the chemical component of these medications can be found in the body even after 10 years. That is why the duration of the treatment is considered a risk factor for BRONJ [61].

In general, the risk of developing osteonecrosis of the jaw due to medication intake is very low, it is multifactorial and is related to trauma or injury of the bone. Patients exposed to treatment with intravenous bisphosphonate are assumed to have an incidence of approximately 0.5-0.8% of developing BRONJ in the first year, 0.9-1.8% in the second year, and 1.1-1.8% after three years of intake. The incidence of BRONJ for patients being treated with biphosphonates orally is however lower: 0% in the first year, 0.05% in the second and third year and 0.2% after four years of intake. In general, a 0.5% risk of developing BRONJ is considered following a dental extraction [18,21].

It is vital for the clinician to have a clear medical history of the patient, especially if they are taking bisphosphonates, before carrying out any type of treatment.

References

1. WHO. *Preamble to the Constitution of WHO as adopted by the International Health Conference, New York, 19-22 July 1946; signed on 22 July 1946 by the representatives of 61 States (Official Records of WHO, n. 2, p. 100) and entered into force on 7 April; 1948.* pp. 119-38.
2. Winkler S. *Symposium on complete dentures.* Vol. 21. Saunders; 1977. pp. 197-8
3. ISTAT. *Condizioni di salute e ricorso ai servizi sanitari.* ISTAT; 2008.
4. Douglass CW, Shih A, Ostry L. Will there be a need for complete dentures in the United States in 2020? *J Prosthet Dent.* 2002;87(1):5-8.
5. Naharro M, Carlsson GE. What are the prevalence and incidence of tooth loss in the adult and elderly population in Europe? *Clin Oral Implants Res.* 2007;18(3):2-14.
6. ISTAT. *Il ricorso alle cure odontoiatriche.* ISTAT; 2015.
7. Yven C, Bonnet L, Cormier D et al. Impaired mastication modifies the dynamics of bolus formation. *Eur J Oral Sci.* 2006;114(3):184-90.
8. Emami E, De Souza RF, Kabawat M, Feine JS. The impact of edentulism on oral and general health. *Int J Dent.* 2013;2013:498305 epub.
9. Musacchio E, Perissinotto E, Binotto P et al. Tooth loss in the elderly and its association with nutritional status, socio-economic and lifestyle factors. *Acta Odontol Scand.* 2007;65(2):78-86.
10. Bitetti E, Senna A, Strohmenger L. Oral health comparison between the institutionalized and non institutionalized elderly. *Minerva Stomatol.* 2004;53(9):507-16.
11. Cunha-Cruz J, Hujoel PP, Nadanovsky P. Secular trends in socioeconomic disparities in edentulism. *J Dent Res.* 2007;86:131-6.
12. The Prevalence of Dental Caries in Europe 1990-1995. *Caries Res.* 1996;30:237-55.
13. Passarelli PC, Pagnoni S, Piccirillo GB et al. Reasons for tooth extractions and related risk factors in adult patients: a cohort study. *Int J Environ Res Public Health.* 2020;17(7):2575.
14. Lamont RJ, Egland PG. Dental caries. *Mol Med Microbiol Second Ed.* 2014;2-3(4):945-55.
15. Bollero P, Grassi F, Federici A et al. *Linee guida nazionali per la promozione della salute orale e la prevenzione delle patologie orali in età adulta.* Ministero Della Salute; 2009. pp. 6-13.
16. Tramini P, Montal S, Valcarcel J. Tooth loss and associated factors in long-term institutionalised elderly patients. *Gerodontology.* 2007;24(4): 196-203.
17. Hamasha AAH. Medical conditions associated with missing teeth and edentulism in the institutionalized elderly. *Spec Care Dent.* 1998;18(3): 123-7.
18. Alves C, Casqueiro J, Casqueiro J. Infections in patients with diabetes mellitus: A review of pathogenesis. *Indian J Endocrinol Metab.* 2012;16 (7):27.
19. Tallgren A. Positional changes of complete dentures a 7-year longitudinal study. *Acta Odontol Scand.* 1969;27(5):539-61.
20. Malheiros AS, Carvalhal ST, Pereira TL et al. Association between tooth loss and degree of temporomandibular disorders: A comparative study. *J Contemp Dent Pract.* 2016;17(3):235-9.
21. Manfredini D, Lombardo L, Siciliani G. Temporomandibular disorders and dental occlusion. A systematic review of association studies: end of an era. *Evid Based Dent.* 2017;18(3):86-7.
22. Wayler AH, Chauncey HH. Impact of complete dentures and impaired natural dentition on masticatory performance and food choice in healthy aging men. *J Prosthet Dent.* 1983;49(3):427-33.
23. Österberg T, Carlsson GE, Sundh V. Trends and prognoses of dental status in the Swedish population: Analysis based on interviews in 1975 to 1997 by Statistics Sweden. *Acta Odontol Scand.* 2000;58(4):177-82.
24. Helkimo E, Carlsson GE, Helkimo M. Bite force and state denticion. *Acta Odont Scand.* 1977;35: 297-303.
25. Haraldson T, Karlsson U, Carlsson GE. Bite force and oral function in complete denture wearers. *J Oral Rehabil.* 1979;6(1):41-8.
26. Michael CG, Javid NS, Colaizzi FA, Gibbs CH. Biting strength and chewing forces in complete denture wearers. *J Prosthet Dent.* 1990;63(5):549-53.
27. Kapur KK, Soman SD. Masticatory performance and efficiency in denture wearers. *J Prosthet Dent.* 2004;92(2):107-11.

28. Liedberg B, Stoltze K, Owall B. The masticatory handicap of wearing removable dentures in elderly men. *Gerodontology*. 2005;22(1):10-6.
29. Geertman ME, Slagter AP, Van Waas MAJ, Kalk W. Comminution of food with mandibular implant-retained overdentures. *J Dent Res*. 1994;73(12):1858-64.
30. Geertman ME, Slagter AP, Thof M et al. Masticatory performance and chewing experience with implant-retained mandibular overdentures. *J Oral Rehabil*. 1999;26(1):7-13.
31. Sandström B, Lindquist LW. The effect of different prosthetic restorations on the dietary selection in edentulous patients: A longitudinal study of patients initially treated with optimal complete dentures and finally with tissue-integrated prostheses. *Acta Odontol Scand*. 1987;45(6):423-8.
32. Sebring NG, Guckes AD, Li SH, McCarthy GR. Nutritional adequacy of reported intake of edentulous subjects treated with new conventional or implant-supported mandibular dentures. *J Prosthet Dent*. 1995;74(4):358-63.
33. Ellis JS, Thomason JM, Jepson NJ et al. A randomized-controlled trial of food choices made by edentulous adults. *Clin Oral Implants Res*. 2008;19(4):356-61.
34. Allen F, McMillan A. Food selection and perceptions of chewing ability following provision of implant and conventional prostheses in complete denture wearers. *Clin Oral Implants Res*. 2002;13(3):320-6.
35. Shepherd R. Influences on food choice and dietary behavior. *Forum Nutr*. 2005;57:36-43.
36. Bradbury J, Thomason JM, Jepson NJA et al. Perceived chewing ability and intake of fruit and vegetables. *J Dent Res*. 2008;87(8):720-5.
37. Shinkai RSA, Hatch JP, Sakai S et al. Oral function and diet quality in a community-based sample. *J Dent Res*. 2001;80(7):1625-30.
38. Shinkai RSA, Hatch JP, Rugh JD et al. Dietary intake in edentulous subjects with good and poor quality complete dentures. *J Prosthet Dent*. 2015;72(6):495-8.
39. Pierce JP, Newman VA, Natarajan L et al. Telephone counseling helps maintain long-term adherence to a high-vegetable dietary pattern. *J Nutr*. 2007;137(10):2291-6.
40. Bradbury J, Thomason JM, Jepson NJA et al. Fruit and vegetable intake in the edentulous. *J Dent Res*. 2006;85(5):463-8.
41. Cademartori MG, Gastal MT, Nascimento GG et al. Is depression associated with oral health outcomes in adults and elders ? A systematic review and meta-analysis. *Clinical Oral Investigations*. 2018;22(8):2685-702.
42. Sko K, Malicka B, Zie M, Kaczmarek U. Oral health condition and occurrence of depression in the elderly. *Med*. 2018;97(41):e12490.
43. Tyrovolas S, Koyanagi A, Panagiotakos DB et al. Population prevalence of edentulism and its association with depression and self-rated health. *Sci Rep*. 2016;6(1):1-9.
44. Wideman TH, Sullivan MJL, Inada S et al. Brief symptom inventory. *Encycl Behav Med*. 2013;269-70.
45. Sesti G. Il diabete in Italia. A cura di Enzo Bonora e Giorgio Sesti. Bologna: Bononia University Press; 2016.
46. Pearson ER. Type 2 diabetes: a multifaceted disease. *Diabetologia*. 2019;62:1107-12.
47. Hansson S, Halldin A. Alveolar ridge resorption after tooth extraction: a consequence of a fundamental principle of bone physiology. *J Dent Biomech*. 2012;3:1758736012456543.
48. Chappuis Vi, Araujo MG, Buser D. Clinical relevance of dimensional bone and soft tissue alterations post-extraction in esthetic sites PM. *Periodontol* 2000. 2017;73:73-83.
49. Clementini M, Agostinelli A, Castelluzzo W, et al. The effect of immediate implant placement on alveolar ridge preservation compared to spontaneous healing after tooth extraction: Radiographic results of a randomized controlled clinical trial. *J Clin Periodontol*. 2019; 46(7):776-86.
50. Tompkins KA. The osteoimmunology of alveolar bone loss The osteoimmunology of alveolar bone loss. *Connect Tissue Res*. 2016;57(2):69-90.
51. Cawood JI, Howell RA. A classificationof the edentulous jaws. *Int J Oral Maxillofac Surg*. 1988;(13):232-6.

52. Misch CE, Judy K. Classification of partially edentulous arches for implant dentistry. *Int J Oral Implantol.* 1987;4(2):7-13.

53. Ruscin JM, Linnebur SA. *Farmaci problematici negli anziani.* Manuale MSD. 2018.

54. Besdine RW. *Valutazione del paziente anziano.* Manuale MSD. 2019.

55. Zheng Y, Ley SH, Hu FB. Global aetiology and epidemiology of type 2 diabetes mellitus and its complications. *Nat Publ Gr.* 2017;14(2):88-98.

56. International Diabetes Federation IDF. *IDF Diabetes Atlas.* 7th ed. Bruxelles; 2015.

57. Collin HL, Niskanen L, Uusitupa M et al. Oral symptoms and signs in elderly patients with type 2 diabetes mellitus: a focus on diabetic neuropathy. *Oral Surg Oral Med Oral Pathol Oral Radiol Endod.* 2000;90(3):299-305.

58. Parbhakar KK, Rosella LC, Singhal S, Quiñonez CR. Acute and chronic diabetes complications associated with self-reported oral health : a retrospective cohort study. *BMC Oral Health.* 2020; 20(1):1-9.

59. Lamster IB, Lalla E, Borgnakke WS, Taylor GW. The Relationship Between Oral Health and Diabetes Mellitus. *J Am Dent Assoc.* 2008;139:19S-24S.

60. Pawlowicz A, Tymczyna-borowicz B, Ptasiewicz M. The state of the oral health in patients with type 2 diabetes. *Pol Merkur Lekarski.* 2020;48(283):27-31.

61. Wang H, Weber D, Mccauley LK. Effect of long-term oral bisphosphonates on implant wound healing: literature review and a case report. *J Periodontol.* 2007;78(3):584-94.

62. Eleutherakis-Papaiakovou E, Bamias A. Antiresorptive treatment-associated ONJ. *Eur J Cancer Care (Engl).* 2017;1-11.

63. Coleman RE, Marshall H, Cameron D et al. Breast-cancer adjuvant therapy with zoledronic acid. *N Engl J Med.* 2011;365(15):1396-405.

64. Gnant M, Mlineritsch B, Stoeger H et al. Adjuvant endocrine therapy plus zoledronic acid in premenopausal women with early-stage breast cancer: 62-month follow-up from the ABCSG-12 randomised trial. *Lancet Oncol.* 2011;12(7):631-41.

65. Wan JT, Sheeley DM, Somerman MJ, Lee JS. Mitigating osteonecrosis of the jaw (ONJ) through preventive dental care and understanding of risk factors. *Bone Res.* 2020;8:14.

66. Nicolatou-galitis O, Kouri M, Papadopoulou E et al. Osteonecrosis of the jaw related to non-antiresorptive medications: a systematic review. *Support Care Cancer.* 2019;27(2):383-94.

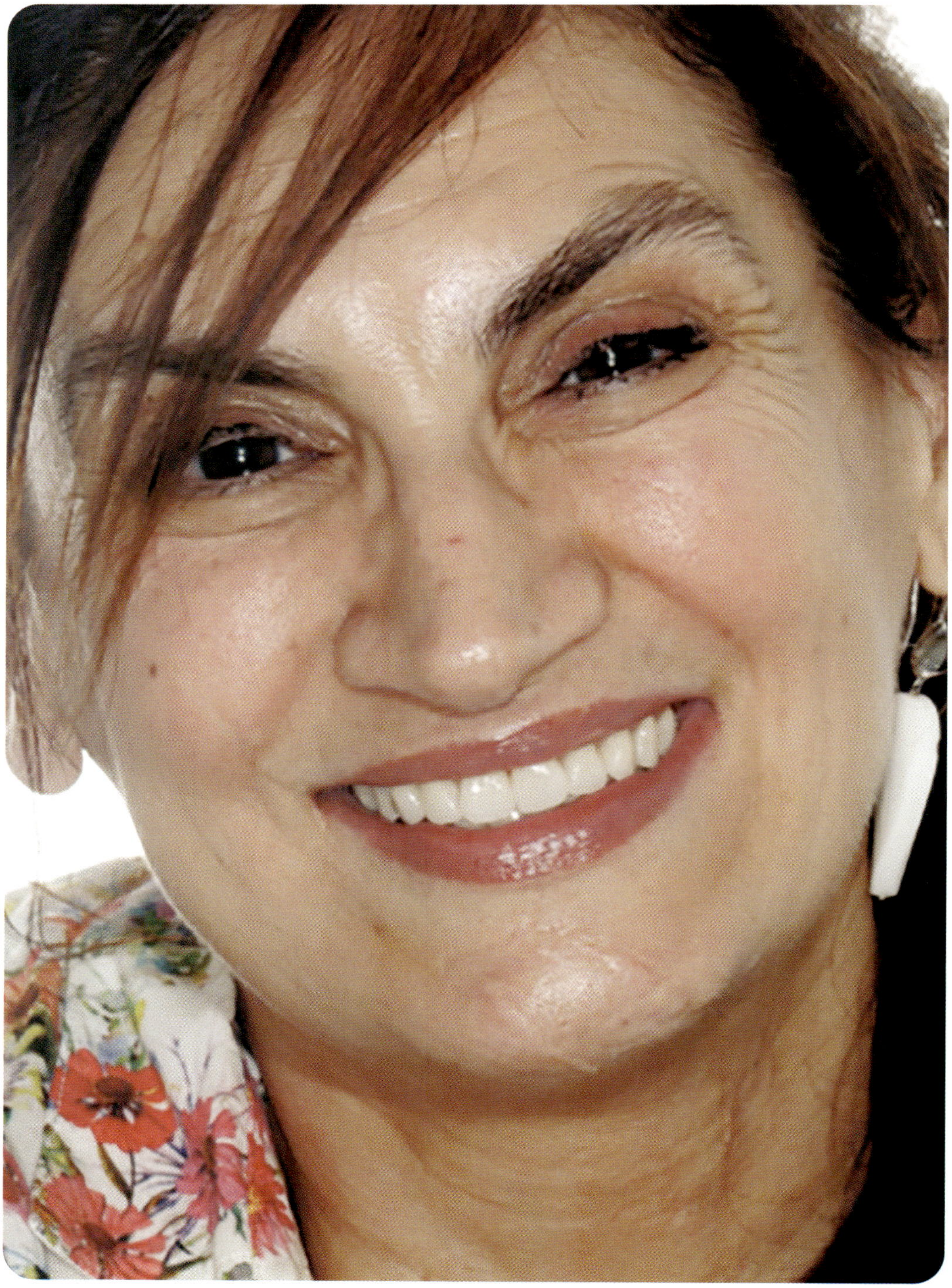

CHAPTER 2

P. VENEZIA

Biomimetic approach to complete prostheses

The purpose of all prosthetic rehabilitations is to provide phonetic and esthetic function to patients (at the end of the treatment). The reference that has best described the "esthetic" approach to fixed prosthetic rehabilitation is the work by Mauro Fradeani [1].

Other criteria have been proposed, somehow linked to mathematical evaluations of dental and facial proportions.

One of the most interesting ones is that suggested by Spear [2] who defined facially generated treatment planning (FGTP) as the guided prosthetic treatment that starts from esthetics then goes on with the function and structure of the rehabilitation.

The starting point of all prosthetic rehabilitations, either fixed or removable, is establishing the three-dimensionally ideal position of the central upper incisors.

The analysis must be performed in the frontal and sagittal direction and must inevitably take into account the relationships of the upper teeth with the lower ones and with the perioral tissues and, above all, the correlation between the position of the teeth and the vertical dimension (VD). The analysis must be both static and dynamic.

The first evaluation concerns precisely the facial proportion.

The face is divided into three thirds, each measuring between 62 and 75 mm vertically, depending on the patient's face morphology **(Figure 2.1)** [3].

Remaining within the sphere of dental competence, the lower third of the face can in its turn be divided into two parts: the first goes from the base of the nose to the commissural line of the lips and the second from there to the point that defines the outermost part of the chin (*gnation*) (**Figure 2.2**). The second part of the lower third is on average twice the first part. A decreased height of the lower face third is generally associated to a loss in VD.

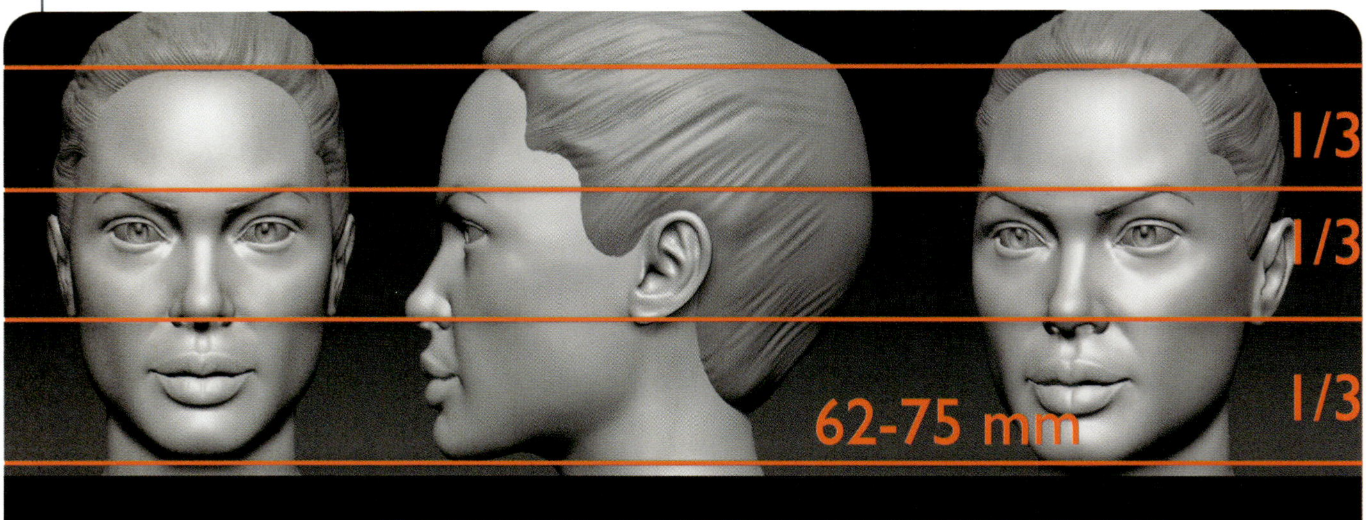

Figure 2.1 • The face can be divided into three thirds, each one measuring approximately 62-75 mm.

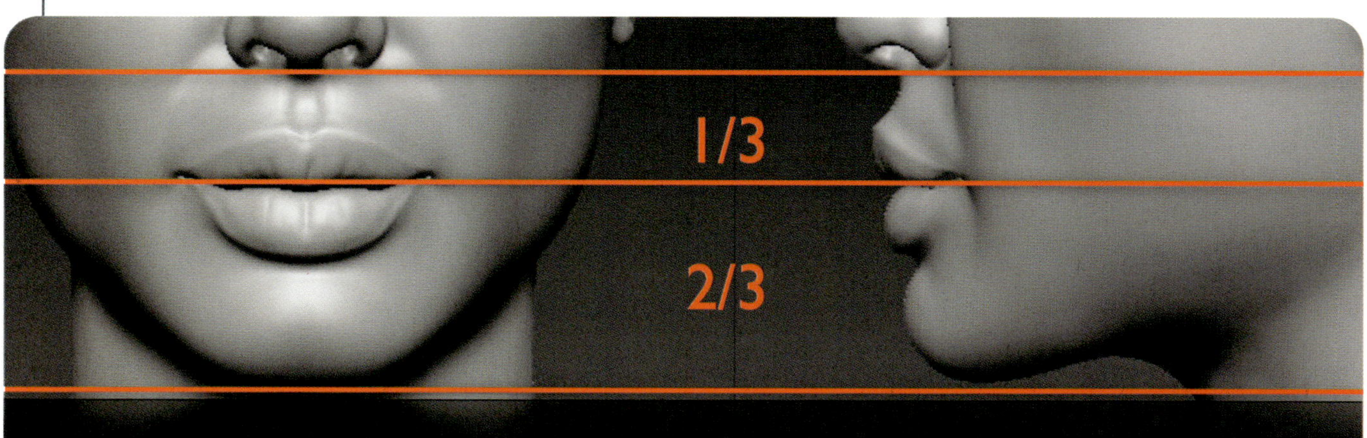

Figure 2.2 • The lower third of the face can be divided into two parts.

Vertical dimension

The resting vertical dimension (RVD) must be distinguished from the occlusion vertical dimension (OVD).

The RVD equals the distance between two arbitrary points taken one above and the other below the lip line when the mandible is in a resting position with the elevator and depressing muscles in a balanced state and with the condyles in a non-forced joint position.

The OVD equals the distance between two arbitrary points, one above and the other below the lip line, when the teeth are in maximum intercuspation.

The distance between the antagonist dental arches when the mandible is at rest is referred to as occlusal free way space [4] and is the result of the difference between RVD and OVD.

On average it measures 1-3 mm. This figure may vary from patient to patient and even in the same individual at different times during the day [5].

A decrease in OVD can be observed in patients, due to wear, loss or migration of the teeth.

This evidence may concern even young patients who present with genetic disorders, such as ectodermal dysplasia [6] **(Figure 2.3)**.

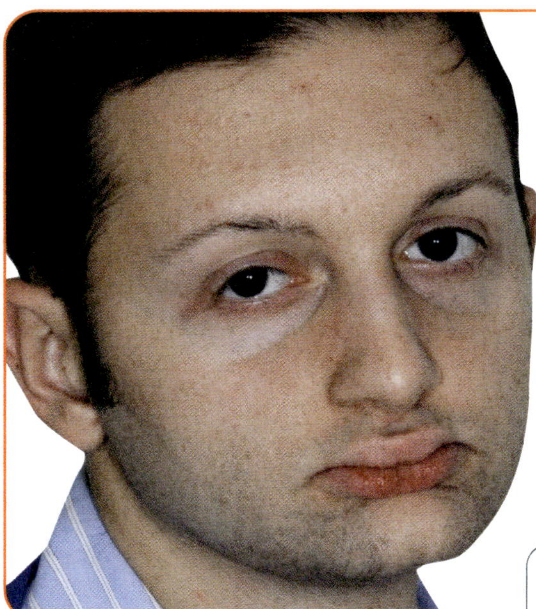

- Angular cheilitis
- Deepened crease between lower lip and chin
- Decreased height of the face lower third
- "Thinning" of the lips
- "Sliding" forwards and upwards towards the maxilla

Figure 2.3 • Signs of loss of vertical dimension in a young patient.

The signs of VD loss are:

- angular cheilitis;
- deepened mentolabial crease;
- vertical decrease of the face lower third;
- forward and upward sliding of the mandible [7].

The implant-prosthetic treatment of patients who show severe atrophy of the maxilla and mandible must often include a preliminary diagnostic stage with the use of removable prostheses that will allow the volume and space of the bone reconstruction to be quantified (**Figures 2.4** and **2.5**).

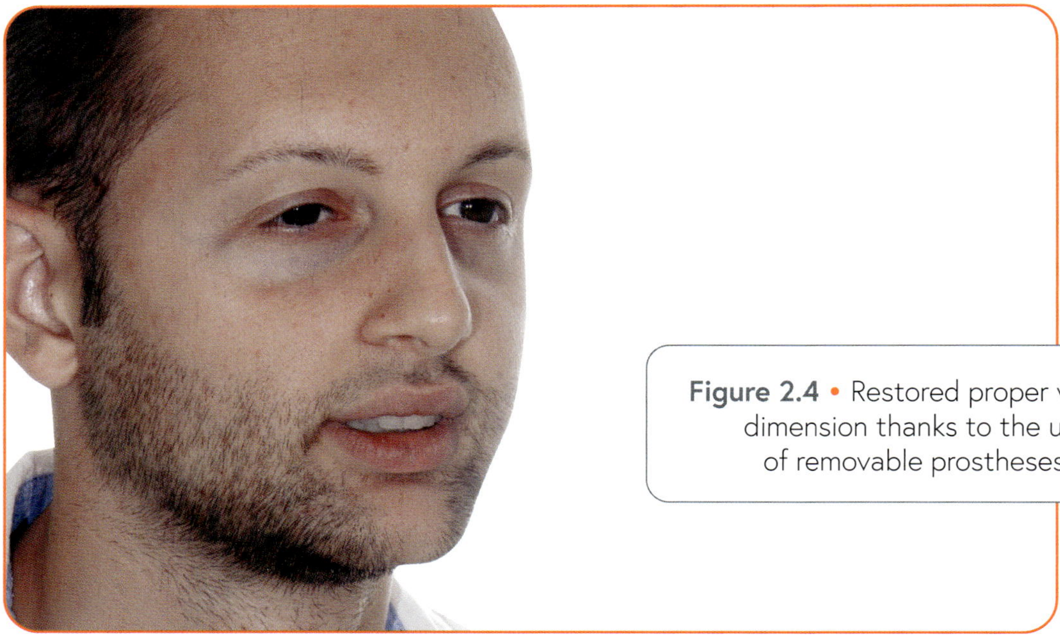

Figure 2.4 • Restored proper vertical dimension thanks to the use of removable prostheses.

This diagnostic approach will make it possible to evaluate the ideal relationship between teeth and bone bases and therefore allow any reconstructive and/or regenerative surgery preliminary to the implant-prosthetic treatment to be thoroughly planned.

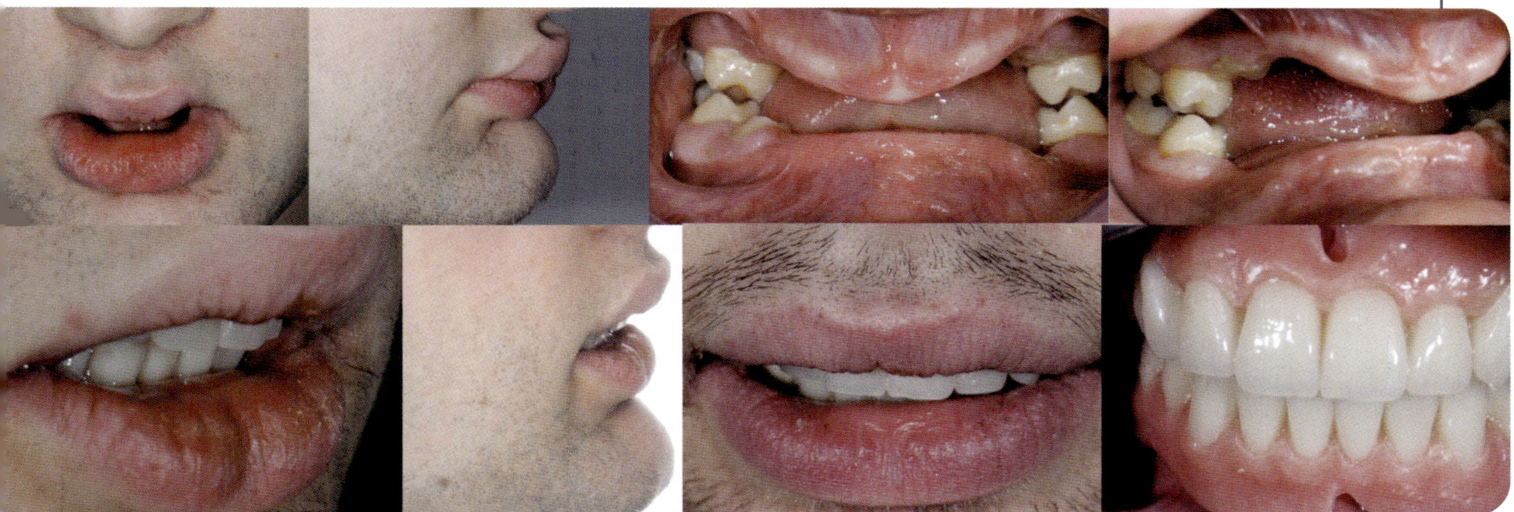

Figure 2.5 • Restored face proportions and esthetics after the prosthetic rehabilitation.

One of the primary goals of the rehabilitation therapy is therefore careful VD assessment (**Figures 2.6** and **2.7**).

In frontal view, after evaluating the proportions between the three thirds of the face, the horizontal reference lines on which to orient the prosthetic rehabilitation must be analysed.

Ideally, the incisal edge should be parallel to all horizontal reference lines.

The bipupillary line, frequently cited as an important horizontal reference line, is very rarely parallel to the other lines (ophriac, commissural and interalar). It is more appropriate to refer to the horizon line [8].

In frontal view, the facial midline should be perpendicular to the horizontal lines (**Figures 2.8** and **2.9**).

It is important to remember that the facial midline goes through three fixed points:

- glabella;
- philtrum;
- chin.

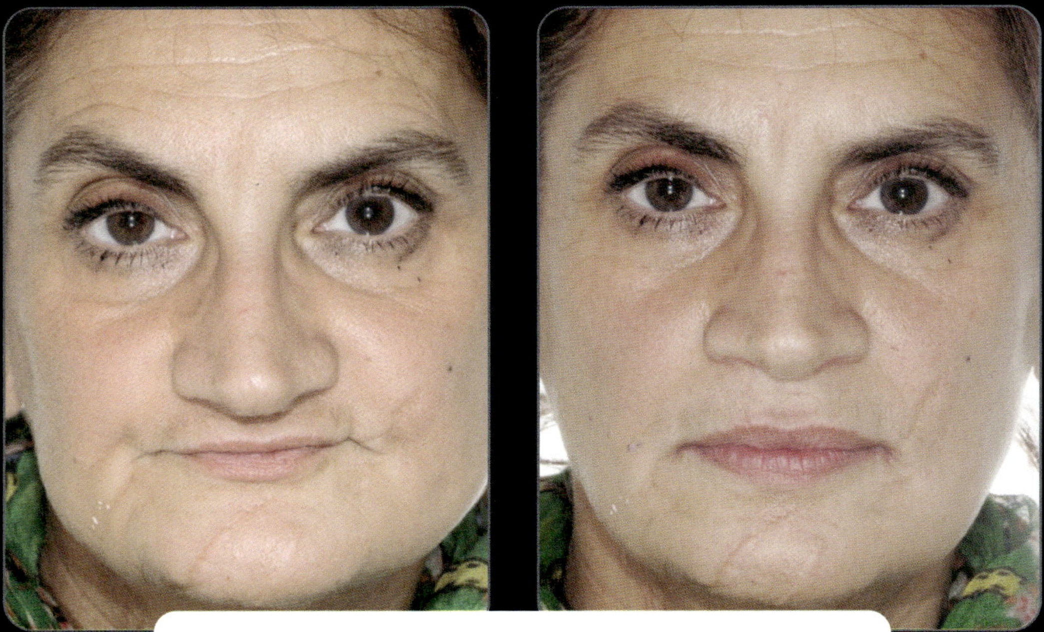

Figure 2.6 • The rehabilitation treatment plan must be guided by the patient's face. Front view.

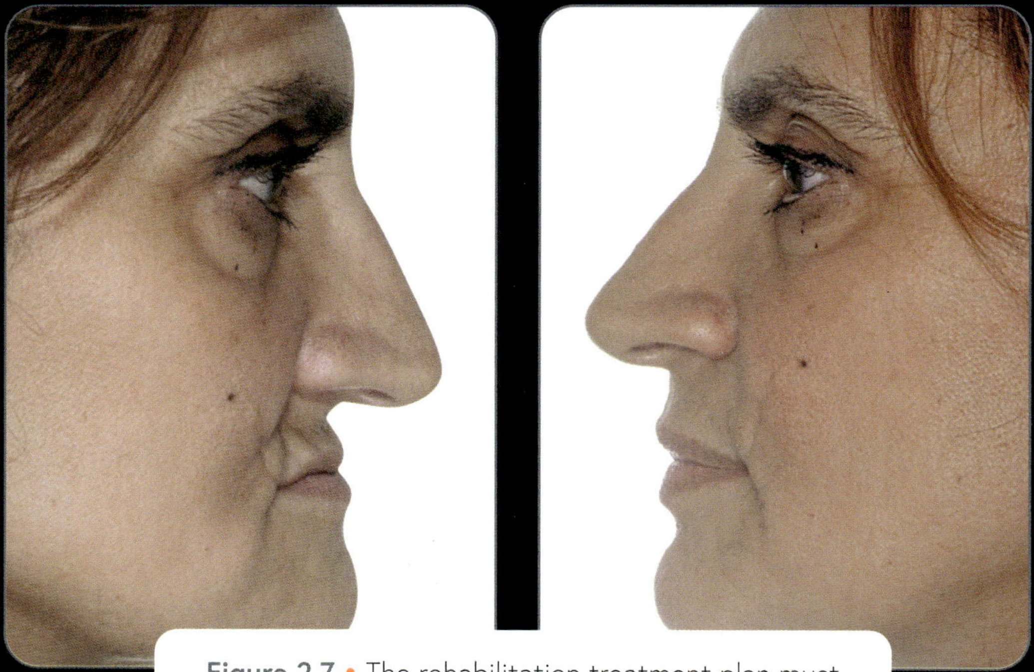

Figure 2.7 • The rehabilitation treatment plan must be guided by the patient's face. Side view.

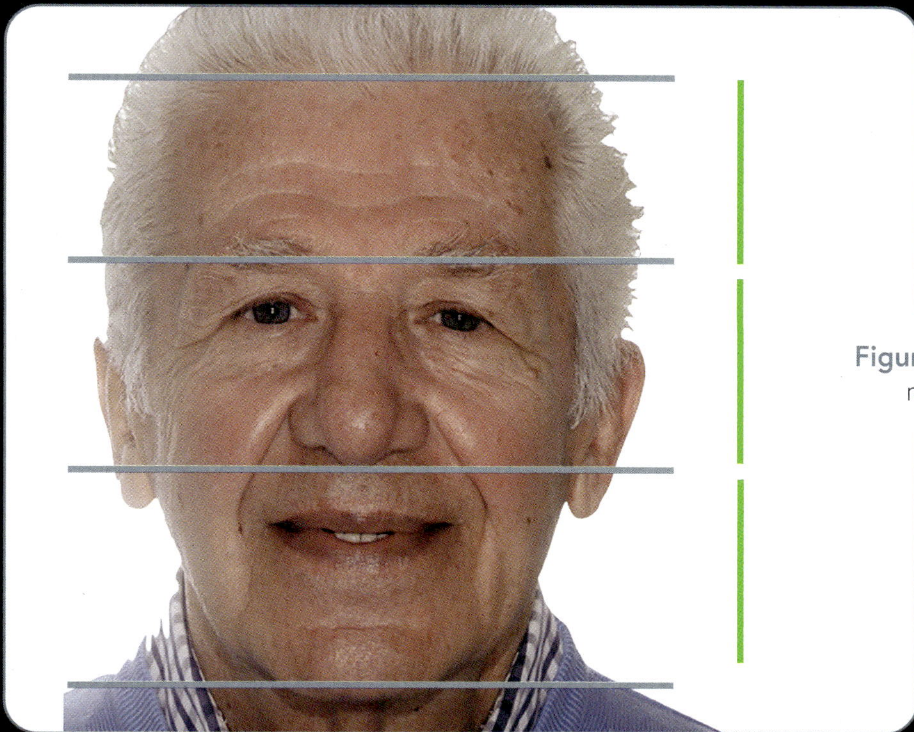

Figure 2.8 • Horizontal reference lines.

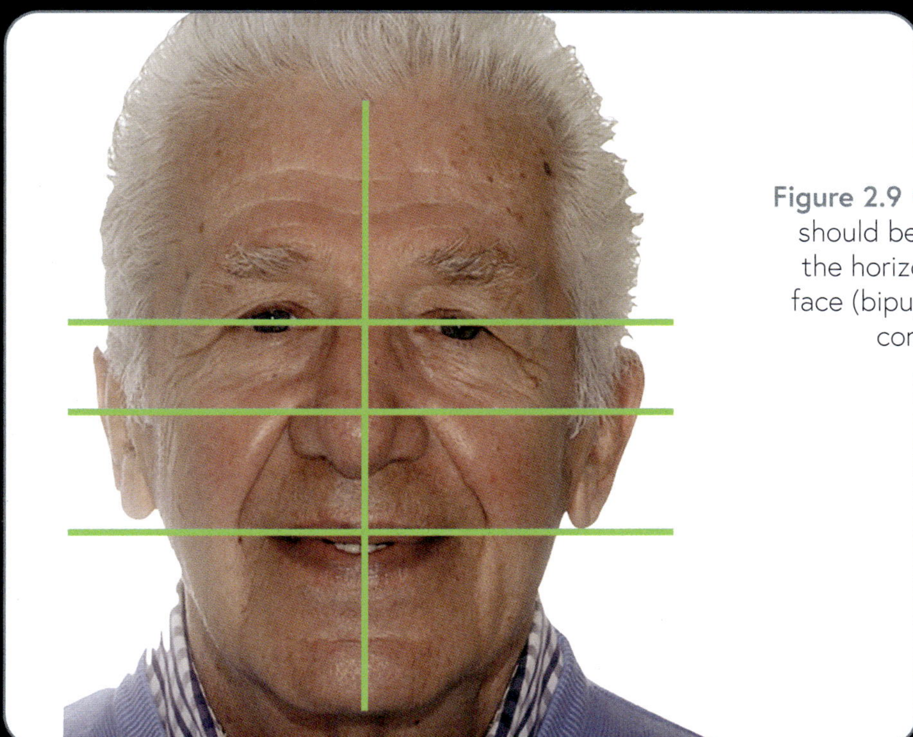

Figure 2.9 • The facial midline should be perpendicularto the horizontal lines of the face (bipupillary, horizontal, commissural).

Ideally, the facial midline should coincide with the dental interincisal midline of the maxilla (**Figure 2.10**).

In actual fact, the frontal discrepancy even up to 4 mm between the two lines is not perceived by the general population or even by general dentists. However, even a minimal variation in the inclination of the clinical crown axis of the upper central incisors with respect to the facial midline is very evident even for small angular variations (**Figure 2.11**) [9,10].

The anterior teeth are essential in supporting perioral tissues (**Figure 2.12**).

From a side view, it is possible to measure the extent of the perioral tissue support. One of the most commonly used reference lines is the E-line (Esthetic-line) which was defined by Rickets in 1968 [11]. This line indicates the ideal distance of the lips from the line joining the tip of the nose to the most prominent point of the chin; the distance of the upper lip from the E-line should be 4 mm, while that of the lower lip should be about 2 mm (**Figure 2.13**).

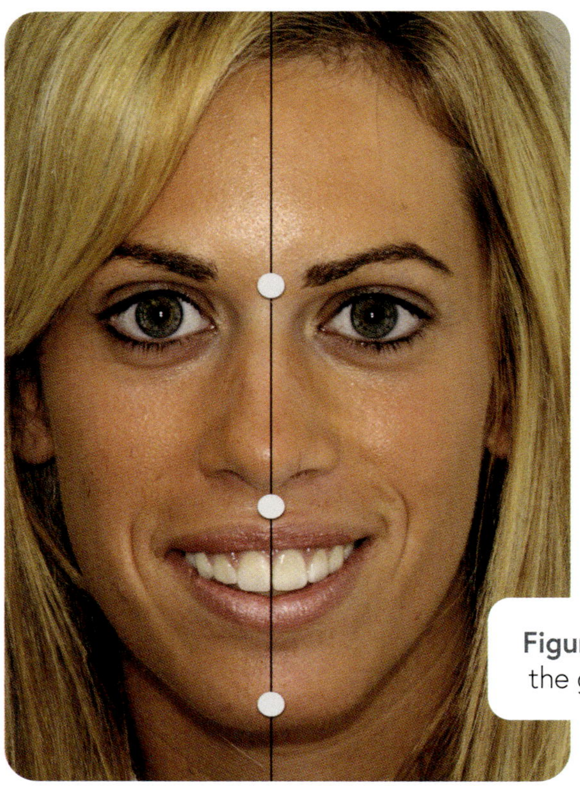

Figure 2.10 • The midline goes through the glabella, the philtrum and the chin.

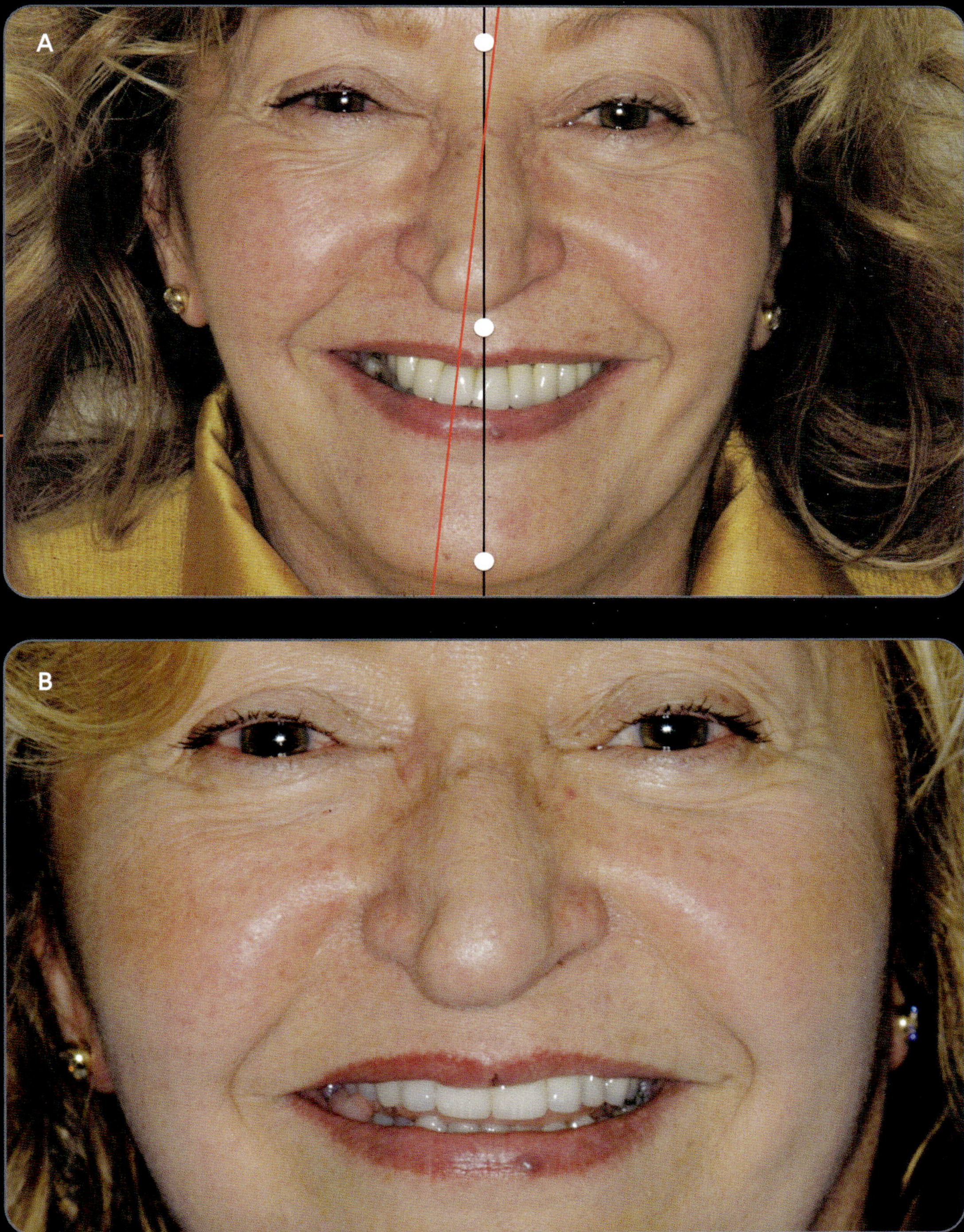

Figure 2.11 • (**A**) A slight inconsistency between the dental and facial midline is not perceived by patients, unlike incorrect inclination of the incisal plane.
(**B**) Photograph of the patient after the prosthetic rehabilitation.

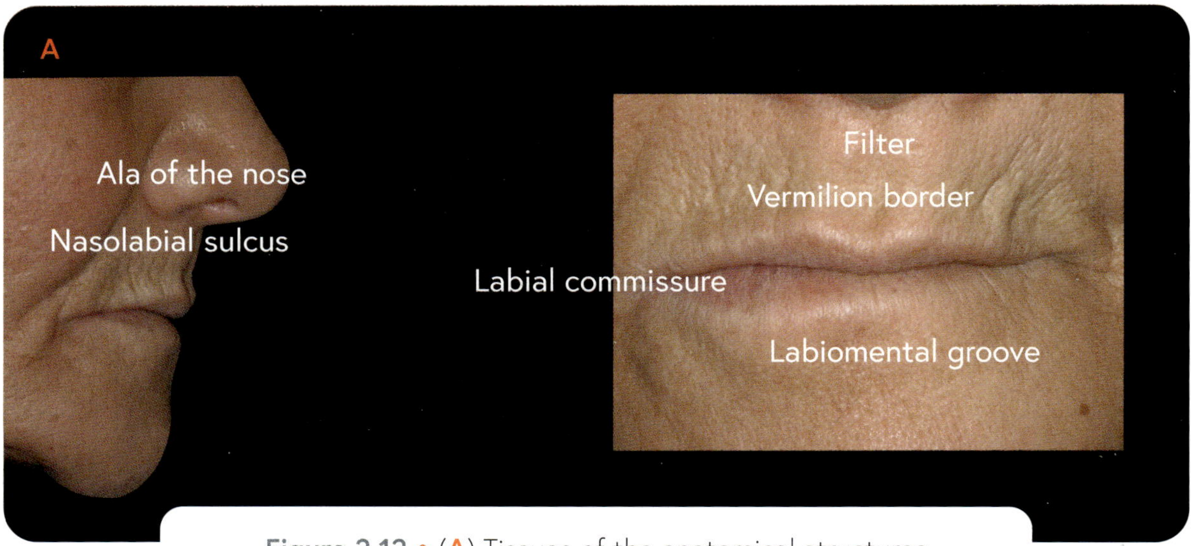

Figure 2.12 • (**A**) Tissues of the anatomical structures supported by the teeth and by the alveolar process. (**B**) Tissues of the anatomical structures that benefit from the support of the removable prosthesis.

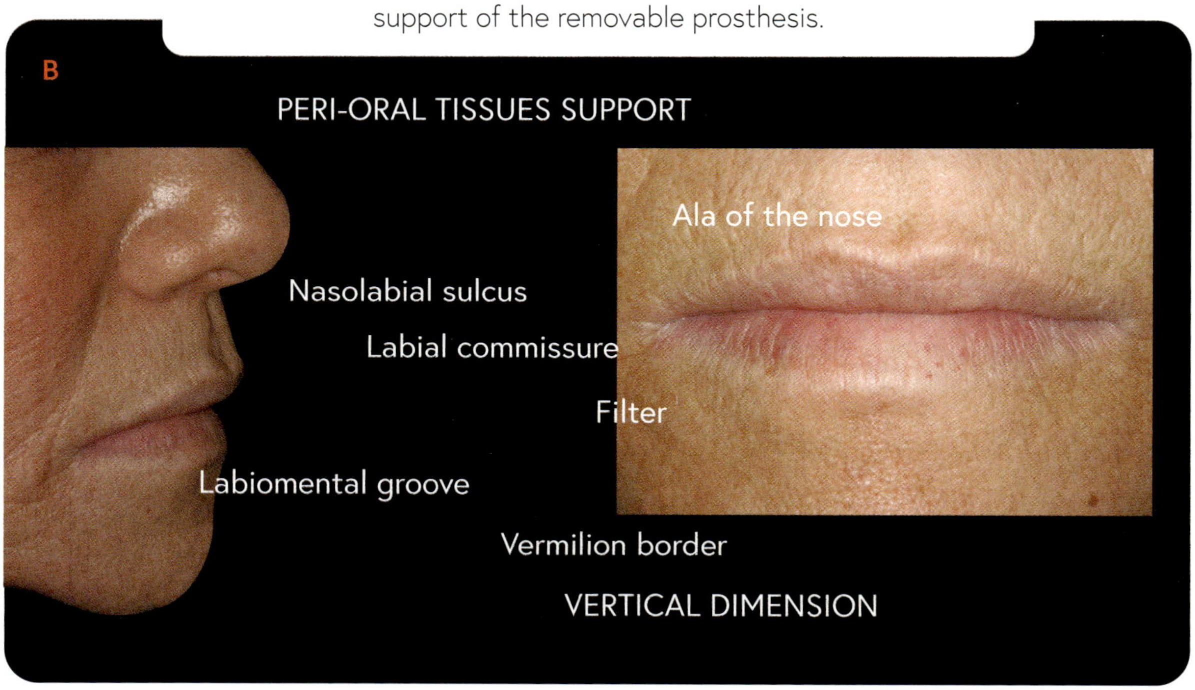

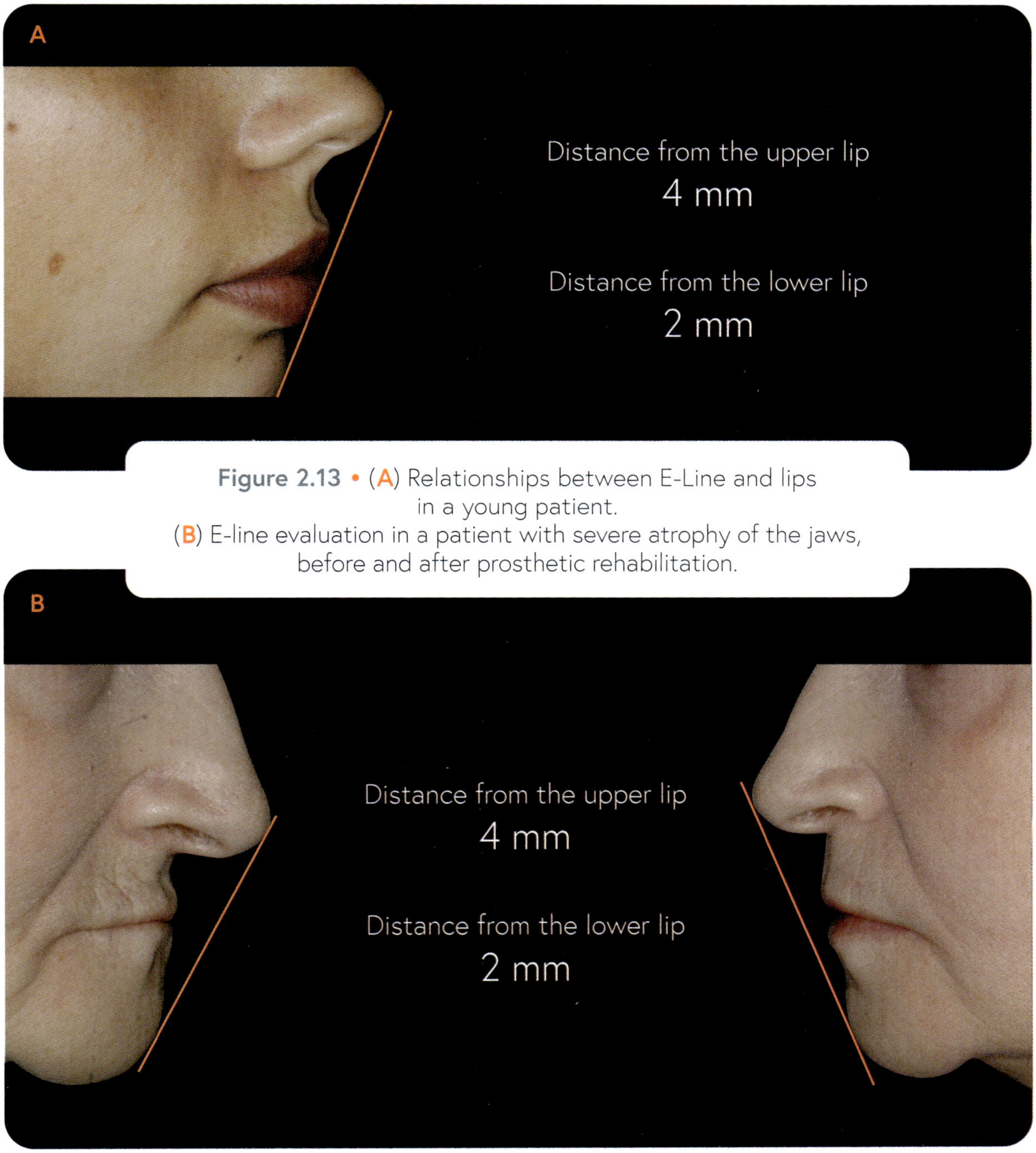

Figure 2.13 • (**A**) Relationships between E-Line and lips in a young patient.
(**B**) E-line evaluation in a patient with severe atrophy of the jaws, before and after prosthetic rehabilitation.

These relationships are needed in the fixed prosthetic approach and have an additional value in the removable prosthesis, as they allow the need for the prosthetic flange to be assessed. A second parameter that is considered in esthetic rehabilitations with removable prosthesis is the width of the nasolabial angle: this angle should be between 100° and 105° in women, and between 90 and 95° in men [12] (**Figure 2.14**).

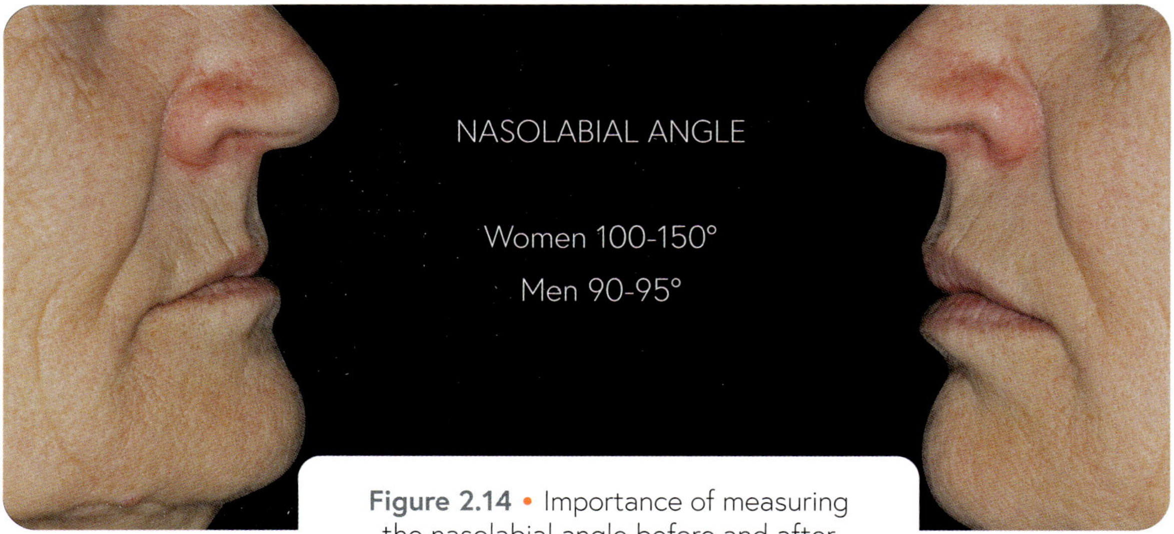

Figure 2.14 • Importance of measuring the nasolabial angle before and after prosthetic rehabilitation.

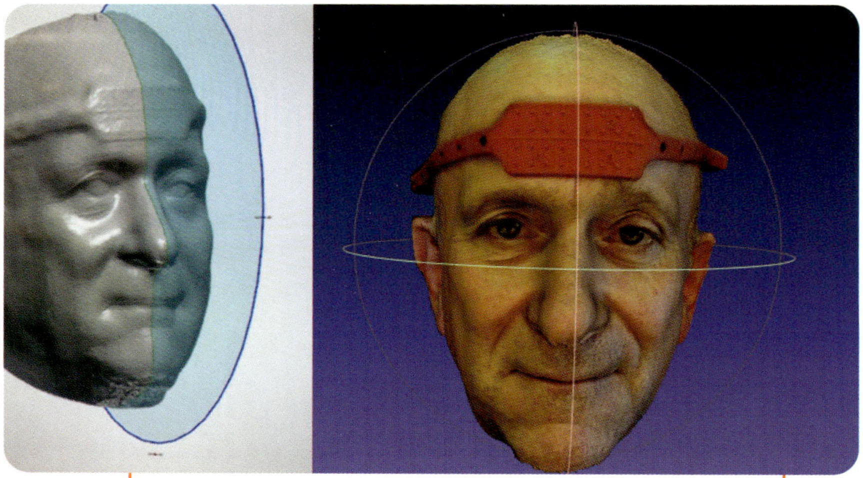

Figure 2.15 • Possibility of evaluating the support of perioral tissues with digital instruments.

In the case of the removable prosthesis, the prosthetic flange may dramatically change the width of this angle.

A new possibility to evaluate the extent of perioral tissue support to be provided to the patient is to perform facial scans. The files can be exported in STL format and be superimposed to perform sagittal comparisons **(Figure 2.15)**.

Certain anatomical determinants must be taken into consideration in order to perform adequate positioning of the front anterior teeth on the horizontal plane. One of them is the incisive papilla, always present in dentate as well as wholly edentulous patients.

The atrophy of the upper jaw causes vestibularisation of the papilla **(Figure 2.16)**.

The distance on the horizontal plane between the centre of the papilla and the vestibular surface of the upper central incisors is 8-10 mm on average [13,14] **(Figure 2.17)**.

As we will see in Chapter 4, the correct positioning of the front teeth according to a setting defined as "harmonic" (which entails correct positioning of the frontal incisors 8-10 mm from the centre of the incisive papilla) on the one hand ensures adequate support of the perioral tissues, on the other it ensures the space for prosthetic functionality.

This setting also influences the volume of the posterior teeth.

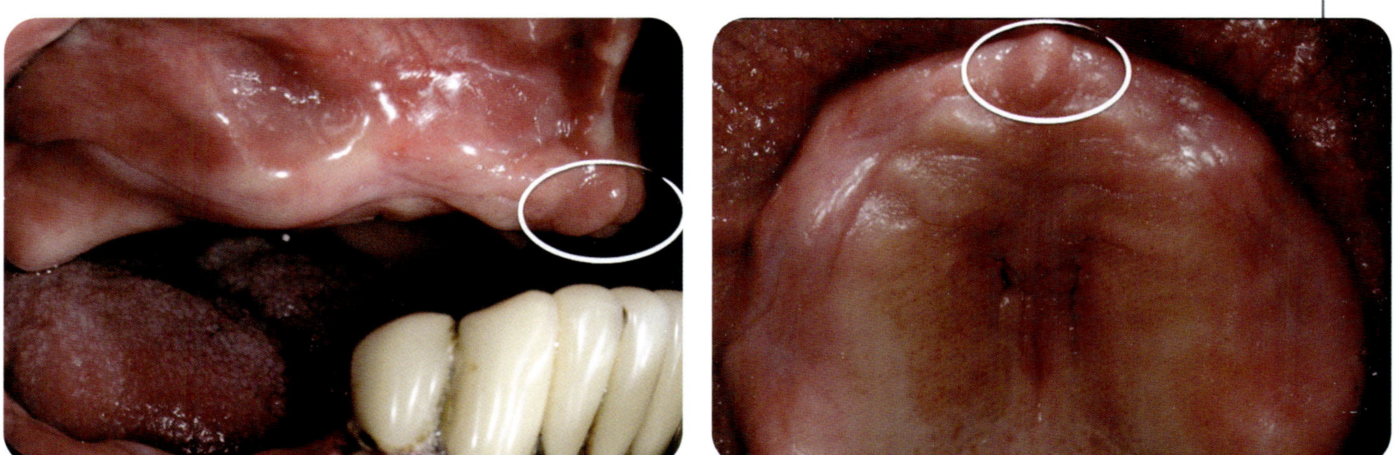

Figure 2.16 • Vestibularisation of the upper incisive papilla in case of atrophy of the upper jaw.

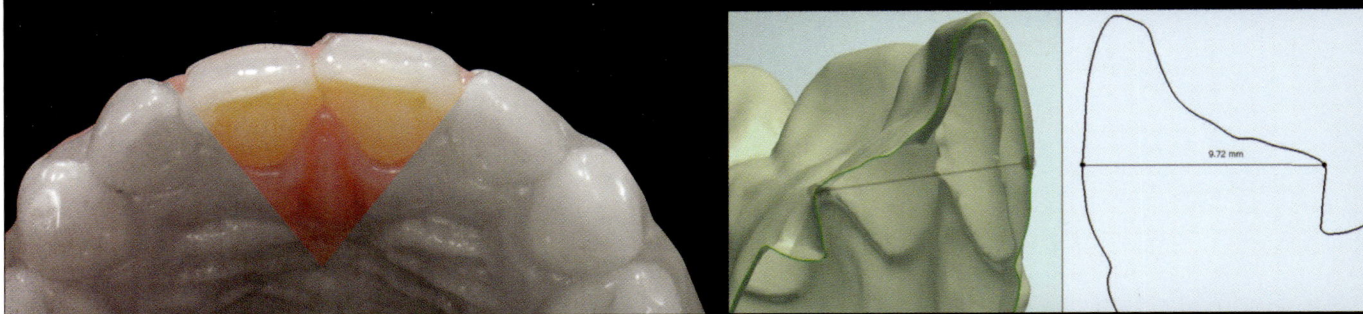

Figure 2.17 • The distance on the horizontal plane between the incisive papilla and the vestibular surface of the upper central incisors is approximately 8-10 mm.

A centre-crestal setting of the artificial teeth in the anterior sector will lead to the development of a contracted arch, with disastrous consequences regarding maintenance of the space required by the prosthetic item to operate properly [15] **(Figure 2.18)**.

The positioning of the front teeth is also guided by the relationship with the lips at rest, during speech and when smiling.

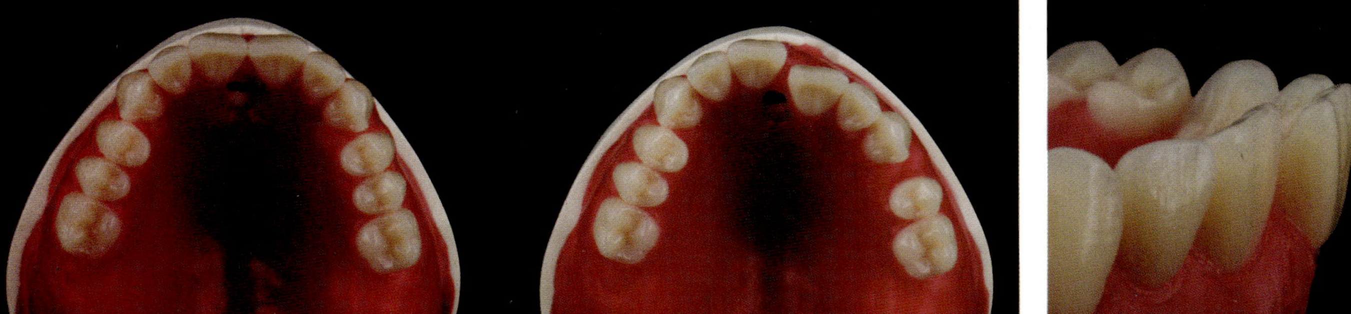

Figure 2.18 • Difference between harmonic and centre-crestal setting of the upper anterior sector.

Dental display at rest is the portion of the teeth that the patient uncovers when the lip is at rest. In the literature, this value ranges between 1 and 5 mm and changes according to gender and age [16] (**Figures 2.19** and **2.20**).

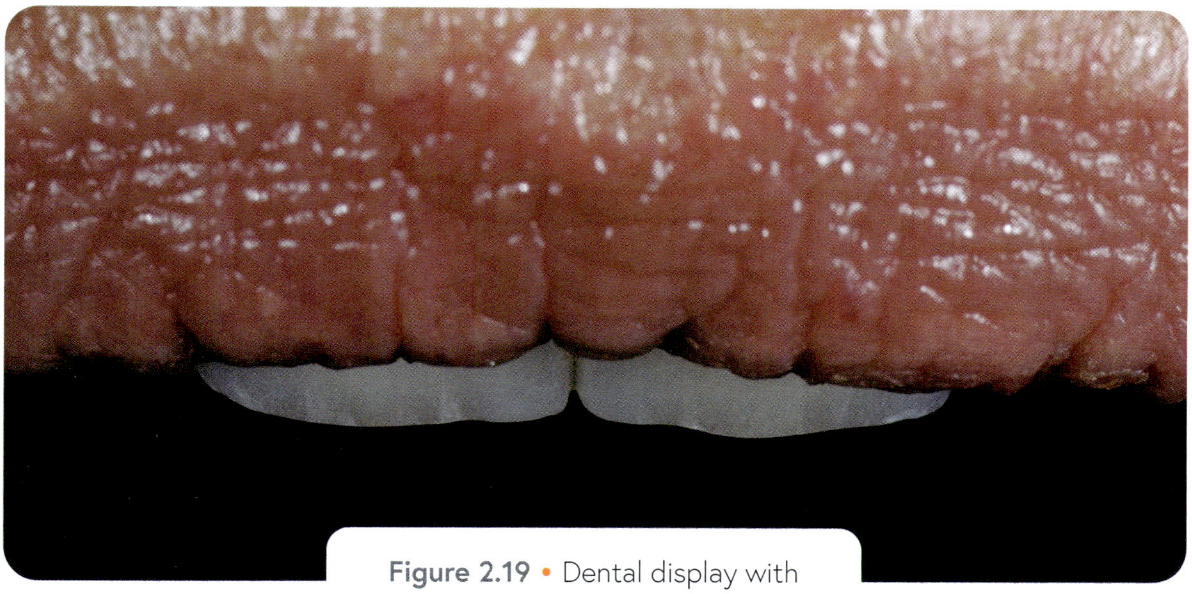

Figure 2.19 • Dental display with lips at rest

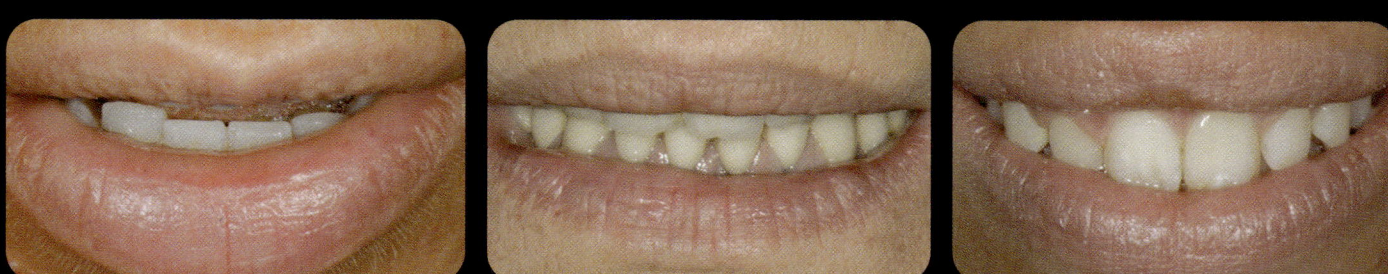

1 mm

2 mm

5 mm

Figure 2.20 • Dental display at rest may range between 1 and 5 mm.

Very often, in totally edentulous patients with inadequate total prostheses, the value may even be negative: the incisal edge in these cases is located more apically with respect to the upper lip, and therefore, certainly, the visibility of the anterior teeth must increase [16] **(Figure 2.21)**.

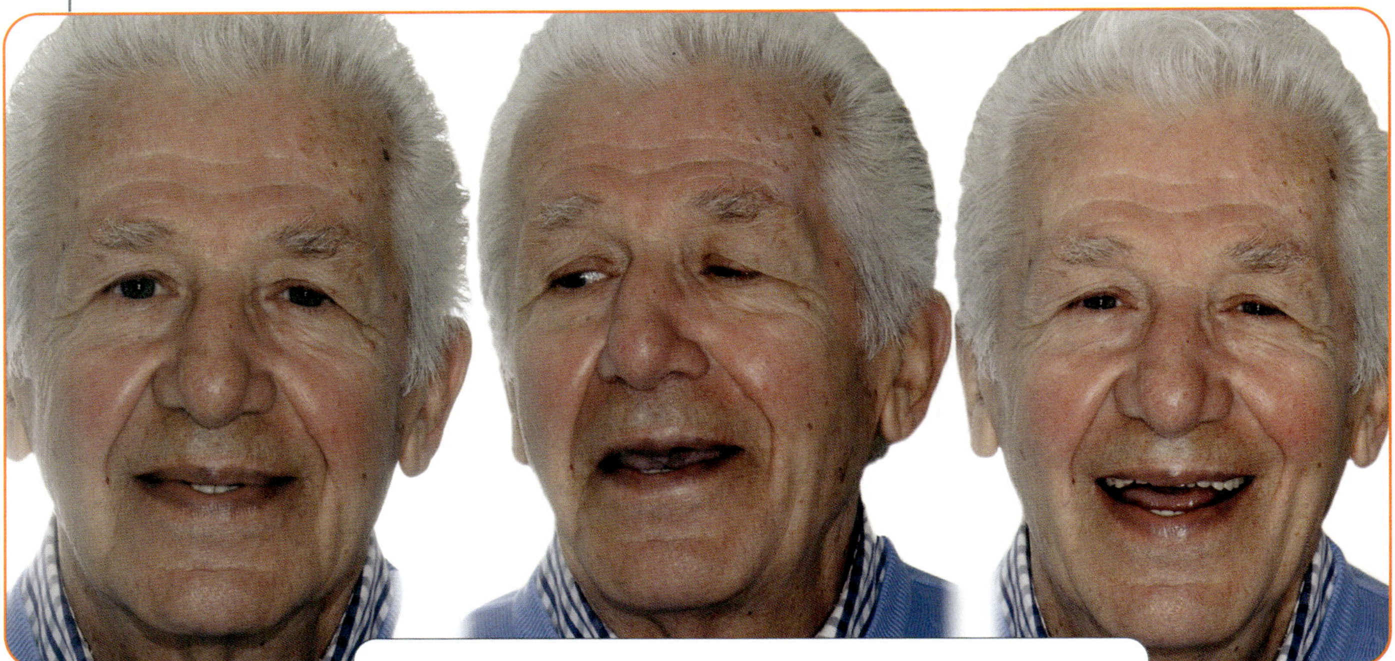

Figure 2.21 • In patients with inadequate prostheses the dentolabial relationship may be esthetically unfavourable.

These esthetic assessments are essential in the registration session of the occlusion bases (Chapter 4): a 1-2 mm resting dental display of the wax bite rim will be established, compatibly with the patient's phonetics and function.

Smile line

The smile line can be classified as low, medium or high **(Figure 2.22)**:

- it is "low" when, in a full "smile", the patient displays up to 75% of the clinical crown of the anterior teeth;
- it is "medium" when the patient displays the whole clinical crown and the interproximal papillae as well;
- it is "high" when the patient displays the whole clinical crown and a band of attached gingiva ("gummy smile") [17].

According to a study by Tjan [17] involving 454 candidates, 20% of the subjects have a low smile line, 69% a medium smile line and 11% a high smile line.

The prevalence of a high smile line is twice as much in female patients [18].

The causes of a gummy smile can be manifold:

- length of the upper lip;
- length of the clinical crowns of the upper teeth;
- dental extrusion due to lack of the antagonists and/or due to periodontal issues;
- hypermobility of the upper lip;
- excessive upper jaw verticality.

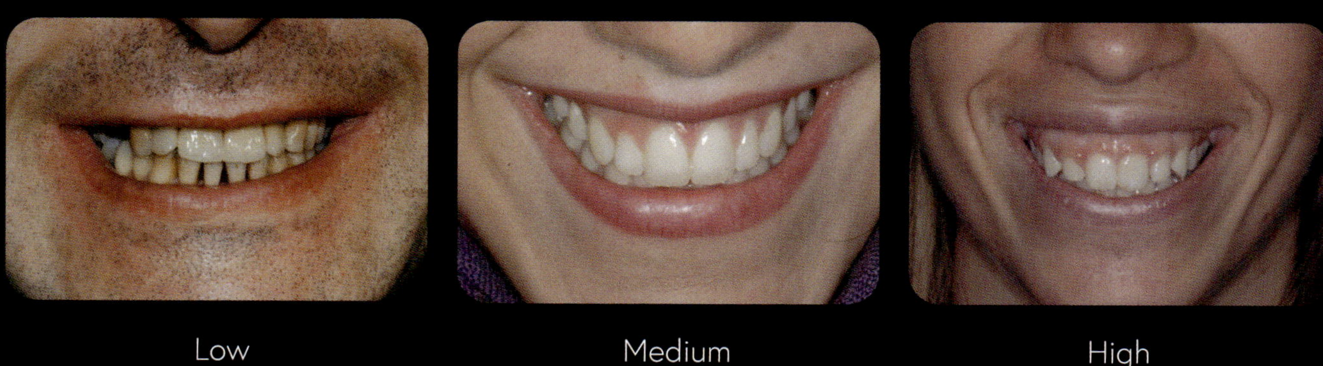

Figure 2.22 • Smile line.

The latter parameter must be carefully evaluated by the dentist: the proper solution to the case might require the intervention of the maxillofacial surgeon as conventional implant-prosthetic therapies might easily lead to serious esthetic failures.

Patients with excessive verticality of the upper jaw would need rehabilitations with very long teeth and would not enable finalisation with hybrid prostheses as the displayed transition area between the prosthesis and the mucosa would be unacceptable (**Figure 2.23**).

The most appropriate solution, in many of these cases, is to perform a thorough study with removable prosthesis before the implant-prosthetic therapy.

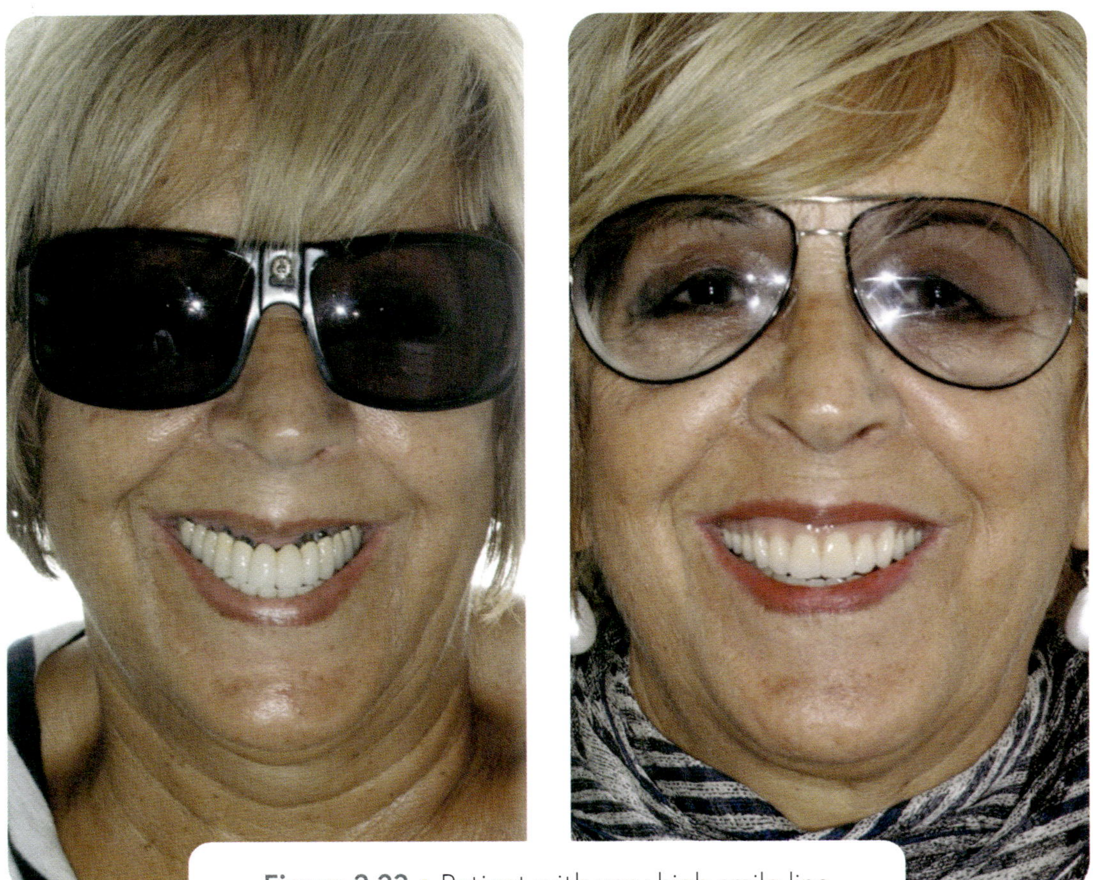

Figure 2.23 • Patient with very high smile line rehabilitated with removable prosthesis.

Position of the incisal edge with respect to the lower lip

With respect to the lower lip, the incisal edge should be parallel and might be spaced, touching or covering [3] (**Figures 2.24** and **2.25**).

The aim of prosthetic rehabilitation is to achieve a touching smile, with the incisal edge parallel to the lower lip, thereby tracing a convex curve [18].

In the sagittal direction, the incisal edge, in addition to touching the lower lip, should fall within the vermillion of the lower lip, in the wet-dry border area.

The best way to evaluate proper positioning of the upper central incisors with respect to the lower lip is to have the patient utter the phoneme /f/ with an appropriate word (**Figure 2.26**). The incisal edge of the upper incisors must touch the wet-dry border line.

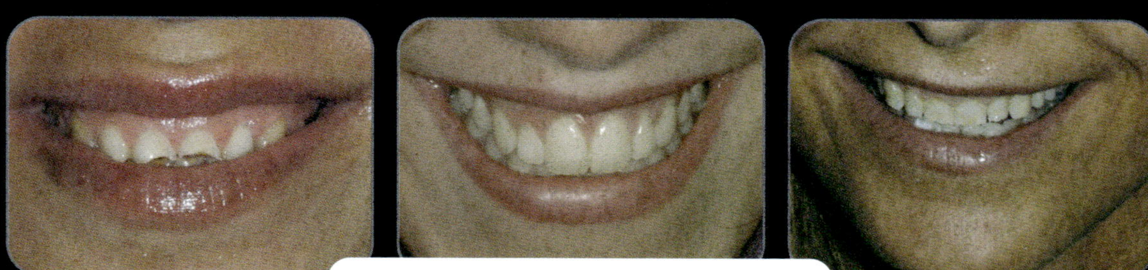

Figure 2.24 • Incisal edge position.

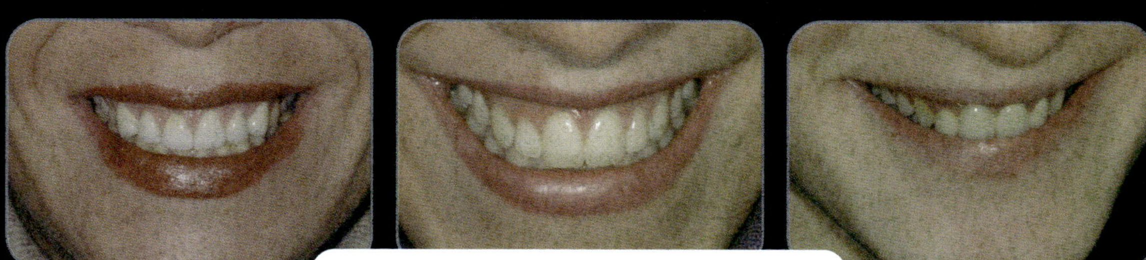

Figure 2.25 • Position of the incisal edge with respect to the lower lip.

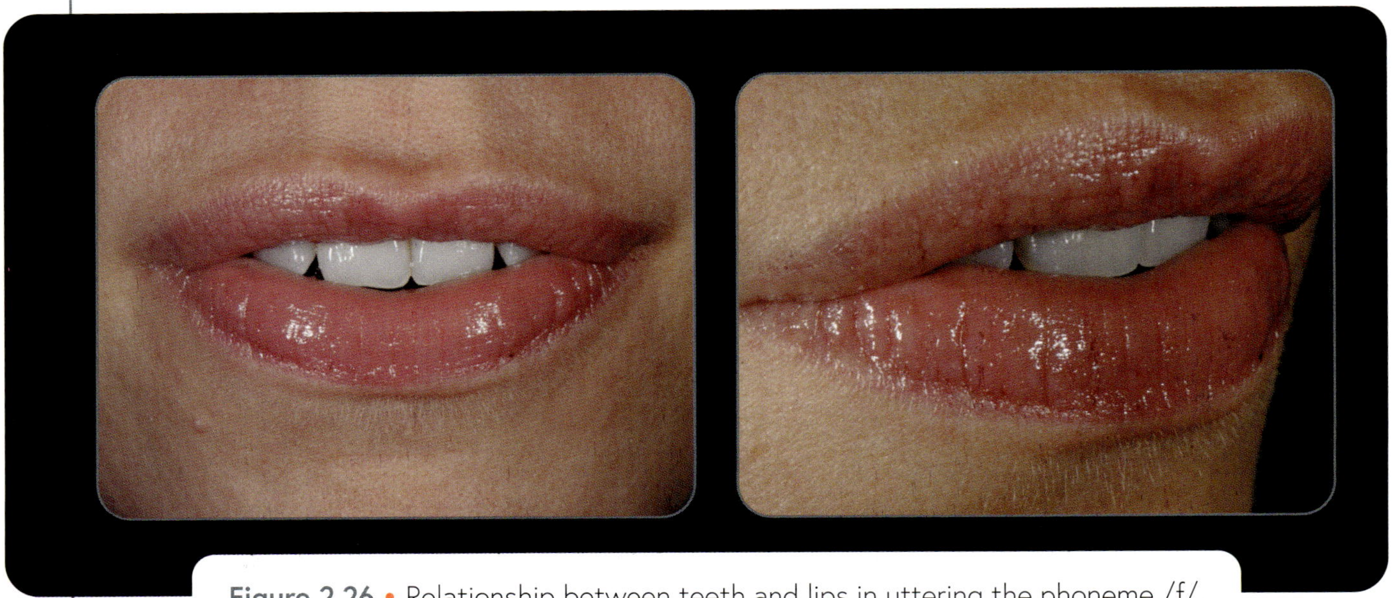

Figure 2.26 • Relationship between teeth and lips in uttering the phoneme /f/.

There are other phonemes used in prosthetics as indicators of the proper dynamic relationships between teeth and perioral tissues. The phoneme /i/ **(Figure 2.27)** is used to evaluate the interlabial gap which will be partly taken up by the upper incisors. In younger patients, these take up approximately 80% of the interlabial gap during phonation.

The evaluation of the phoneme /s/ makes it possible to evaluate the position of the upper incisors with respect to the lower ones. To voice the sound of the typical letter "S" **(Figure 2.28)**, the space between the front teeth is reduced to 1-1.5 mm (S closest speaking space). If the space is small the patient will voice a hissing /s/ phoneme; if, however, the space is excessive the /s/ sound will be "lisping".

The phoneme /s/ also provides useful indications for the evaluation of a proper OVD, on average 1 mm lower than that measured when the patient achieves the ideal phonetic space.

The phoneme /m/ **(Figure 2.29)** makes it possible to measure the RVD and also calculate the occlusal free way space by measuring between the arches in the premolar region [17-19].

Applying all these parameters when designing the edentulous space makes it possible to solve extremely complex cases thanks to the use of removable full dentures **(Figure 2.30)**.

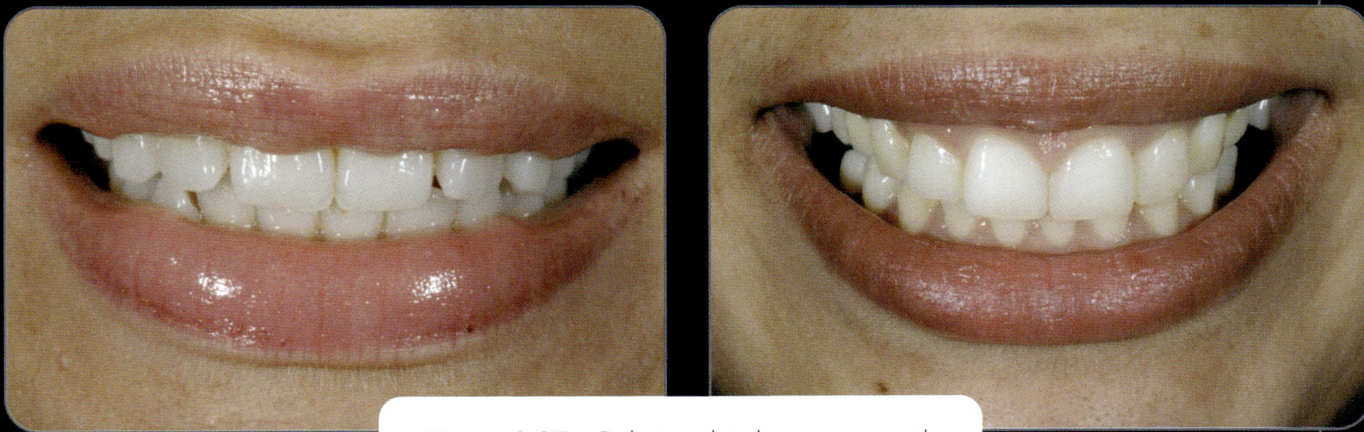

Figure 2.27 • Relationship between teeth and lips in uttering the phoneme /i/.

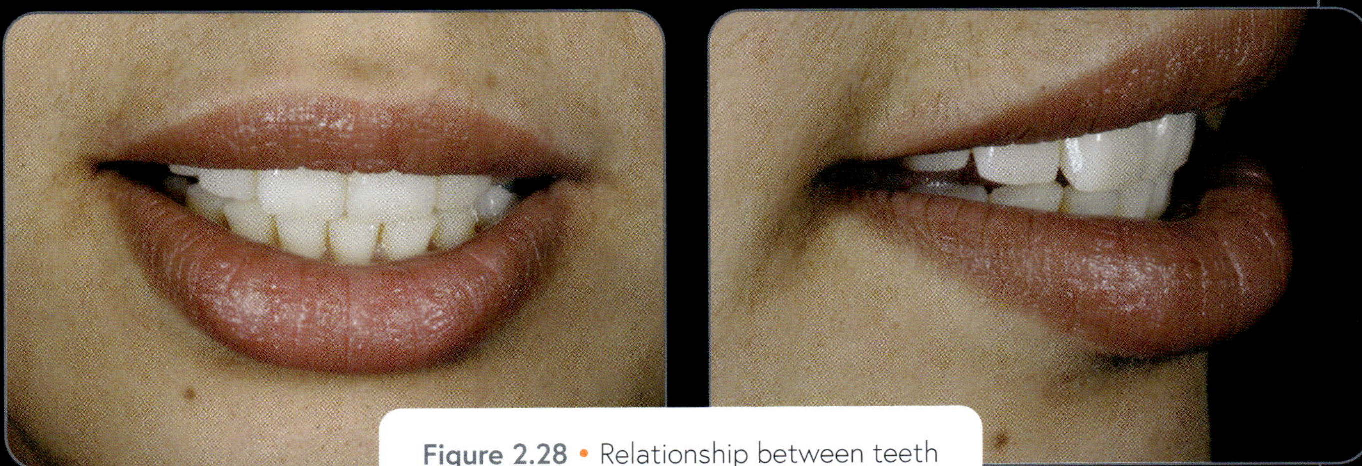

Figure 2.28 • Relationship between teeth and lips in uttering the phoneme /s/.

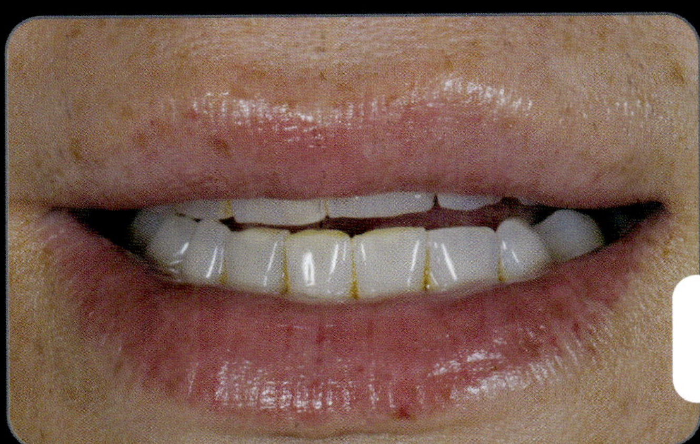

Figure 2.29 • Relationship between teeth and lips in uttering the phoneme /m/.

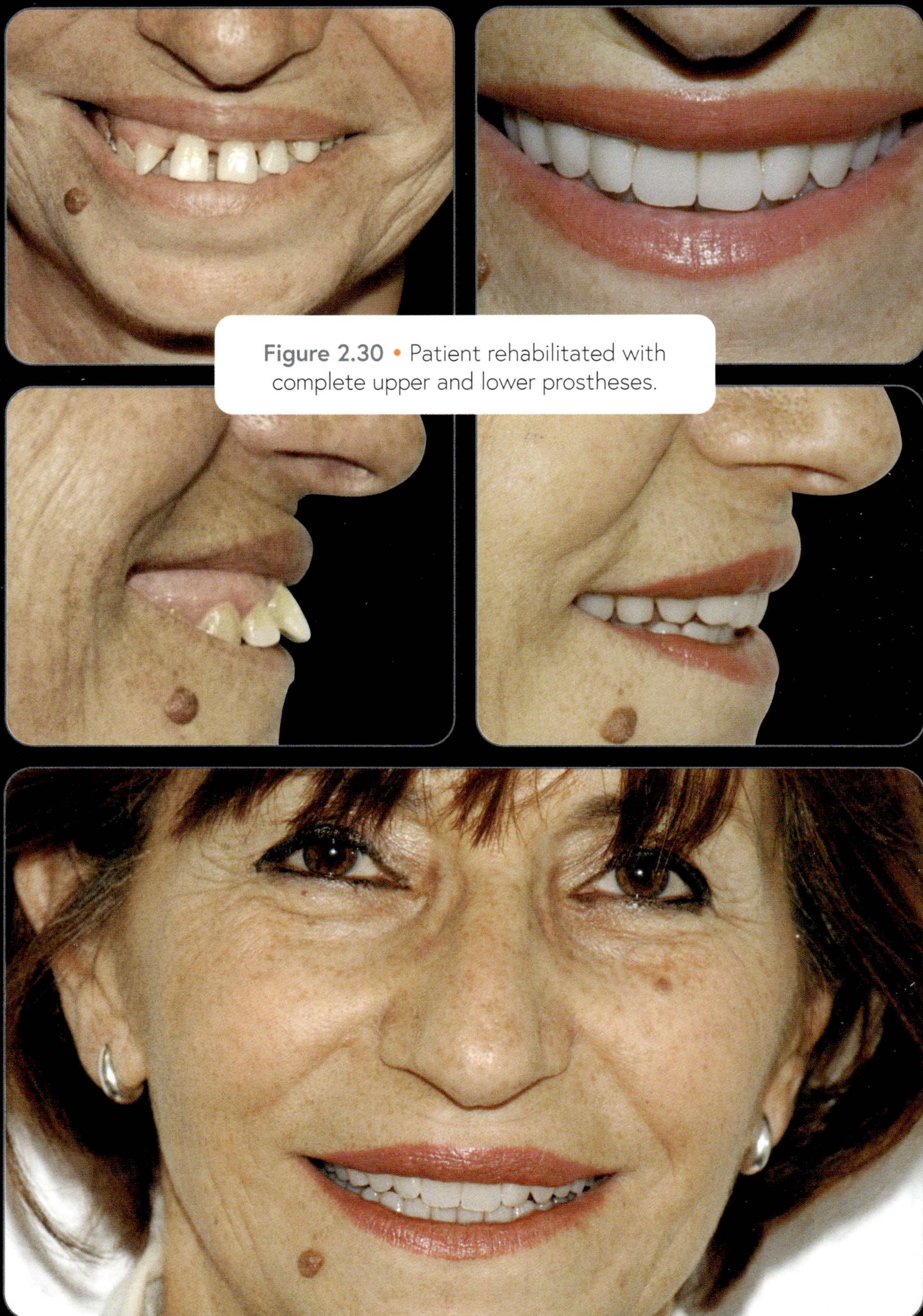

Figure 2.30 • Patient rehabilitated with complete upper and lower prostheses.

Dental composition

The esthetic optimisation of prosthetic rehabilitations, in the upper anterior region, must include compliance with certain parameters such as, for example, the dental proportions, the zenith and the gingival level. On average, the central upper incisors are 10.5 mm long (H) and 8 mm wide (W), with a W/H ratio of 75/80% [22,23] **(Figure 2.31)**.

Figure 2.31 • Mean dental proportions in the central upper incisors.

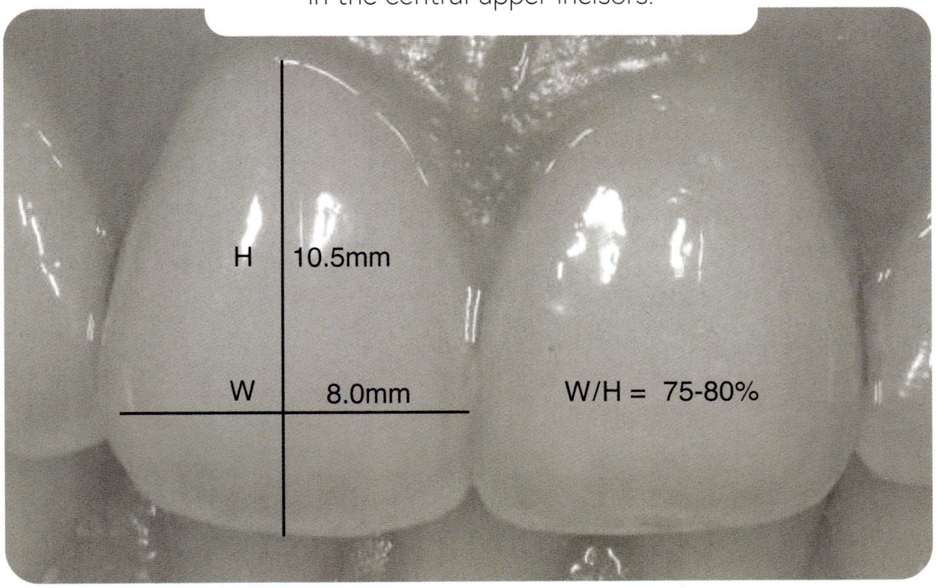

Figure 2.32 • Interdental closure.

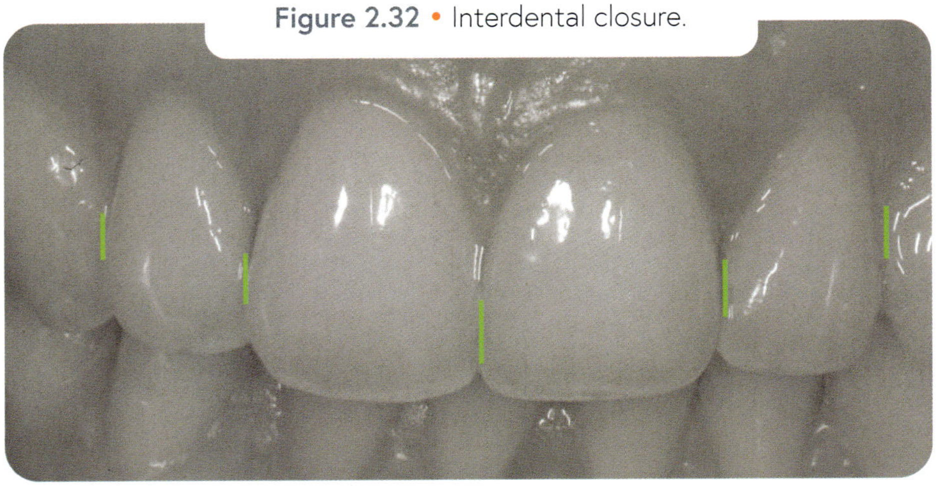

The composition of the upper anterior teeth is harmonious when there are no diastemas **(Figure 2.32)**.

The dental axes are not perpendicular to the incisal plane, but are inclined increasingly more distally from the central to the canine **(Figure 2.33)**. The most apical part of the clinical crown (zenith) is located distally with respect to the centre of the tooth **(Figure 2.34)**.

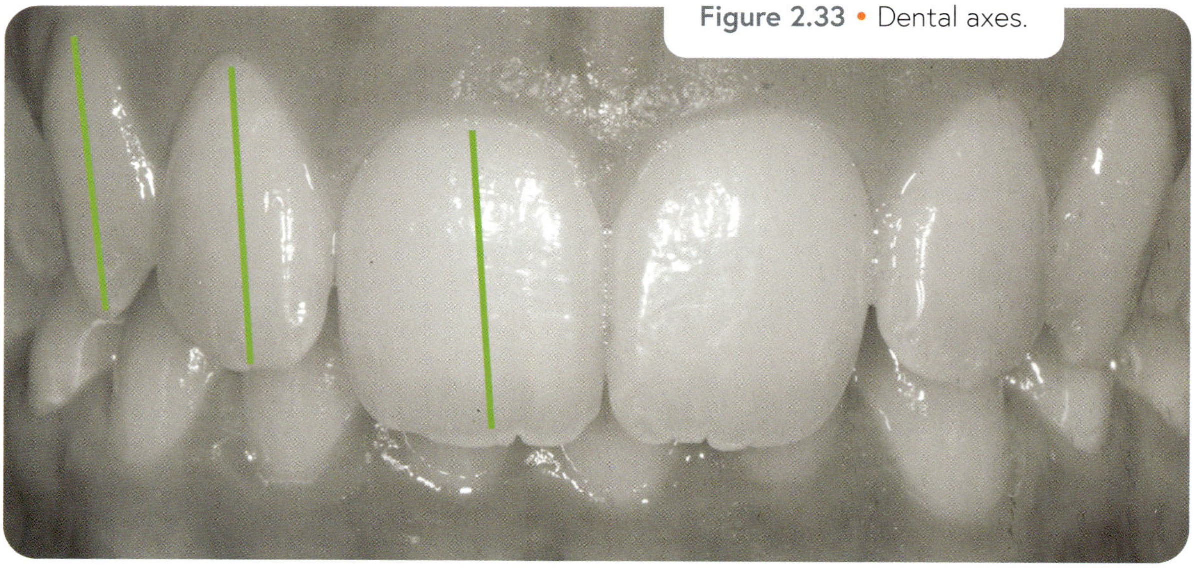

Figure 2.33 • Dental axes.

Figure 2.34 • The gingival zenith is always distal with respect to the centre of the central incisor.

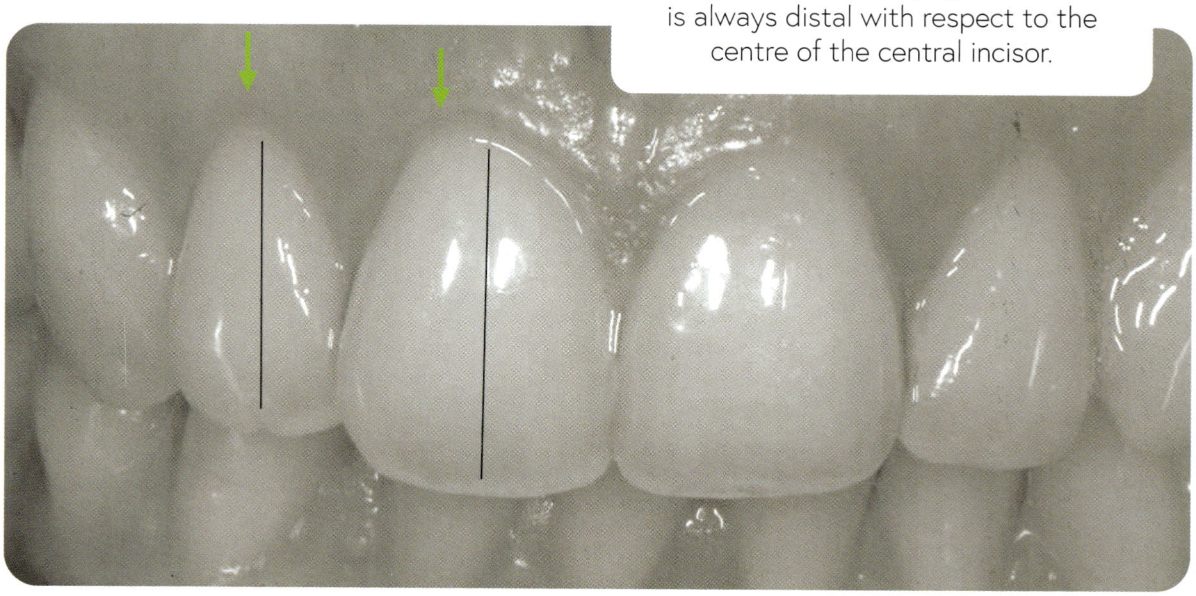

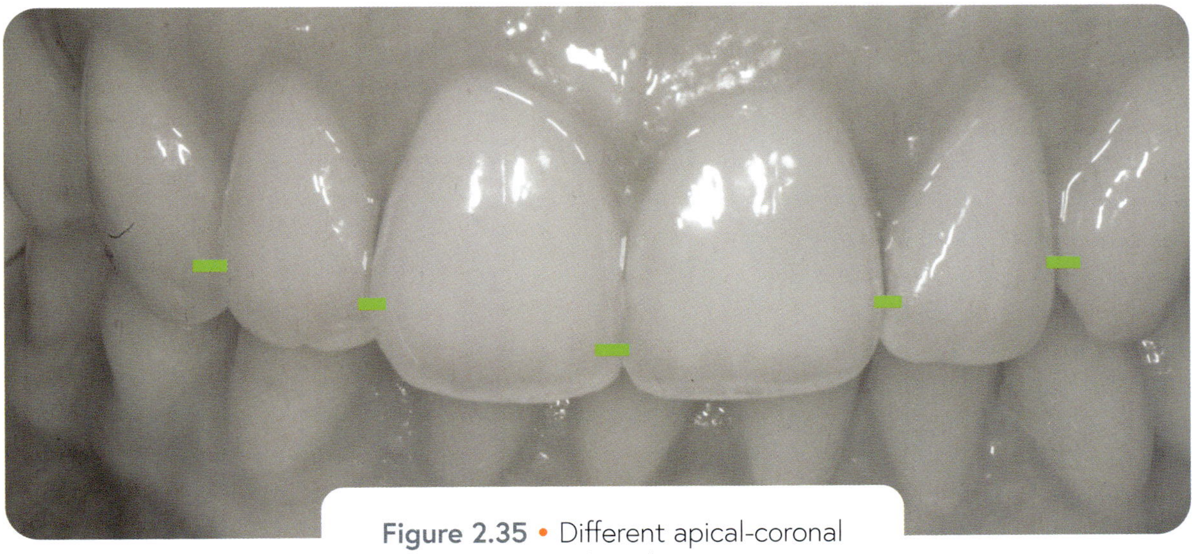

Figure 2.35 • Different apical-coronal level of the interdental contact points.

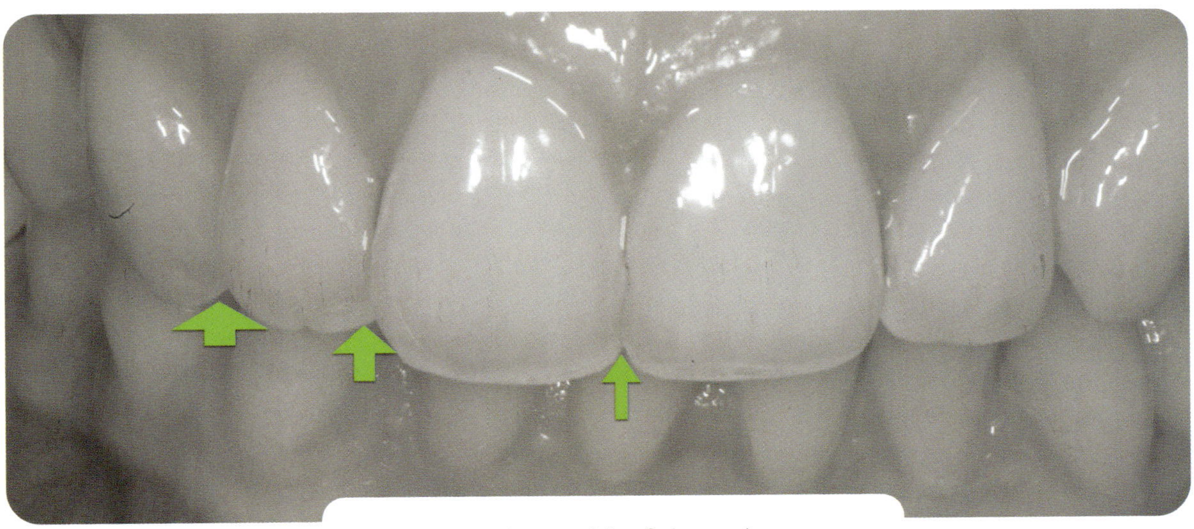

Figure 2.36 • Width of the embrasures.

The interdental contacts are closer to the incisal margin between the two upper central incisors and more coronal between central incisor and lateral incisor. The contact between lateral incisor and canine is even more apical, as can be noted in **Figure 2.35**. The width of the embrasures is minimal between the two central incisors, wider between central and lateral incisor and the widest between lateral incisor and canine **(Figure 2.36)**.

In natural dentition, esthetic optimisation must include a regularisation of gingival levels **(Figure 2.37)**. The gingival level depends directly on the presence of bone [24]. The zenith of the lateral incisor should be below, and more coronally, the line that joins the zenith of the canine and of the central incisor. A balance of the gingival levels is therefore achieved [25] **(Figures 2.38** and **2.39)**.

All these criteria are sometimes applied with the utmost difficulty in prostheses on natural teeth **(Figure 2.40)**.

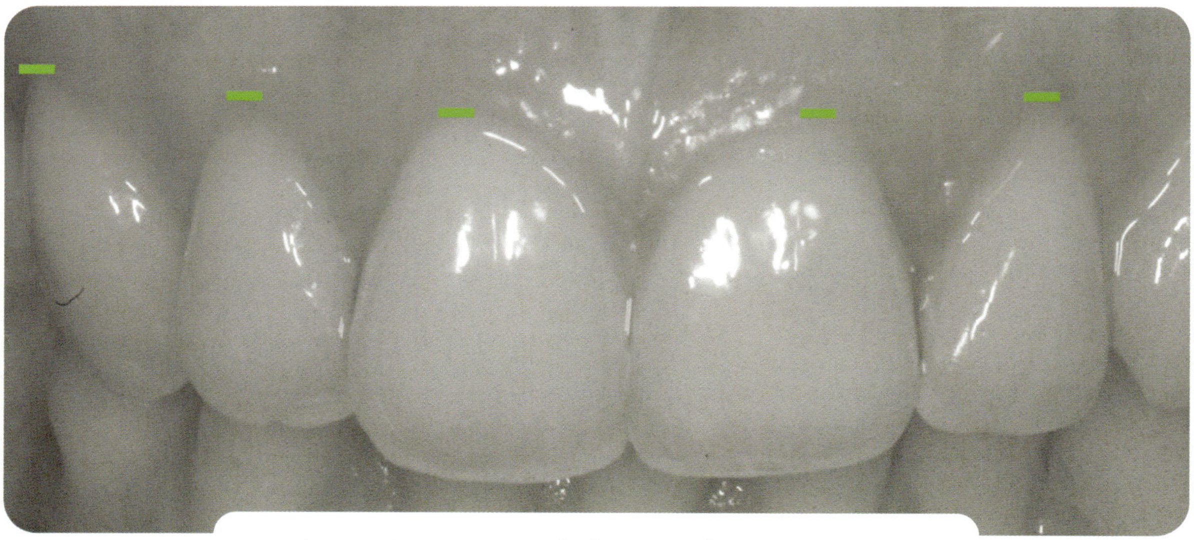

Figure 2.37 • Proper balancing of gingival levels.

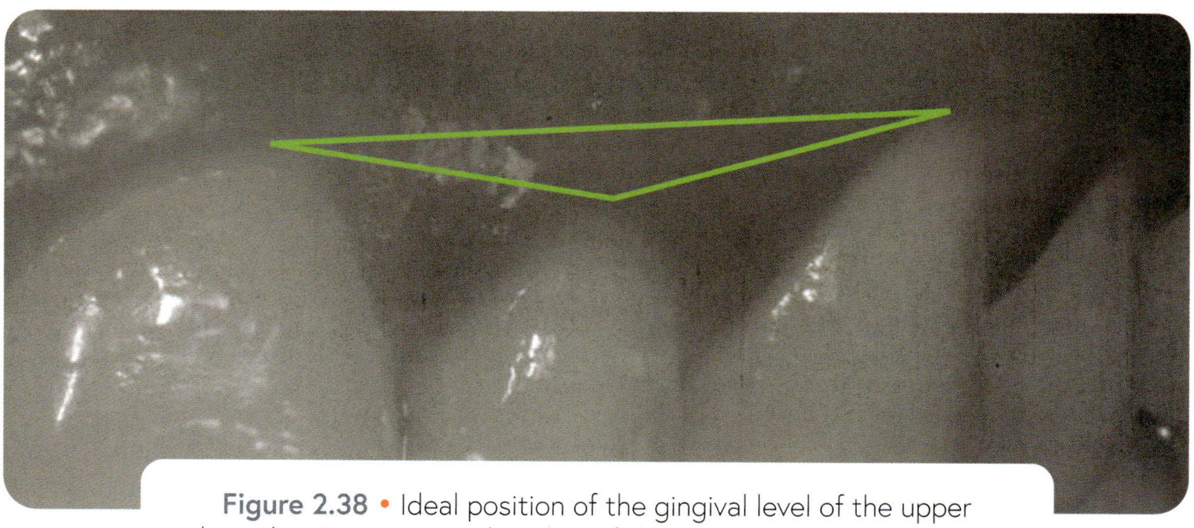

Figure 2.38 • Ideal position of the gingival level of the upper lateral incisor compared to that of the central incisor and canine.

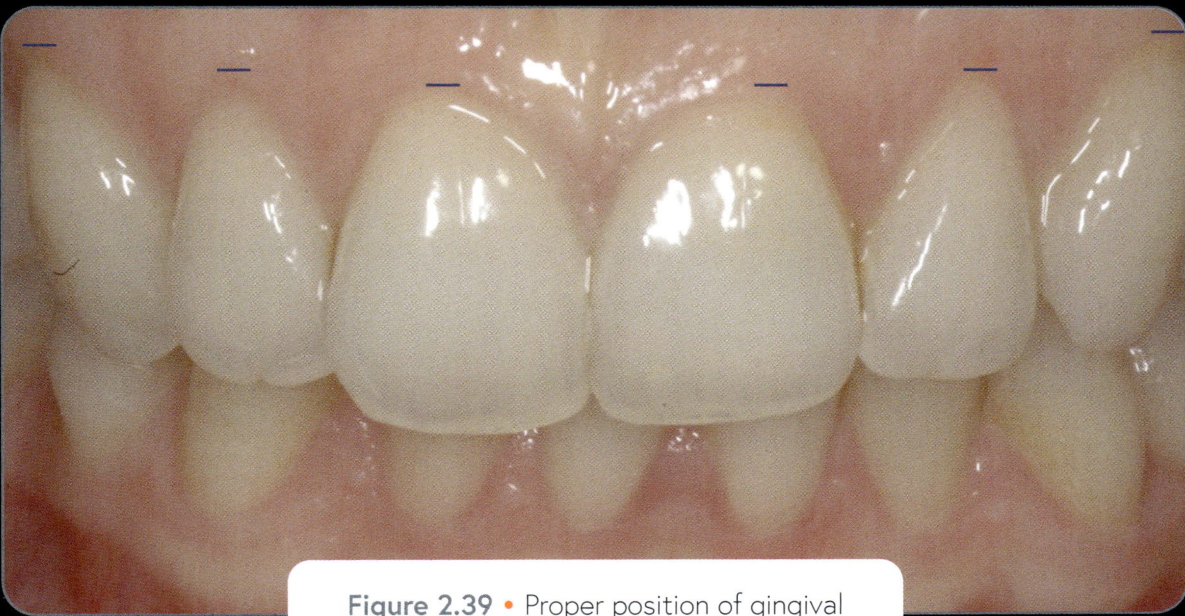

Figure 2.39 • Proper position of gingival levels in a young female patient.

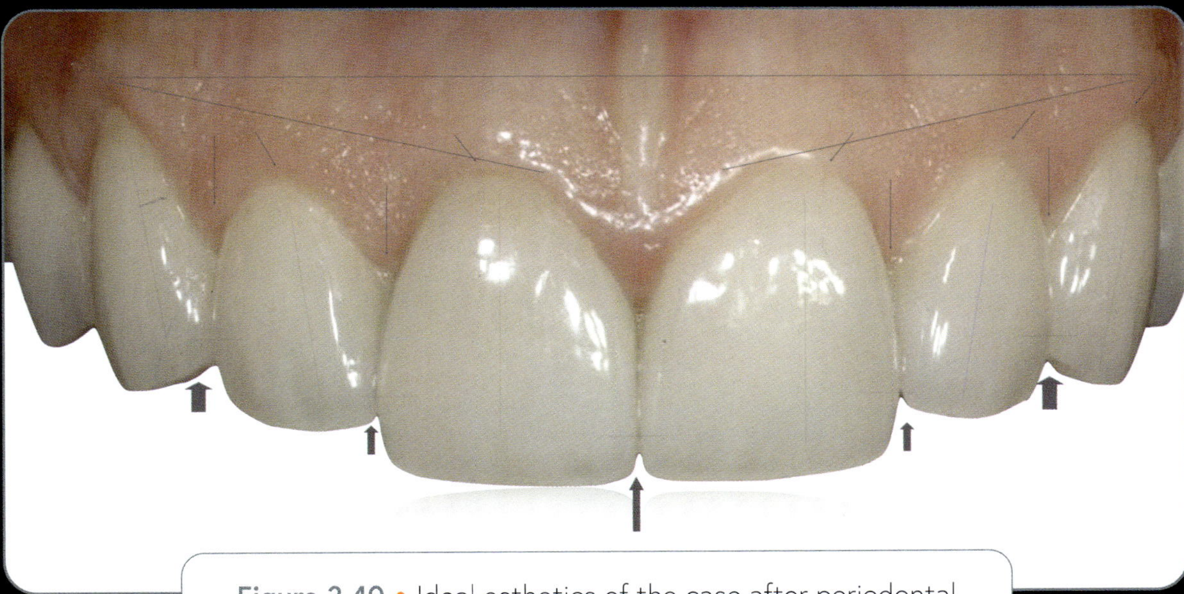

Figure 2.40 • Ideal esthetics of the case after periodontal surgery and prosthetic rehabilitation with ceramic veneers.

The Authors believe that a modern approach to full dentures must combine their functionality – the main goal of all prosthetic rehabilitation – to the mimesis principles (**Figures 2.41** and **2.42**).

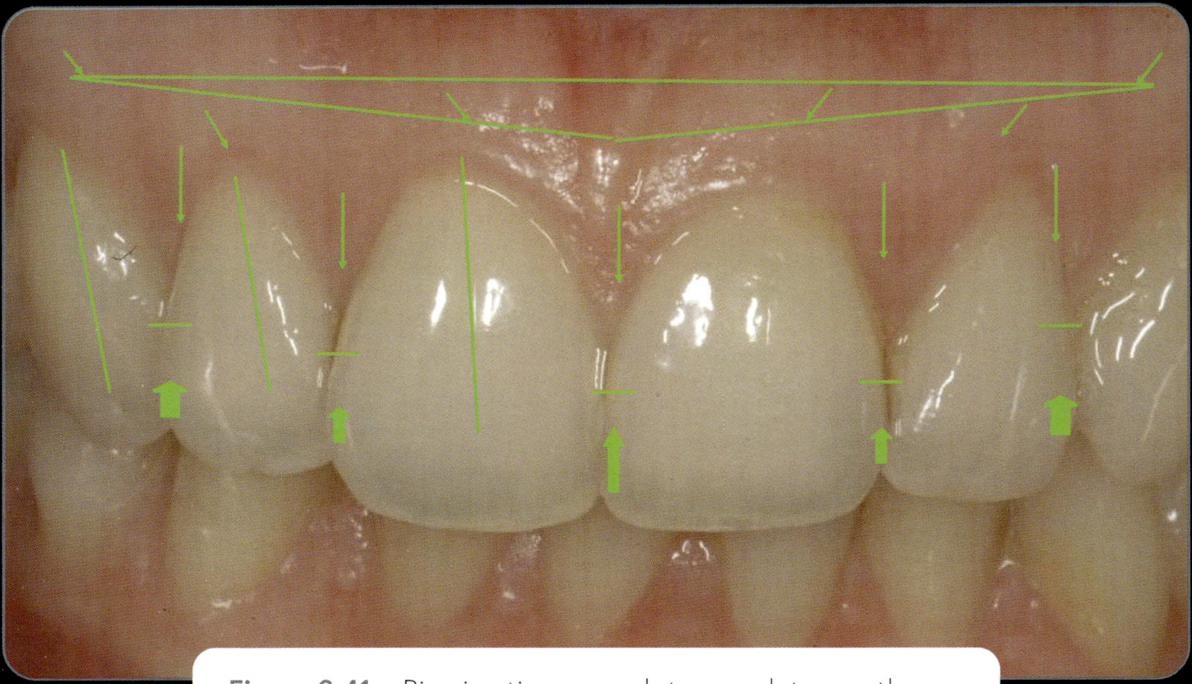

Figure 2.41 • Biomimetic approach to complete prostheses.

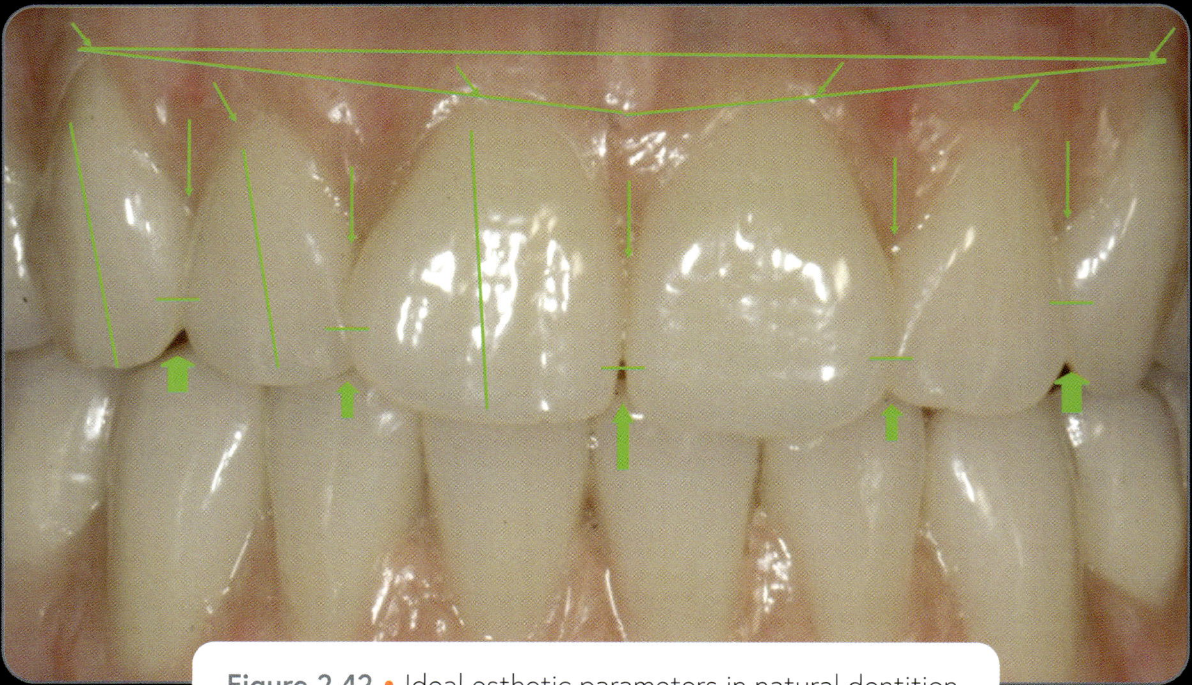

Figure 2.42 • Ideal esthetic parameters in natural dentition.

References

1. Fradeani M. *La riabilitazione estetica in protesi fissa*. Quintessenza Edizioni; 2004.
2. Spear FM, Kokich VG. A Multidisciplinary approach to esthetic dentistry. *Dent Clin North Am*. 2007;51(2):487-505.
3. McLaughlin RP, Arnett WG. Pianificazione estetica e programmazione ortodontica in chirurgia ortognatica. Elsevier; 2006. p. 336.
4. Johnson A, Wildgoose DG, Wood DJ. The determination of freeway space using two different methods. *J Oral Rehabil*. 2002;29(10):1010-3.
5. Silverman MM. The speaking method in measuring vertical dimension. 1952. *J Prosthet Dent*. 2001;85(5):427-31.
6. Nakayama Y, Baba Y, Tsuji M et al. Dentomaxillofacial characteristics of ectodermal dysplasia. *Congenit Anom (Kyoto)*. 2015;55(1):42-8.
7. Preti G, Gassino G. Approccio biologico al trattamento del paziente edentulo. Quintessenza Edizioni; 2007. p. 274.
8. Rifkin R. Facial analysis: a comprehensive approach to treatment planning in aesthetic dentistry. *Pract Periodontics Aesthet Dent*. 2000; 12(9):865-71.
9. Mavani S, TR R, Patel N, Patel. V. Evaluation of coincidence of facial midline to dental midline and maxillary midline to mandibular midline in undergraduate students. *Int J Adv Res*. 2017; 5(2):2364-9.
10. Kokich ViJ, Kiyak A, Shapiro P. Comparing the Perception of Dentists and Lay People to Altered Dental Esthetics. *J Esthet Dent*. 1999;1(6):311-24.
11. Ricketts RM. Esthetics, environment, and the law of lip relation. *Am J Orthod*. 1968;54(4):272-89.
12. Armijo BS, Brown M, Guyuron B. Defining the ideal nasolabial angle. *Plast Reconstr Surg*. 2012; 129(3):759-64.
13. Ortman HR, Tsao DH. Relationship of the incisive papilla to the maxillary central incisors. *J Prosthet Dent*. 1979;42(5):492-6.
14. Schiffman P. Relation of the maxillary canines to the incisive papilla. *J Prosthet Dent*. 1964;14(3): 469-72.
15. McGEE GF. Use of facial measurements in determining vertical dimension. *J Am Dent Assoc*. 1947;35(5):342-50.
16. Vig RG, Brundo GC. The kinetics of anterior tooth display. *J Prosthet Dent*. 1978;39(5):502-4.
17. Tjan AHL, Miller GD, The JGP. Some esthetic factors in a smile. *J Prosthet Dent*. 1984;51(1):24-8.
18. Passia N, Blatz M, Strub JR. Is the smile line a valid parameter for esthetic evaluation? A systematic literature review. *Eur J Esthet Dent*. 2011;6(3):314-27.
19. Pound E. Let /S/ be your guide. *J Prosthet Dent*. 1977;38(5): 482-9.
20. Dawson P. Evaluation, diagnosis, and treatment of occlusal problems. 2nd ed. St. Louis: Company M; 1974.
21. Showa J. The use of phonetics in determining the vertical dimension of occlusion. *J Showa Univ Dent Soc*. 1983;2(2):139-47.
22. Magne P, Gallucci GO, Belser UC. Anatomic crown width/length ratios of unworn and worn maxillary teeth in white subjects. *J Prosthet Dent*. 2003;89(5):453-61.
23. Sandeep N, Satwalekar P, Srinivas S et al. An analysis of maxillary anterior teeth dimensions for the existence of golden proportion: clinical study. *J Int oral Heal JIOH*. 2015;7(9):18-21.
24. Pini NIP, De-Marchi LM, Gribel BF, et al. Analysis of width/height ratio and gingival zenith in patients with bilateral agenesis of maxillary lateral incisor. *Dental Press J Orthod*. 2012;17(5):87-93.
25. Nomura S, Freitas KMS, da Silva PPC, et al. Evaluation of the attractiveness of different gingival zeniths in smile esthetics. *Dental Press J Orthod*. 2018;23(5):47-57.

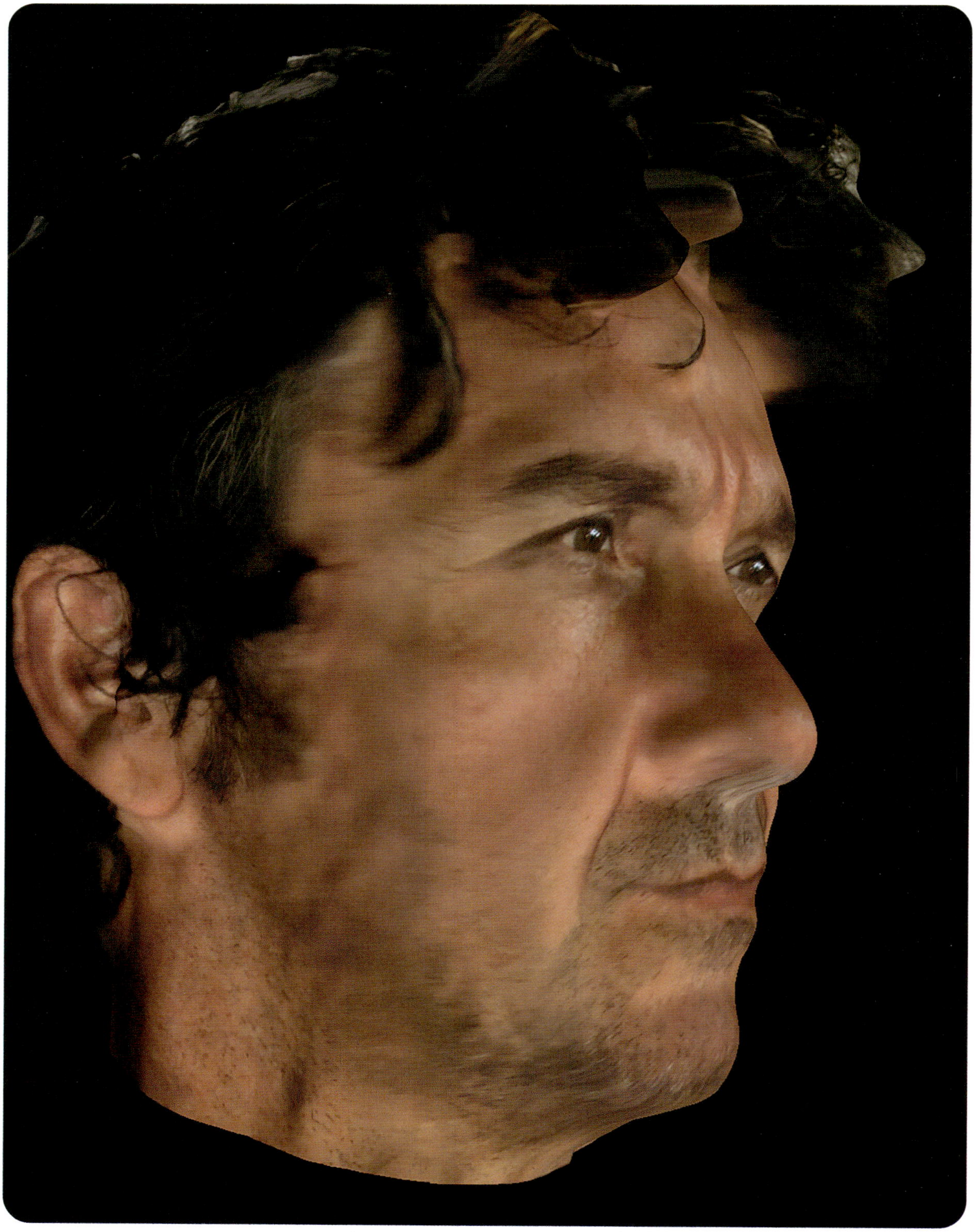

CHAPTER 3

P. VENEZIA, V. SANTOMAURO

New diagnostic instruments: the digital edentulous patient

Digital technology in the dentistry sector is making work flows on average more accurate, faster and more predictable.

The treatment of fully edentulous patients can benefit from the use of digital technologies at various levels:

- data acquisition (intraoral scanners, face scanners, radiology, photography);
- processing of the data acquired with specific software;
- virtual prosthetic design (CAD, Computer Aided Designing);
- production of the final prosthesis with CAM (Computer Aided Manufacturing) flows.

Intraoral scanners (IOS)

Intraoral scanners make it possible to obtain a virtual 3D model of the patient's mouth; with these technologies it is in fact not only possible to make single restorations but also extensive rehabilitations on teeth and implants, on partial or total removable prostheses, on bites and surgical matrices.

The 3D acquisition of oral tissues and subsequent data processing allow the clinician to diagnose, plan implant surgery, plan and design orthodontic treatment plans.

The basic principle of a 3D intraoral scanner

The 3D scanner consists of a light source, one or more video cameras and a movement system that can support multiple axes for positioning the scanned object towards the light source and the video camera(s). The light source projects clearly defined lines on the surface of the object, while the video cameras acquire images of the lines. Based on the ascertained angle and distance between the video camera and the light source (which together form the scanning head), the three-dimensional position on which the projected light is reflected can be calculated, using trigonometry. This measurement principle is referred to as "triangulation".

A depth image is therefore obtained from the scan, which stores the 3D coordinates of the object's surface. Although the basic principle can be met by using a single video camera, the use of two or more video cameras can lead to an improvement in the scanning speed, the degree of accuracy and coverage of the scannable area. Each projected light line produces a three-dimensional line by adapting to the object. Therefore, the consequent movement of the "scanning head" and of the object produces several lines and, consequently, more three-dimensional contours. Laser scanners generate more lines by moving the scanning head along a precise linear axis **(Figure 3.1A)**, while white light scanners are equipped with a fixed scanning head, projecting several divided beams of lines in sequence, starting from a central position **(Figure 3.1B)**. Evidently, laser scanners and white light ones use the same basic principles. Therefore, it is not possible to establish which technology, laser or white light, should be preferred, simply on the basis of the general scanning principle.

Therefore, one may identify the following main scanner parts **(Figure 3.2)**:

- a light projection device (laser or LED light);
- one or more sensors or micro video cameras;
- a mechanical component (which moves the optical parts and the sensors).

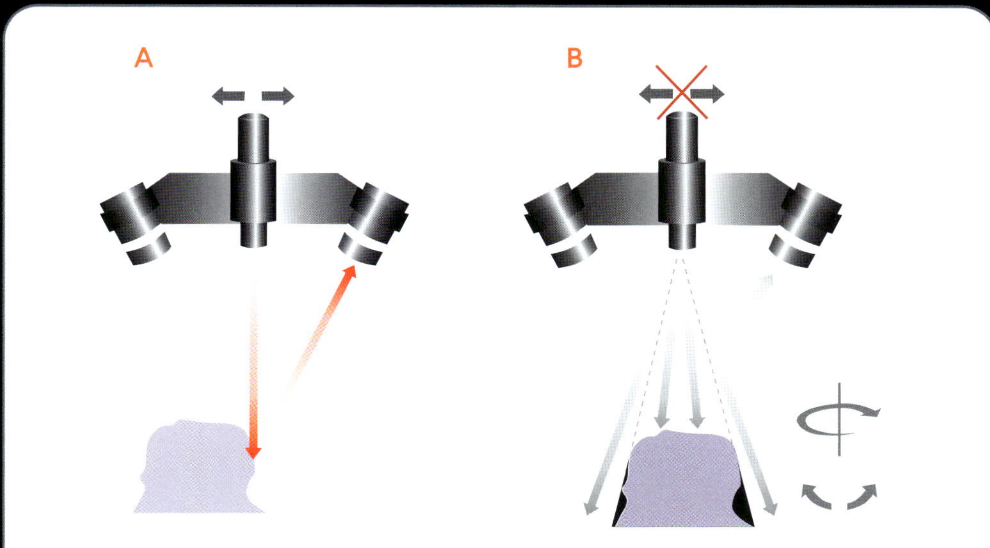

Figure 3.1 • The three-dimensional scanning principle. (**A**) 3D laser scanner with two rotational axes and one linear axis. The laser scanner generates a line of light that is moved along the object with the linear axes. (**B**) White light scanner with two rotational axes. The light source generates multiple lines of light and, consequently, provides an overview from a single position.

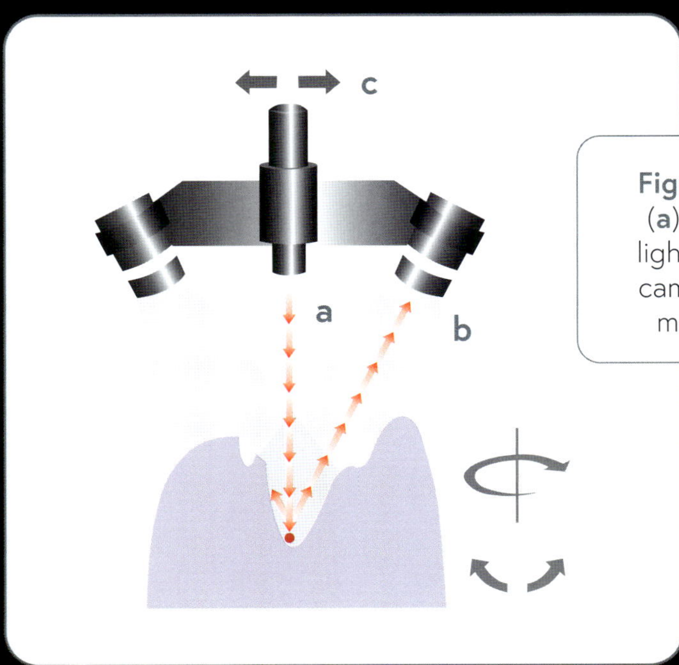

Figure 3.2 • Main parts of the scanner: (**a**) light emission device (laser or LCD light); (**b**) one or more sensors or micro-cameras; (**c**) mechanical component (to move the optical parts and sensors).

The combined action of the three parts is coordinated by software. Since the scans are very many and are taken on the entire circumference of the object to be scanned, the result obtained is a point cloud which, like a pointillist painting, reproduces the morphology of the scanned object **(Figure 3.3)**.

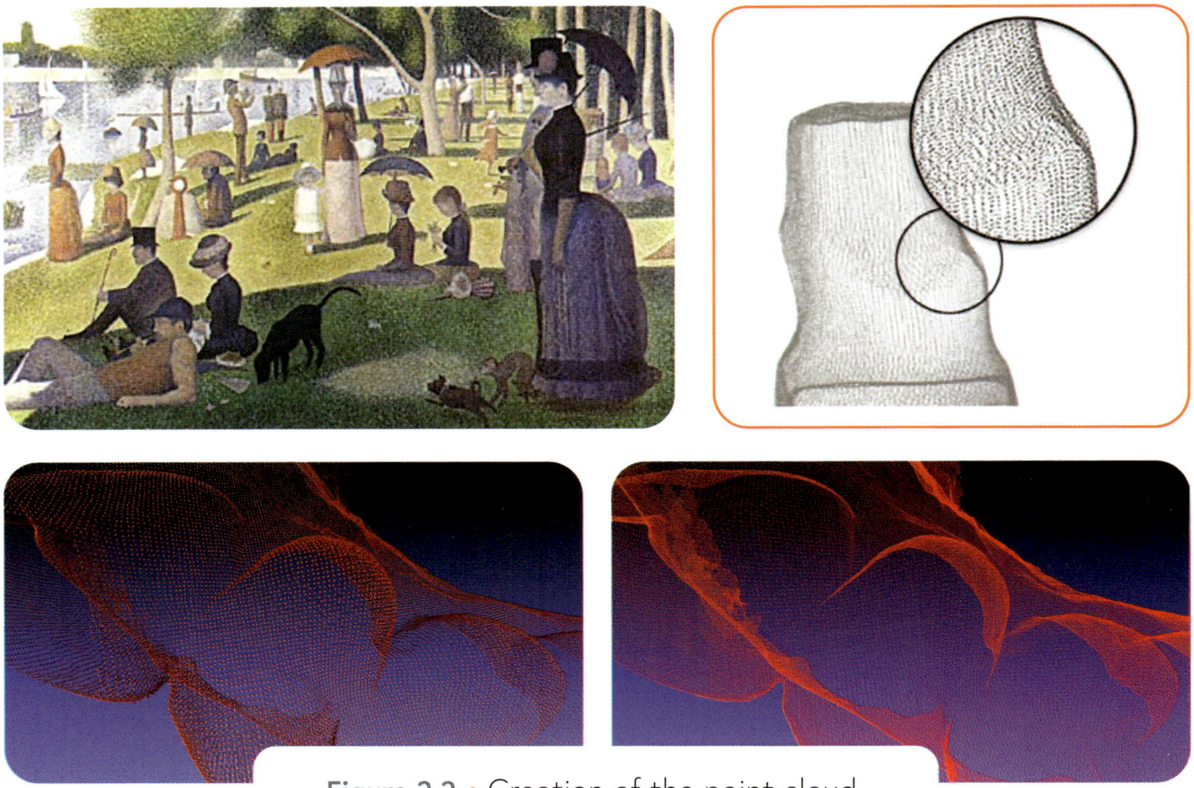

Figure 3.3 • Creation of the point cloud.

At this stage, the point cloud must be turned into a surface. To do so, the software connects individual points according to a mathematical formula, by measuring the distances between them and reconstructing a lattice formed by a series of tiny polygons (generally, triangles) **(Figure 3.4)**.

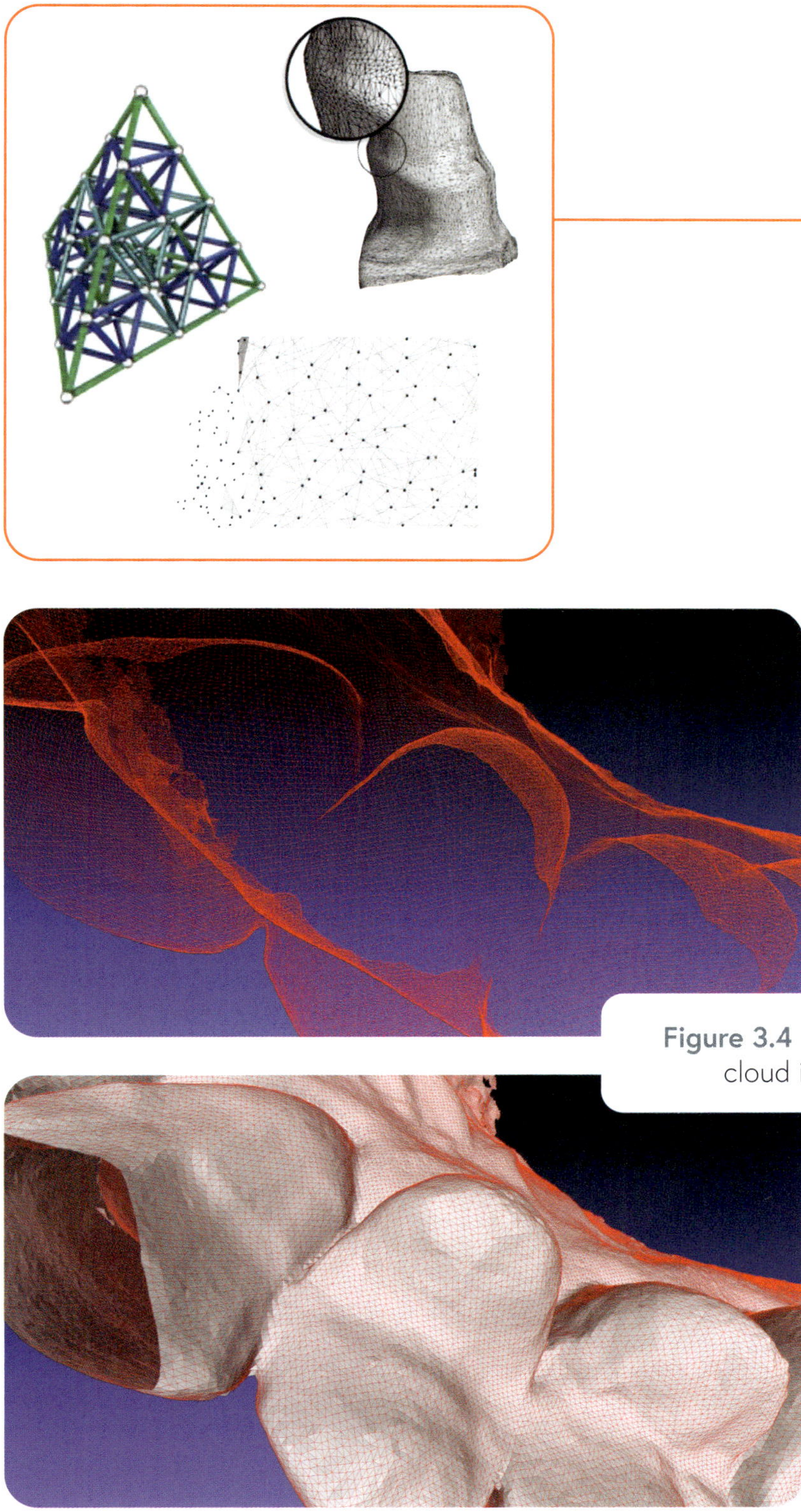

Figure 3.4 • Turning the point cloud into a surface.

With the series of polygons provided by the wireframe, the software is able to calculate the area of the individual triangles and define their filling. The solid figure that forms the virtual model (Shade) has thus been obtained, whose fidelity of reproduction depends mainly on the size and number of triangles and, therefore, on the number of reference points initially recorded by the scanner **(Figure 3.5)**

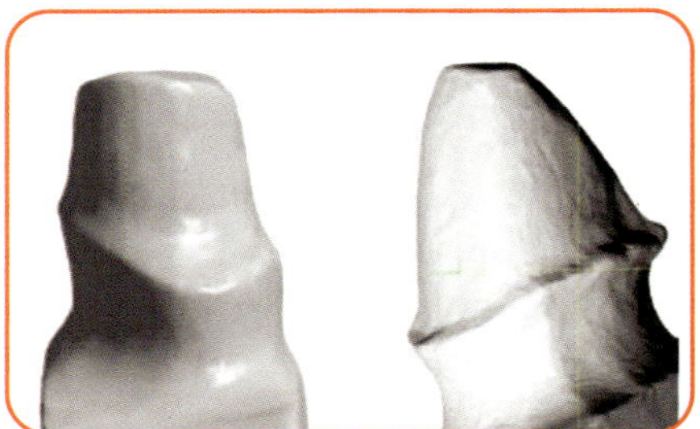

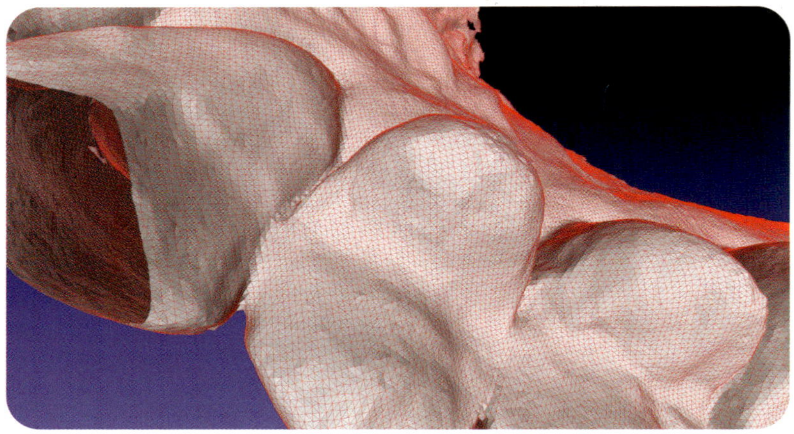

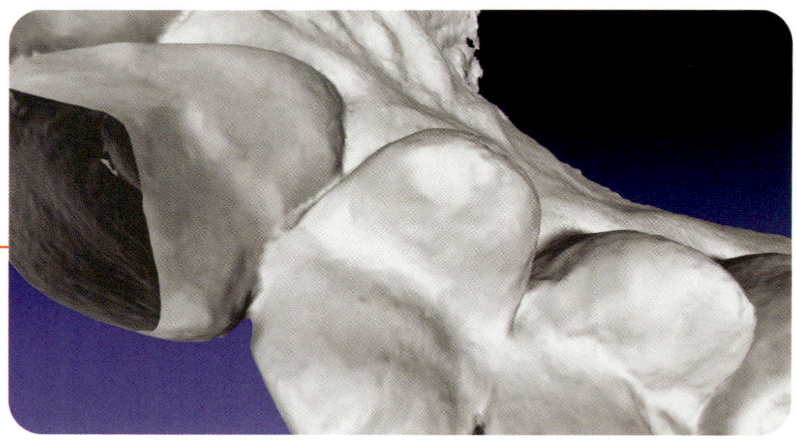

Figure 3.5 • Creation of the virtual model.

In the final processing step, the set of points obtained from all views is converted into a 3D surface made up of regular triangles. The more detailed the scan, the heavier the output file. The most commonly used type of file is currently the STL file, which aptly stands for Standard Triangulation Language.

The set of points is used to generate the triangle-based surface. Smart triangle reduction algorithms can be used to reduce the number of unnecessary triangles as they keep the finish line crisp and legible **(Figure 3.6)**.

Therefore, in the dental sector, one of the most critical components of the CAD/CAM production chain regards the first component of the digital workflow, that is, the scanner. The software design precision is limited by the precision of the data captured by the scanner and subsequently imported into the processor [1].

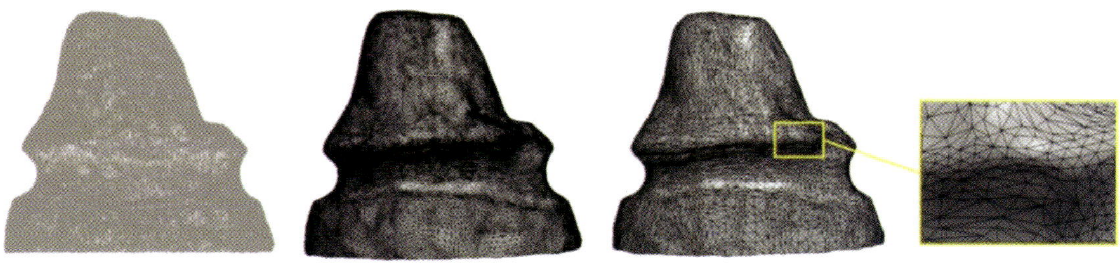

Figure 3.6 • Streamlining the scan file by reducing the number of triangles.

The intraoral scanner makes it possible to avoid some of the errors associated to the conventional impression (warping linked to storage and transport) [2]. The information on shape and dimensions of the arches is immediately available and can therefore be entered into a digital workflow.

All 3D scanners are essentially measurement instruments that use light and specific sensors to convert optical data, the so-called "point cloud", into a 3D virtual model.

Nowadays, a variety of intra- or extraoral scanners/scanning systems are available on the market. In general, these scanners seek to deal with the issues and disadvantages deriving from the conventional impression taking process and its plaster development [3].

The main advantages provided by these devices are: the option of creating high fidelity virtual models, the reduction of the steps in the work flow and the reduction of times and costs. Since scanners can be considered measurement instruments, they should undergo periodic calibration, set-up and inspections. Calibration is performed immediately after manufacturing the instrument; set-up is carried out each time the scanner is used to measure an object. A periodic inspection is also required to check the condition of the instrument. Dental scanners perform automatic set-up of the instrument.

Parameters and clinical choice criteria of scanners

The essential parameters to be taken into account when considering an intraoral scanner are:

- accuracy, precision and resolution **(Figure 3.7)**;
- clinical operability (including the option of producing colour images or otherwise);
- open/closed system.

Accuracy, precision, resolution

Resolution (maximum): it generally consists in the smallest variation of the measurand that can be measured. In the case of optical scanners, the resolution corresponds to the resolution of the optical sensor (CMOS, CCD etc). The density of the point cloud is proportional to the resolution: it affects the mutual distance of the acquired points and therefore the ability to describe small geometric details. This condition of higher resolution is desirable in the dental field for the areas of the closing edges of the stumps. Although it defines a scanned area better, a higher number of points does not ensure accuracy and precision.

Accuracy: it represents the error between the measurement taken and its value (accepted as true). In other words, it is an error that overlaps with the measured data; in the case of repeated measurements of the same value, it can be determined as the distance between the average of the measured data and the real data. Accuracy means how close the average of the measurements is to reality: from a mathematical point of view, in fact, the more the average of the measurements approximates the true value of the quantity, the more accurate a measurement. An intraoral scanner should therefore be as accurate as possible, that is, be able to record every detail of the impression and process a virtual 3D model as similar as possible to the real one and which deviates little or not at all from reality.

Precision: it is represented by the dispersion of the measurements around their average. Therefore, it makes it possible to estimate the random component of the error by considering several repeated measurements; it is evaluated by the mean square deviation between the individual measurements and their average.

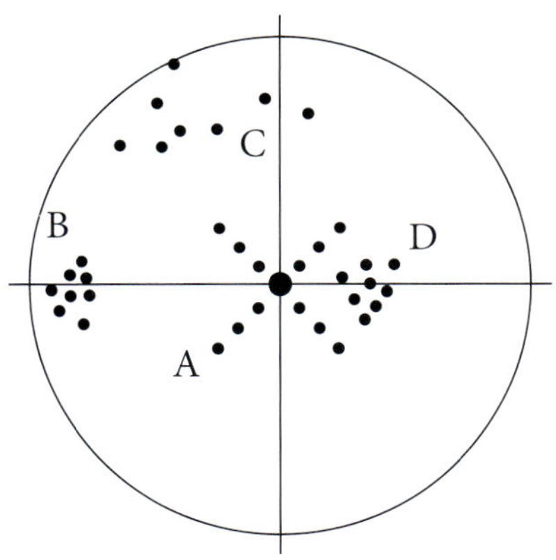

Scanner A, B, C, D with different degrees of precision and accuracy

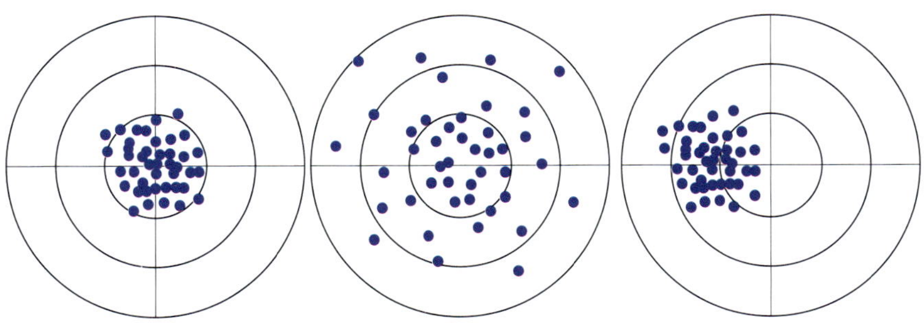

High accuracy
High precision

High accuracy
Low precision

Low accuracy
High precision

Figure 3.7 • Accuracy and precision of intraoral scanners.

Precision refers to the scanner's ability to ensure a repeatable result when it is used for different measurements of the same object. The constant repeatability of the result is crucial: different measurements of the same object must necessarily be superimposable and minimally deviate from each other.

One can easily understand how, jointly accuracy and precision are the main characteristics that an intraoral scanner must have. Theoretically, a scanner might be very accurate and not very precise, or very precise but not very accurate: in either case, this would adversely affect the quality of the optical impression.

The accuracy and precision of a scanner largely depend on the processing software it comes with, which performs the most difficult task, by "building" the virtual model.

The international standard pertaining to the sector of measurement instruments is ISO 10360-1-9 2013 [7] Geometrical Product Specifications (GPS) – Acceptance and reverification tests for coordinate measuring systems (CMS); while for the dental sector, there is standard ISO 12836:2012 [8] (Dentistry, Digitizing devices for CAD-CAM systems for indirect dental restorations – Test methods for assessing accuracy).

Currently, there is no common standard to measure and validate the precision of dental scanners. For the most part, the scanner manufacturers do not disclose the method supporting the degree of precision they claim. Therefore, the stated degree of precision, normally at 20 μm [9], cannot be compared nor confirmed.

The science of precision measurement, i.e. metrology, refers to objects whose degree of precision is far higher than that provided by a scanner. A number of studies are currently appearing in the literature on the accuracy of scanners [10] but unfortunately, few of them are in vivo. In recent years, some systematic literature revisions have been published [11,12] which came to the conclusion that intraoral scanners have a good degree of accuracy.

In 2019, the 6th Consensus Conference ITI [13] concluded in a systematic review and meta-analysis that:

- limited high quality tests are available for the study of conventional and digital implant impressions (**Table 3.1**);
- conventional and digital impressions give similar results for parallel implants;

Table 3.1 Synthesis of the type and number of the studies included in the accuracy evaluation of digital and analogue impressions

TYPE OF TRIAL	NUMBER OF TRIALS
Controlled randomised	1
Controlled clinical non randomised	–
Experimental	77
Retrospective	1
Series of cases	77
TRIAL SETTING	**NUMBER OF TRIALS**
In vitro	75
In vivo	4
TECHNOLOGY USED	**NUMBER OF TRIALS**
Digital impression	11
Digital impression vs conventional impression	9
Conventional impression	59

From: Flügge T, Meer WJ, Gonzalez BG et al. The accuracy of different dental impression techniques for implant-supported dental prostheses: A systematic review and meta-analysis. Clin Oral Impl Res. 2018;29(Suppl. 16):374-92.

- the conventional impression loses in precision when the implants are angled between them, while the digital impression remains precise;
- there is evidence showing that the scanning protocol and the operator's experience have an impact on the precision of digital impressions;
- further trials are required centred upon the in vivo use of conventional and digital implant impressions with study protocols to reliably evaluate the accuracy of the impressions;
- the accuracy of digital impressions with intraoral scanners of individual or adjacent implants in partially edentulous jaws and multiple implants in edentulous jaws is comparable to the accuracy of impressions of conventional implants under laboratory conditions. This conclusion is based on six in vitro trials;
- the precision of the digital impressions is adversely affected by the increase in the inter-implant interval between implants in partially as well as fully edentulous situations. This conclusion is based on three in vitro trials;

- the scanning protocol that uses intraoral scanners has a significant influence on the precision of the digital impression of the implant in the edentulous jaw. This conclusion is based on four in vitro trials that use the same control method;
- the precision of the digital implant impressions in edentulous jaws varies when different intraoral scanners are used. This conclusion is based on four in vitro trials.

Clinical operability

The essential parameters to be taken under consideration are the scanning speed, the size of the tip and the ability to take colour impressions or otherwise [14].

Scanning speed: this is certainly a very important aspect for an intra-oral scanner. The scanner must be efficient and must not stop while scanning, as this would excessively slow it down, especially where a whole arch needs to be scanned. There are probably differences in the speed of use of the various scanners available today: the speed in performing the scan mostly depends on the clinician's experience and on the learning curve.

Tip size: it plays an important role. A scanner with a small tip size would be preferable for patient comfort during scanning; however, a scanner with larger tips allows the posterior areas to be scanned as well. A scanner with a small tip size would be preferable for patient comfort and manoeuvrability (**Figure 3.8**).

Colour images yes/no: to date, almost all intraoral scanners allow a colour impression to be taken. In actual fact, colour is simply added to the three-dimensional model that derives from scanning, superimposing on it the information obtained by taking high-definition photographs. Currently, colour is processed through the presence of either a spectrophotometer or RGB cameras present within the handpiece. Therefore, it is a software artefact (**Figures 3.9** and **3.10**).

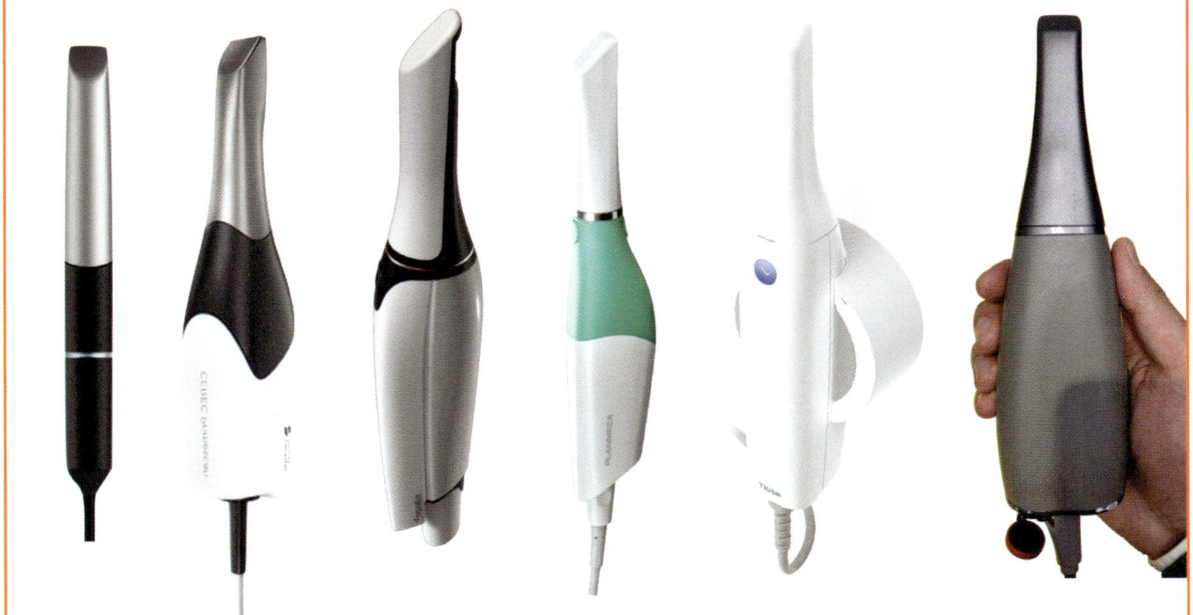

Figure 3.8 • Different models of intraoral scanners.

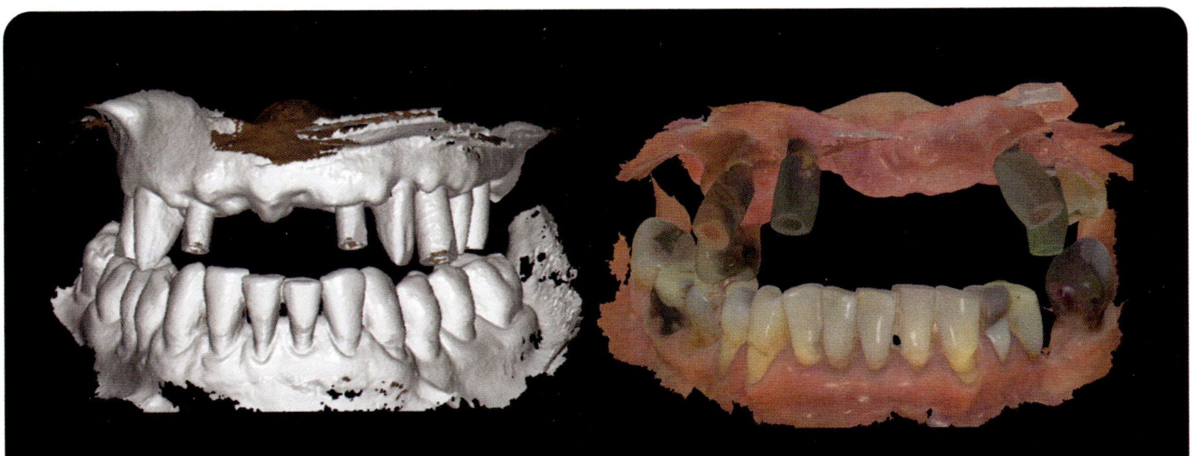

Figure 3.9 • Difference between a black and white and colour image between intraoral scanners.

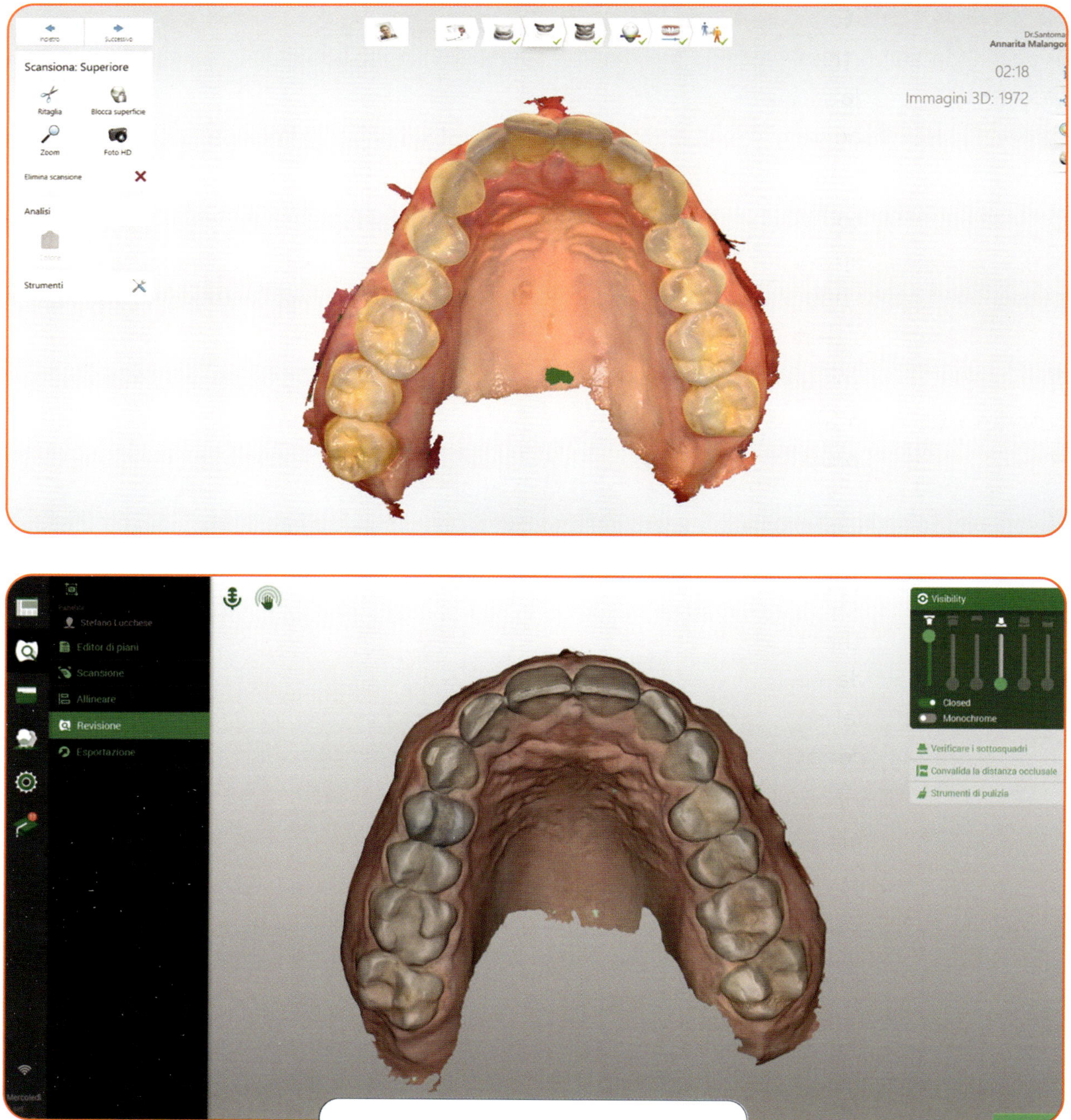

Figure 3.10 • Colour scan.

Open/Closed system

In some systems, the user must pay definite fees to perform a digital scan. In many cases, the scan data are then sent to cloud-based storage systems owned by the company; since the data are in encoded file format, one speaks of a closed system in this case.

Open STL data export for further processing using any CAD software is often, if not only, possible after exporting the file from this platform. Recently, a growing number of manufacturers has been offering systems that are referred to as open, that is, intraoral scanners that allow STL files to be exported directly.

The output of an intraoral scanner should ideally be, in addition to the legally valid proprietary file, an STL (*Solid-To-Layer*) file, i.e. one that can be opened immediately and used by any prosthetic CAD system.

Capture techniques with intraoral scanners

With regard to the scanning technique, to date there is still no universal and scientifically validated technique as to the most correct operational sequence to achieve an optimal scan. Sometimes, the manufacturer recommends an optimised scanning sequence for their own instrument (**Figure 3.11A**).

However, as mentioned above, there is a procedure that has not been fully verified yet, and is generally recommended for many types of scanners. For example, when scanning an entire arch, one starts distally from the last tooth of the arch, right or left, with a first rough scan.

A fluid and continuous scan of the occlusal and lingual surfaces of the teeth is performed, paying attention to the anterior area of the incisors, where, due to its small size, it is also required to scan a portion of the vestibular surface. When the last contralateral tooth is reached in this manner, you go back to the vestibular surfaces, while always maintaining an occlusal reference, so that the scan overlaps the one previously acquired. Then you go back to where you had started scanning to close the workflow of the data collected continuously. At this point you can switch to higher definition of the areas where, for example, there are scanning voids, in order to improve its quality and definition.

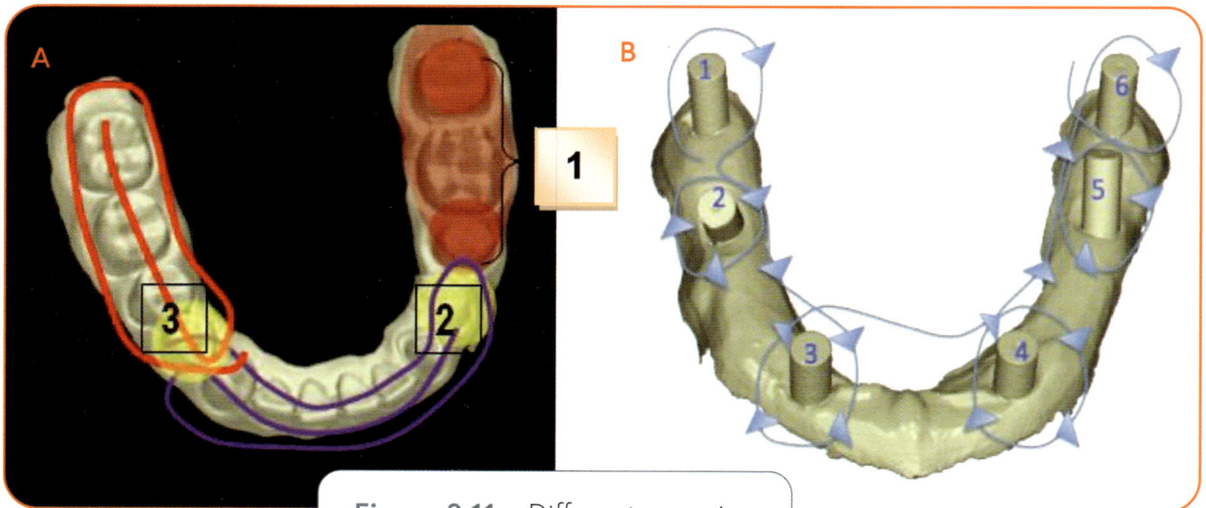

Figure 3.11 • Different scanning protocols.

Another recommended procedure [15] **(Figure 3.11B)** also entails starting from the distal end of an arch and to continuously scan mesially, occlusally and distally each tooth, with a rotating movement all around the tooth or the scanbody, trying to obtain as much information as possible, then switch to the next tooth always scanning continuously and smoothly. Only at the end, in the case of prepared teeth or around scanbodies, as also in the previous technique, is it possible to go back to these areas to obtain the maximum definition of the final preparation margins and, in any case, of the entire stump.

In principle, there is no universal scanning technique, but each manufacturer indicates their own for their product. In this respect, the article by Medina-Sotomayor et al. [16] is extremely interesting, as it highlights how the accuracy and precision of scanners Trios® (3Shape), Omnicam® (Sirona) and True Definition® (3M) is not affected by the different scanning strategies in recording complete arches. This is very likely because the software algorithm intervenes correcting the errors due to the scanning technique.

Mangano et al. [17] in an in vitro trial, compared the accuracy of reproduction and reliability of five different IOS (PRIMESCAN®, Sirona; CS 3700®, Carestream; MEDIT i-500®

and ITERO ELEMENTS 5D®, Align; Emerald S®, Planmeca) in capturing scanbodies of the implant and verified the dimensional consistency between the scanbody meshes and corresponding LF (Library File).

At the end of the quantitative evaluation, statistically different levels of consistency were found in the meshes of the scanbodies captured with the different IOS and the corresponding CAD LF.

Many studies have examined and compared the accuracy of the various implant impression techniques [18-19]. To date, in particular, the few studies support the use of IOS to capture the impression on multiple implants, aimed at making extensive implant supported restorations such as full arches.

In particular, the study by Monaco et al. [20] highlights, through a 3D position analysis, that not all scanners are suitable for digital impressions in fixed dental prostheses supported by full arch implants and the quality of the final file depends on the precision of the IOS.

This limitation is caused by the IOS capture method hence by the difficulty in reconstructing large surfaces [21].

It is particularly difficult to obtain accurate digital scans of the arch where there are large homogeneous areas (such as the spaces between implants in the edentulous arches); such difficulties are due to the absence of anatomical unevenness in the area to be scanned [22].

The scanner is unable to get its bearings especially when there is a lack of attached gingiva, this is because, by moving during the intraoral scan, the mucosa creates areas with ever changeable geometries and with different reflection planes.

The precision of the digital scans of the complete arch of edentulous patients can be improved by using a prefabricated resin ancillary device that simulated a dental prosthesis. As this device has the shape and superficial geometries of a typical dental arch, it makes digitalisation of the complete edentulous arch easier because it allows the scanner to capture areas with a clearly defined and stable geometry and therefore ensures more precise triangulation [23-24].

Intraoral scans in totally edentulous patients

Currently, several studies have highlighted the accuracy of IOS devices in scanning edentulous patients.

One of the first researches was that by Patzelt, in 2013 [22], which highlighted that only one of the intraoral scanners tested enabled accurate scans of the wholly edentulous arches.

The study by Osnes et al. [25] examined the precision of various IOS using two in vitro measurement methods. The study reached the conclusion that both the conventional method of average deviation and the maximum deviation method revealed a significant difference between the precision of some of the six intraoral scanners examined.

The greatest global average errors were produced by Emerald®, Planmeca and DWIO® (Dental Wings) but dropped just below the clinically significant threshold of 0.3 mm

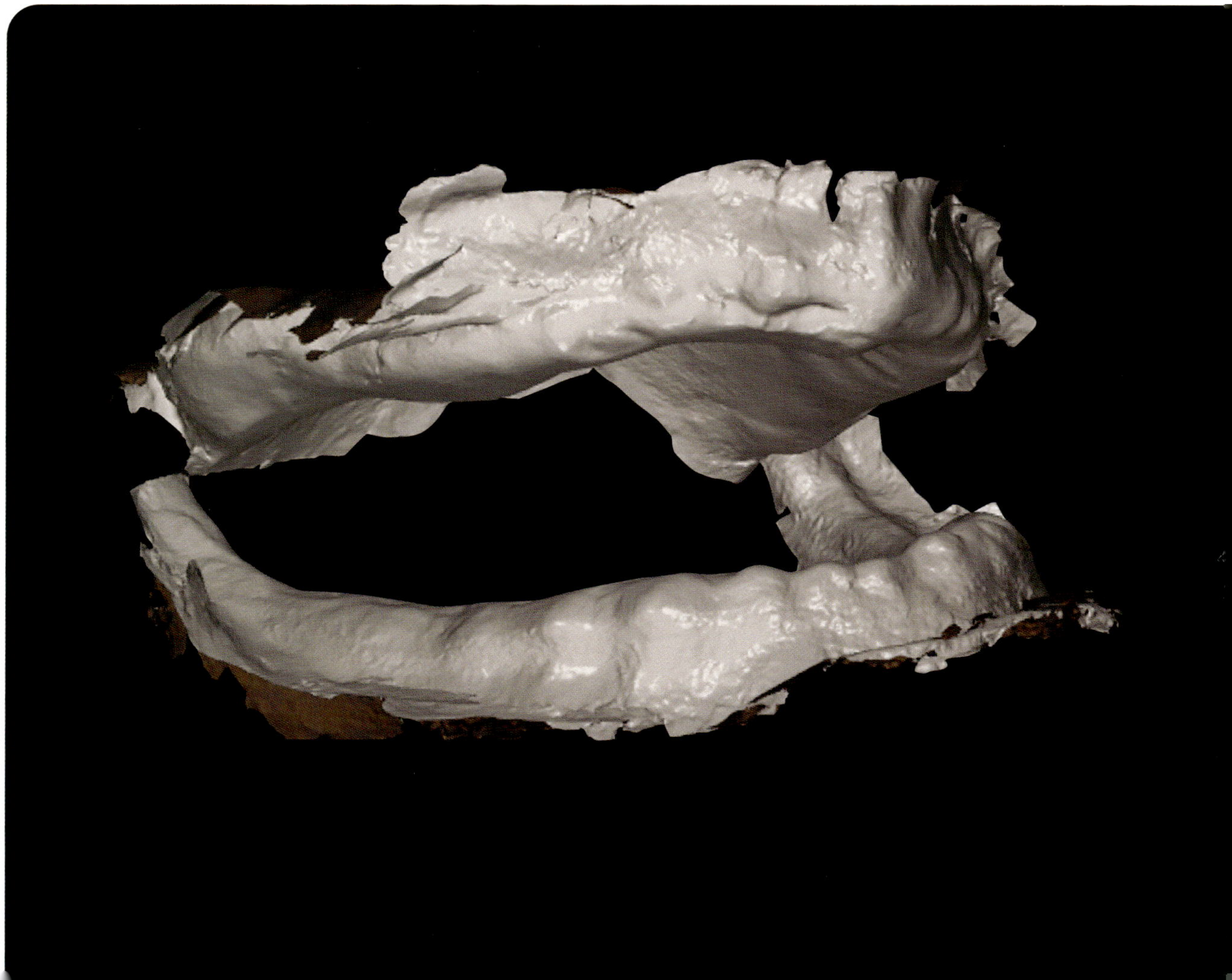

under optimal measurement conditions. The deviations of the upper limit of both scanners produced clinically significant errors higher than 0.3 mm. Trios® (3Shape), CEREC Omnicam (Sirona) and TDS (3M) produced clinically acceptable scans based on both metrics. The researchers suggest that future studies should report average distance measurements as well as upper limit deviation to ensure comparability between studies and promote clinically significant investigations.

Fully edentulous patients are still the most complex to be treated using fully digital workflows.

In the IOS use difficulty pyramid defined by Derksen in 2015 [26], the possibility of producing total removable prostheses from intraoral scans is considered extremely difficult both for the registration of the intermaxillary relationships and for the impossibility of registering the muscular activity at the peripheral joint level (edging procedure of the analogue procedures) **(Figure 3.12)**.

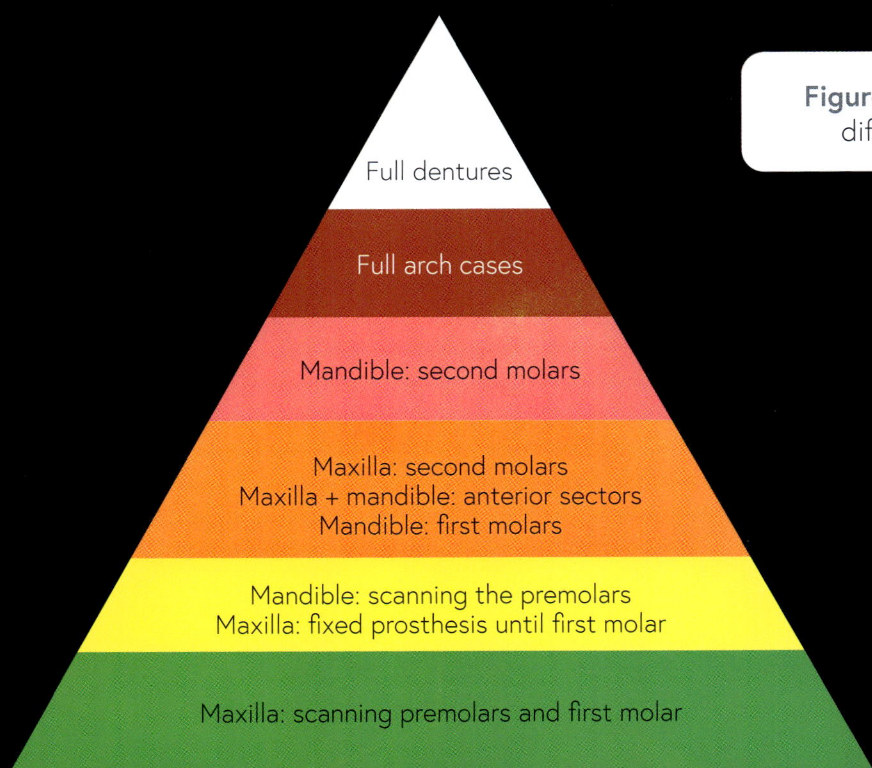

Figure 3.12 • Derksen's difficulty pyramid.

The problems related to occlusal registration, thanks to the use of new software, have been solved, while it is still impossible to perform accurate total prostheses with fully digital flows, as it remains impossible to record (with current instruments) the patient's muscle activity. The treatment of patients in terminal dentition or fully edentulous ones who must undergo implant therapy can however benefit from the use of intraoral scanners (see Chapters 6 and 7).

Face scanners

The transfer of extra- and intraoral clinical information into the virtual environment is required in order to streamline planning of the prosthetic treatment.

With the increasingly frequent use of virtual articulators, digital face bow techniques have been developed for the transfer of virtual maxillary models into virtual simulators of mandibular movements. It is possible to use different scanning methods to obtain 3D facial scans, but the influence these methods have on the precision with which a digital jaw scan is transferred to a 3D facial scan is unknown.

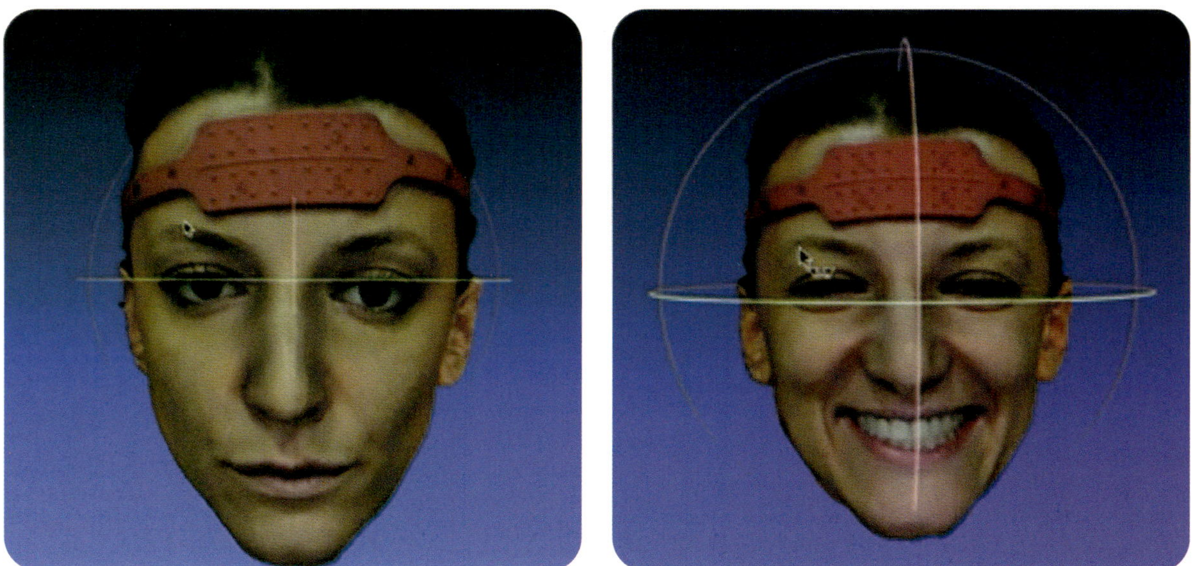

Figure 3.13 • Example of scan with structured light scanner.

Facial scanners **(Figures 3.13 and 3.14)** are used for planning the prosthetic treatment but also for planning orthognathic surgery.

Several 3D facial scanning methods have been introduced: photogrammetry, stereophotogrammetry, laser beam scanning and structured light scanning.

The first two are passive facial scanning methods and are based on taking two or more photographs from different views with similar common points to obtain facial reconstruction through a reverse engineering software program.

Laser beam scanning and structured light scanning, on the other hand, use active 3D sensors that project light patterns onto the patient's extraoral soft face tissues which are then captured by one or more high resolution cameras using active triangulation.

A face digitiser generates a specific digital file format such as standard tessellation language (STL), Polygonal Face Tessellation (OBJ), or Stanford triangle (PLY) file. An STL file only describes the geometric surface of a digitised object with no representation of colour, texture or other CAD attributes. On the contrary, OBJ and PLY files store information on surface, colour and texture.

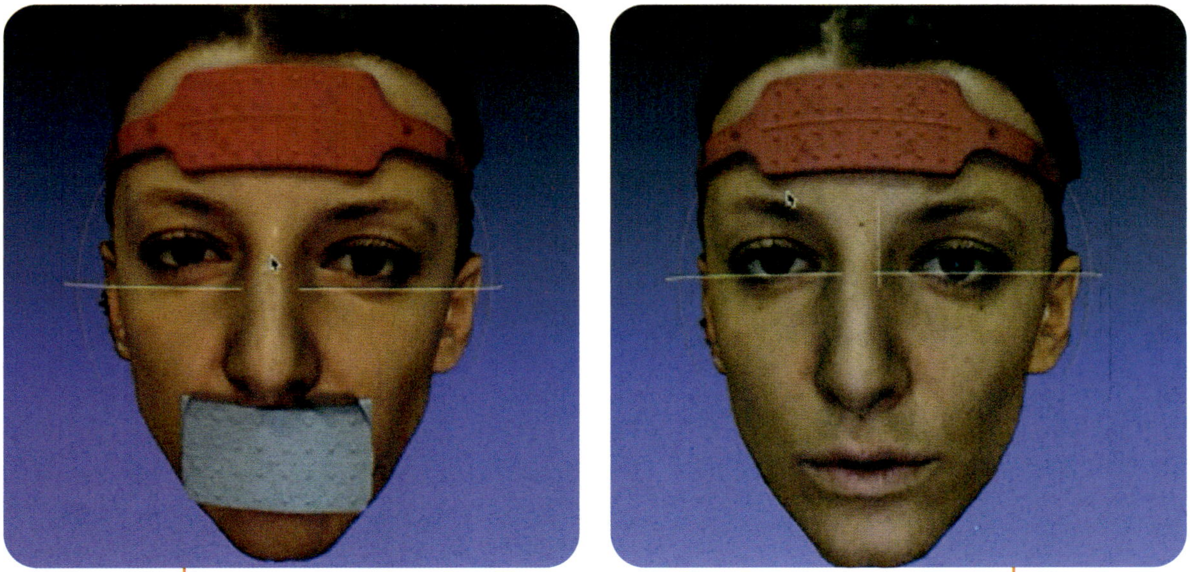

Figure 3.14 • Another example of scan with structured light scanner.

Literature reviews regarding the accuracy of facial scans show that mobile device compatible facial scanners do not perform as well as professional face capture 3D scanning systems, but that deviations fall within the clinically acceptable range of less than 1.5 mm. Significant differences in results were observed when 3D facial scans were performed on inanimate facial objects and when performed on the faces of real participants.

Different technologies were compared: stereophotogrammetry and white light scanners show a similar level of accuracy, higher than infrared scanners [27-31].

Virtual articulators

The virtual articulator is software capable of reproducing the intermaxillary relationship between virtual models of the dental arches and simulating mandibular movements.

Over the past ten years, interest in this instrument has grown increasingly in dentistry.

In prosthetics, the virtual articulator should be considered as a diagnostic and planning instrument for the treatment plan and complementing the mechanical articulator, to be used especially in complex prosthetic cases in which there are significant alterations of the vertical occlusion dimension and of the intermaxillary spatial relationships.

In order to properly simulate the mandibular movement, virtual models must be digitised and mounted properly in the virtual articulator. There are currently two main types: individual (IA) and mathematically simulated virtual articulator (MS).

The IA type reproduces the exact moving pathways of the mandible by using digital accessories. The main indication for the IA type involves complex cases where the morphology of the occlusal plane must be evaluated during mandible movements to avoid occlusal dynamic interference.

The MS type is a mean value articulator that requires adjusting additional settings in order to reproduce mandible movements.

The main clinical indication for the MS type involves cases in which reproducing the static relationship between the models is sufficient to plan the occlusal morphology of the prosthesis. The main disadvantage of the MS type is that it is not possible to obtain the patient's individualised movements. However, the MS type is easier to use and more affordable than the CA type and therefore more widespread.

Four steps are required to use the virtual articulator: (1) impression of the arches; (2) occlusal registration; (3) transfer of the jaw position with respect to the cranium (FV); (4) virtual mounting.

Technological developments in the devices and software will lead to switching from 3D to 4D over time.

The animation of mandible movements will ensure accurate simulation of the occlusion dynamics in the virtual patient. The digital approach to the use of the virtual articulator is promising and should be further developed to promote its use in interdisciplinary cases that require it.

In the future, the use of virtual articulators will probably be routine in everyday clinical practice **(Figures 3.15-3.17)** [32-41].

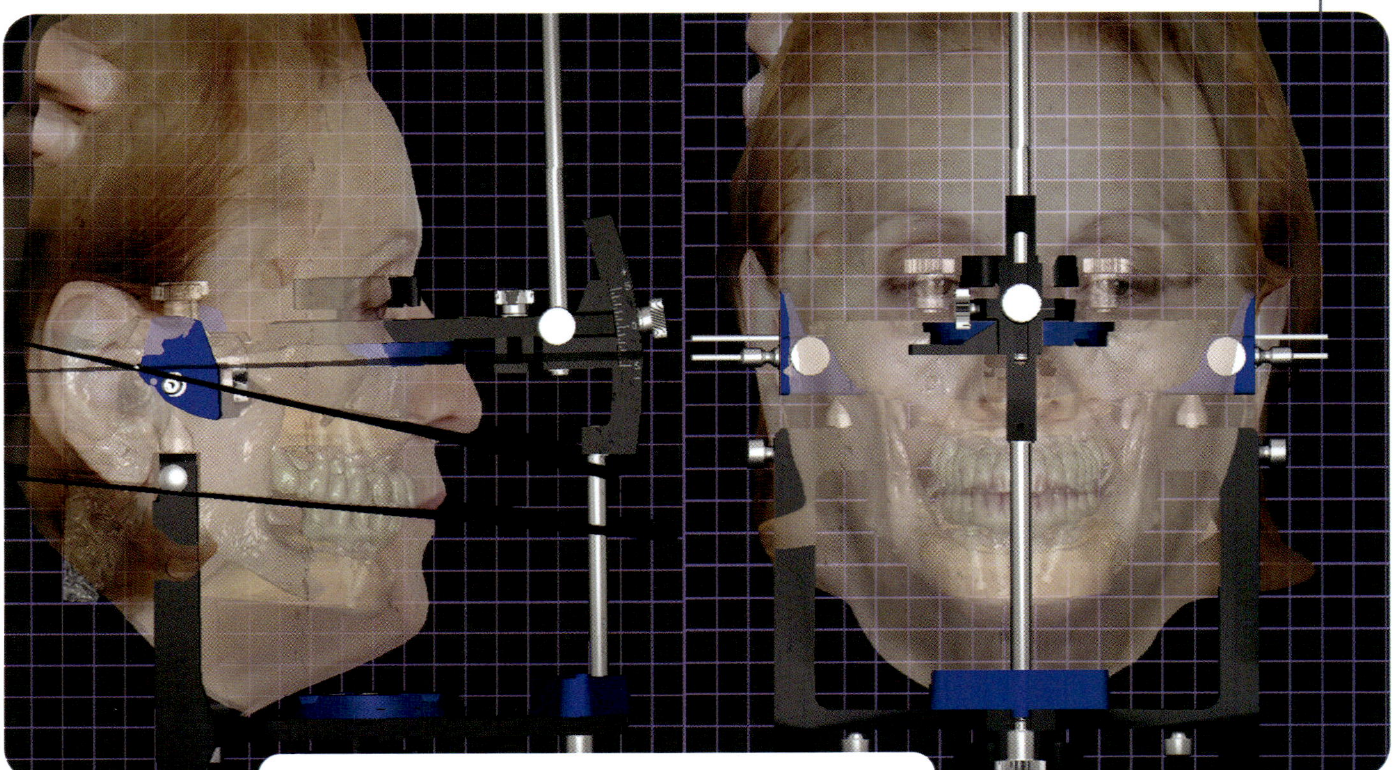

Figure 3.15 • Use of the digital diagnostic instruments in digital patient management.

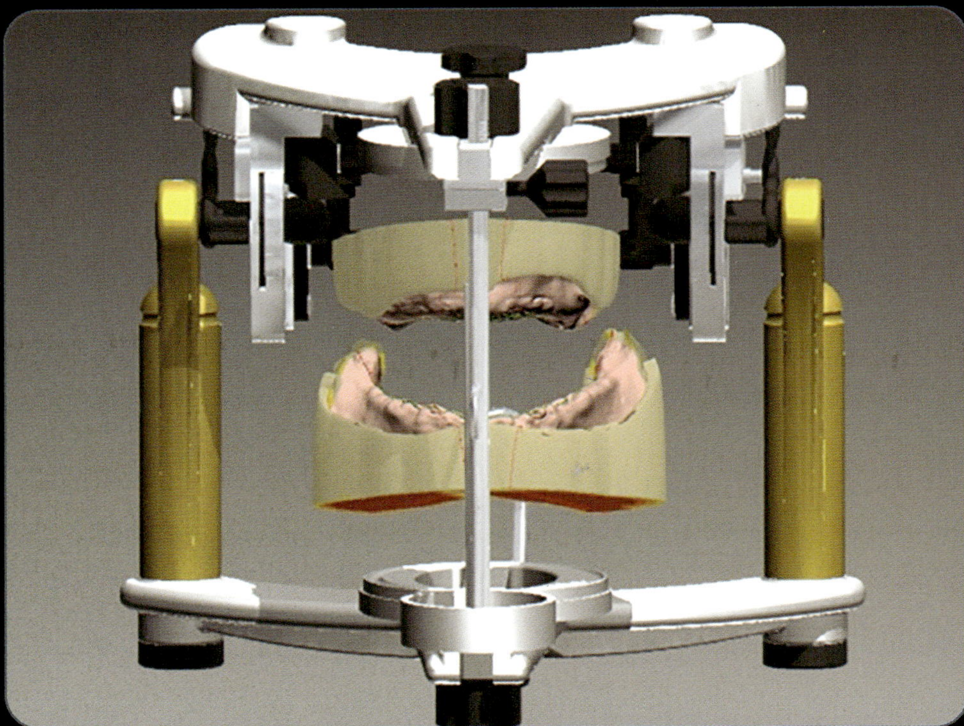

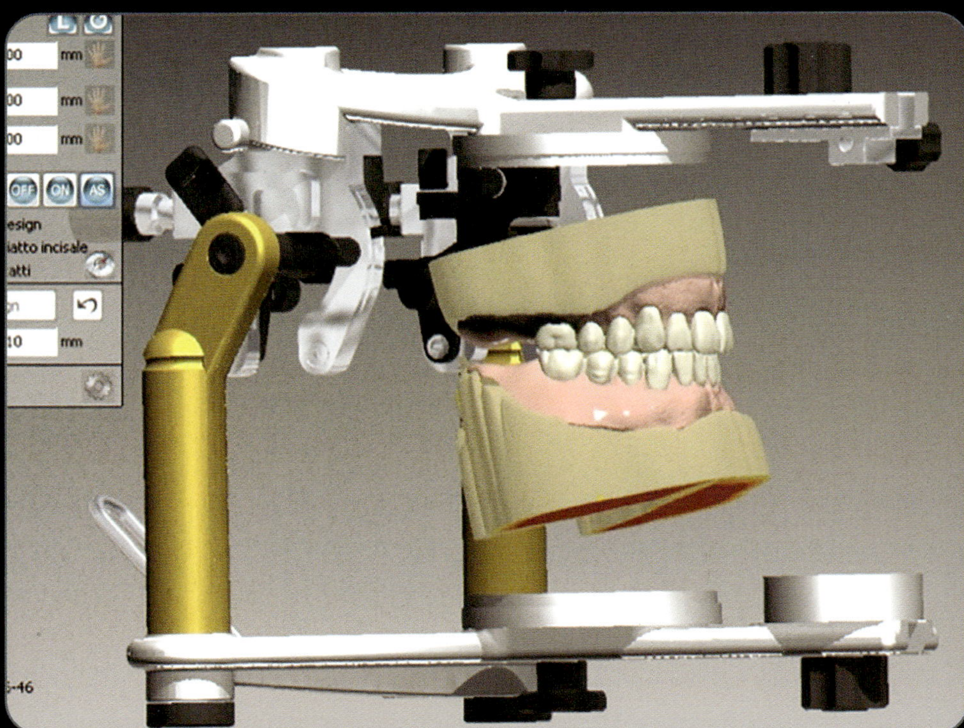
mm
mm
mm
OFF
ON
AS
esign
iatto incisale
atti
10
mm
6-46

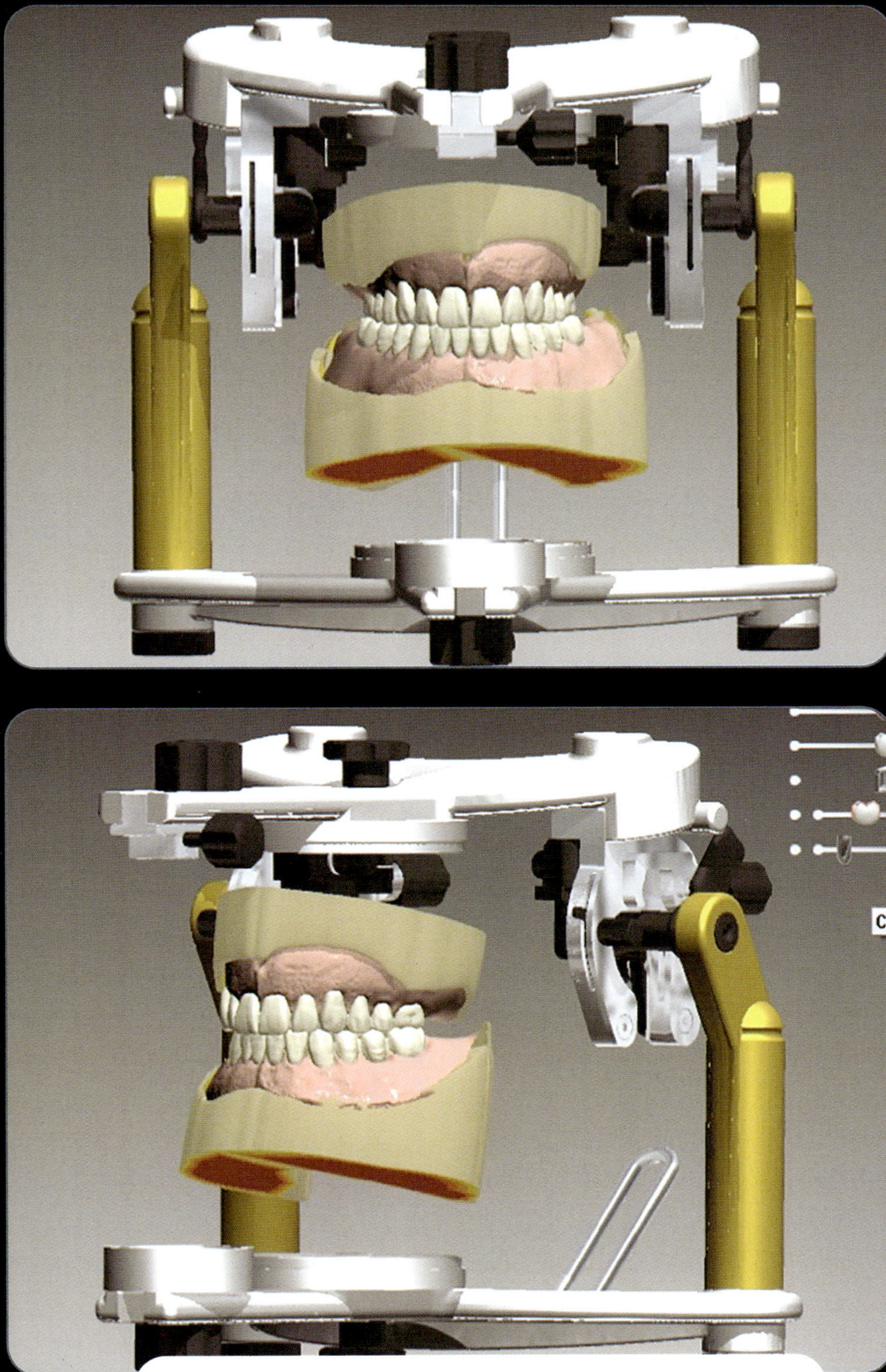

Figure 3.16 • Use of the virtual articulator in the design of the total removable prosthesis.

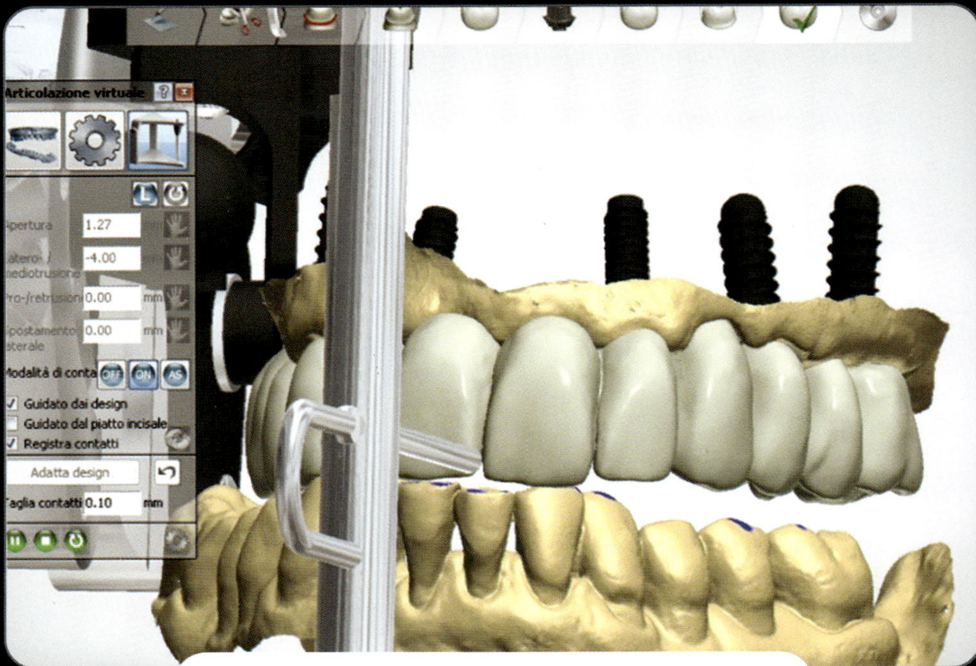

Figure 3.17 • Use of the virtual articulator in the design of the fixed prosthesis.

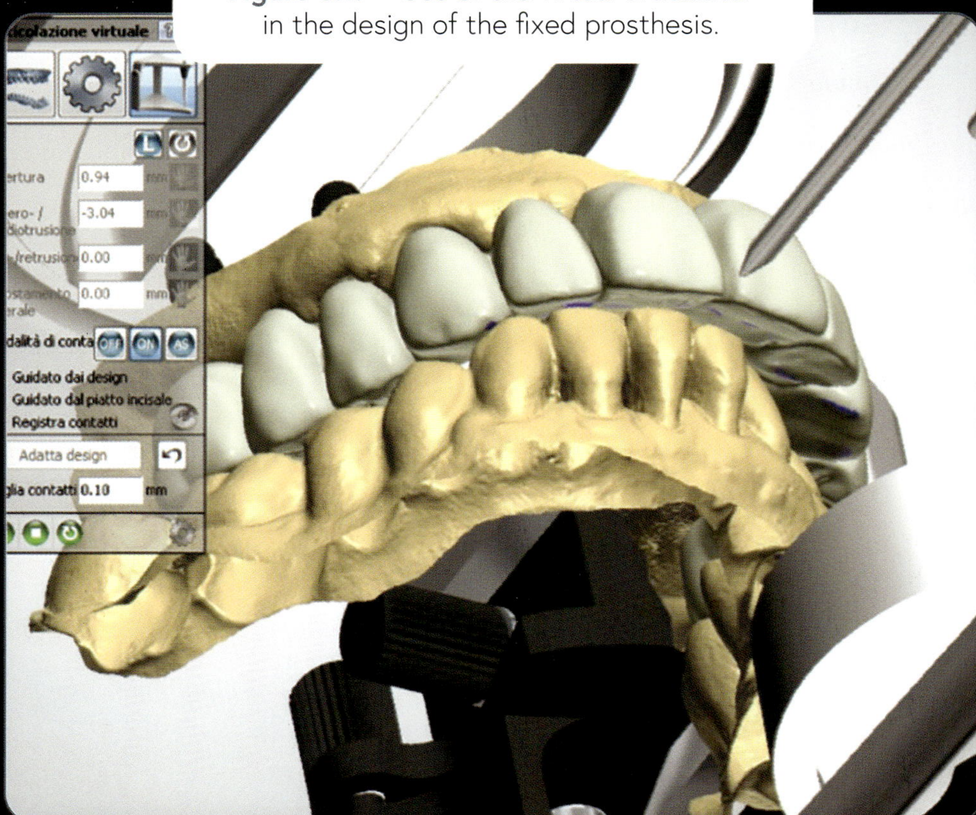

Application of digital technologies in removable complete prostheses

The concept of "digital patient" in which all the acquisition of the prosthetic coordinates and their processing involves the use of digital tools is close to being exhaustively defined.

In complete digital prostheses, after checking the bite plates (see Chapter 5), it is possible to perform facial scans of the patient, assessing the dental exposure at rest, minimum and maximum display of the smile, in addition to support of the perioral tissues and esthetic assessment of the face.

In the same session, a facial scan is also performed using extra-oral landmarks that allow the facial scans to be superimposed on those of the plates in a virtual environment and thus to preview the final prosthetic design in the patient's face.

The first landmark consists of a fork on which scannable silicone is spread for occlusal registration which the patient is asked to clench between the registration plates **(Figures 3.18-3.20)**.

The second extraoral landmark is positioned on the forehead **(Figure 3.21)** and the facial scan is then performed and all the material is sent to the laboratory **(Figure 3.22)**.

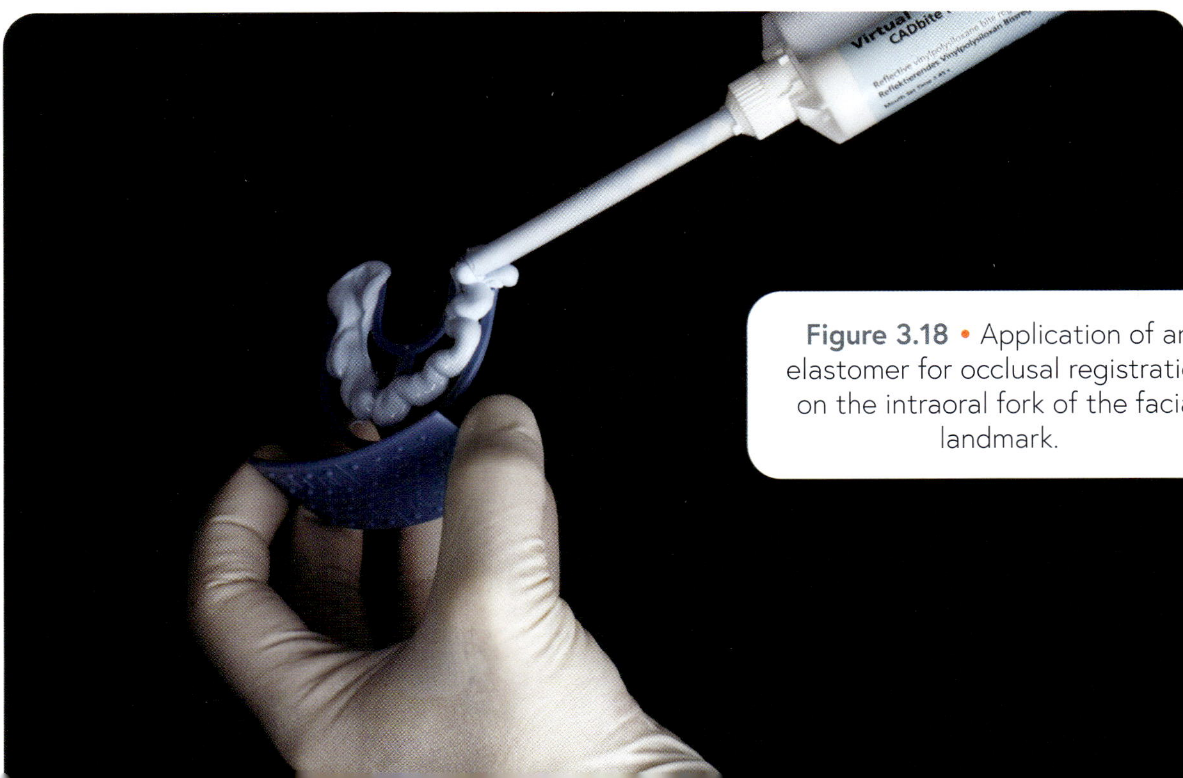

Figure 3.18 • Application of an elastomer for occlusal registration on the intraoral fork of the facial landmark.

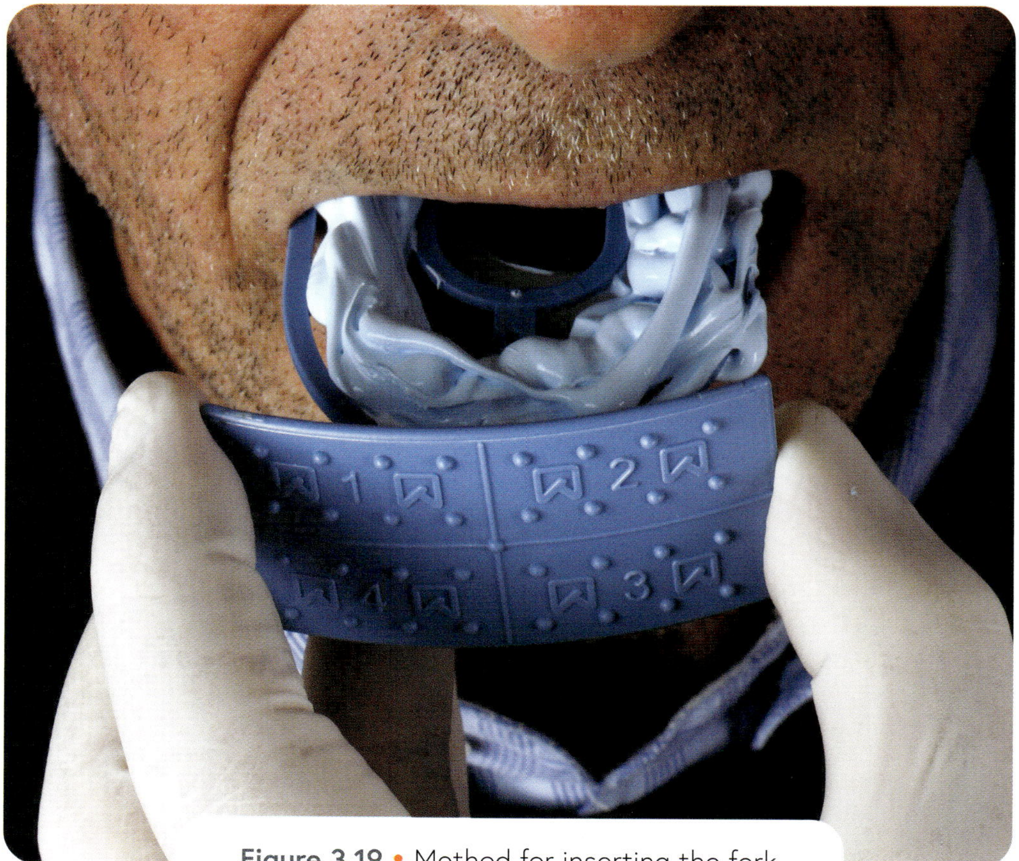

Figure 3.19 • Method for inserting the fork between the occlusal registration bases.

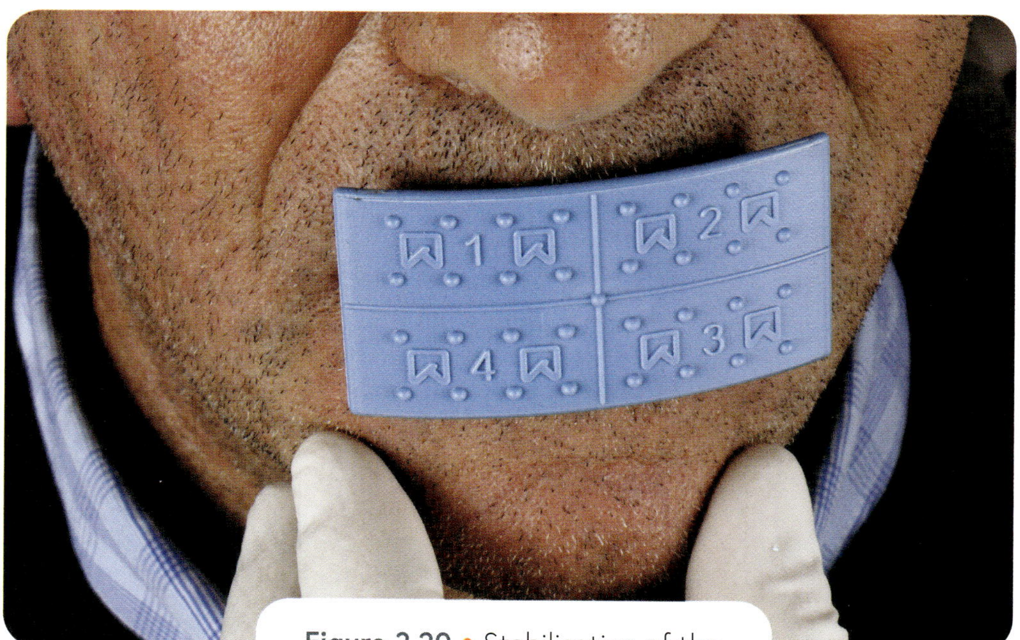

Figure 3.20 • Stabilisation of the extraoral landmark.

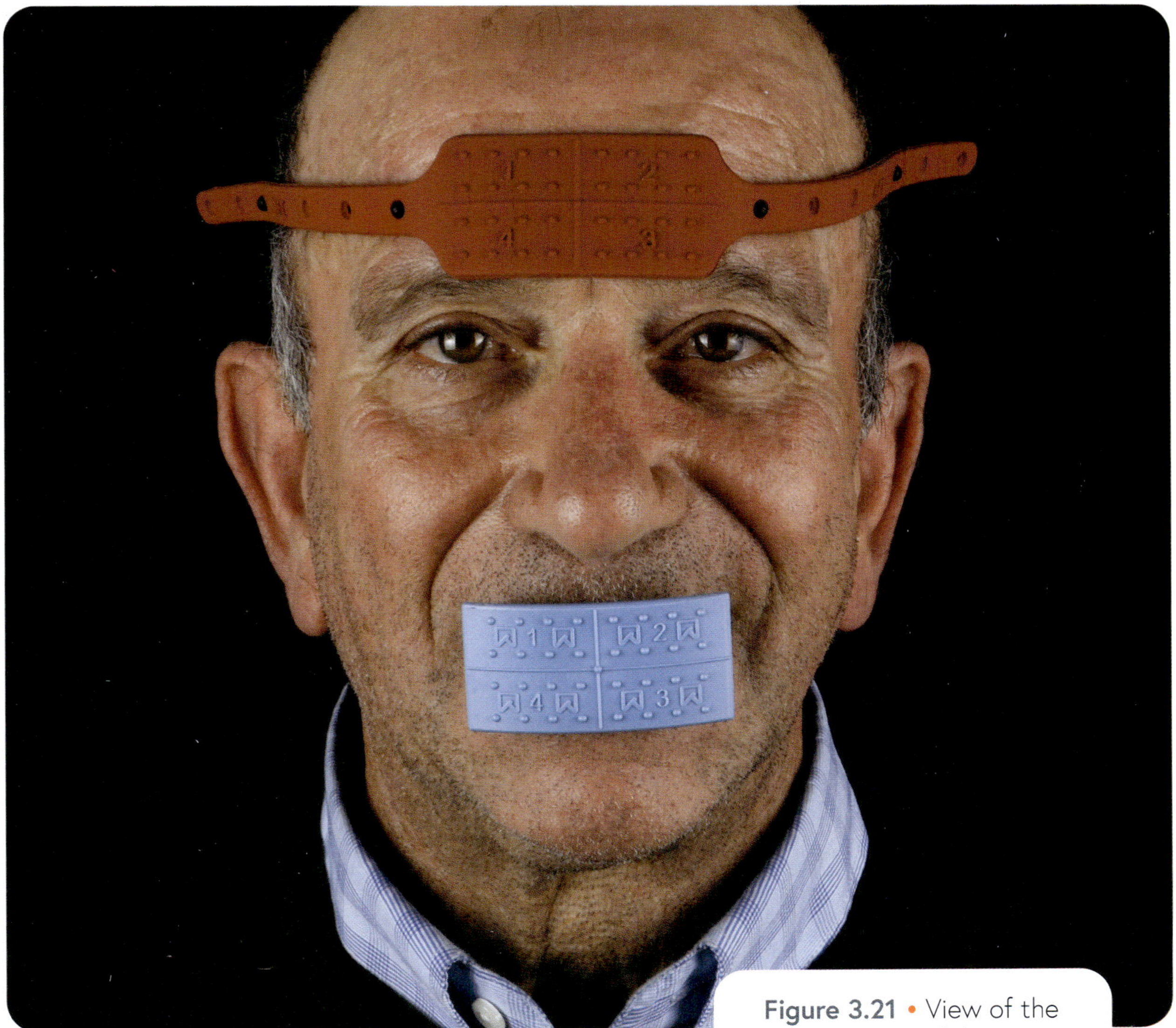

Figure 3.21 • View of the patient and of the two scanning landmarks (frontal and oral).

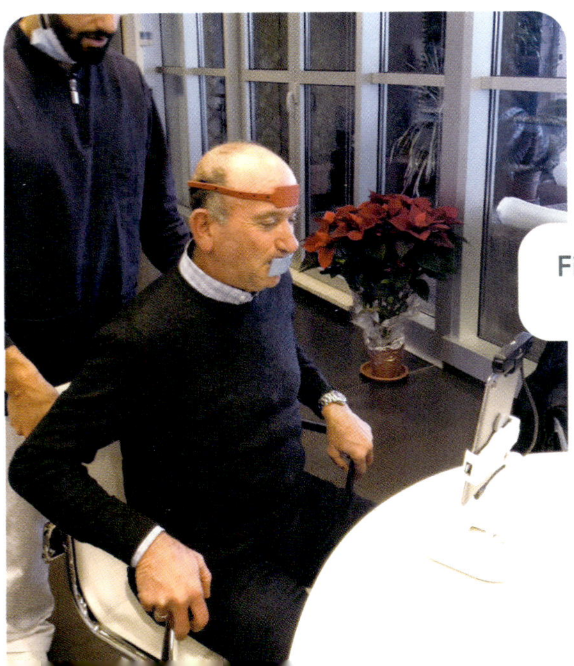

Figure 3.22 • Performing the facial scan.

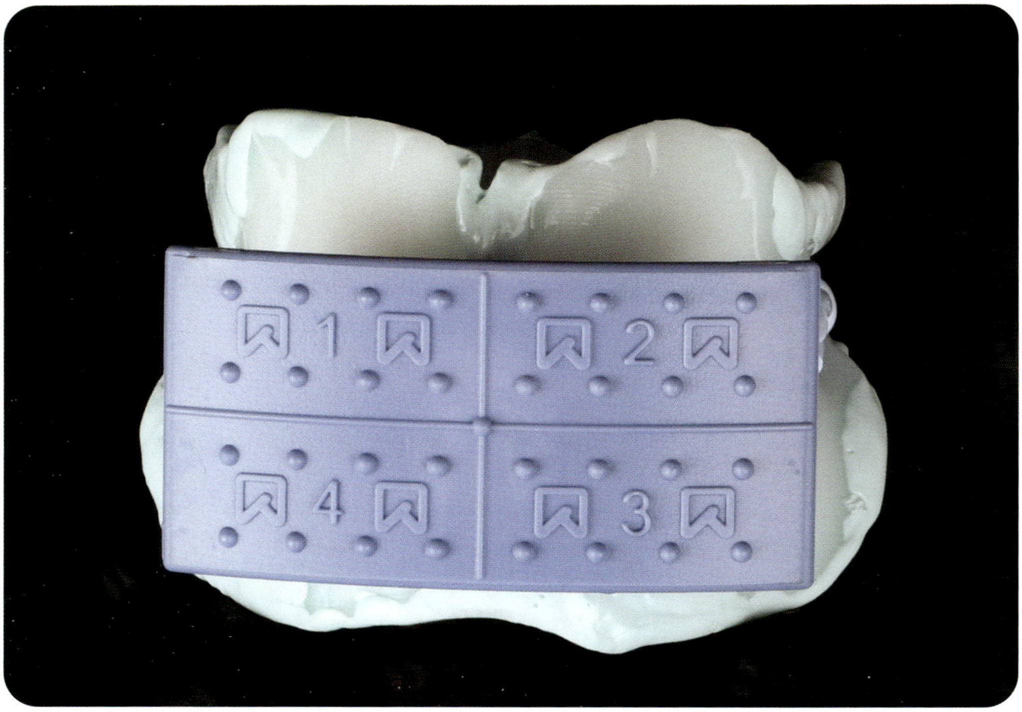
1
2
4
3

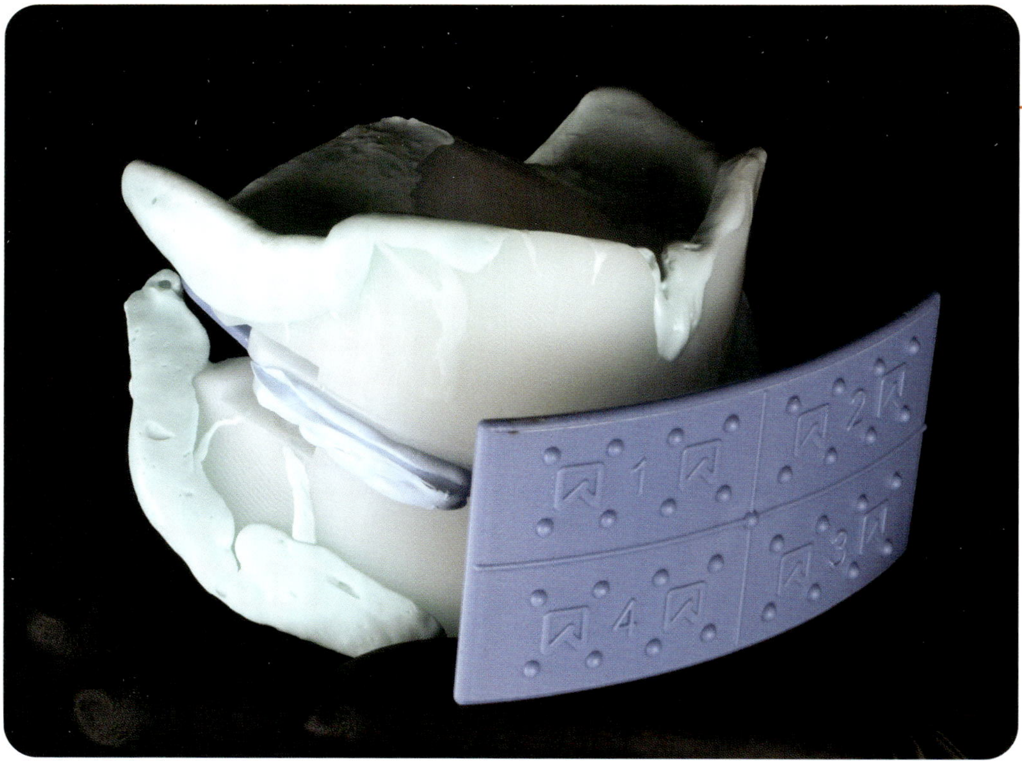
1
2
4
3

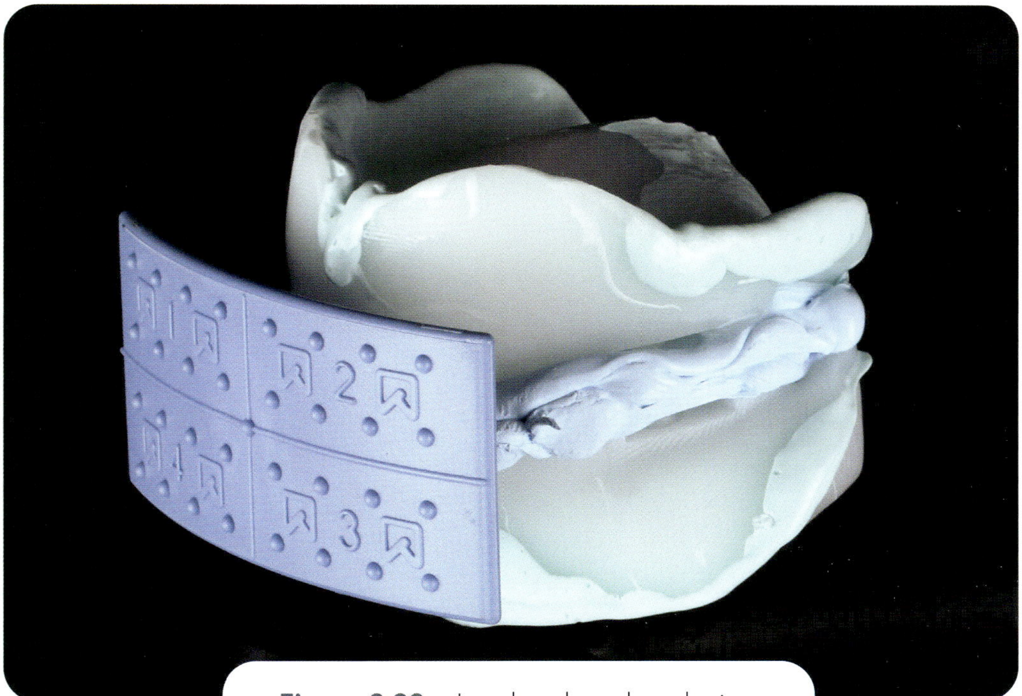

Figure 3.23 • Landmark and occlusion bases before scanning in the laboratory.

At the laboratory, scans are performed of the plates in occlusion with the interposed landmark **(Figure 3.23)**. The impression landmark of both the intra- and extraoral portion is then completely scanned and the scan files can be superimposed.

It is therefore possible to obtain in a virtual environment the three-dimensional reconstruction of the edentulous arches, spatially oriented in relation to occlusal registration and properly positioned in the virtual patient's face **(Figures 3.24** and **3.25)**.

The prosthetic design can therefore be previewed in the patient's face to assess its esthetic adequacy.

It is also possible to assess the various degrees of the smile by superposing the various face scans thanks to the forehead landmark **(Figures 3.26-3.28)**.

The validation of the virtual design is followed by the CAM step, when the prototype of the final prosthesis will be milled or moulded **(Figure 3.29)** (see Chapter 5).

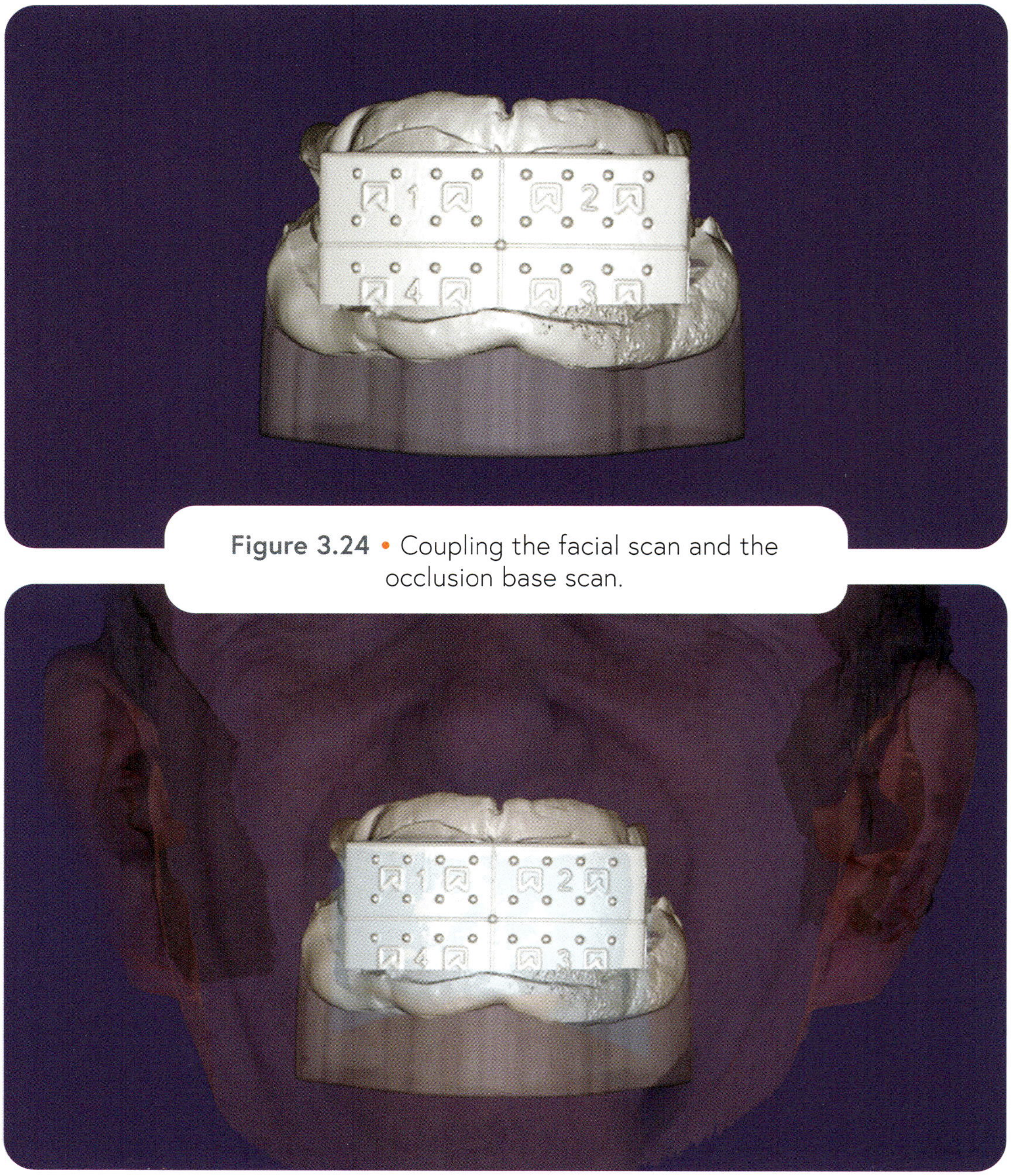

Figure 3.24 • Coupling the facial scan and the occlusion base scan.

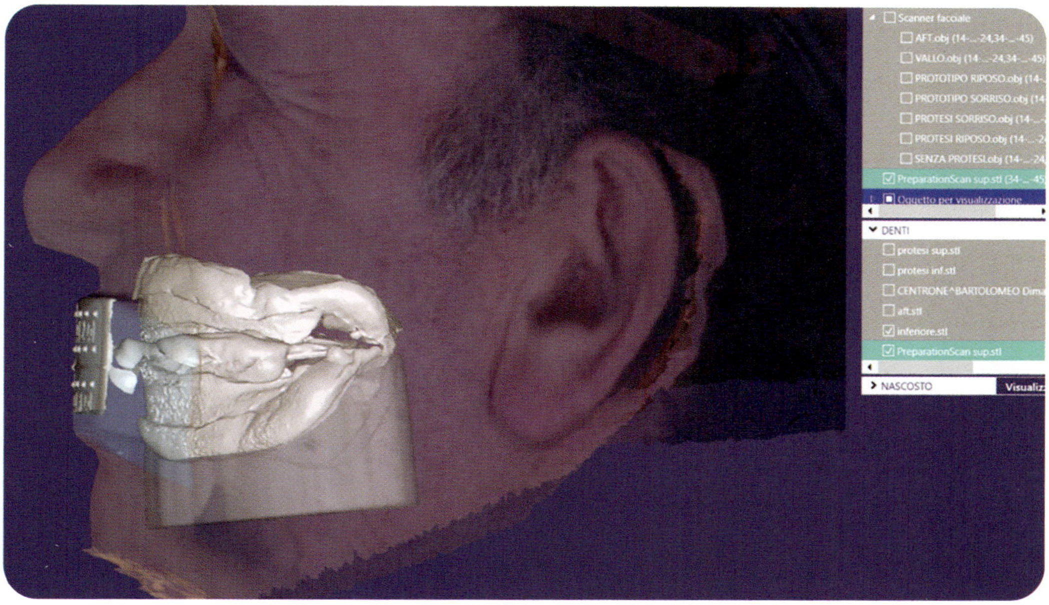

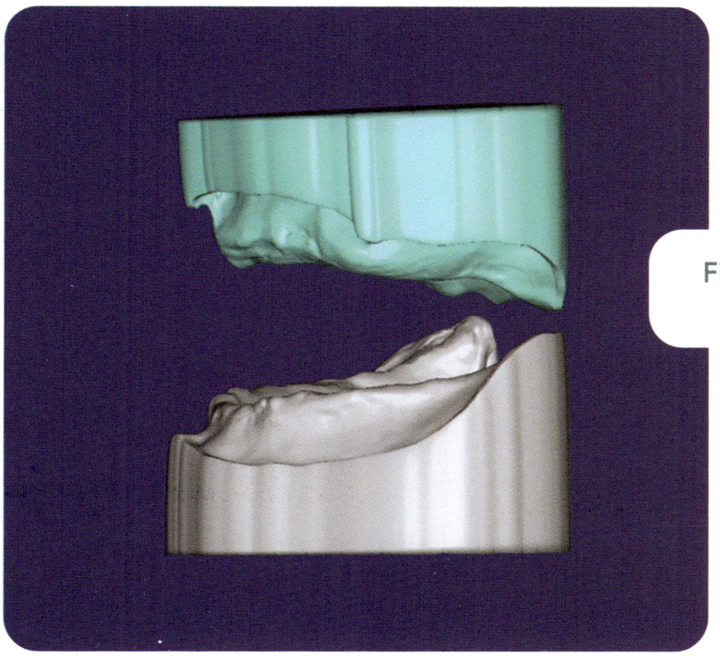

Figure 3.25 • Positioning the virtual models in space.

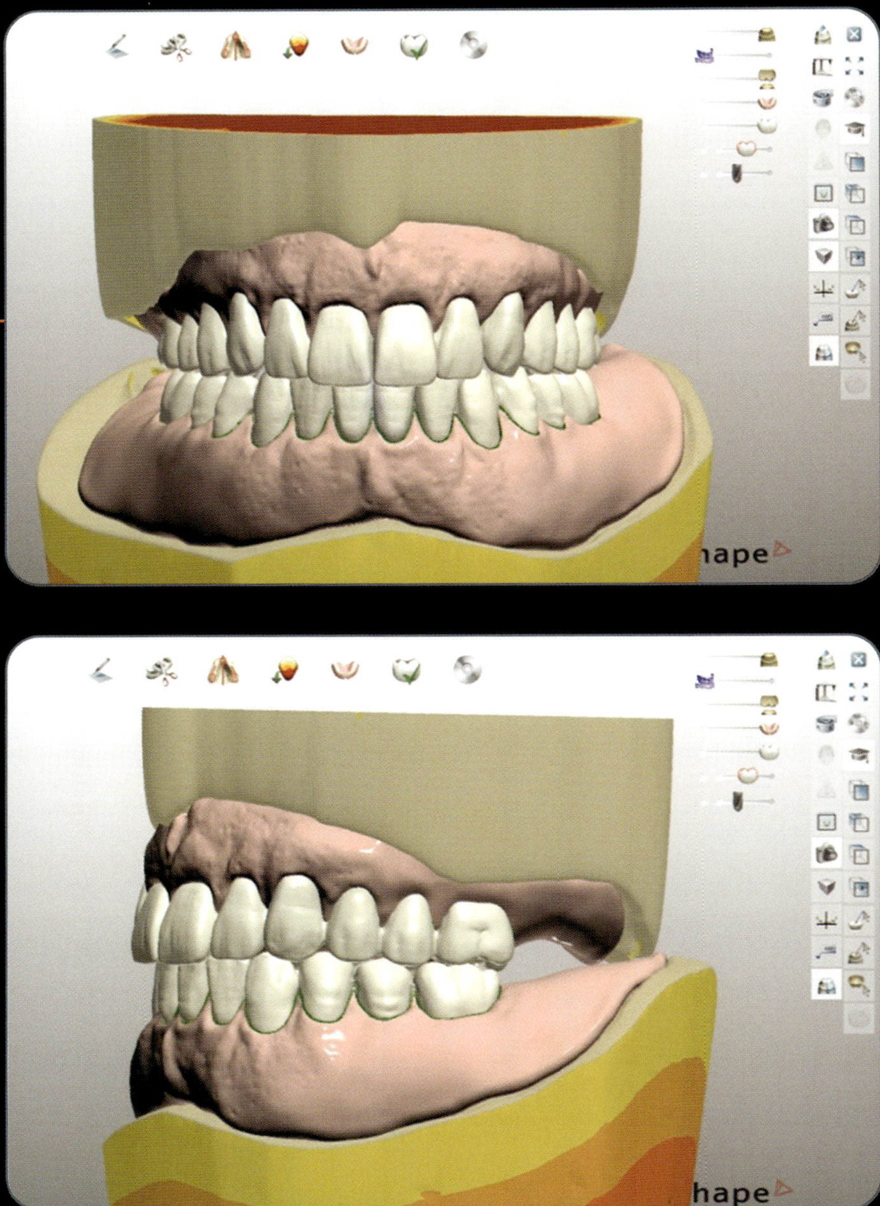

Figure 3.26 • CAD design of the complete prosthesis.

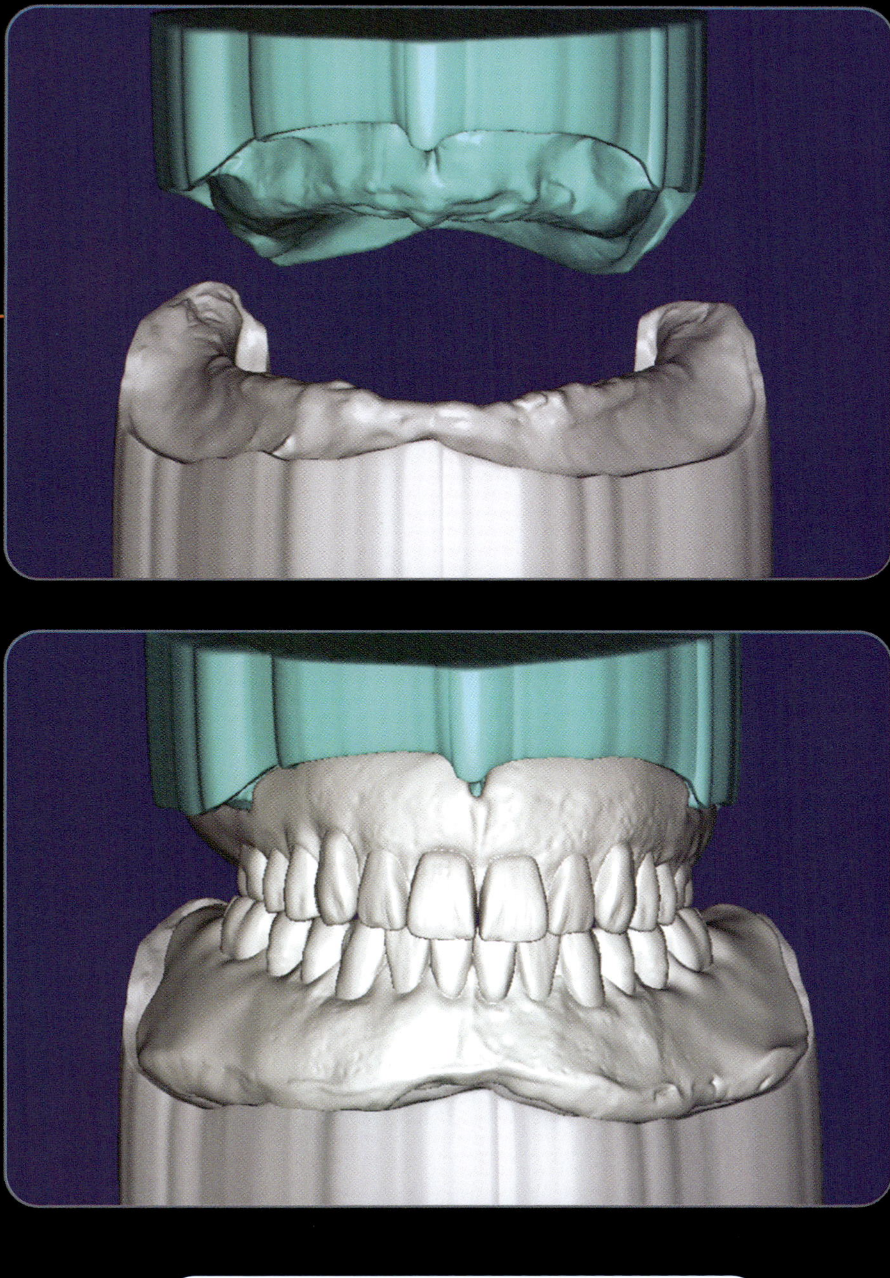

Figure 3.27 • Virtual models of the edentulous arches and prosthetic design.

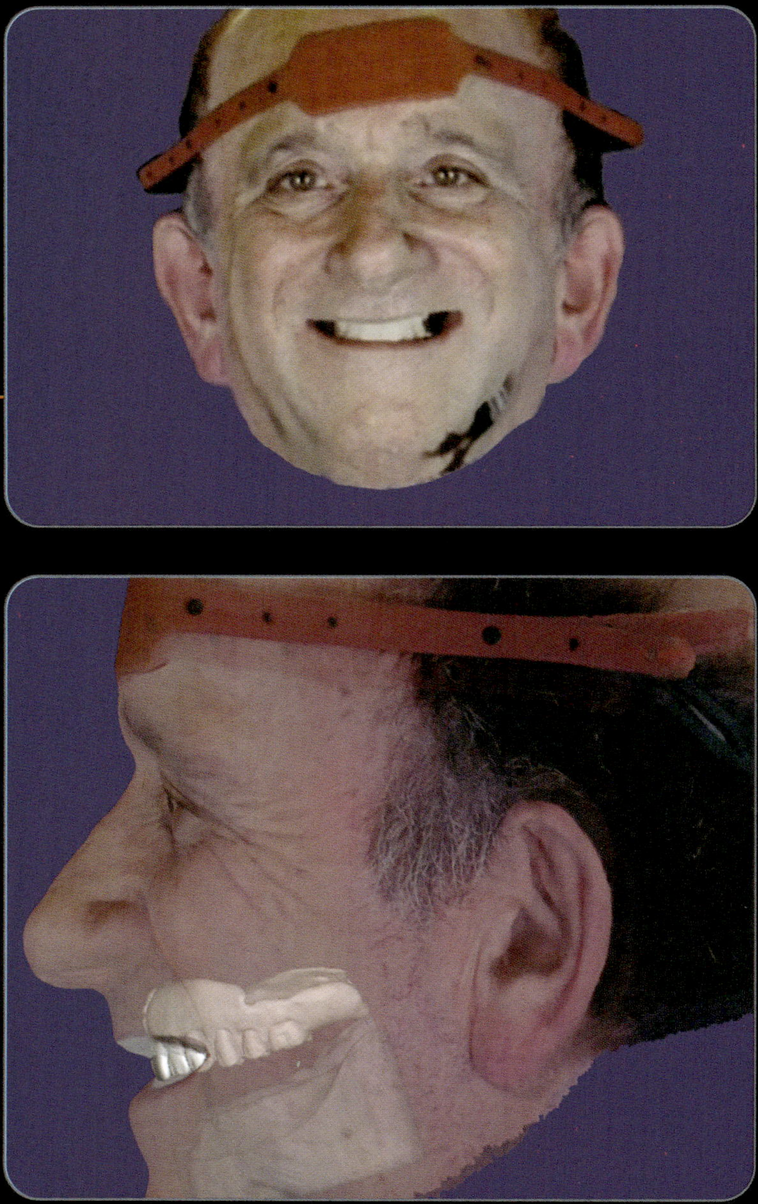

Figure 3.28 • Esthetic assessment of the prosthetic design in the patient's face.

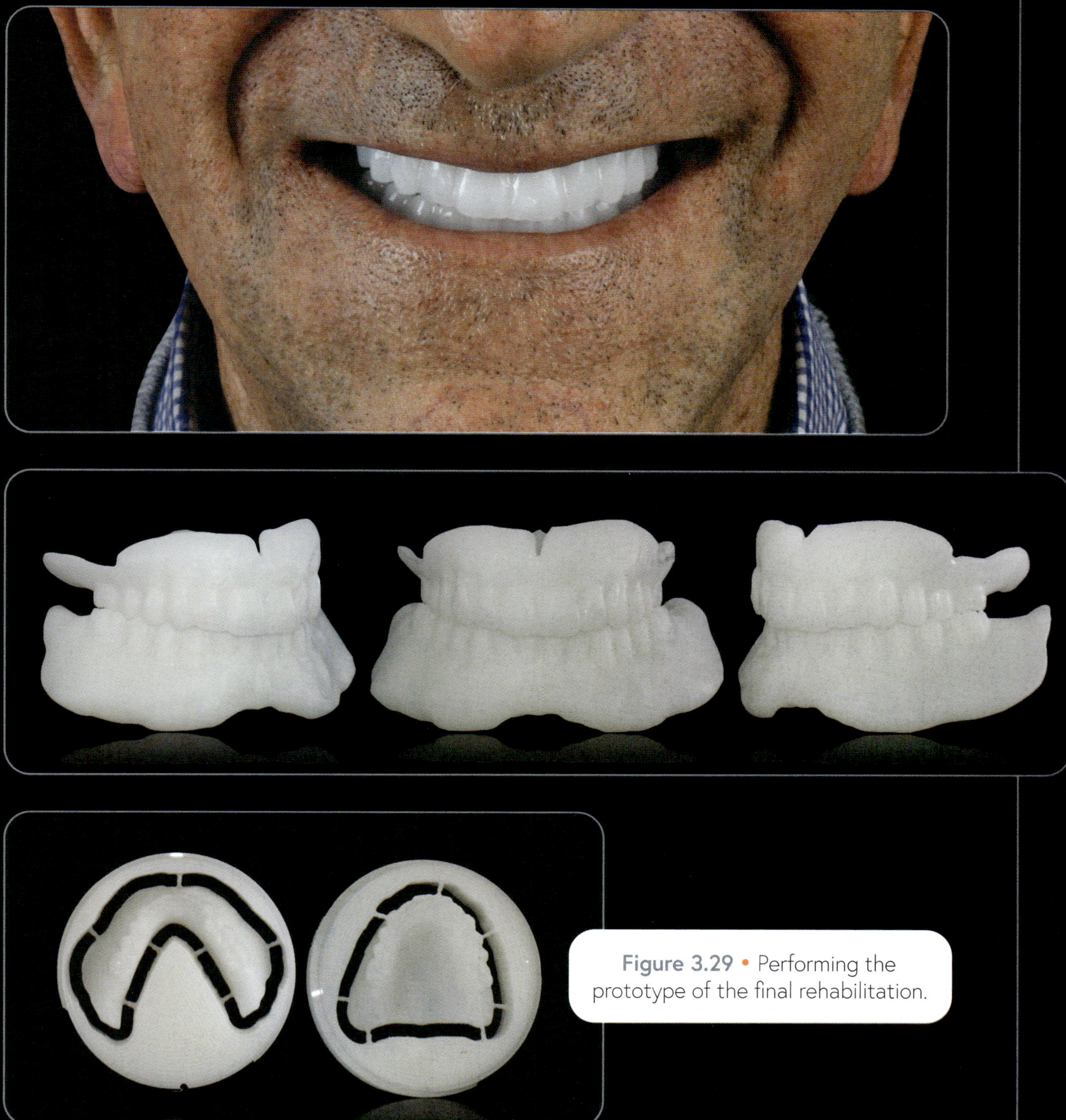

Figure 3.29 • Performing the prototype of the final rehabilitation.

References

1. Fasbinder DJ. Digital dentistry: innovation for restorative treatment. *Compend Contin Educ Dent.* 2010;31(4):2-11.
2. Christensen GJ. The challenge to conventional impressions. *J Am Dent Assoc.* 2008;139:347-9.
3. Christensen GJ. Will digital impressions eliminate the current problems with conventional impressions? *J Am Dent Assoc.* 2008;139(6):761-3.
4. Kim JH, Kim KB, Kim SH et al. Quantitative evaluation of common errors in digital impression obtained by using an LED blue light in-office CAD/CAM system. Quintessence Int. 2015;46(5):401-7.
5. Flugge TV, Schlager S, Nelson K et al. Precision of intraoral digital dental impressions with iTero and extraoral digitization with the iTero and a model scanner. *Am J Orthod Dentofac Orthop.* 2013;144(3).
6. Logozzo S, Zanetti EM, Franceschini G. Recent advances in dental optics. Part I: 3D intraoral scanners for restorative dentistry. *Optics and Lasers in Engineering.* 2014;54:203-21.
7. ISO 10360-9:2013 Geometrical product specifications (GPS) – Acceptance and reverification tests for coordinate measuring systems (CMS) – Part 9: CMMs with multiple probing systems.
8. ISO 12836:2012 specifies test methods for the assessment of the accuracy of digitizing devices for computer-aided design/computer-aided manufacturing (CAD/CAM) systems for indirect dental restorations.
9. Hollenbeck K, Allin T, van der Poel M. Dental Lab 3D Scanners – How they work and what works best 3Shape Technology Research, Copenhagen 2012.
10. Nedelcu RG, Persson AS. Scanning accuracy and precision in 4 intraoral scanners: an in vitro comparison based on 3-dimensional analysis. *J Prosthet Dent.* 2014;112(6):1461-71.
11. Wulfman C, Naveau A, Rignon-Bret C. Digital scanning for complete-arch implant-supported restorations: A systematic review. *J Prosthet Dent.* 2020;124(2):161-7.
12. Kihara H, Hatakeyama W, Komine F et al. Accuracy and practicality of intraoral scanner in dentistry: A literature review. *J Prosthodont Res.* 2020;64(2):109-113.
13. Flügge T, van der Meer WJ, Gonzalez BG et al. The accuracy of different dental impression techniques for implant-supported dental prostheses: A systematic review and meta-analysis. *Clin Oral Implants Res.* 2018;29(16):374-92.
14 Mangano F, Bosetti M. Conoscere la nuova odontoiatria digitale: gli scanner intraorali. *Il Dentista Moderno.* Monografia gennaio 2016.
15. Giménez B, Özcan M, Martínez-Rus F, Pradíes G. Accuracy of a digital impression system based on active wavefront sampling technology for implants considering operator experience, implant angulation, and depth. *Clin Implant Dent Relat Res.* 2015;17:e54-e64.
16. Medina-Sotomayor P, Pascual-Moscardó A, Camps I. Accuracy of four digital scanners according to scanning strategy in complete-arch impressions. *PLoS One.* 2018;13(9):e0202916.
17. Mangano F, Lerner H, Margiani B et al. Congruence between meshes and library files of implant scanbodies: an in vitro study comparing five intraoral scanners. *J Clin Med.* 2020;9(7):2174.
18. Flügge T, Meer WJ, Gonzalez BG et al. The accuracy of different dental impression techniques for implant-supported dental prostheses: A systematic review and meta-analysis. *Clin Oral Impl Res.* 2018;29(Suppl. 16):374-92.
19. Richert R, Goujat A, Venet L et al. Intraoral Scanner Technologies: A Review to Make a Successful Impression. *J Healthc Eng.* 2017;1-9.
20. Di Fiore A, Meneghello R, Graiff L, Savio G, Vigolo P, Monaco C, Stellini E. Full arch digital scanning systems performances for implant-supported fixed dental prostheses: a comparative study of 8 intraoral scanners. *J Prosthodont Res.* 2019;63(4):396-403.
21. Mangano F, Hauschild U, Veronesi G et al. Trueness and precision of 5 intraoral scanners in the impressions of single and multiple implants: a comparative in vitro study. *BMC Oral Health.* 2019;19:101.

22. Patzelt S, Vonau S, Stampf S; Att W. Assessing the feasibility and accuracy of digitizing edentulous jaws. *JADA*. 2013;144(8).

23. Iturrate, Mikel et al. Obtaining reliable intraoral digital scans for an implant-supported complete-arch prosthesis: A dental technique. *J Prosthet Dent*. 2019;121(2):237-41.

24. Iturrate, Mikel et al. Accuracy analysis of complete-arch digital scans in edentulous arches when using an auxiliary geometric device. *J Prosthet Dent*. 2019;121(3):447-54.

25. Osnes CA, Wu JH, Venezia P. et al. Full arch precision of six intraoral scanners in vitro. *J Prosthodont Res*. 2019.

26. Derksen W, Wismeijer D, Hanssen S, Tahmaseb S. Dental technician of the future. Forum Implantologicum 2015;11(1):12-20.

27. Bohner L et al. Accuracy of digital technologies for the scanning of facial, skeletal, and intraoral tissues: A systematic review. *J Prosthet Dent*. 2019;121(2):246-51.

28. Junying L et al. Creating a virtual patient for completely edentulous computer-aided implant surgery: A dental technique. *J Prosthet Dent*. 2021;125(4):564-8

29. Lepidi L et al. Digital fixed complete-arch rehabilitation: From virtual articulator mounting to clinical delivery. *J Prosthet Dent*.

30. Granata S et al. Incorporating a facial scanner into the digital workflow: A dental technique. *J Prosthet Dent*. 2020;123(6):781-5.

31. Papaspyridakos P, Gallucci GO, Chen CJ et al. Digital versus conventional implant impressions for edentulous patients: accuracy outcomes. *Clin Oral Impl Res*. 2016;27:465-72.

32. Lepidi L, Galli M, Mastrangelo F et al. Virtual articulators and virtual mounting procedures: where do we stand? *J Prosthodont*. 2020;1-12.

33. Solaberrieta E, Otegi JR, Goicoechea N et al. Comparison of a conventional and virtual occlusal record. *J Prosthet Dent*. 2015;114:92-7.

34. Edher F, Hannam AG, Tobias DL et al. The accuracy of virtual interocclusal registration during intraoral scanning. *J Prosthet Dent*. 2018;120:904-12.

35. Solaberrieta E, Garmendia A, Brizuela A et al. Intraoral digital impressions for virtual occlusal records: section quantity and dimensions. *Biomed Res Int*. 2016;2016:7173824.

36. Ahlholm P, Sipila K, Vallittu P et al. Digital versus conventional impressions in fixed prosthodontics: a review. *J Prosthodont*. 2018;27:35-41.

37. Seo JM, Oh WS, Lee JJ. A technique for verifying the accuracy of the virtual mounting of digital scans against the actual occlusal contacts. *J Prosthet Dent*. 2019;121:729-32.

38. Hsu MR, Driscoll CF, Romberg E et al. Accuracy of dynamic virtual articulation: trueness and precision. *J Prosthodont*. 2019;28:436-43.

39. Yee SHX, Esguerra RJ, Chew AAQ et al: Three-dimensional static articulation accuracy of virtual models – Part I: system trueness and precision. *J Prosthodont*. 2018;27:129-36.

40. Yee SHX, Esguerra RJ, Chew AAQ et al: Three-dimensional static articulation accuracy of virtual models-part II: effect of model scanner-CAD systems and articulation method. *J Prosthodont*. 2018;27:137-44.

41. Radu M, Radu D, Abboud M. Digital recording of a conventionally determined centric relation: a technique using an intraoral scanner. *J Prosthet Dent*. 2020;123(2):228-31.

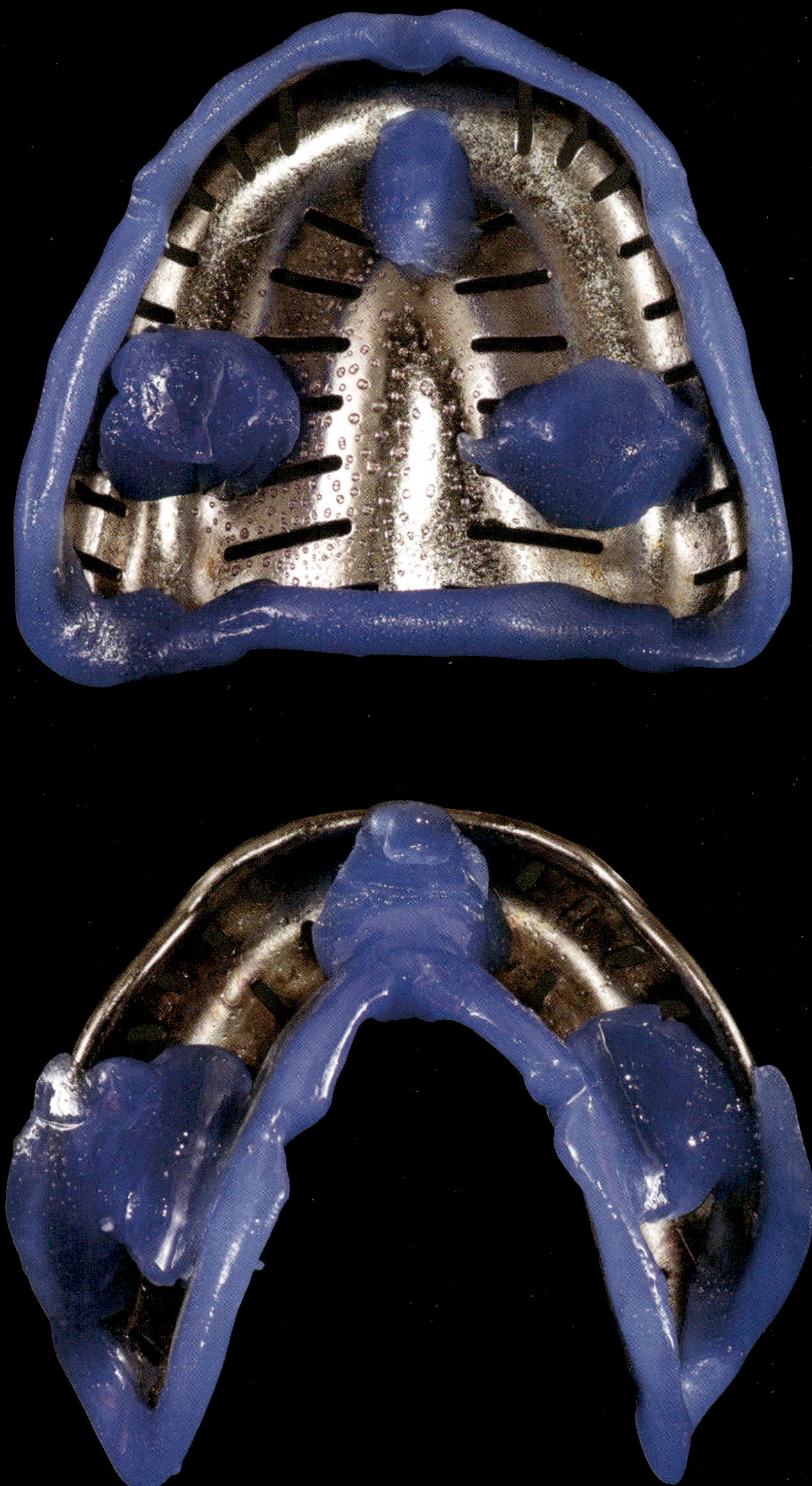

CHAPTER 4

A. CASUCCI, A. IELASI

The complete prosthesis with analogue protocol

Preliminary analysis

A careful analysis of the patient is required in order to be able to properly carry out all the following steps.

During the first visit it is essential to establish what the patient's real rehabilitation needs are, in order to choose the best solution corresponding to their needs, whether it is a new prosthetic reconstruction or any re-adaptation of the existing one. In the stage prior to the treatment, the clinician must evaluate the deficient aspects of the patient's rehabilitation and try to understand what changes must be made in order to improve their oral condition and the resulting quality of life [1,2].

In the event that the history factors are negative and the prognosis of any rehabilitation with full prosthesis is poor, one should clarify with the patient what the actual treatment options are and in the event that these do not meet their requests, schedule a different one, most likely using implants [2]. This section illustrates all the clinical and laboratory steps with the aim of rehabilitating a patient with full prosthesis, following a purely analogue protocol.

In the full prosthetic rehabilitation it can be underlined how the possibility of simplifying the patient's rehabilitation pathway is by now a well documented procedure in the literature and indicated in many cases [3].

Specifically, in setting up the rehabilitation process, the dentistry clinician must take into account the specific needs of older patients, who do not always have the possibility of reaching the office independently or may have particular general medical conditions that hinder the possibility to operate. Under these circumstances, pathways that include the use of replicas of the old prostheses or the closed mouth impression technique can be especially suitable [3-5].

Esthetic and phonetic assessments

A proper esthetic and phonetic analysis of the patient with the existing prostheses allows the clinician to obtain a lot of useful information for the future rehabilitation. These data must be documented with photos and videos of the patient during the dynamic phase, at rest and maximum display. Front, side and three-quarter view images of the patient's face are acquired, which can be shared with both the patient and the laboratory during the rehabilitation process [2] **(Figure 4.1)**.

The esthetics must assess multiple aspects of the teeth, such as: length, display at rest and when smiling, medial-distal dimensions of the anterior ones and their position in relation to the lip support. The general principles of bio-esthetics may be applied [2,6]. In this stage, phonetic criteria can help understand whether the position of the teeth and the vertical occlusion dimension (OVD) are correct.

Normally, the OVD is approximately 2-4 mm smaller than the resting vertical dimension (RVD). Establishing the exact OVD in an edentulous patient is a challenge for the clinician. One of the essential principles to bear in mind is that when producing sounds, neither the natural teeth nor the ones on dental prostheses must occlude. This space between the arches is referred to as "closest speaking space" [7-9] **(Figure 4.2)**.

From a clinical point of view, one might find that there is no closest speaking space in the patient's existing rehabilitations. In this case, the patient's comfort will be impaired, as during phonation the teeth often come into contact and swallowing requires considerable effort. This parameter indicates the need to reduce the OVD.

In the event that the patient has been using a total prosthesis for some time, it is common to find an increased freeway space (FWS) (greater than 4-5 mm), the possible causes for this are to be found in the construction of the prosthesis with reduced OVD, but often they are due to the wear of the dental surfaces or resorption of the residual bone crests.

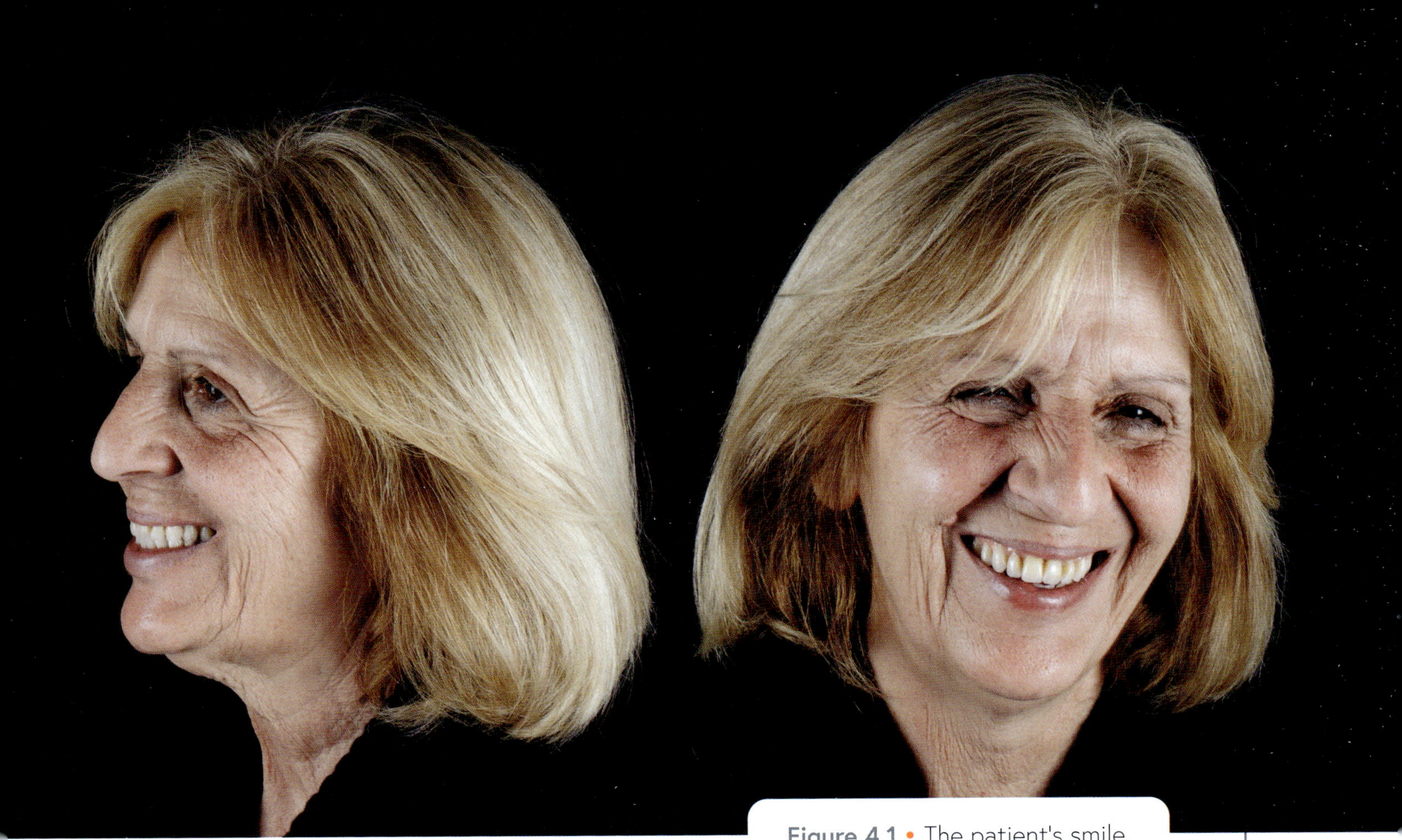

Figure 4.1 • The patient's smile.

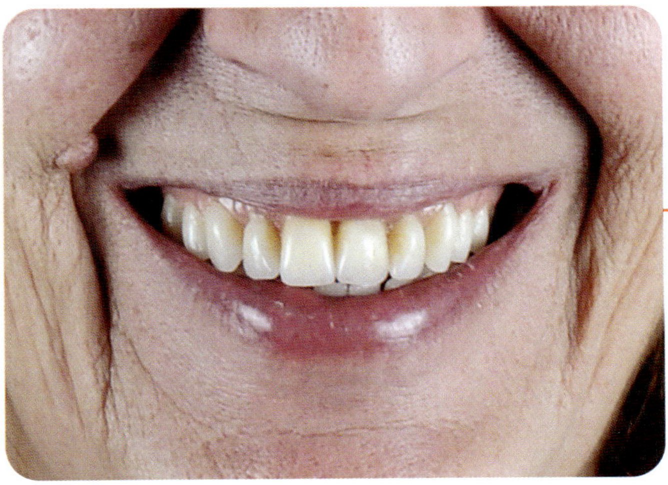

In any case, there is a considerable range between the arches when switching from the rest position to that of occlusion, which is also reflected in a change in the support at the level of the lower third of the face. A smaller OVD will cause problems when chewing and speaking due to the small space for the tongue; all the conditions listed above point to the need to raise the OVD [9,10].

The acquisition of photographs and videos of the patient during the dynamic phases of phonation and the analysis of dental exposure at rest and the minimum and maximum display while smiling are essential for a proper esthetic assessment.

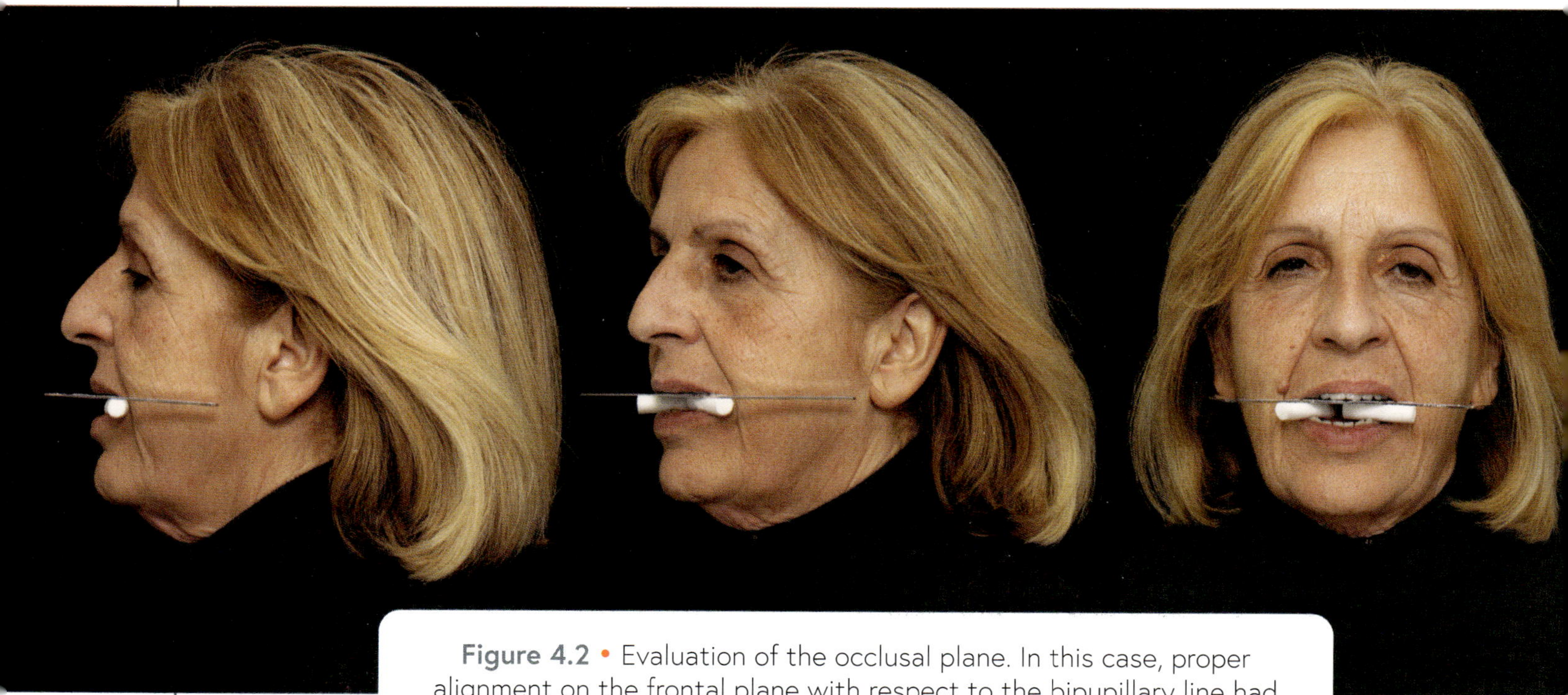

Figure 4.2 • Evaluation of the occlusal plane. In this case, proper alignment on the frontal plane with respect to the bipupillary line had been verified, while on the sagittal plane the correspondence with respect to the Camper's plane both on the right and left was poor.

A Fox plane is used to assess the occlusal plane by placing it between the patient's arches and using cotton rolls to stabilise it.

Another factor to be considered is the occlusal plane, in fact, it has been reported how it is significant in order to be able to manage occlusal loads. For this assessment, just use a Fox plane, placing it between the patient's arches and using cotton rolls to stabilise it as shown in the clinical case described in this chapter. The ideal occlusal plane should have an orientation on the frontal plane parallel to the bipupillary line, or in the case it is not orthogonal to the midline of the face, bring the incisal margins of the upper teeth back in

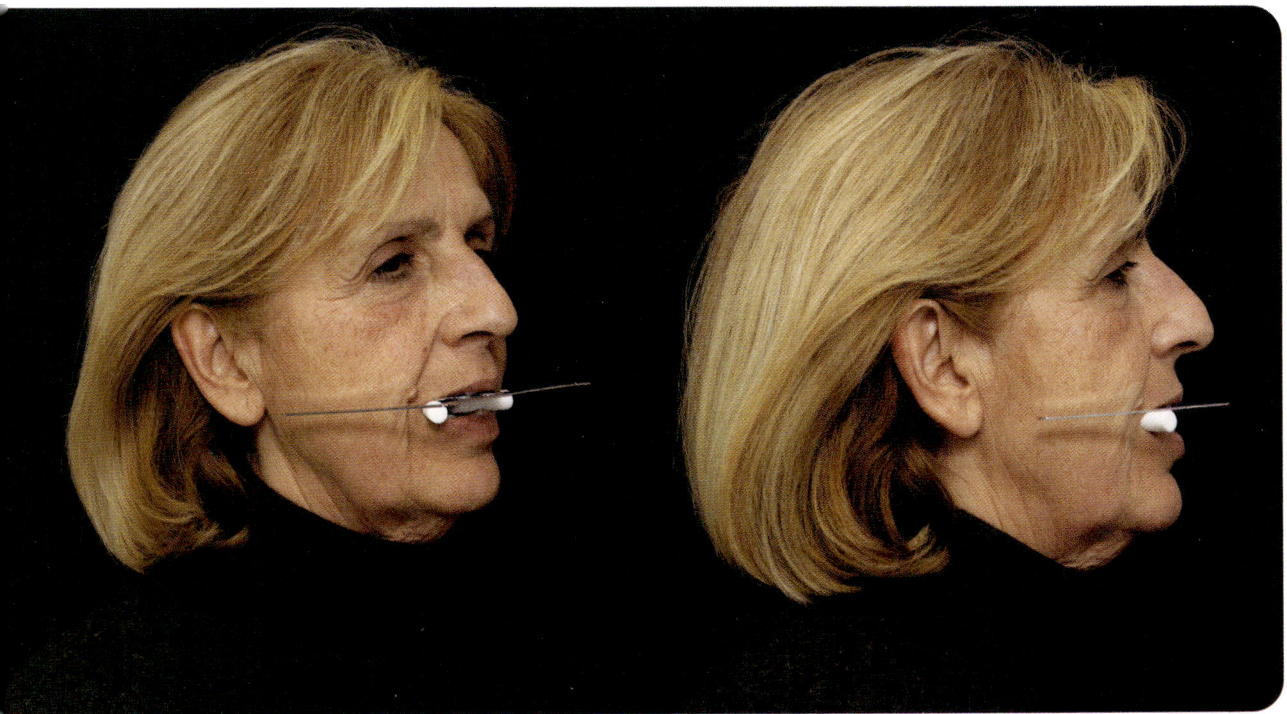

harmony with the lower lip and the corners of the mouth. On the sagittal aspect, the occlusal plane should be parallel to Camper's plane, considered as the line running between the root of the nose ala and the middle of the tragus. This plane is often taken as a reference for the fabrication of the full prosthesis, as it is believed to be the one closest to the occlusal plane in the dentate patient and is the one closest among those used to the residual bone structures (palatal vault and residual alveolar ridges) [1,11,12] **(Figure 4.2)**.

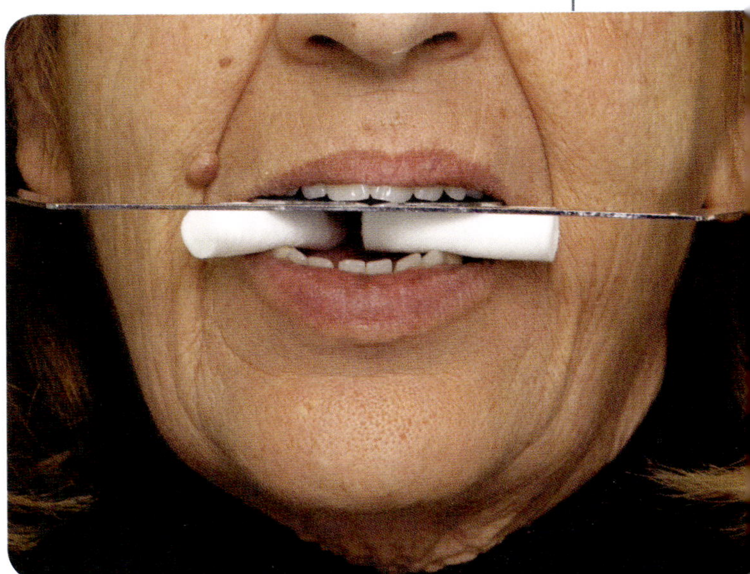

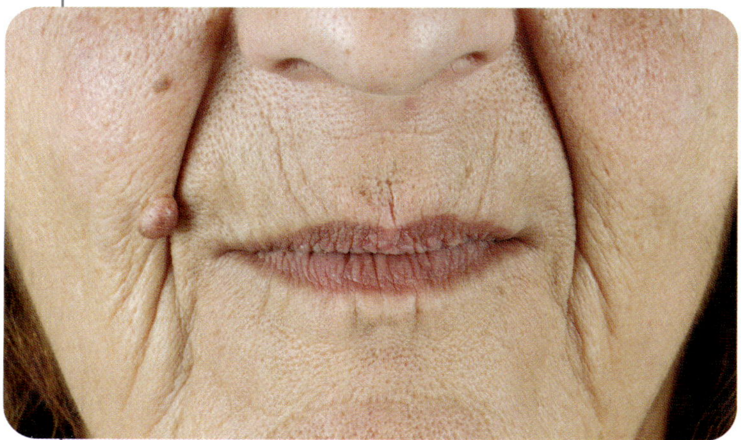

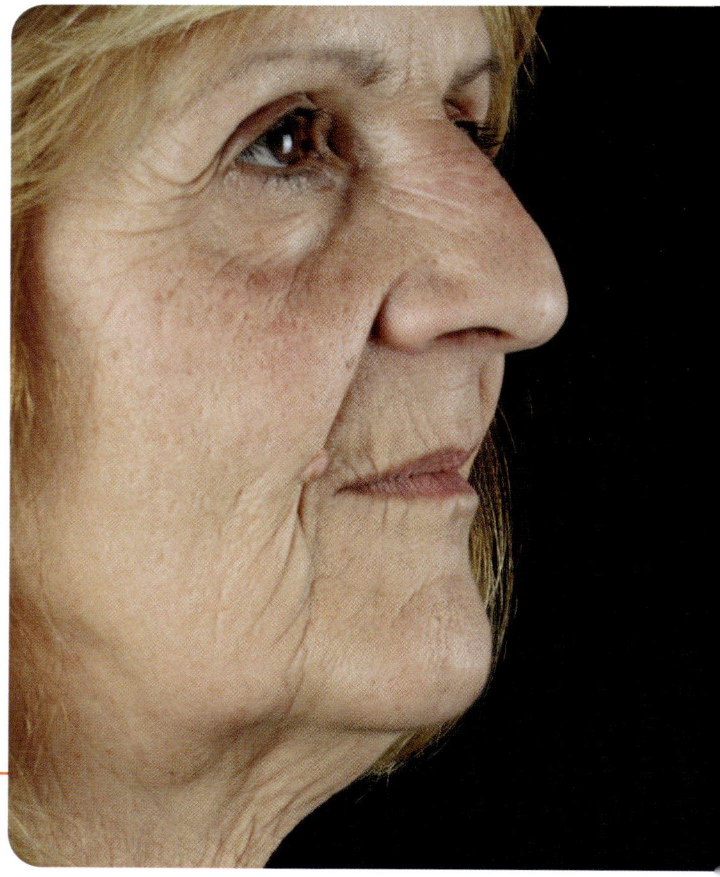

Figure 4.3 • Evaluation of the lower third of the face without prosthesis.
Front and side view.

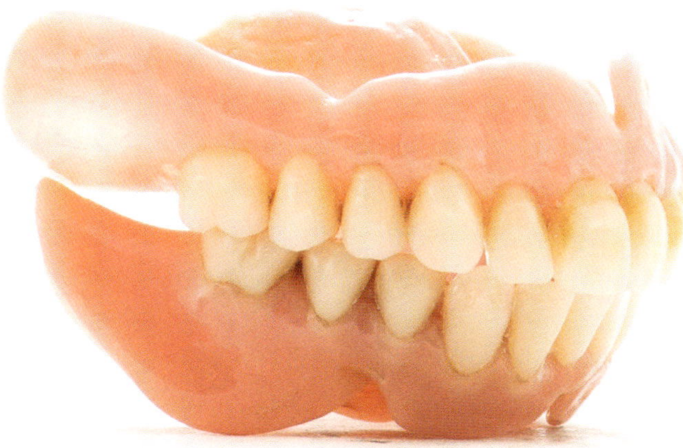

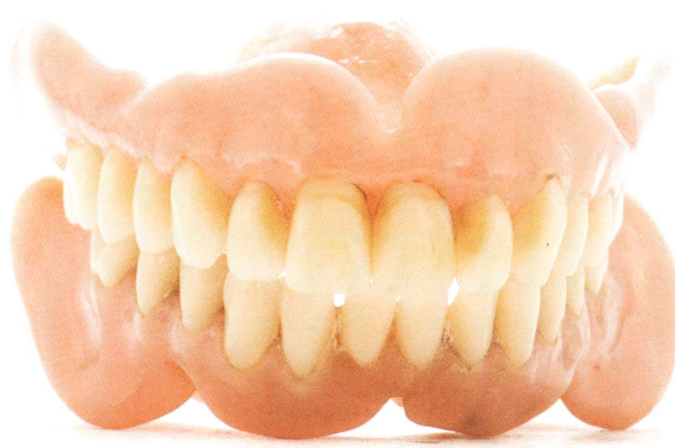

An interesting estimate can be carried out of the impact of losing teeth and their supporting tissues on the perioral soft tissues. This can be done simply by evaluating the patient after removing the prostheses from the oral cavity [13] **(Figure 4.3)**.

Assessment of the existing prostheses

The evaluation of the patient's prostheses can make it possible to collect a lot of data before the treatment and to establish whether the discomfort reported by the patient can be related to issues to do with prosthesis construction [14,15] **(Figure 4.4)**.

Figure 4.4 • Pre-existing prostheses.

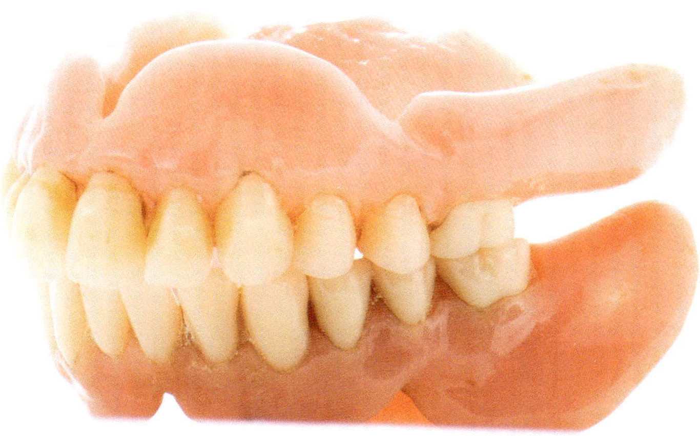

The degree of atrophy and relevant loss of perioral tissue support can be evaluated by removing the prosthesis from the oral cavity.

To begin with, the position of the teeth with respect to the loading areas must be checked. This assessment is based on checking the prosthesis stability when it is loaded on one side. This test, also known as static stability, requires the clinician to exert considerable force on the back teeth on one side, while on the other, by moving the cheek away from the prosthesis, he/she tries to break the peripheral seal so that the prosthesis retention, if any, does not alter the stability assessment. This empirical assessment can highlight a rotating motion of the prosthesis with a dislodgement, which is especially risky for the patient at the beginning of chewing, that is, when the bolus is hard [14] **(Figure 4.5)**.

After checking the behaviour of the prosthesis under load, its fit to the underlying tissues and the length of the edges are also analysed. This step can be carried out with low viscosity silicone paste, which is placed on the entire support base. The prosthe-

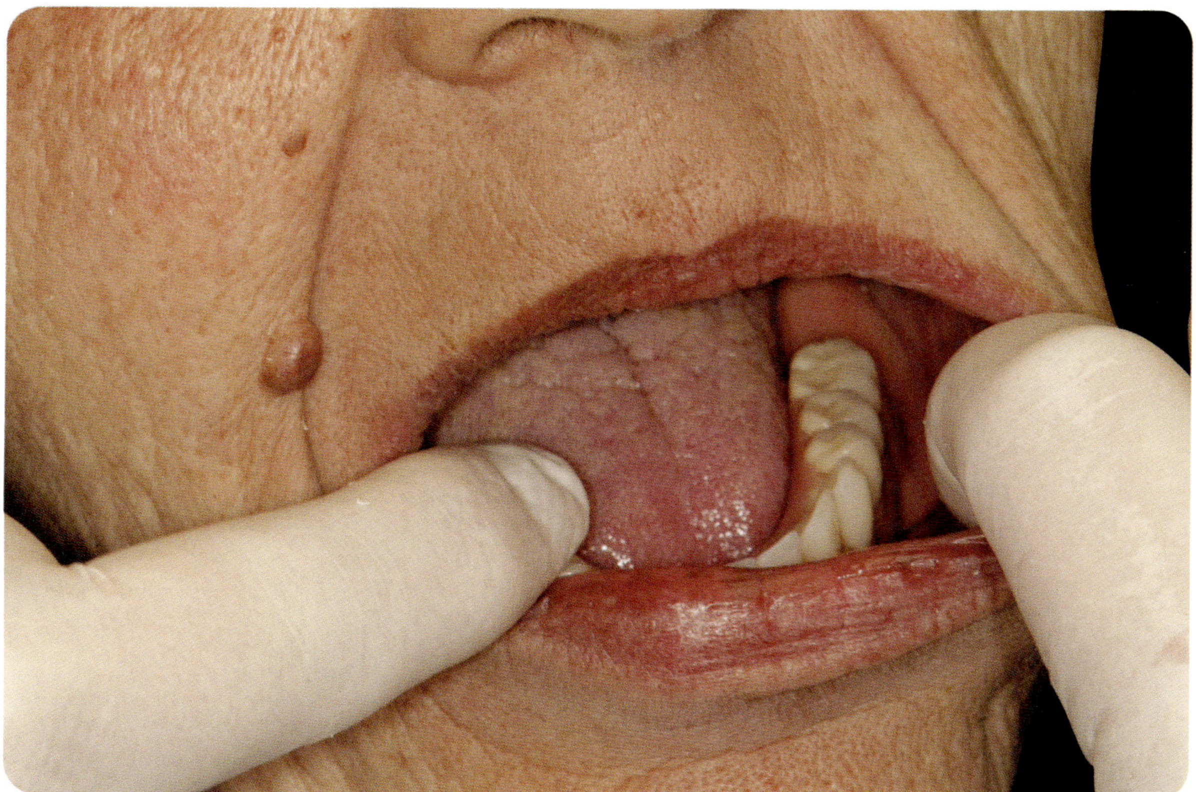

sis must be placed in the oral cavity and the clinician must apply considerable pressure towards the supporting tissues or as an alternative, use cotton rolls to achieve the same result. Both methods make it therefore possible, ruling out the variable related to the occlusion of the existing prostheses, to only assess the fit of the bases regardless of the thrust that the prosthetic plates receive from the occlusal contacts. Furthermore, the patient must be instructed to perform some functional movements with the tongue, cheeks and lips and will be asked to swallow [13,16,17].

In addition to the silicone paste it is possible to use touch, by feeling the patient's cheek from the outside to try and perceive any over-extensions. It is likely, in fact, that by running the pointer finger over the area of the buccal shelf it can be perceived from the outside, if the prosthesis accesses significantly from the external oblique line **(Figure 4.6)**.

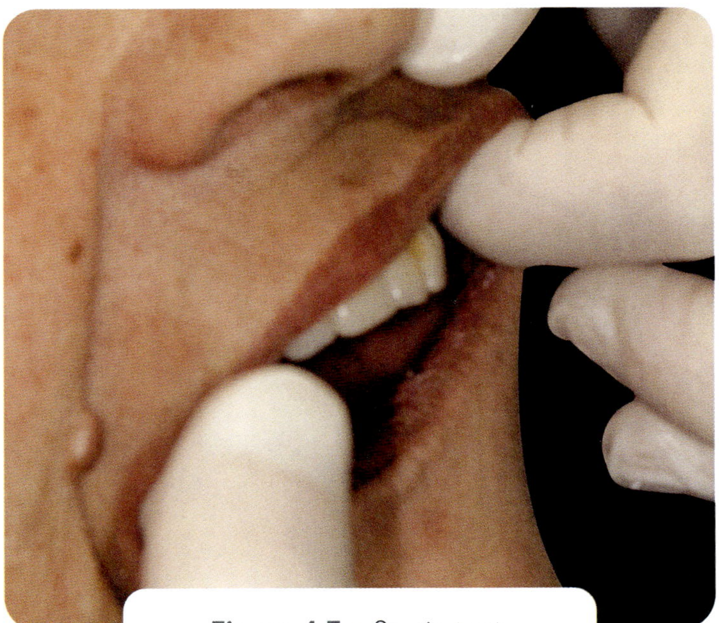

Figure 4.5 • Static test.

Obviously, in case of over-extension the prosthesis might be dislodged by the musculature during functional movements or while opening [17].

Furthermore, the prosthesis can provide the clinician with important information on the patient's occlusion by assessing the occlusal tables, their level of wear and the existing contacts, or simply provide a starting OVD. In some cases, especially when the patient has got used to the prosthesis for some time, a sudden change in these parameters can reduce the possibility of adapting to the new one, especially in the early stages after fitting it [15,18].

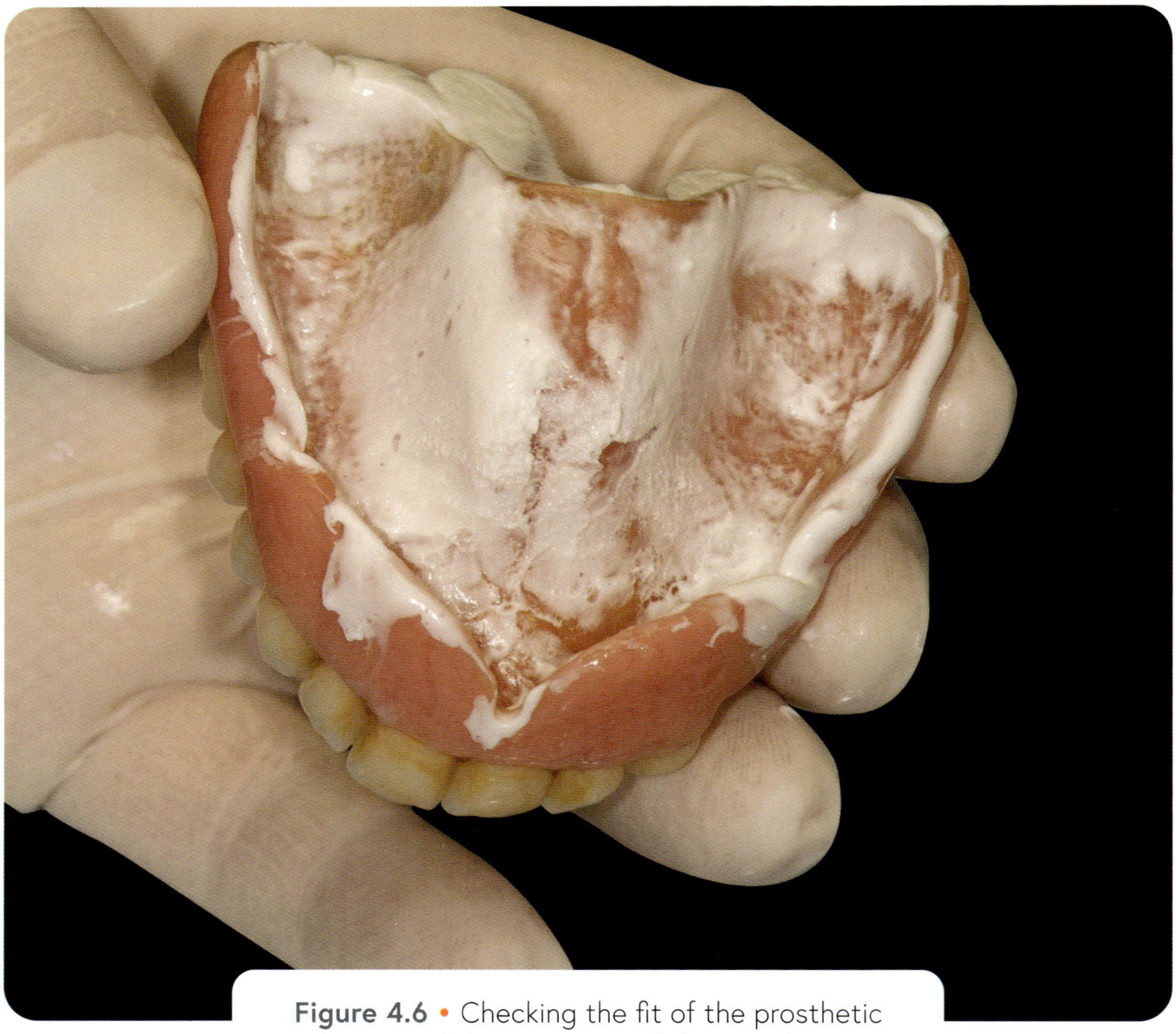

Figure 4.6 • Checking the fit of the prosthetic bases and the extension of the prosthesis.

Intraoral assessments

In addition to adapting perfectly to the supporting tissues, a primary goal of the prosthesis is not to interfere with the musculature and with the movements of the frenula. That is why it is very important to define the design of the prosthesis at the level of the edge as well as on the surfaces of the prosthetic body that connect it to the teeth. In this regard, one often speaks of certain rules that make it possible not to violate the vital space of the tongue during swallowing or phonation. The study of the neutral zone can be used to register this space, which will be described below in this chapter [2,19,20].

Before removing the prostheses from the oral cavity, it may be useful to assess centric relation stability and repeatability. It is in fact essential for the proper functioning of the prosthesis to have a centric relation with the aforementioned features, which allows the base of the prosthesis to adapt perfectly to the tissues. Therefore, thanks to the mediation by the salivary film, the adhesion and cohesion forces that result in retention are obtained [10,21,22].

Once all these parameters have been evaluated, it is possible to have important information for the prognosis of the future prosthesis, also from the analysis of the residual

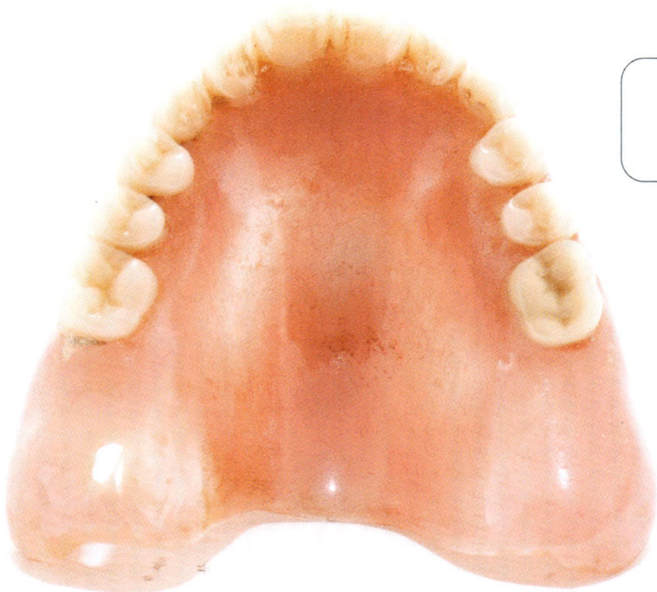

Figure 4.7 • Presence of a hole on the prosthetic base.

alveolar ridges, the quality of the mucosa, the muscle insertions present and the quality of saliva.

Clinical success with a full prosthesis depends on many factors such as: the possibility of the patient to manage the prosthetic item thanks to good neuromuscular control, their attitude towards the prosthesis and the relationship they establish with the dentist.

Although the literature reports conflicting opinions, one of the main factors to be assessed is undoubtedly related to the anatomical analysis of the residual structures.

When the residual bone structures are well represented, execution of the prosthesis is favourable. However, as in the case presented, in the case of marked undercuts it is an aspect that can make it complicated to obtain a good all-round seal and have enough space for positioning the posterior teeth, or at the same time it might significantly reduce the thickness of the prosthesis [10,23,24]. As shown in **Figure 4.7**, the issue related to the inter-arch prosthetic space is also evidenced by the small thickness of the prosthesis and by the hole on the base.

Maxilla

The primary support structures for the upper arch are the residual alveolar ridge and the hard palate. These areas withstand the functional load of the upper prosthesis.

There are two main areas that cause the upper prosthesis to be retained: (1) the area of the anterior and lateral vestibule in the portion that extends over the muco-gingival line by approximately 2-4 mm, extending into its depth; (2) the posterior seal area also referred to as post-dam on the surface of the prosthesis. Both these areas can be compressed hence create the negative pressure required to assure hold of the prosthesis during function. Obviously, if the support area of the prosthesis is too long, there is the possibility that the patient's muscles, during some functional movements such as swallowing, may dislodge the prosthesis. In the opposite case, that is, when the support base fails to extend to the areas that can be compressed, retention might be very poor.

There are also areas where the functional load must be low, for example, in the event that the interincisal papilla is compressed due to an overload of the prosthesis base, the patient may frequently experience pain or allodynia. Finally, areas where the mucosa is mobile must be discharged. This condition is especially evident in the case of high resorption and chronic inflammatory processes. A fitting example is the presence of mobile tissues often found in the anterior region or in the region of the tuberosities such as palatine rugae and raphe. In fact, their compression during registration of the final impression might cause a defect in the fit of the prosthesis or even a fulcrum point for its rotation. As regards the proper design of the posterior limit of the prosthesis, there has been a succession of techniques over time. The palatine fovea are often used as reference to establish the limit line, however, as they are small depressions due to the confluence of the ancillary salivary gland ducts, these structures have a variable position. Ideally, the upper prosthesis should extend beyond the limit of the hard palate to reach the transition zone with the soft palate.

Therefore, two lines can be identified in this area. The posterior one is identified as the vibrating line, is located at the distal limit of the palate area where movement of the soft palate begins and is the point where compressibility is maximum. The second is the anterior line, where tissue resilience becomes minimal as it is closer to the hard palate. With regard to extension, in the anterior vestibule area the upper prosthesis should normally be under-extended by about 3-4 mm with respect to the maximum fornix depth; this has the aim of promoting its mobility, which is linked to activation of the orbicular, zygomatic, buccinator and risorius muscles. In the area that covers the lateral vestibule comprised from the lateral frenulum up to the hamular notch, the prosthesis can reach up to 2 mm from the fornix depth. This is possible because the buccinator muscle in that area inserts in the area of the zygomatic process of the upper jaw. Its fibres continue posteriorly, inserting onto the pterygomandibular raphe and on the external oblique line of the mandible, and from there, flowing in an anterior direction, they flow into the orbicularis muscle.

The lateral area of the labial vestibule is affected by the maxillary zygomatic process; this area is covered with very thin mucosa and has a very low tolerance to loads, in fact in case of hyperextension of the edge it can easily be subject to injuries and cause pain.

Proceeding distal to the area of the zygomatic crest, the prosthesis can be deepened in the retrozygomatic space to then reach the area of insertion of the pterygomandibular raphe, which is referred to as hamular notch. Thanks to its considerable resilience it can be used to improve the posterior seal of the prosthesis, however, excessive pressure or length of the prosthesis in this area may cause pain and ulceration to the patient **(Figure 4.8)**.

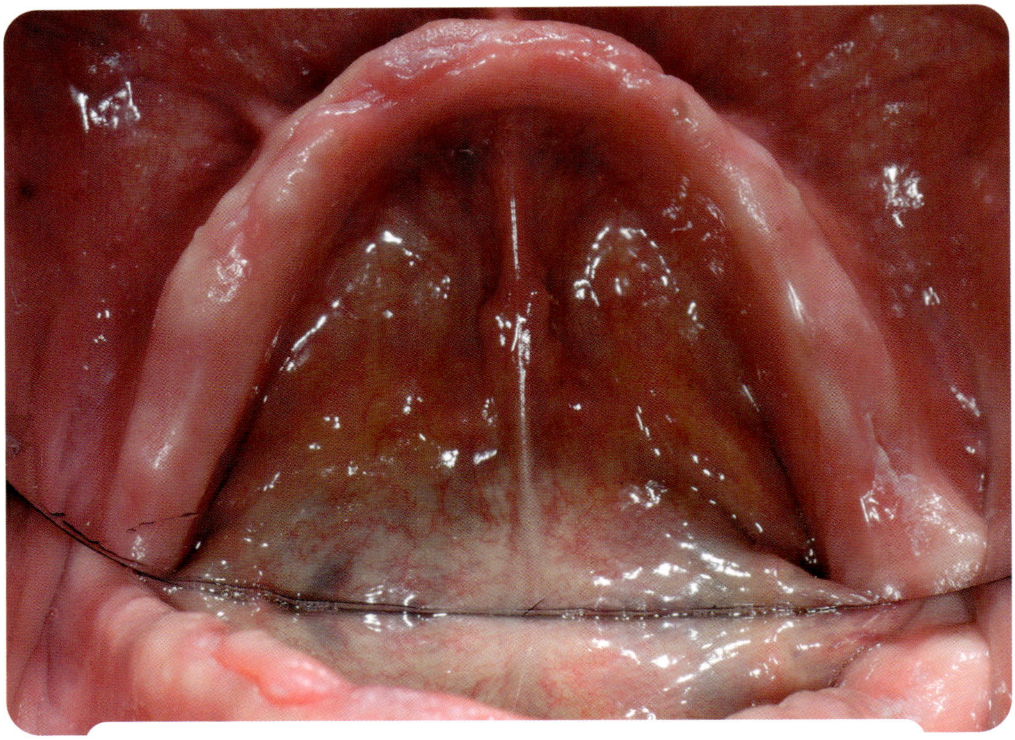

Figure 4.8 • Intraoral view. The crests show low resorption, there are also considerable undercuts in the retrozygomatic space and in the anterior areas of the fornix both above and below.

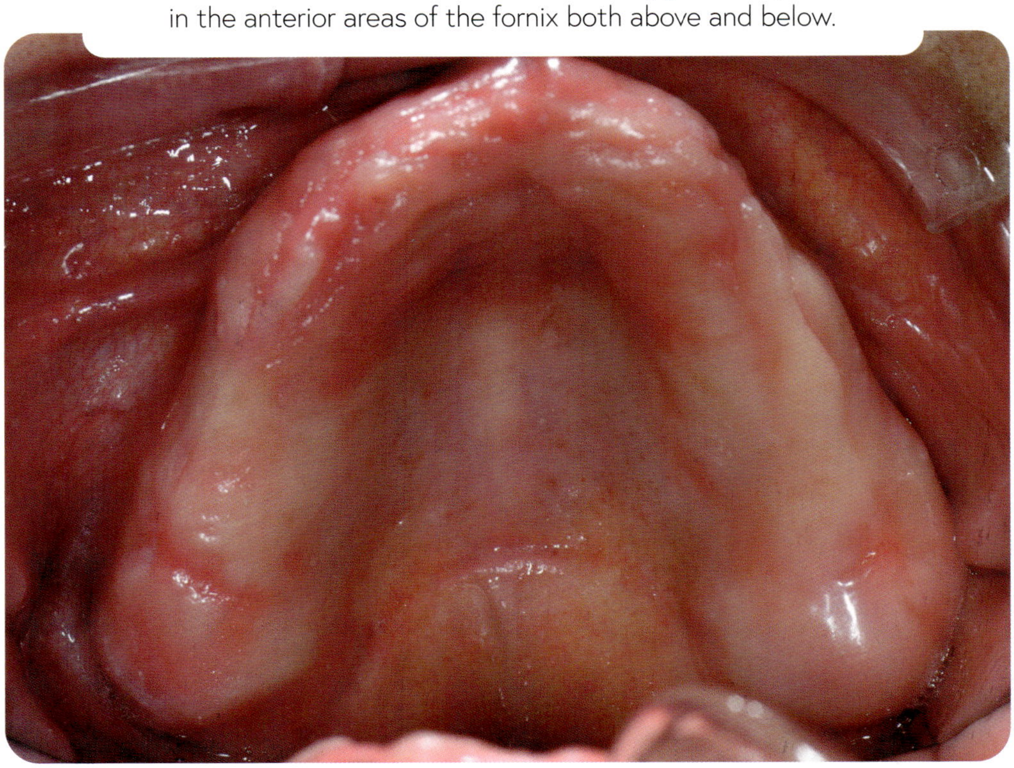

Mandible

The main areas of load resistance of the lower arch are the residual alveolar ridge and the buccal shelf. In the most unfavourable cases, the residual alveolar ridge is both short and narrow; in this condition the amount of keratinised tissue is also often reduced, which is essential for the management of the masticatory loads from the prosthetic base. In fact, the keratinised attached mucosa is able to absorb the forces thanks to the fibrous layer underlying the mucosa.

As regards the limits of the prosthesis, it ought to be considered that, in the anterior area, it cannot extend up to the maximum depth of the fornix, due to the activity of the orbicularis oris muscle and of the depressor labii and of the mentalis which tend to reduce its width and depth.

The buccal shelf is bounded medially by the residual crest, laterally by the external oblique line that corresponds to the insertion of the buccinator muscle and, distally, by a concave line called the masseteric notch that joins the posterior part of the external oblique line with the retromolar trigone and ensures the absence of displacement forces towards the prosthesis, which can however develop when the masseter reaches its maximum contraction. The masseter, in fact, during isometric contraction increases in volume and pushes the buccinator muscle medially and anteriorly. The retromolar trigone is a structure that contains a thick layer of fibrous connective tissue underneath the mucosa. At least half this area must be covered by the extension of the prosthesis, in order to promote the dissipation of loads.

The limits of the prosthesis on the lingual side are a crucial factor for its construction and retention. The anterior area of the lingual sulcus can be compressed, as the sublingual glands are underneath the mucous layer. It must be considered that in this area the genioglossus muscle inserts anteriorly on the genial tubercles or mental spines and can dislodge the prosthesis during its activation.

Proceeding distally towards the area between the first and second premolar, the prosthesis must ensure functional activity to the mylohyoid muscle. This area is defined by Passamonti [25] as "P notch", and is closely related to the insertion and course of the mylohyoid muscle fibres. It is inserted along the mylohyoid crest, which is located on the lingual side of the mandible. Near the region between the first and second premolar, the muscle fibres descend below the sublingual fossa, basically arranged vertically with respect to the previous arrangement.

Preliminary impression

The preliminary impression aims to record all the anatomical structures required for the fabrication of the individual impression tray; therefore, it is an over-extended and panoramic impression [26,27].

Choice of trade tray

In order for the impression material to be able to record all the areas of interest, a suitable impression tray must be chosen: it must be dimensionally stable, stiff and

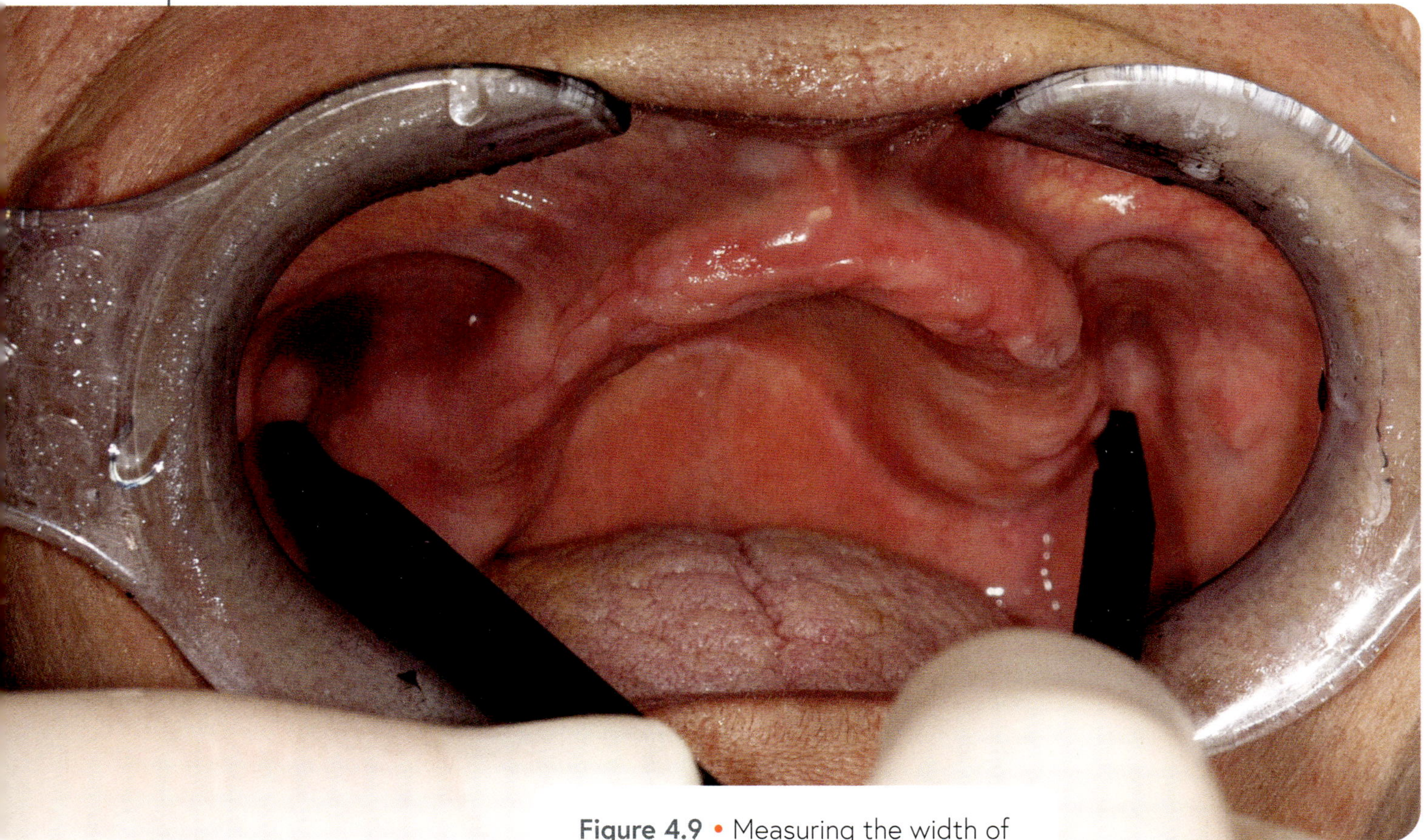

Figure 4.9 • Measuring the width of the upper and lower arch.

cover the entire extension of the arch above as well as below. To select it, you can use a compass placed on the upper arch in the retrozygomatic area in order to fully include the maxillary tuberosities. In the lower arch, the points of the compass must measure the distance between the retromolar trigones or the retromylohyoid areas. Normally, the chosen upper tray must be wider than the measured distance, the lower one must be narrower to allow the material to easily access the retrozygomatic area and sublingual sulcus, which extend from the sublingual to the mylohyoid area to end in the retromilohyoid area. The space required for the material is approximately 4-5 mm [1,27,28] **(Figure 4.9)**.

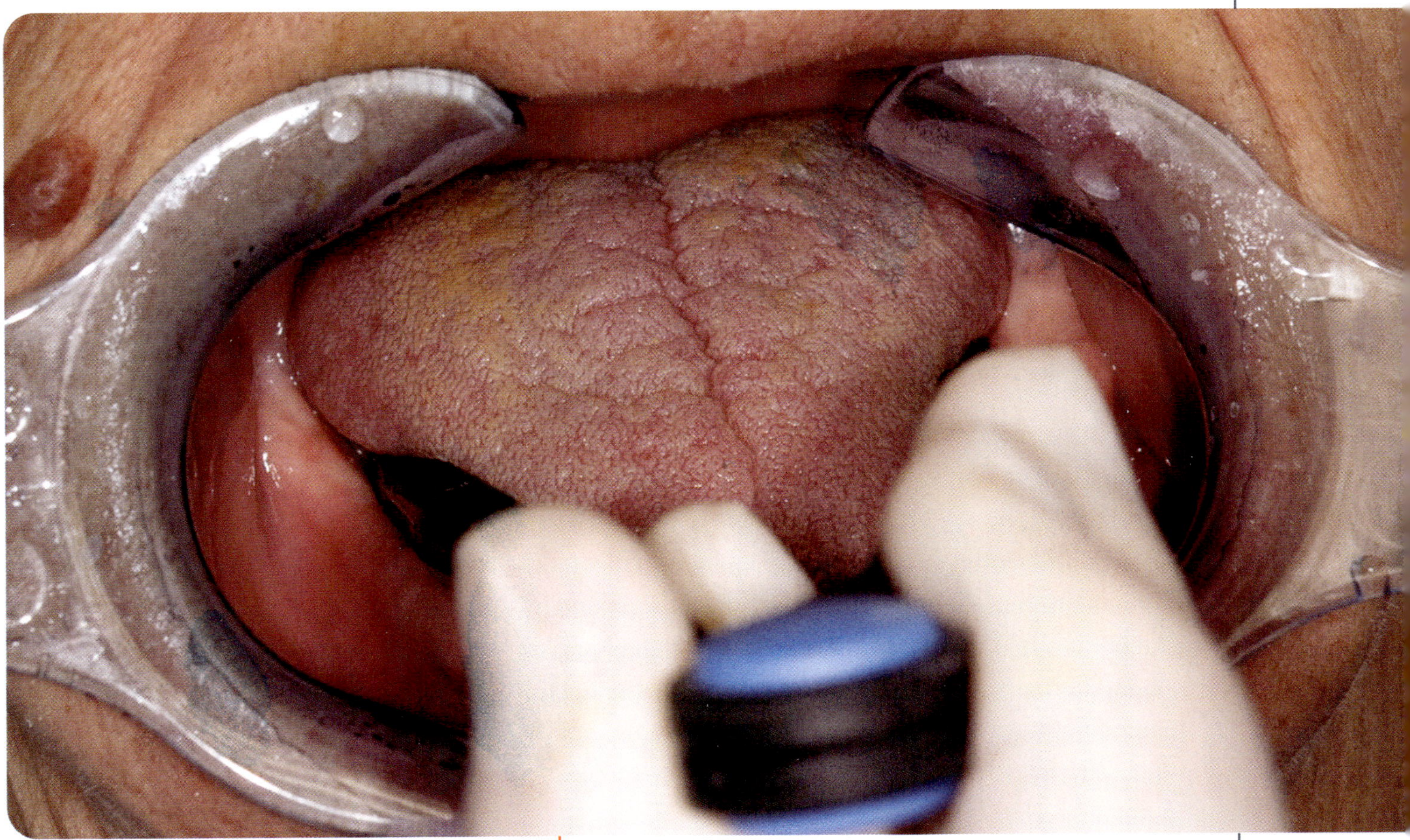

Trying the tray

Before performing registration of the impressions, it is necessary to try the tray in the oral cavity, to check whether it actually covers all the areas of interest and whether the size allows the material to be supported properly. In this stage, the clinician must ensure that the tray can be seated without discomfort for the patient and that the space required for the impression material is sufficient (**Figure 4.10**).

Figure 4.10 • Trying the tray in the oral cavity.

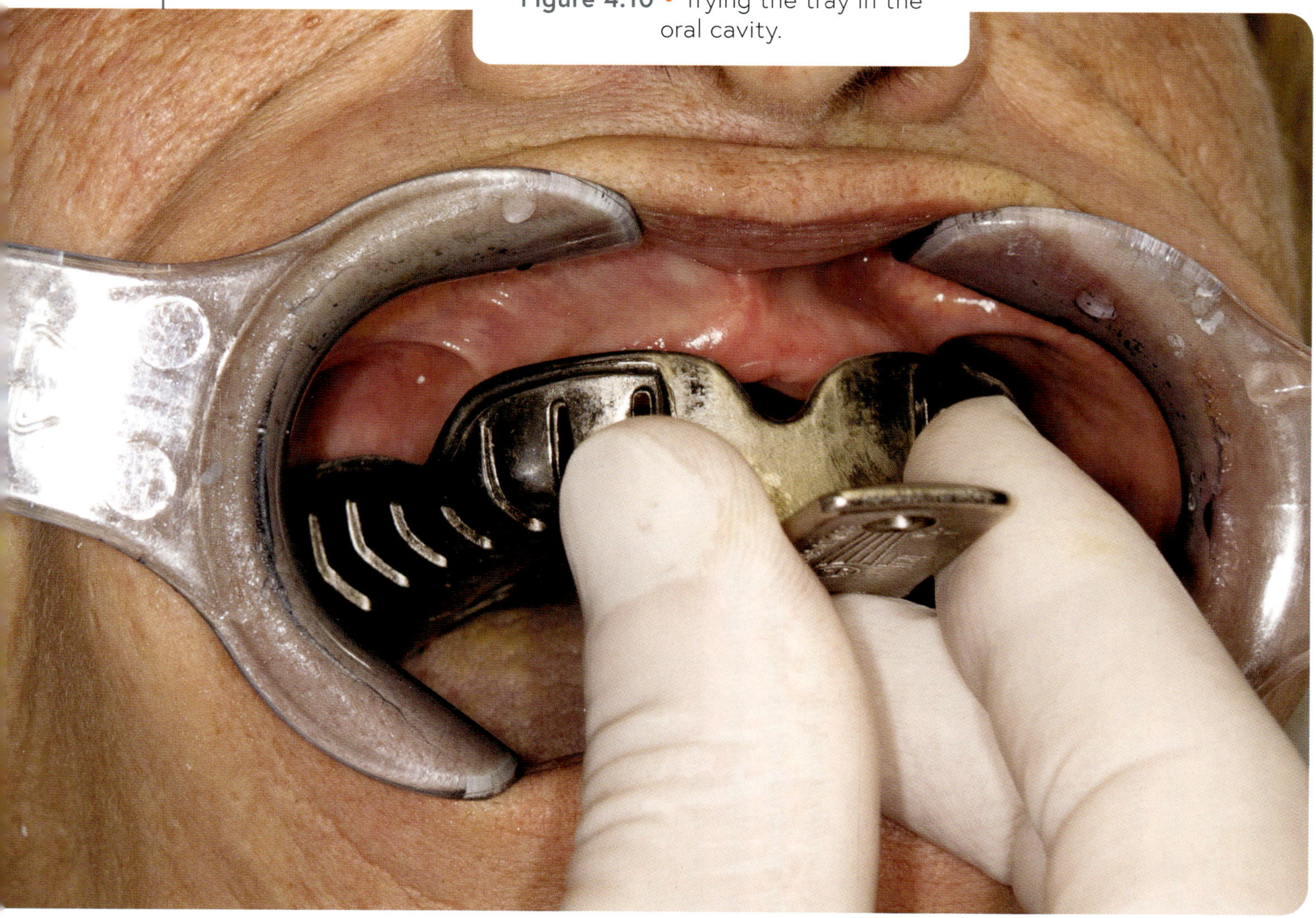

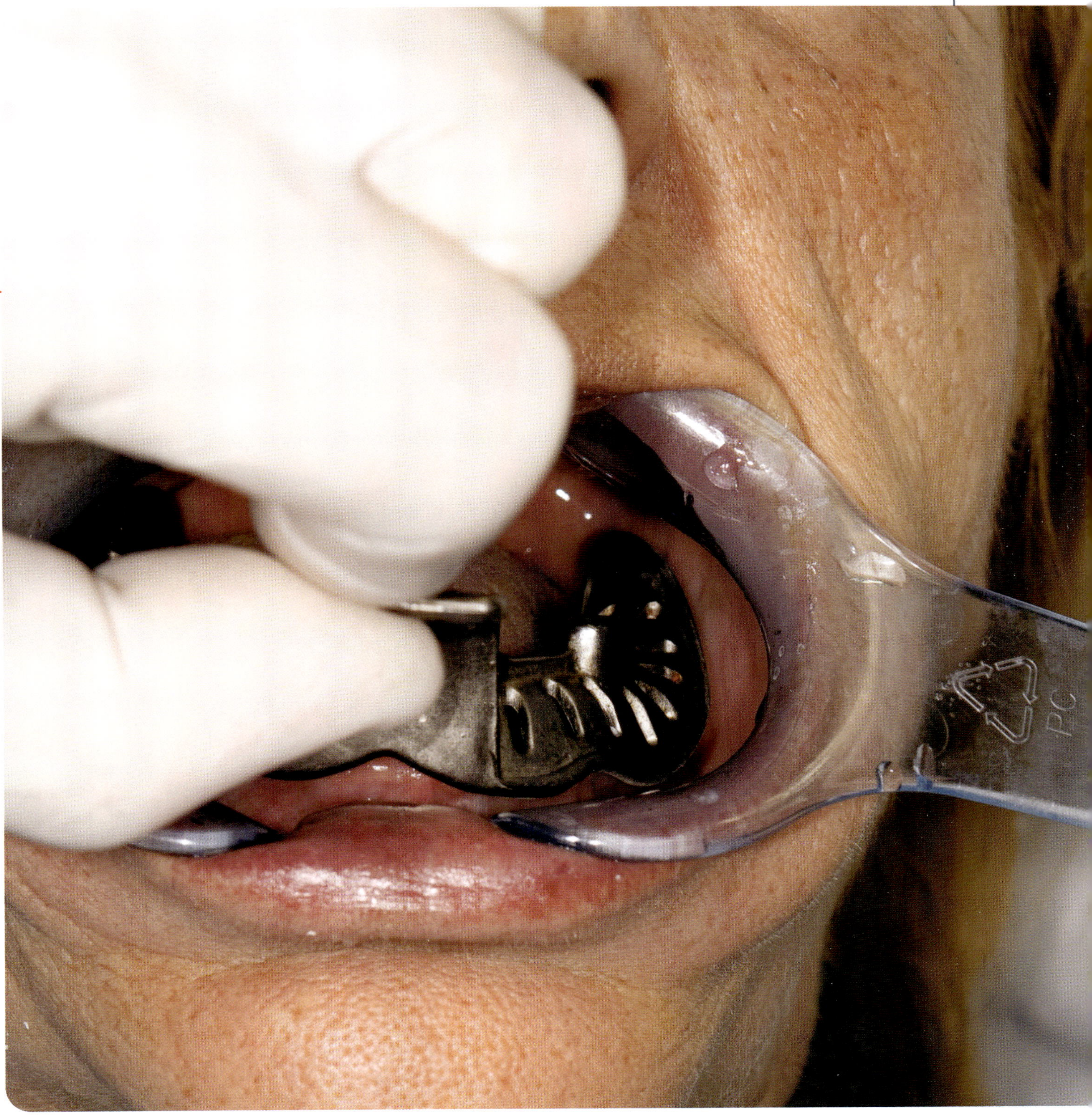
PC

The impression tray is then stabilised with soft wax. The impression trays on the market, although they can be set up for edentulous arches, as in the case presented, are almost never perfectly suited to the patient's anatomy due to the great anatomical variability of the residual alveolar ridges [27,29].

Stabilisation and customisation of the tray

Three small wax stops can be used to stabilise the impression tray, placed in the areas of the incisors and molars. It is useful to temper the wax in lukewarm water to achieve good stabilisation easily and quickly.

Once the impression tray has been stabilised, there is almost always the need to lengthen it on the edges with wax, since the stops prevent contact with the tissues. In this way, stabilisation of the tray as well as proper support for the material on the deeper areas of the fornix or the lingual sulcus are achieved.

The wax must be firmly anchored to the edge of the tray to ensure it remains stable during insertion and removal from the oral cavity. Always at the edge, it may be useful to set the course of the frenula, where present, or to increase the length of the impression tray with wax consistently in the sublingual area [27,30].

A final precaution before registering the preliminary impression is to apply adhesive on the surface of the prepared impression tray. This precaution ensures better adhesion of the impression material during removal of the impression from the oral cavity and in the steps required for building the model (**Figure 4.11**).

Stabilisation of the upper and lower impression tray performed with soft wax. They are then treated with a specific adhesive for the impression material that will be used during removal of the impression and in the subsequent stages.

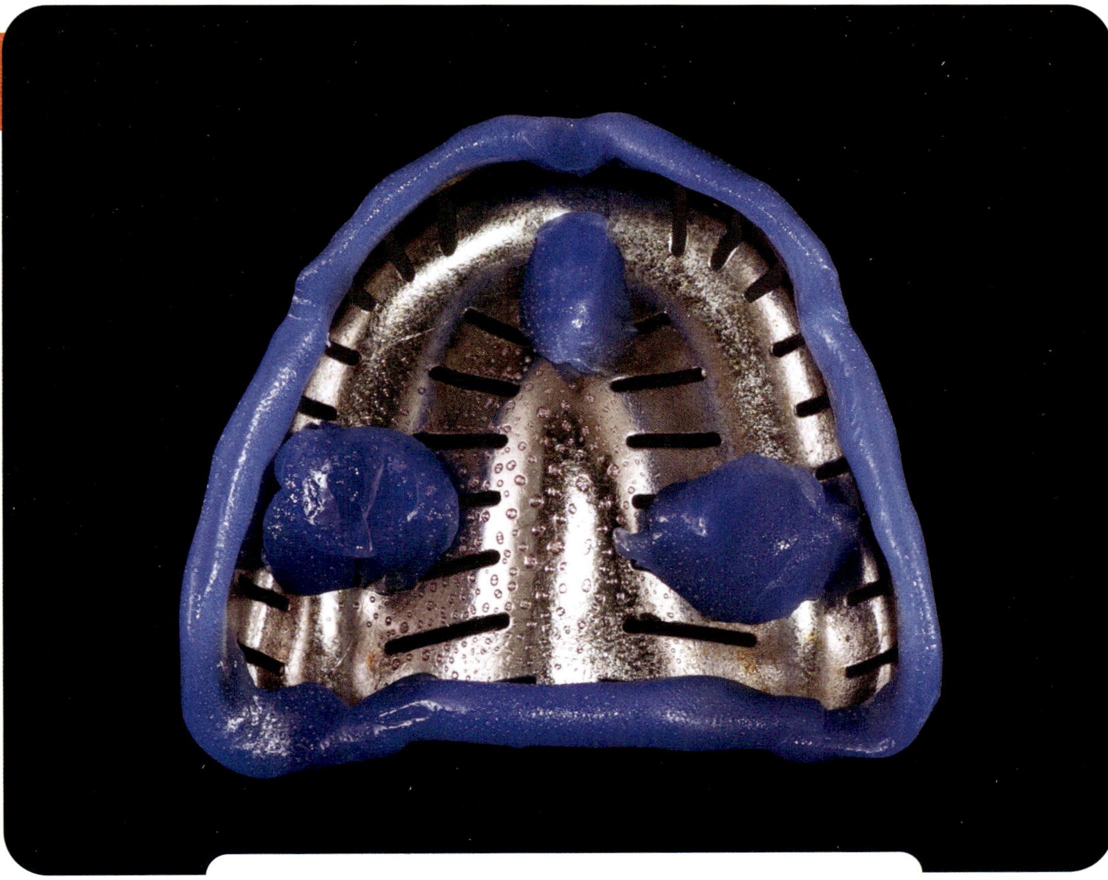

Figure 4.11 • Customising the tray with soft wax.

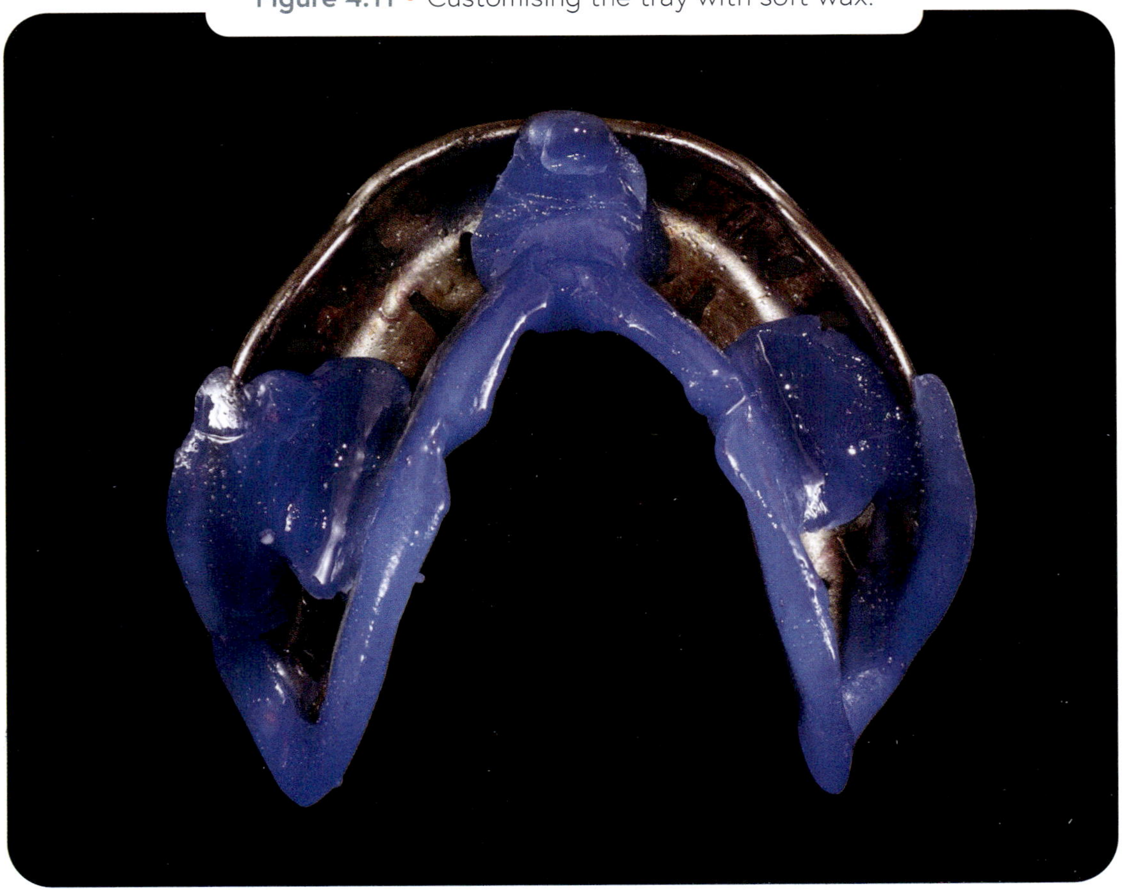

Registering the impression

Various materials can be used for the registration of the preliminary impression, such as alginate or high viscosity silicone. As regards alginates, the so-called *normal setting* ones are particularly useful, since they maintain an adequate working time despite being prepared with a mixture containing more powder than that normally recommended by the manufacturers [27].

The proportions used for the upper arch are normally three measuring cups of powder and just over two parts of water.

An even more viscous material is required in the lower arch, in order to properly register the deeper areas of the lingual sulcus without the risk of it being displaced

Figure 4.12 • Preliminary impression.

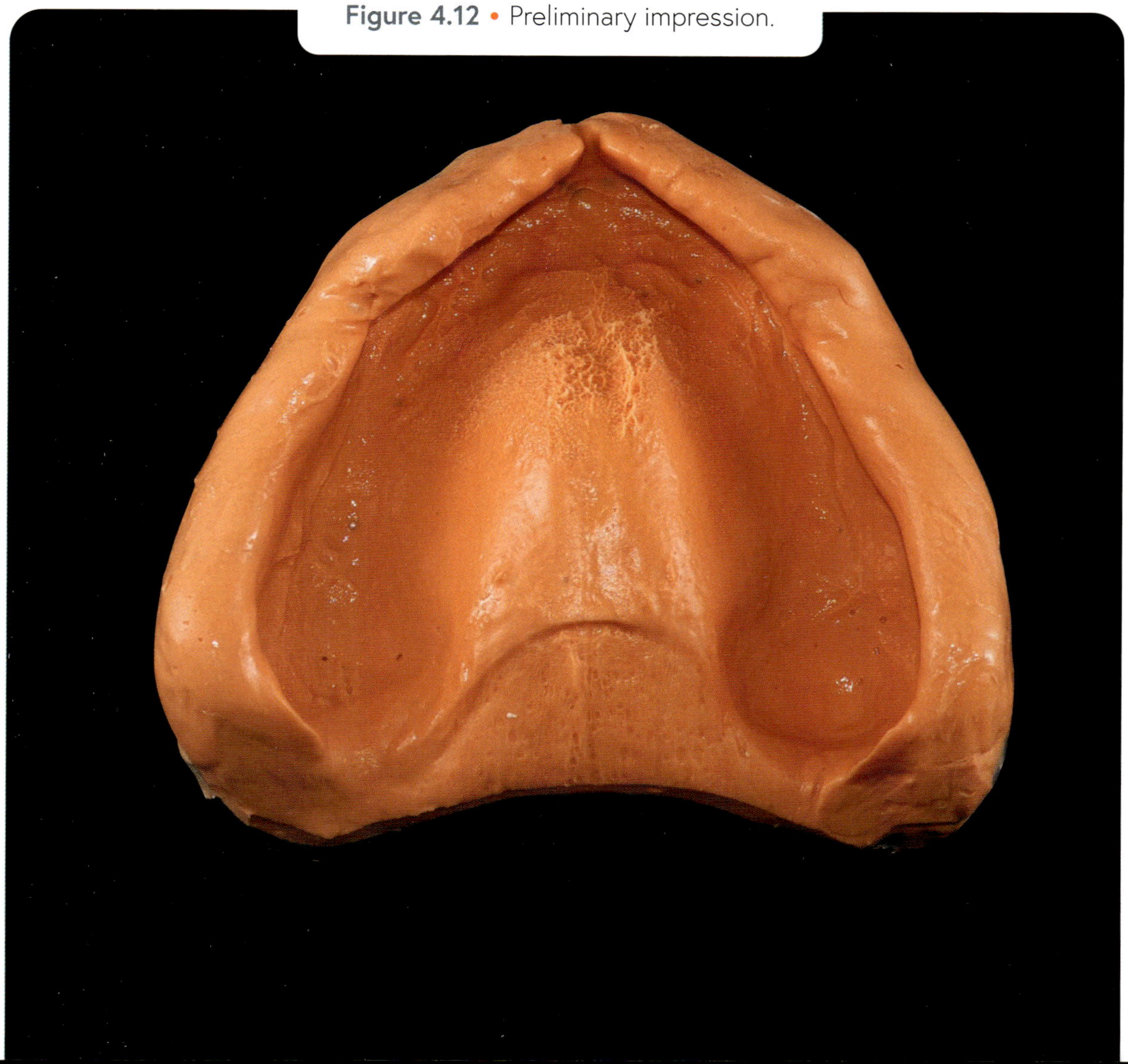

by the musculature of the mouth floor. In this case, two measuring cups of powder and little more than one part of water are used. One of the possible occurrences in the registration of the preliminary impression, owing to the use of a very compact material and a considerable quantity, is trapped air between the material and the tissues, which leads to the formation of bubbles. To make up for this lack of impression precision, it can be rebased. For this operation, the undercuts that may prevent the impression from being repositioned in the mouth are removed and the impression material is dried until it becomes opaque.

Finally, an alginate mixture is prepared, according to the manufacturer's proportions, and applied in a consistent thickness to the entire base [31,32] **(Figure 4.12)**.

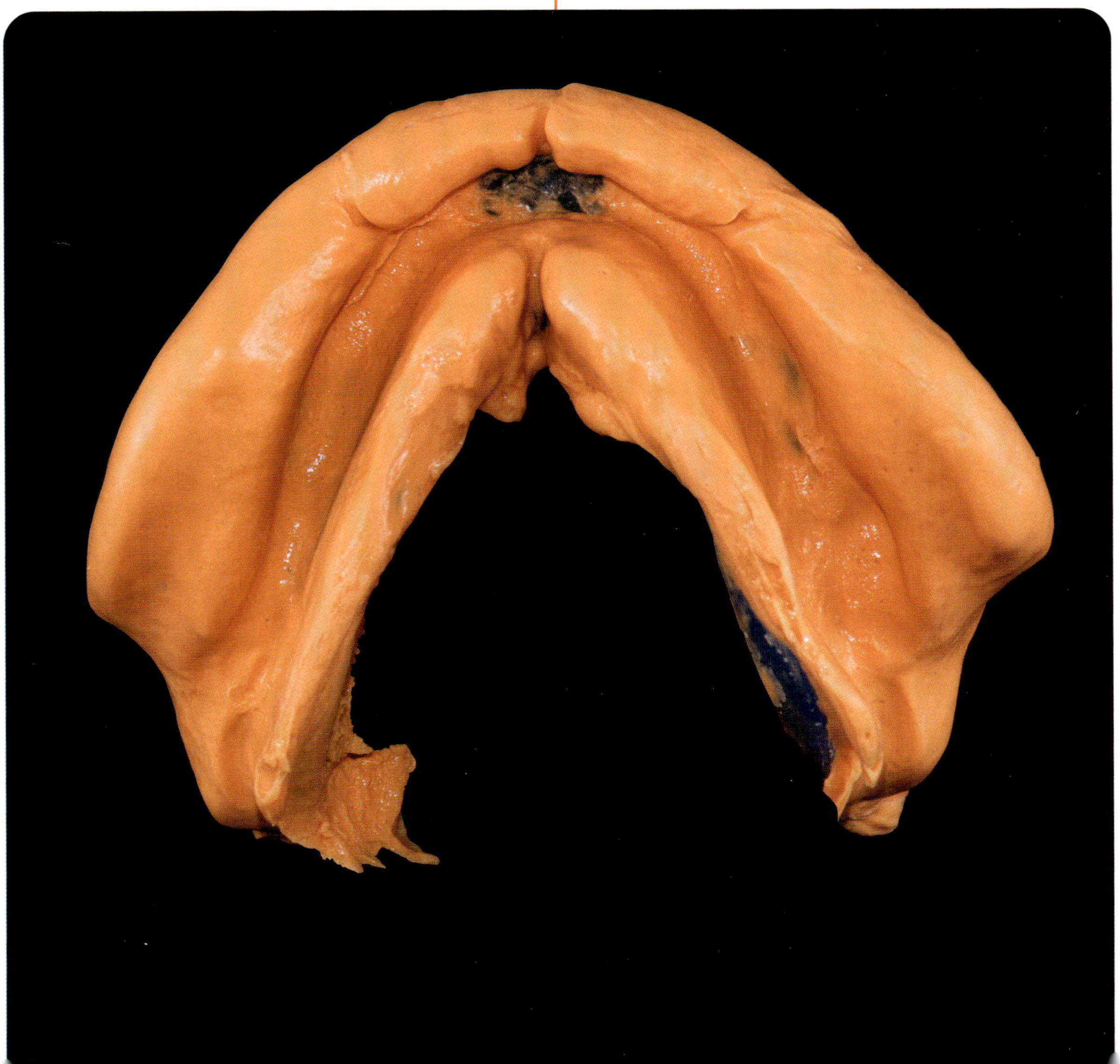

Making the preliminary models

Once any residual saliva has been removed and the impressions have been decontaminated, the plaster powder can be applied to the surface of the impressions to remove any residual alginic acid, then level three plaster is vacuum mixed with distilled water and the models are cast, then, after about 30 minutes, they are squared and finished [27] (**Figure 4.13**)

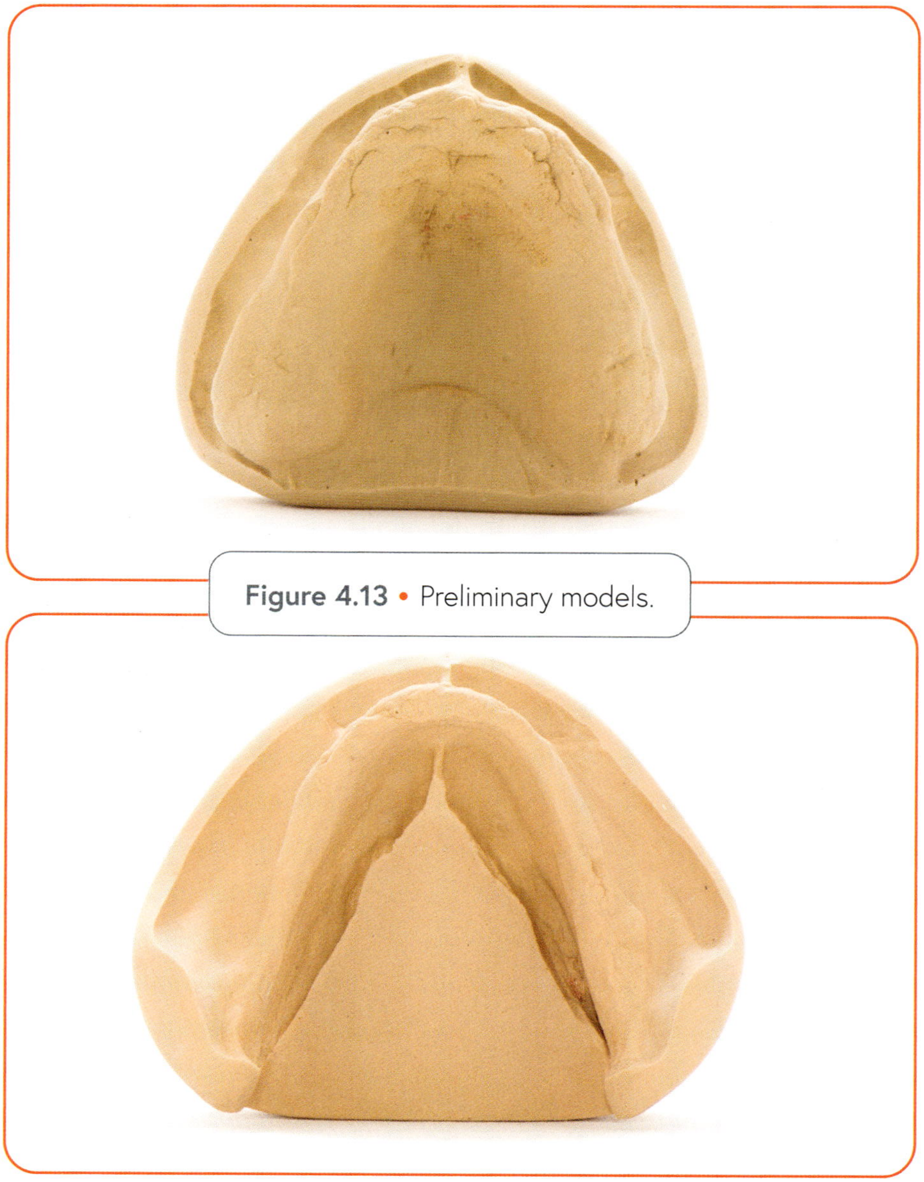

Figure 4.13 • Preliminary models.

Fabrication of the individual trays for closed mouth registration

First of all, certain anatomical landmarks must be identified on the preliminary models. In the upper model, the following must be identified: the palatine fovea, the pterygomandibular ligament, the retromolar tubercle, the retrozygomatic process, the lateral frenula, the vestibular arch, the vestibular frenulum, the palatine arch and the ridges.

In the lower one, the areas to be identified are: the retromolar trigone, the masseteric notch, the buccal shelf, the lateral frenula, the mental process, the central frenulum, the mylohyoid line, the P notch, the sublingual area, the lingual frenulum and the crests. The buccal shelf is an essential part for the stability of the future prosthesis. With this information one is able to start designing the proposed border extension [1,33].

For the upper model, one must keep a couple of millimetres beyond the fovea, continue laterally including part of the pterygomandibular ligament, the retrozygomatic process and the entire area of the retromolar tubercle. The under-extended tracing is prolonged anteriorly to the maximum depth of the fornix by about 2 mm **(Figure 4.14)**. The frenula are discharged by making curves and the vestibular arch is included, remaining under-extended at the maximum depth of the fornix by about 4 mm. Below, one starts from the middle of the retromolar trigone and continues vestibularly, creating a curve that does not interfere with the masseteric notch. The buccal shelf and the mental process are included and the frenula are discharged with curves. Lingually, one goes down from the middle of the trigone to 2 mm beyond the retromilohyoid line. One continues anteriorly and superiorly, paying attention not to include the P notch area. Finally, the entire sublingual area is fully incorporated, which is essential for the retention of the lower prosthesis [33] **(Figure 4.15)**.

Once the trace has been made on the upper model, any undercuts and the rugae area are eliminated with wax **(Figure 4.16)**. The tracing is retraced by making a groove of about 1 mm so as to be able to find a reference for the length of the tray during finishing, then a plaster-resin insulation layer is applied. The impression trays are made using a self-hardening resin prepared according to the proper proportions of polymer and monomer. The bases are finished with a 2 mm thickness, with the exception of the sublingual and retrozygomatic areas where it is set at about 3-4 mm.

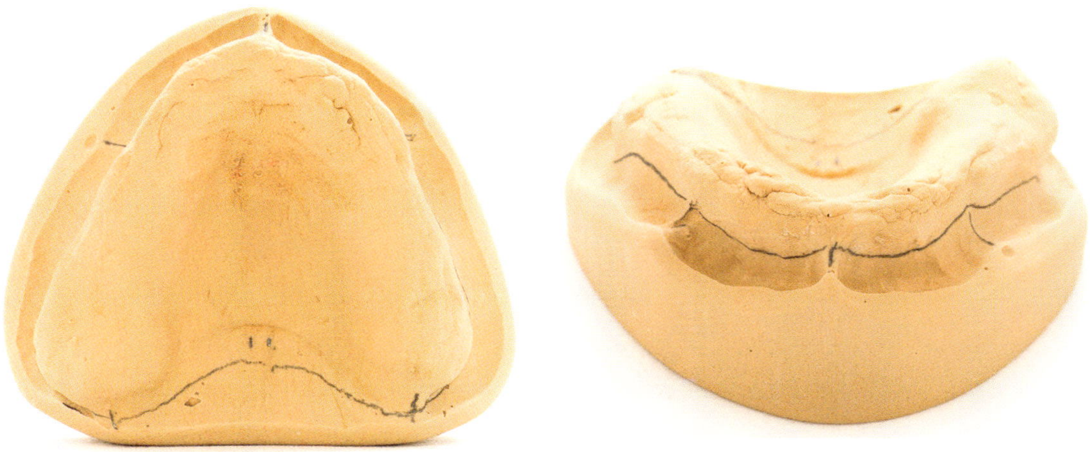

Figure 4.14 • Tracing of the upper tray.

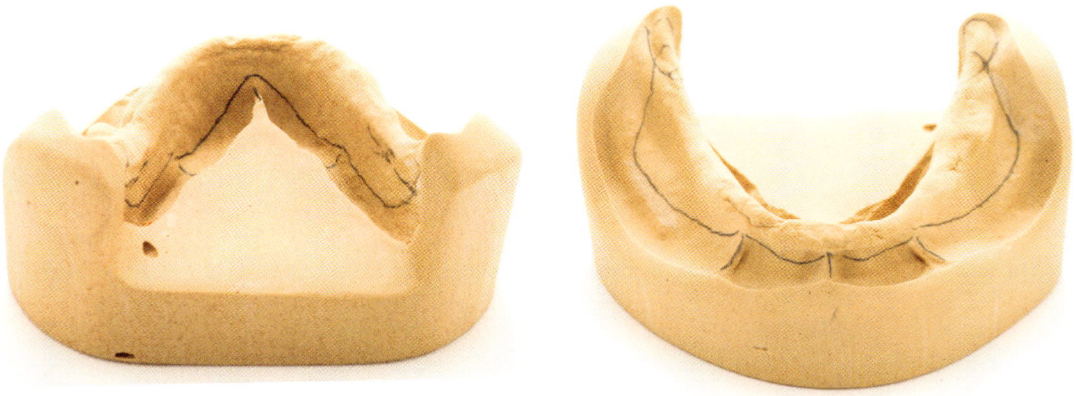

Figure 4.15 • Tracing of the lower tray.

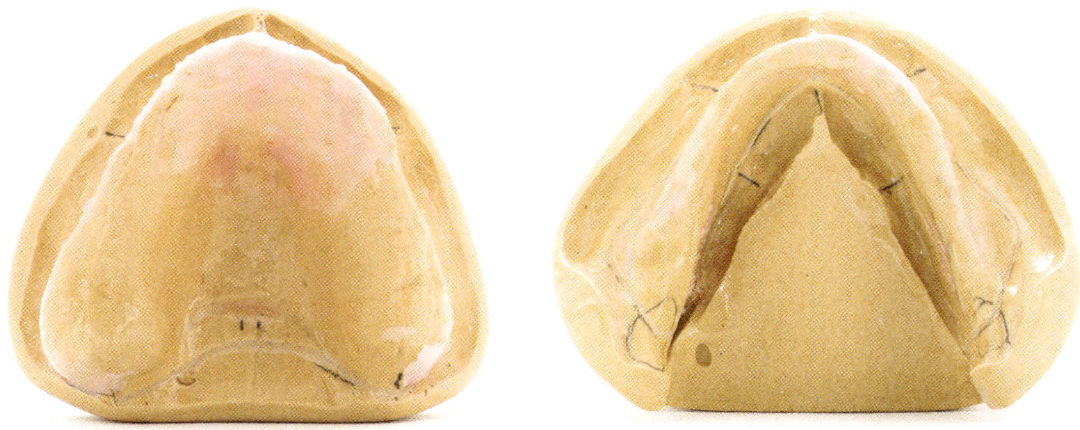

Figure 4.16 • Waxed up and isolated models.

The wax walls are positioned on the base of the impression trays, simulating the design and volume of the dental arches, so as to be used chairside to record the centric relation at the same time as taking the final impressions. This impression technique is referred to as "closed mouth". The upper bite rim is made with a rigid wax while a softer wax is used for the lower one.

For the maxilla, the average distance between the upper labial sulcus and the incisal edge of the central incisors is set at 22 mm and the upper plane is established using the Rim Former. The incisal margin is positioned about 8-10 mm forward, in the centre of the incisive papilla, with an inclination on the sagittal plane of about 12-15°. The posterior limit line is set at the mesial limit of the tuberosity **(Figure 4.17)**. For the lower bite rim, however, the distance between the lower labial sulcus and the margin at the level of the incisors is 18 mm. Posteriorly, the wax occlusal border is set in the middle of the retromolar trigone. The wax is placed on the centre of the alveolar ridge and is inclined anteriorly by 8-10° on the sagittal plane **(Figure 4.18)**. The sulci are moulded by simulating an arch, following the course of the ridges: a thickness of 8-10 mm is left in the molar region, while in the incisal region it is 2-4 mm. Finally, the lower bite rim is extended posteriorly up to the point where the ramus of the mandible starts going up [10,33-36].

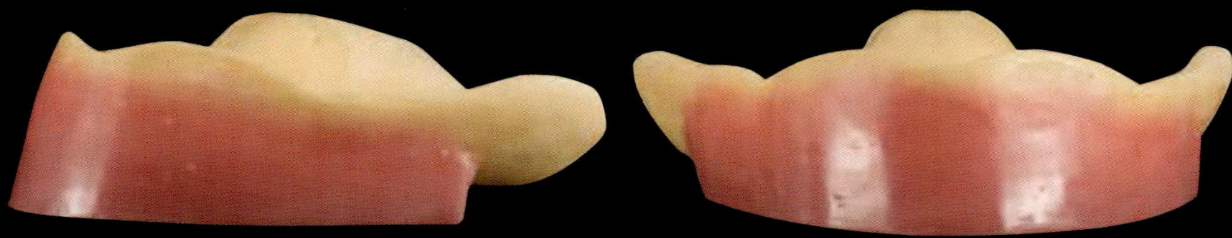

Figure 4.17 • Upper impression tray with bite rim.

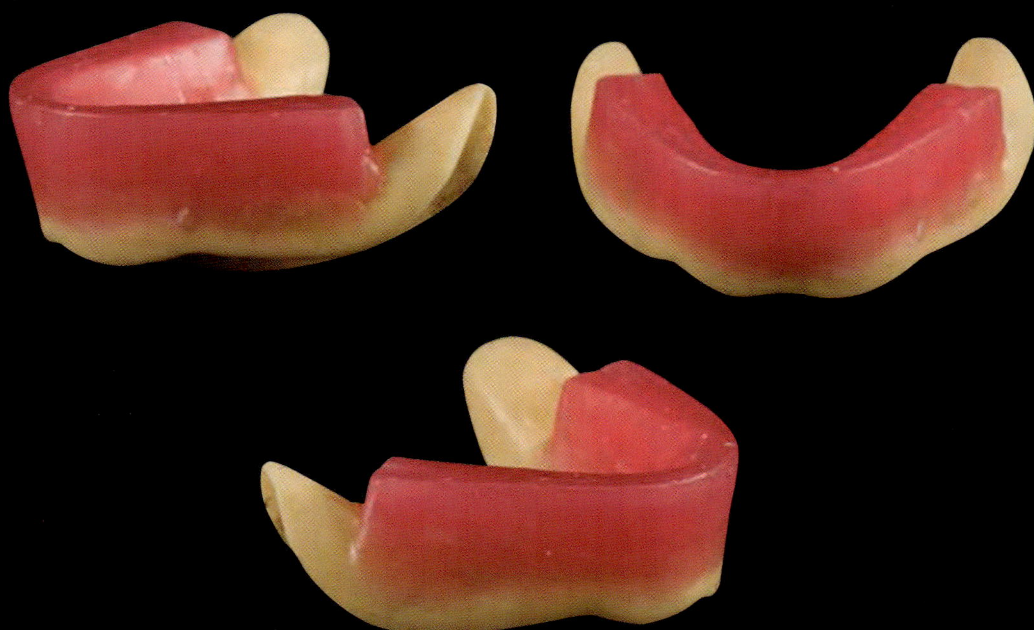

Figure 4.18 • Lower impression tray with bite rim.

Final closed mouth impression

During the second appointment, the final impressions are recorded with the intermaxillary relationship. Therefore, all the information the laboratory needs to mount the teeth is collected in one session only.

The following steps are required, to be arranged in subsequent steps in order to streamline chair time and be more effective in the clinical operations:

- fitting the trays on the tissues, assessing the support base and borders;
- customisation of the wax bite rims to establish the vertical dimension and centric relation;
- edging and registration of the final impression;
- checking the occlusal parameters (occlusal plane, OVD, centric relation, patient photos and video with bite rims in vivo;
- registration of the facebow.

Checking the base of the tray

As already described previously, the first aspect to be assessed is the adaptation of the impression tray bases to the tissues. The assessment is managed using light body silicone-based pastes, which are spread evenly on the support base of the impression trays. Once placed in the oral cavity, considerable pressure must be applied to allow the material to spread evenly. Any compression areas will then be retouched to improve the fit of the impression trays on the tissues **(Figure 4.19)**. Subsequently, the length and thickness of the borders are checked. Initially, the extension of the borders is examined by touch, trying to feel them from the outside or alternatively using a silicone paste again which, in this case, will be placed only on the border in question. The patient will have to make functional movements that involve the lips, cheeks and tongue: for example, they will be asked to speak to activate the muscles and to swallow several times while the material is hardening [30,37].

The upper bite rim is then customised. The antero-posterior position and the length of the rim must meet the needs of upper lip support and phonetic criteria. The upper rim can be corrected by adding wax in the buccal part, in case the lip support is lacking; vice versa, in case of excessive support, it is possible to remove wax until the required result is achieved. Jointly with correcting the lip support, one can act on the length by

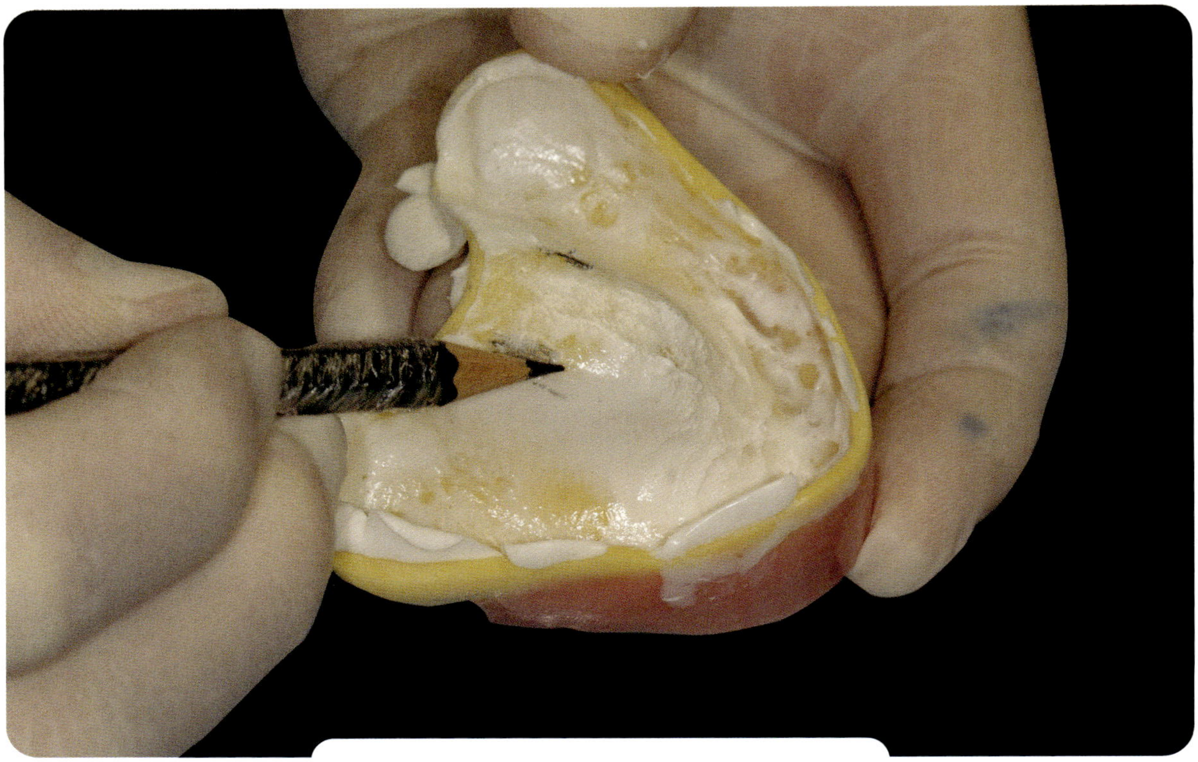

Figure 4.19 • Checking the tray.

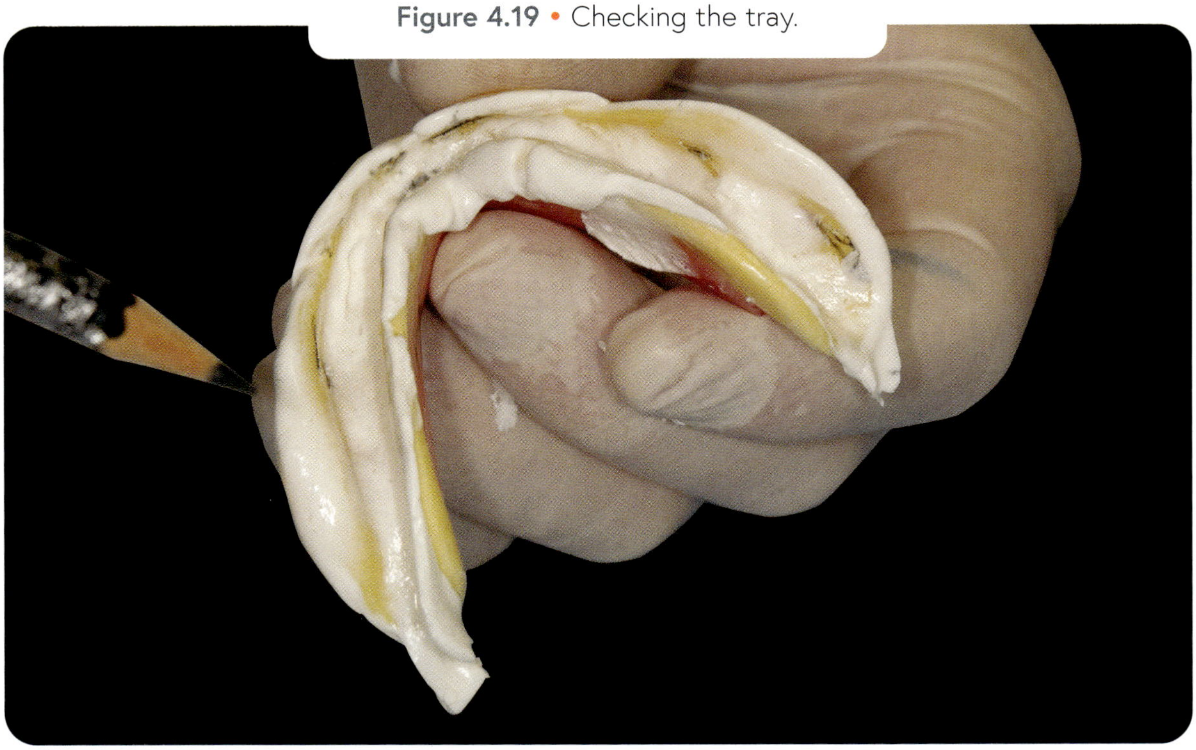

using the phoneme /f/, remembering that the margin of the upper incisors is located on the wet-dry border line of the lower lip when uttering this sound. During this test, it is useful to keep the existing lower prosthesis, in order to help the patient in supporting the lip [30,37].

The second step makes it possible to customise the upper rim, giving it the shape of the future arch with the occlusal plane parallel to the bipupillary line and Camper's plane **(Figure 4.20)**. The correction is performed by adding or removing wax as indicated by rim display when smiling. If the plane is inclined on one side, the wax is removed from that side only if display is excessive; vice versa, if display is insufficient, it will be extended from the contra-lateral side [38]. After customising the upper rim, pivots are made which are required for centric relation registration. This consists of two stages: the first one aims at establishing the OVD, the second one establishes the horizontal relationship between the arches. To establish the OVD of the new prosthesis, the clinician can use various criteria, however the most commonly used ones are esthetic and phonetic criteria. The former assess the support of the lower third of the face seeking to harmonise it with the other parts. The latter mainly exploit the phoneme /s/, which makes it possible to establish the length and inclination of the lower incisors which, after establishing the length of the upper ones, therefore take up the remaining part of the interarch space. Normally, the patient, by uttering the "S" sound, makes an excursion with the mandible forward and upwards with respect to the resting position, thus reaching the upper teeth edge with the incisal edge of the lower incisors. The space between the two arches in this stage is referred to as closest speaking space; in order to ensure it, the OVD must be about 2-4 mm less than the RVD [39-42].

From an operational point of view, two OVD conditions can be observed: high or low. In the former case, the closest speaking space or free space between the arches is not sufficient, therefore the patient, while speaking and especially when uttering the phoneme /s/, will experience a contact between the arches. Because the rims have been fabricated at medium values, it may be observed anteriorly or posteriorly. In any case, the clinician must ensure that the free space between the arches can be restored by reducing the height of the registration rim. When this space is excessive and the patient is therefore unable to close the flow of outgoing air from the upper airways with the anterior part of the rim, the length or vestibular inclination of the wax in this portion must be increased. The clinician will only modify the anterior part because rais-

The wax rim is corrected based on the esthetic and phonetic needs, maintaining proper orientation of the occlusal plane and an adequate thickness to simulate the arch of the future teeth.

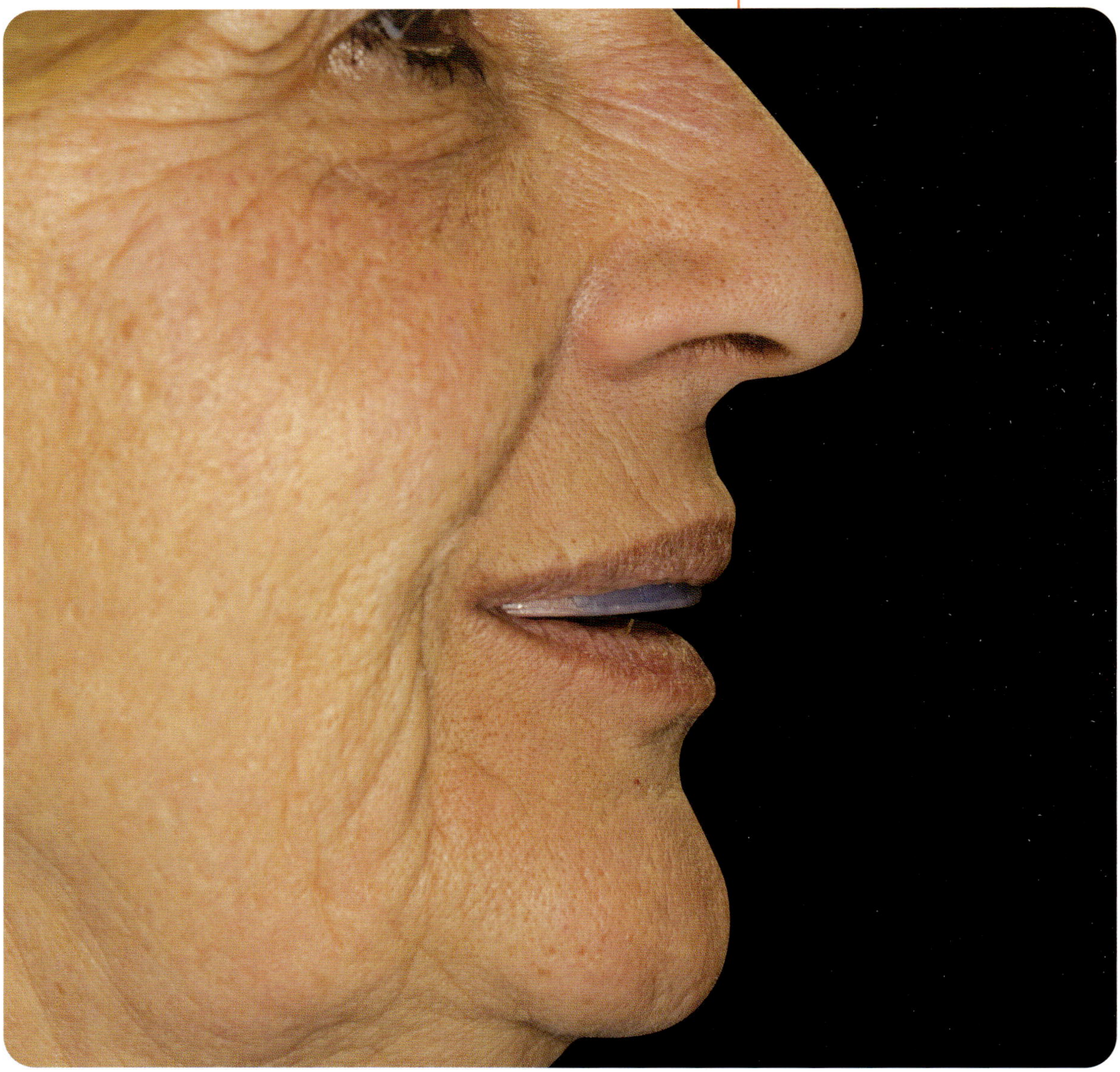

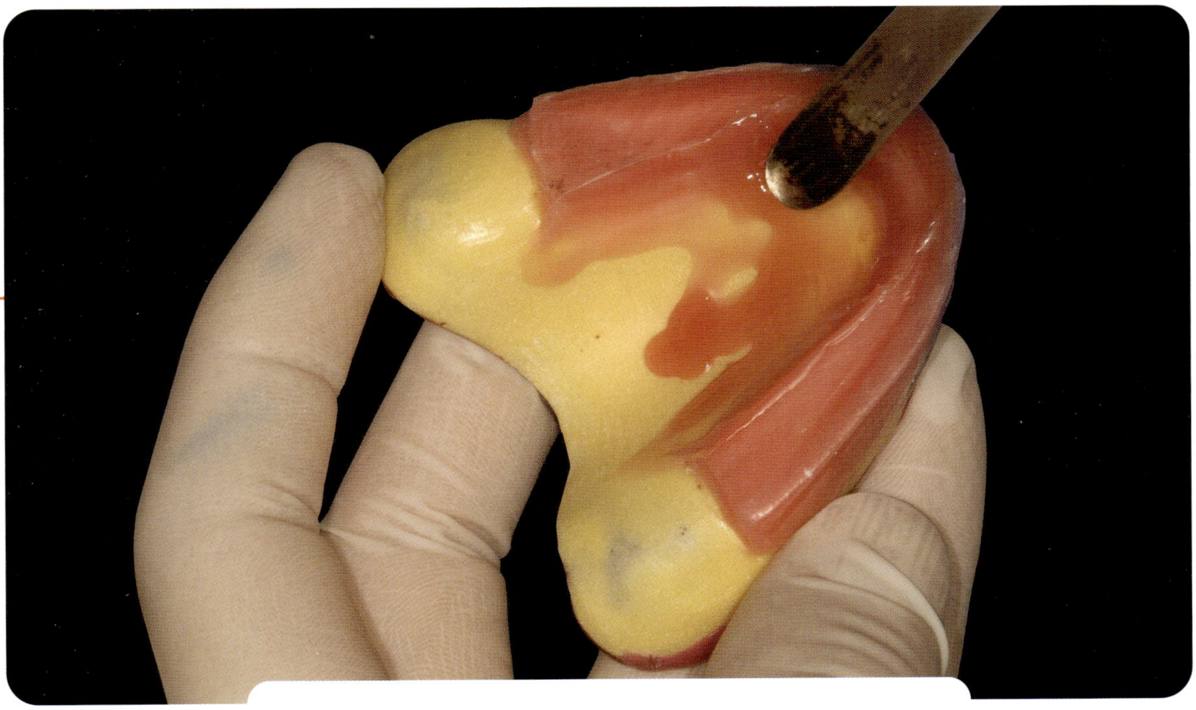

Figure 4.20 • Upper bite rim correction.

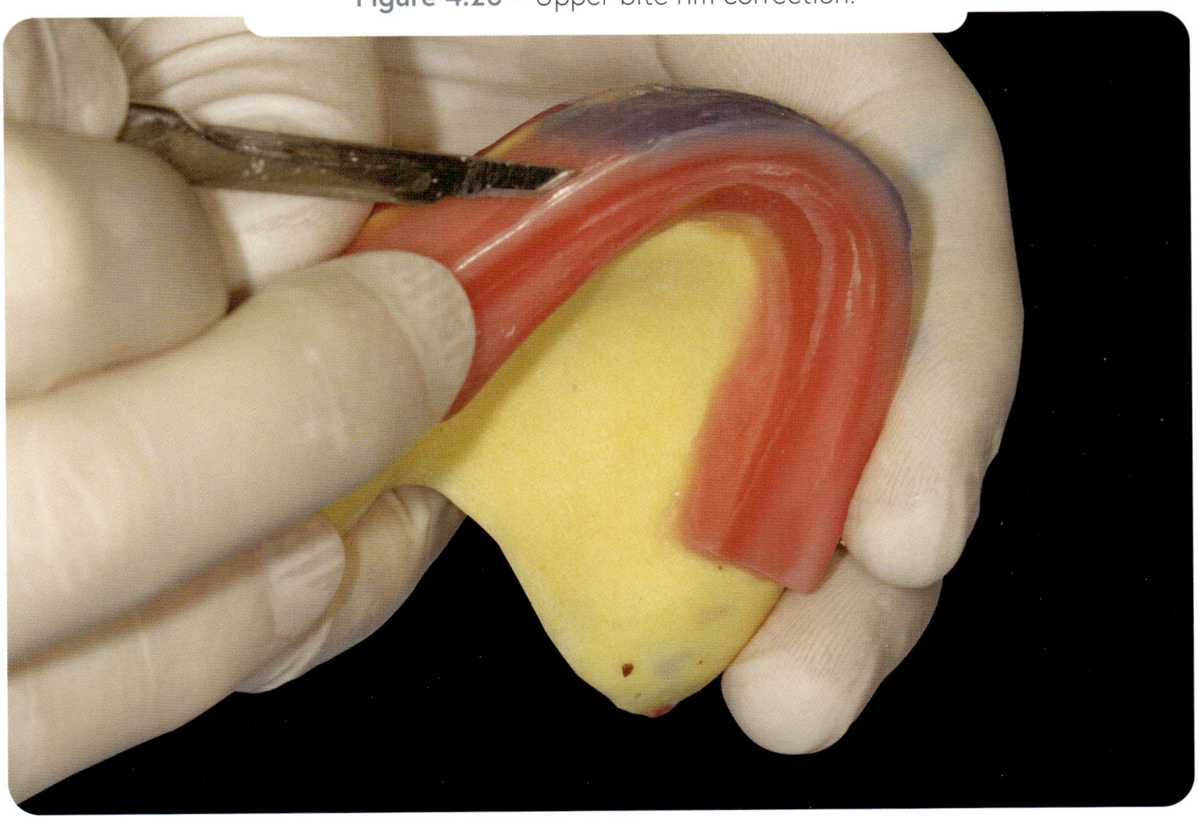

ing the whole rim might lead to a posterior early contact during phonation or centric relation registration.

In the case described here, however, the length of the lower rim, once the upper one is set up, considerably reduced the closest speaking space, therefore it was decided to shorten it (**Figure 4.21**). Therefore, after reducing it, the centric relation was set up by making up for the rim with some soft wax placed in the posterior parts, in order to obtain an even contact between the wax rims.

To check the correct registration of the vertical dimension, it is also possible to compare it with the resting one, which can be obtained by marking two small points on the patient's tip of the nose and chin, in order to have two fairly stable references [7,10,43].

At this stage, it is possible to register the relation between the arches on the horizontal plane. It is essential for the registration to comply with the requirements of stability, repeatability, reproducibility and self-determination by the patient.

Registration is performed by removing 2-4 mm of wax from the lower rim in the area behind the canines, to make sure to rule out any posterior interferences linked to the presence of the wax itself, which might cause forward sliding of the mandible during registration. The posterior inter-arch space that is thus created is filled with low-melting temperature wax, while the anterior rim maintains the OVD (**Figure 4.22**).

Clinically, the rim thus prepared is inserted in the patient's mouth; for registration, one needs to be certain that the plates have been kept in position. Otherwise, there will most certainly be a different position between the patient's mouth and the articulator. The

The reduction in height of the lower rim carried out to reduce the vertical dimension causes a gap between the rims in the posterior sector.

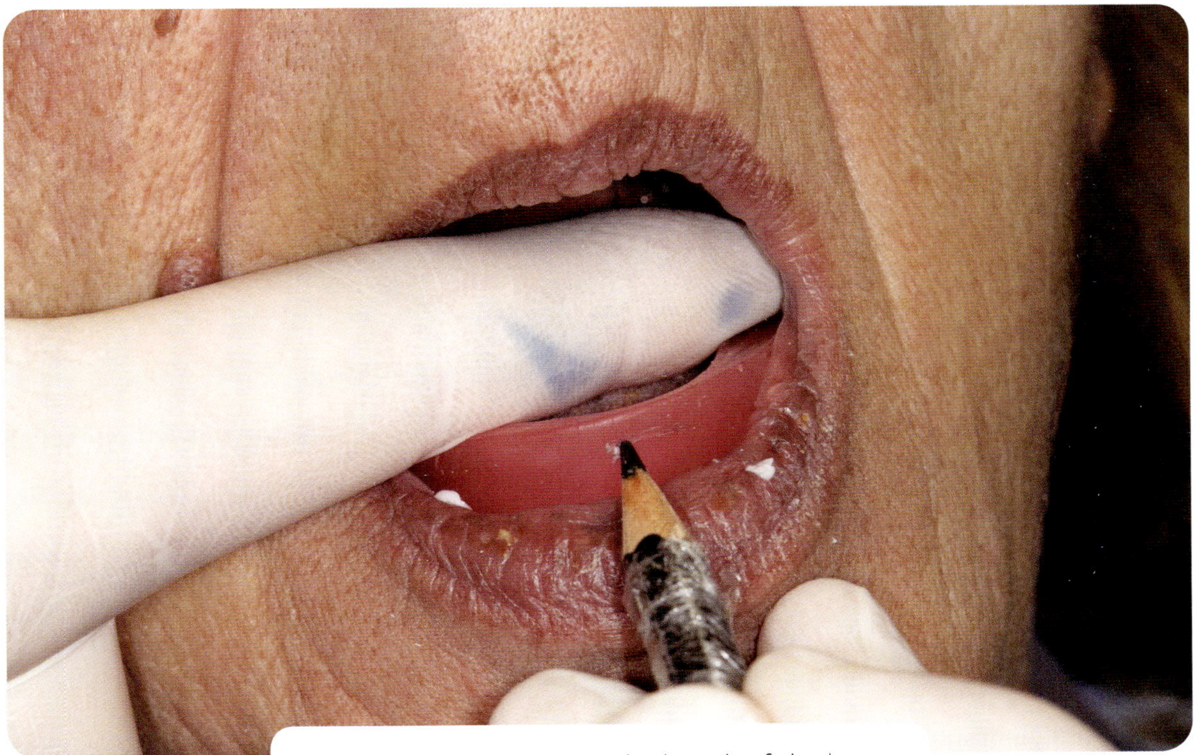

Figure 4.21 • Correcting the length of the lower bite rim and assessing match with the upper one.

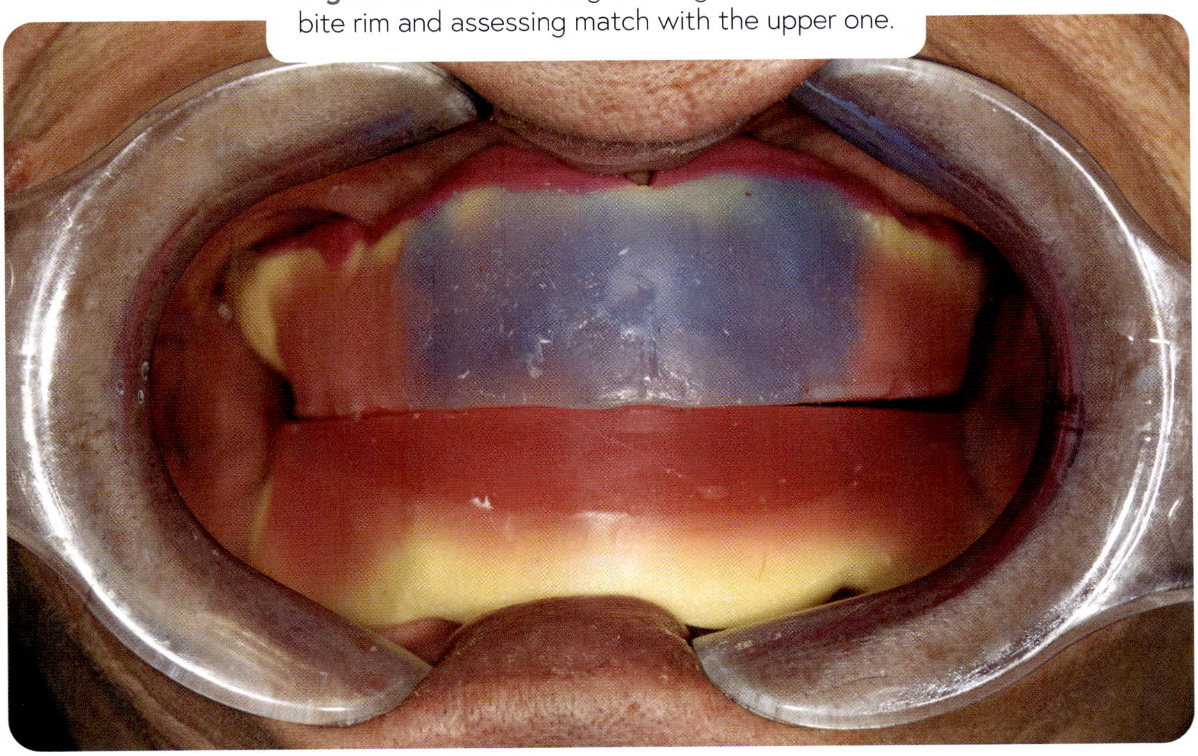

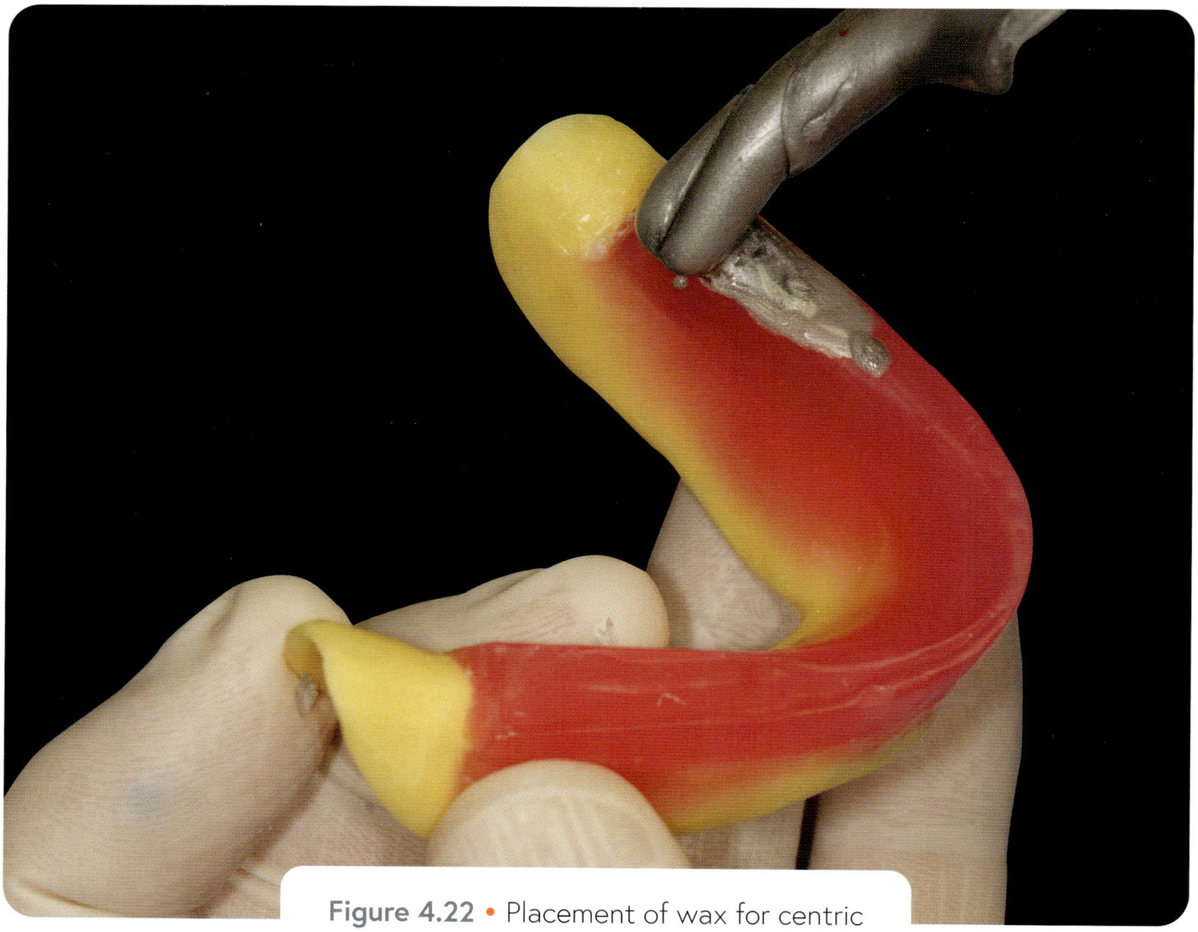

Figure 4.22 • Placement of wax for centric relation registration.

clinician, therefore, must keep the plate firmly in contact with the tissues throughout the whole manual registration, trying to move the mandible back and keeping full control during the closing travel, however without forcing the patient.

The main difficulty of manual registration is to achieve deprogramming of the musculature, so as to rule out its interference during the closing travel. Finally, the patient must repeat the same position between the jaws autonomously through the same closing travel, making the registration stable, repeatable and self-determined, as previously described. The aim is to bring the patient back to the centric relation. This is an important step because in this type of rehabilitation, where all occlusal references have been lost, one must rule out the possibility for the patient's closing position to change during the test stage of the work or after delivery of the prosthesis.

Once the intermaxillary relationship has been established by means of the rims positioned on the impression trays, they are edged and the final impressions are registered.

During these stages, having defined the centric relation position, the patient can easily swallow, which can therefore be used to establish the length and thickness of the prosthetic borders.

Edging of the impression trays starts from the upper area of the post-dam; in this phase, a thermoplastic paste with high melting temperature can be used, since, once tempered, it is able to apply considerable pressure on the tissues and it is easier to improve the seal of the prosthesis. The other areas of the upper prosthetic seal can be edged with a thermoplastic paste having a lower melting temperature **(Figure 4.23)**.

It should be remembered that the aim of peripheral edging is not so much that of over-extending the impression tray, but to make up for any lack of fit. These may be

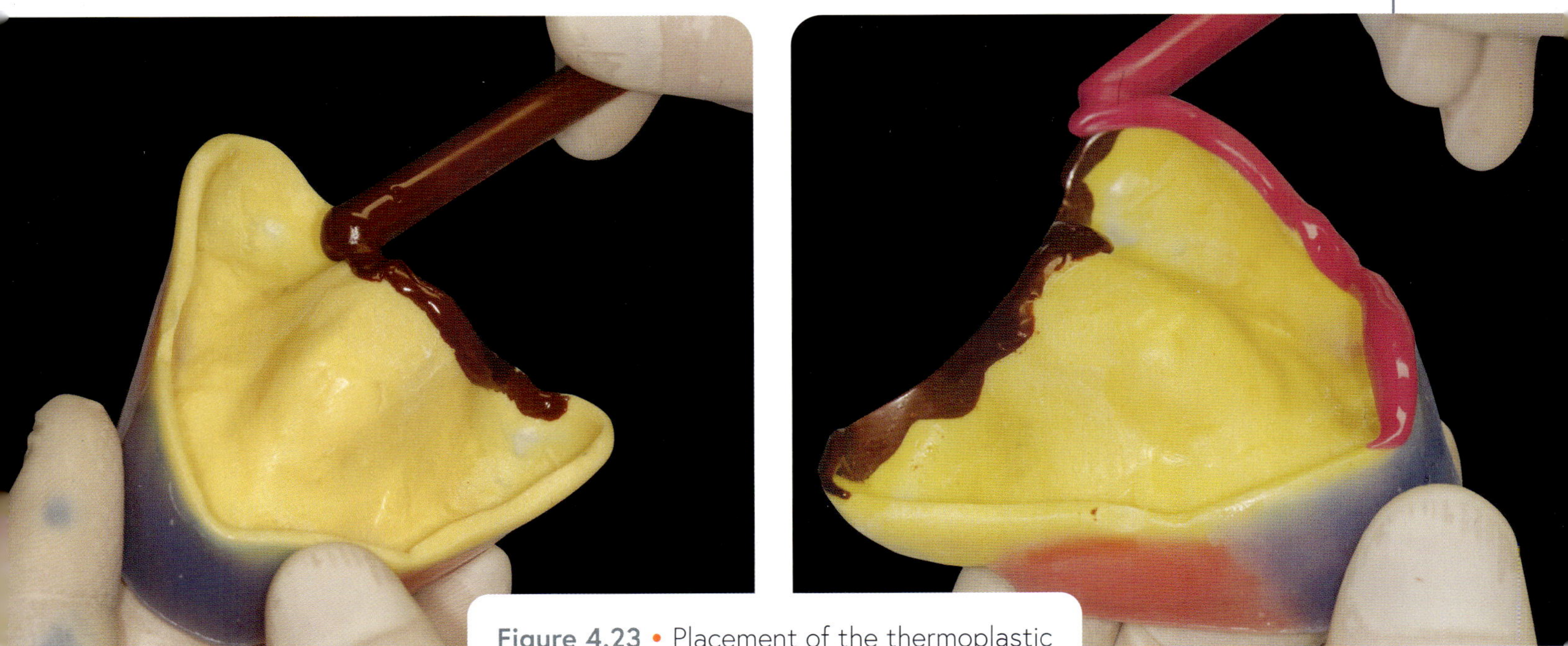

Figure 4.23 • Placement of the thermoplastic paste for peripheral edging.

linked to the reduction of undercuts on the model and it is possible to register the length and thickness of the prosthetic borders considering the impact of the muscles during functional movements.

The overexposed borders and the material that drifts towards the attached mucosa during edging must be removed, in order to reduce the risk of raising the base of the impression tray from the tissues, which might therefore reduce the fit and lose the seal **(Figure 4.24)**.

In the edging stage priority must be given to the patient's active movements. The clinician can promote them at the level of the cheeks and lips, without straining the tissues. The closed mouth impression approach is especially useful to establish the movements made during phonation and swallowing. What is more, the patient can be asked to make normal movements that can be made with the open mouth impression technique, such as protrusion forward or sideways of the tongue.

The sublingual area is essential to obtain retention in the lower area, and it can be edged with a high melting thermoplastic paste. In fact, as in the post-dam area, the presence of glandular tissue through the negative pressure that can be obtained during compression can promote the retention of the future prosthesis. It is very important during edging to ensure that there are no areas of hyperextension or excessive pressure on the tissues; this can be ascertained by using a silicone paste on the areas to be checked **(Figure 4.25)**.

To avoid the risk of overextension of the definitive impression material over the entire prosthetic border, it may be useful to discharge the edging in the deeper and outer areas of the registered border **(Figure 4.26)**.

Once the rims have been customised and edging has been completed, the definitive impressions are registered **(Figure 4.27)**.

Finally, the upper impression and the lower impression are registered, and various materials may be used to do so. The aim of this last step is to make up for the remaining small lacks of fit on the edged individual impression tray. The indication is to use not very viscous materials that reduce pressure on the tissues. In particular, where there are mobile ridges, a sufficient space must be created for the impression material. It is also possible to make holes for the material to leak out to achieve that.

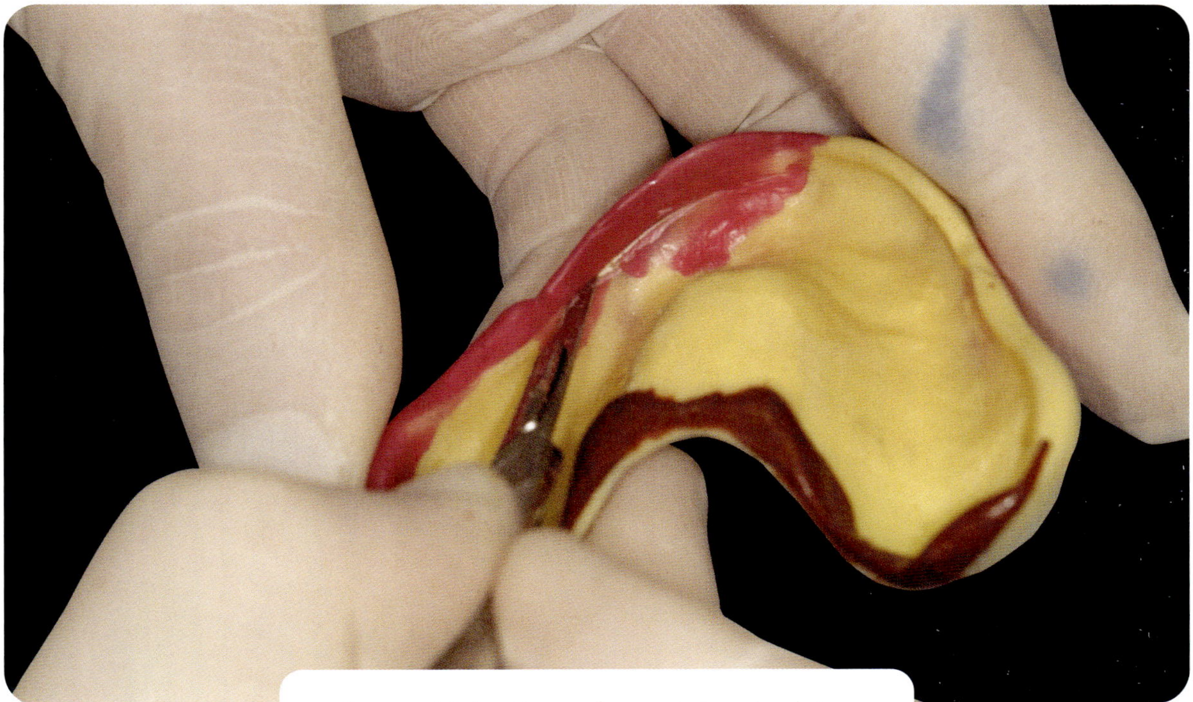

Figure 4.24 • Steps for peripheral edging: removing posterior and internal excesses.

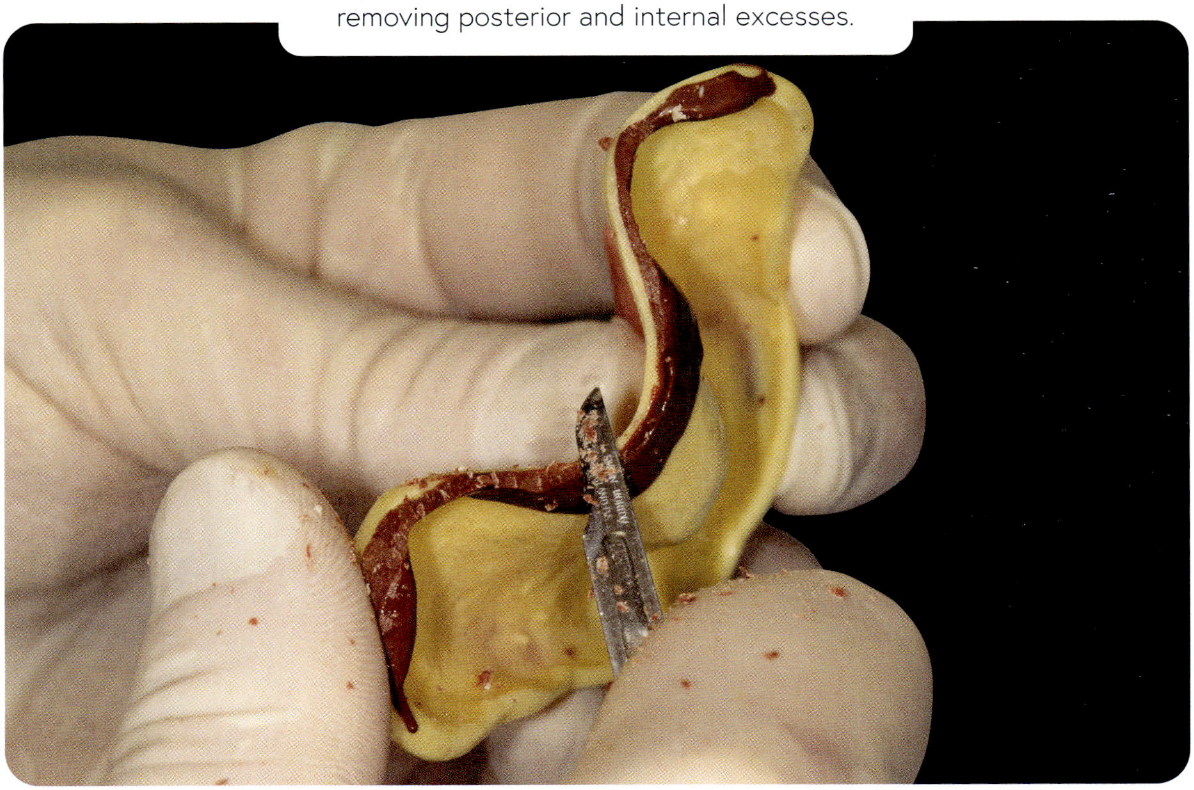

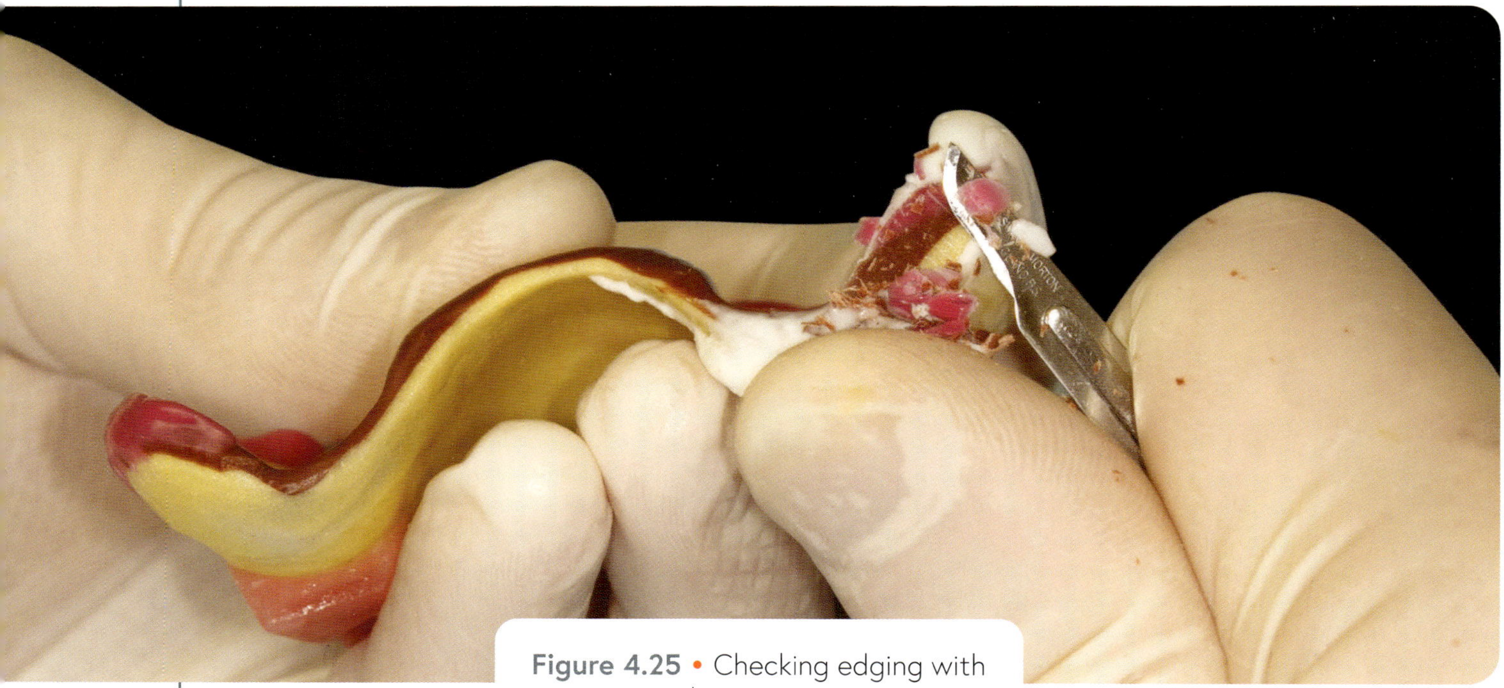

Figure 4.25 • Checking edging with silicone paste.

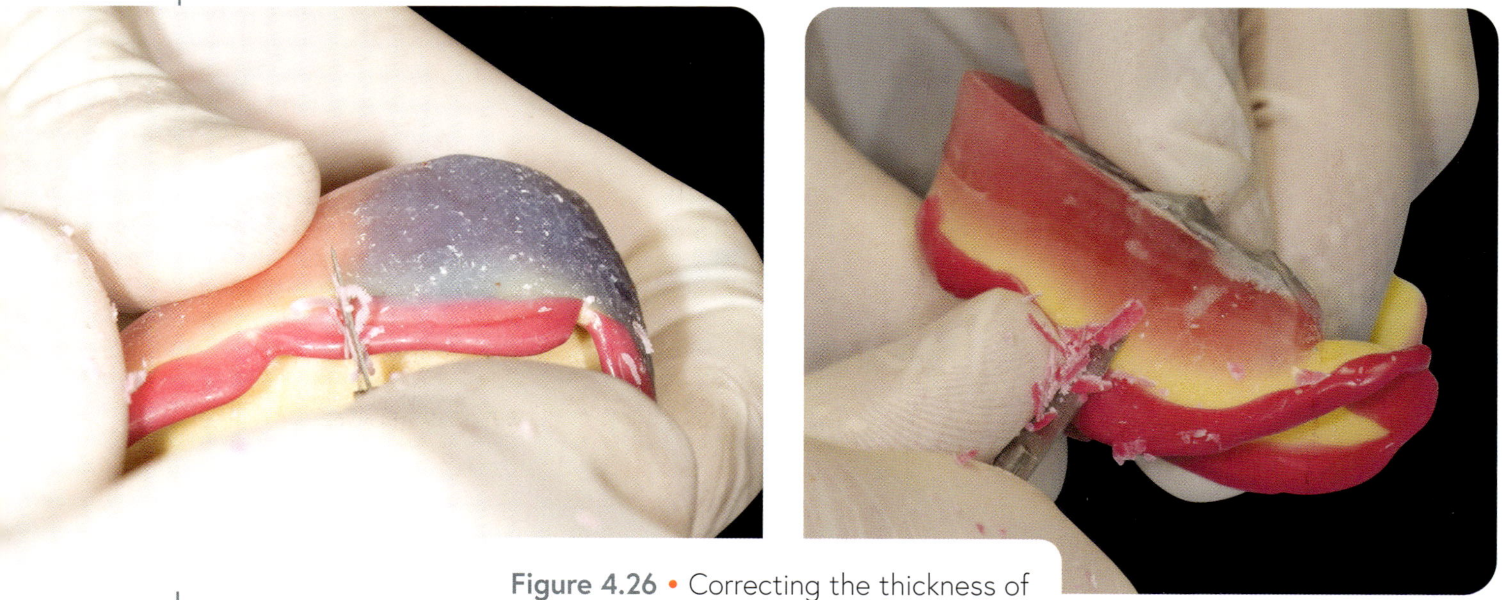

Figure 4.26 • Correcting the thickness of peripheral edging.

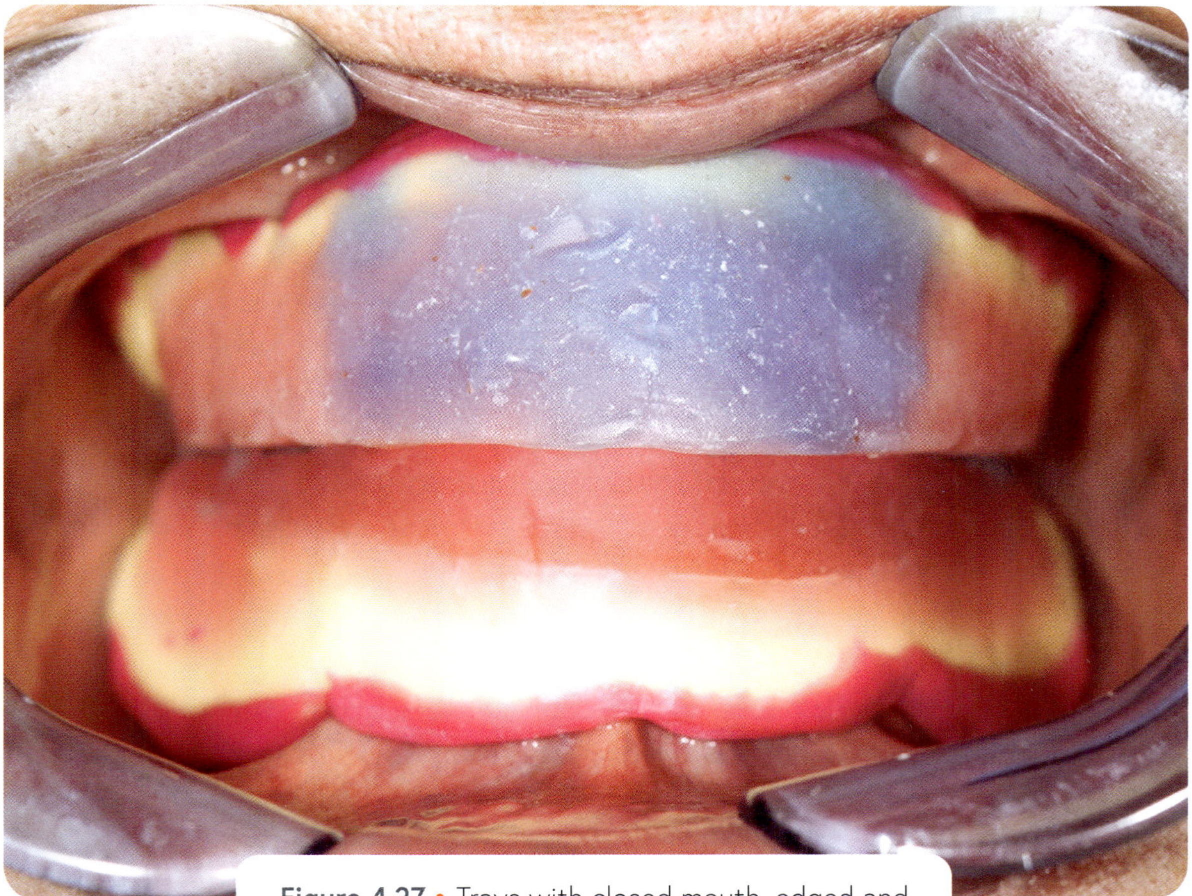

Figure 4.27 • Trays with closed mouth, edged and with registered intermaxillary relationship.

In the case presented in this chapter, polysulfide was used as the material for the definitive impression, for which a specific adhesive must be applied (**Figure 4.28**).

Once the impressions have been registered, it is essential to check the occlusal plane, the vertical dimension and the centric relation again to rule out any errors due to the thickness of the impression material (**Figure 4.29**).

Furthermore, the midline, maximum display line and also the projection of the nose ala must be marked on the upper rim, in order to provide the laboratory with the data required to set up the dentures.

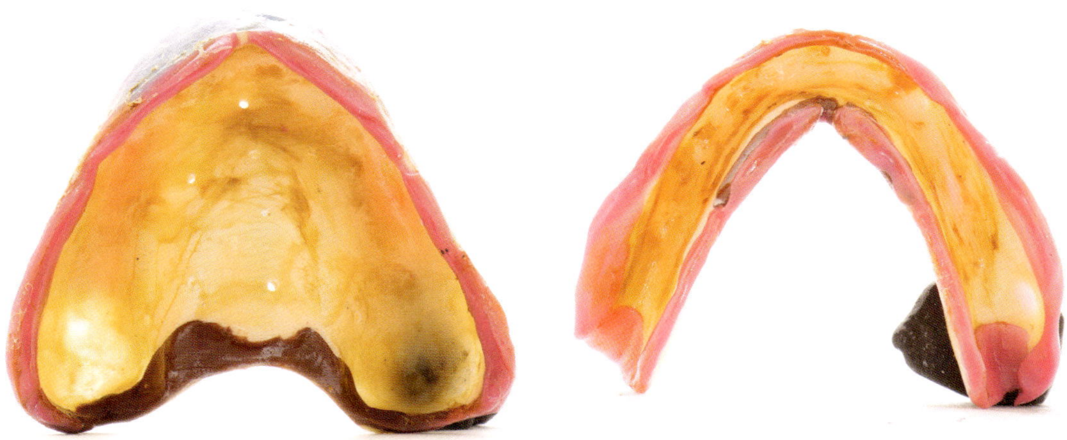

Figure 4.28 • Trays prepared for registration.

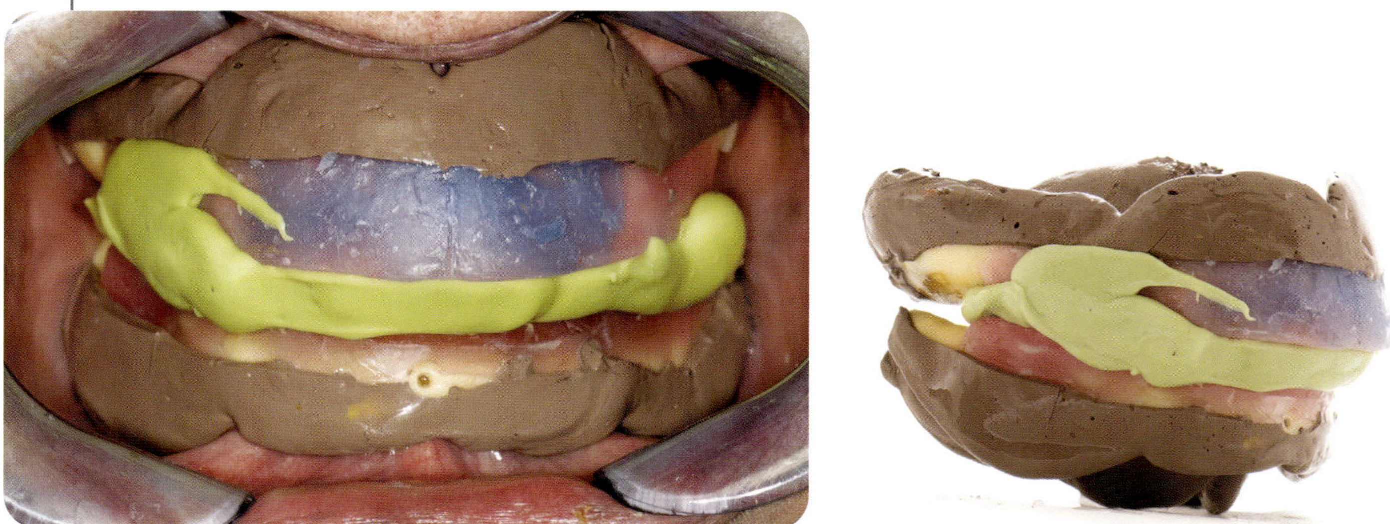

Figure 4.29 • Registered closed mouth impressions.

At this stage, photos are taken of the face and a small video is recorded of the patient with the rims in the oral cavity. These data must be sent to the laboratory together with the previous ones for the subsequent steps **(Figure 4.30)**.

Finally, a face bow is registered, which may not be mandatory in total prostheses, but can be particularly useful if the DVO must be modified by varying the incisal pin of the articulator **(Figure 4.31)**.

As a matter of fact, a modification made in the articulator of 2-3 mm is possible without including occlusal errors if, jointly with registering the centric relation, the maxilla is properly positioned with respect to the condylar axis.

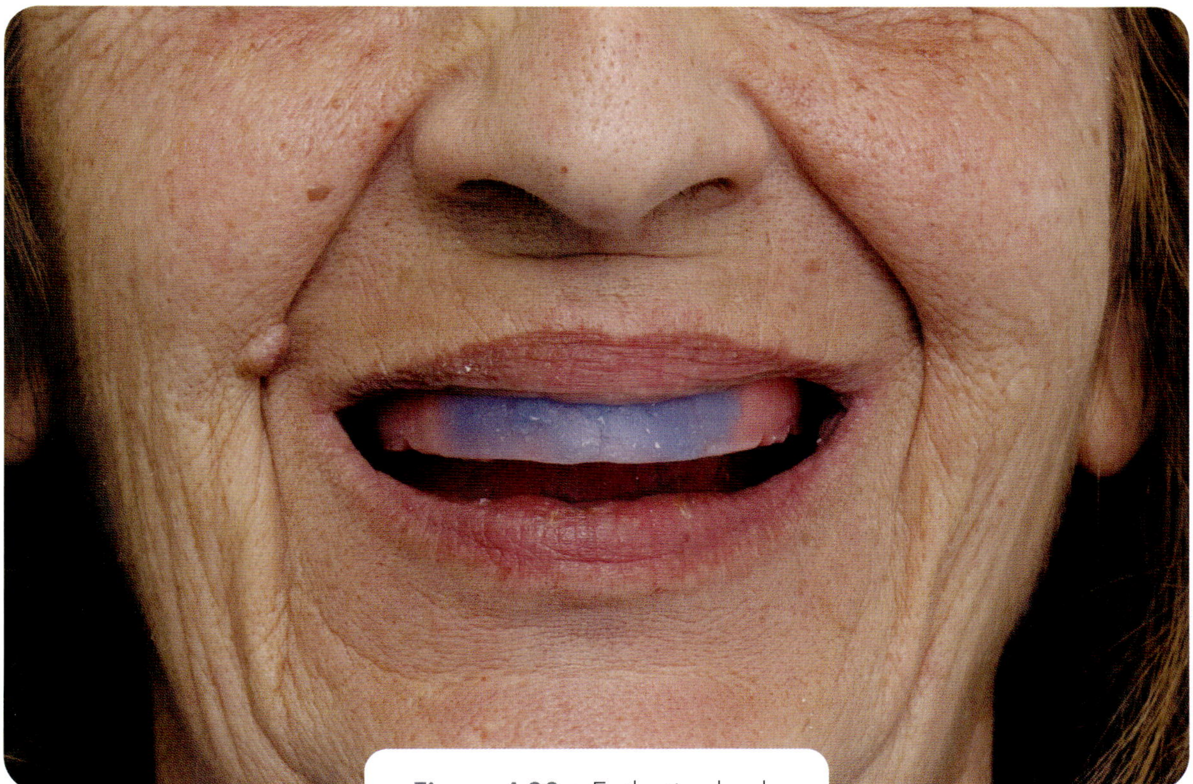

Figure 4.30 • Esthetic check.

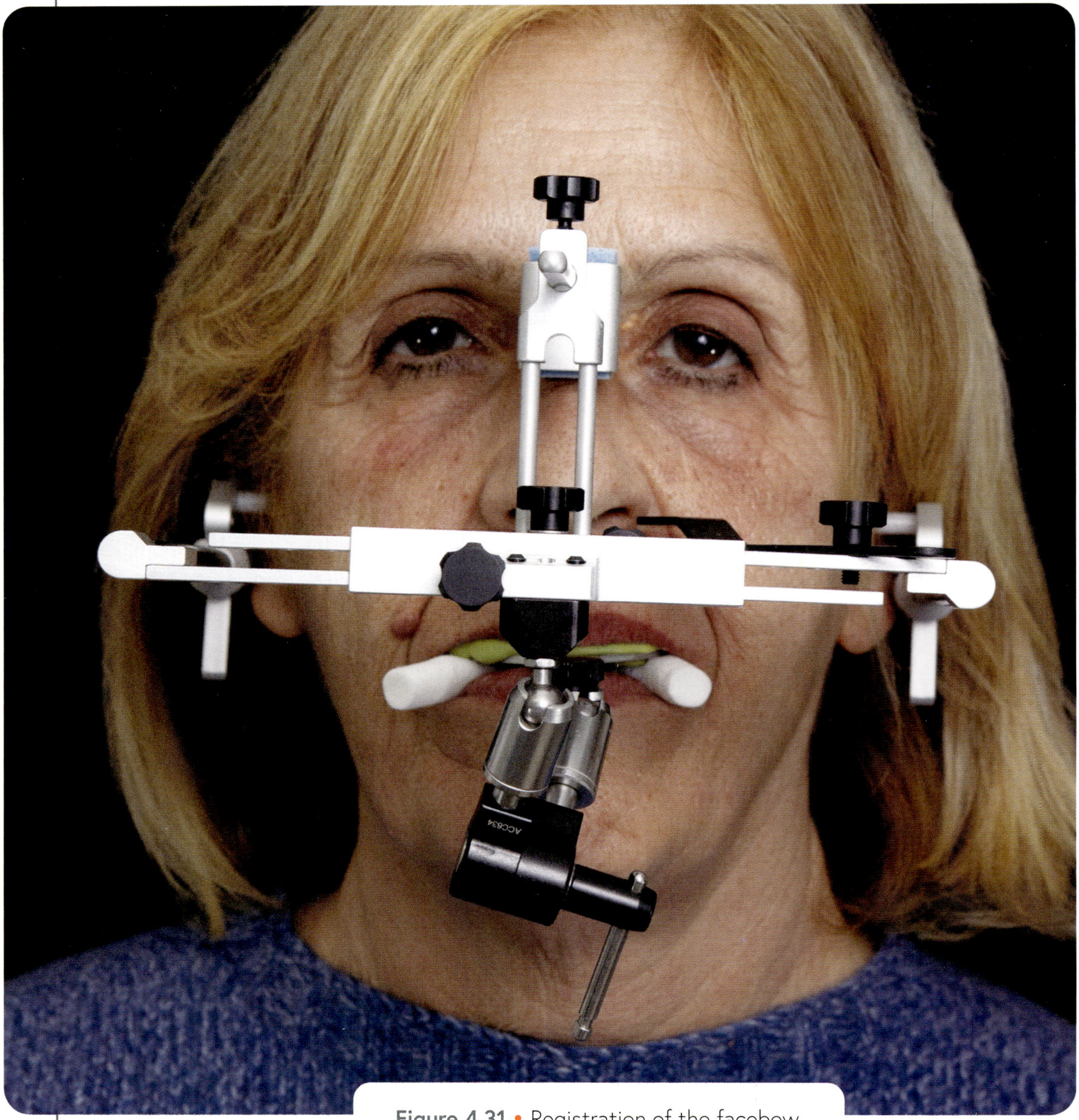

Figure 4.31 • Registration of the facebow.

Making the master models

The accurately defined borders with the second impression and detail of the tissues must be preserved. After washing the impressions with water, decontaminating them and gently drying them, adhesive wax is placed along the outer surface of the impression, 4 mm from the edge of the border. Two round or square section wax sticks are applied perpendicular to the impression. The sticks must be fixed to the adhesive wax so that they do not move while the plaster is cast. On the posterior border of the impression, the sticks should not be fixed directly, but below and distally, to preserve the whole extension of the posterior peripheral edge **(Figure 4.32)**. The impressions are cast using natural level four plaster mixed in vacuum, following the manufacturer's instructions. The models obtained are squared and finished, taking care not to damage the rims [1,36,41,44] **(Figure 4.33)**.

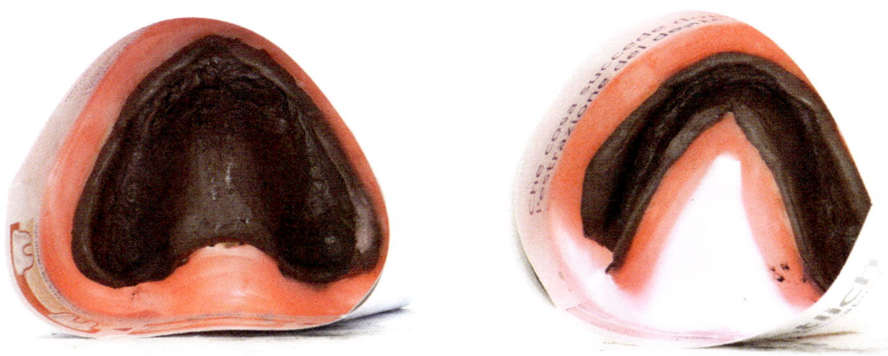

Figure 4.32 • Boxed final impressions.

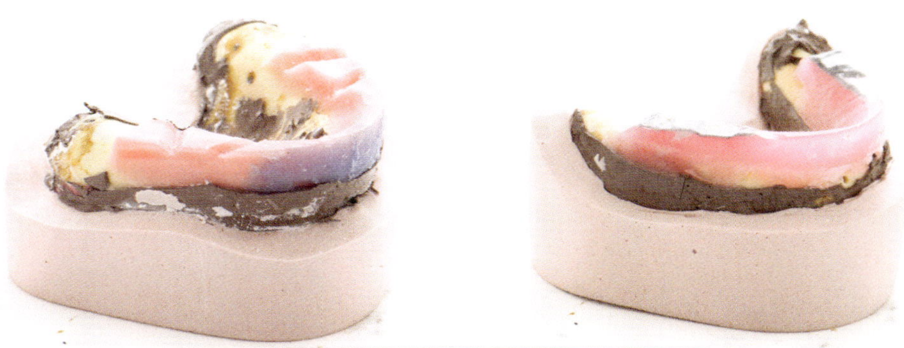

Figure 4.33 • Master models

Setting the models in the articulator

Once the models with the rims still in situ have been squared and finished, the upper model is assembled in the articulator, setting it with the facebow **(Figure 4.34)**.

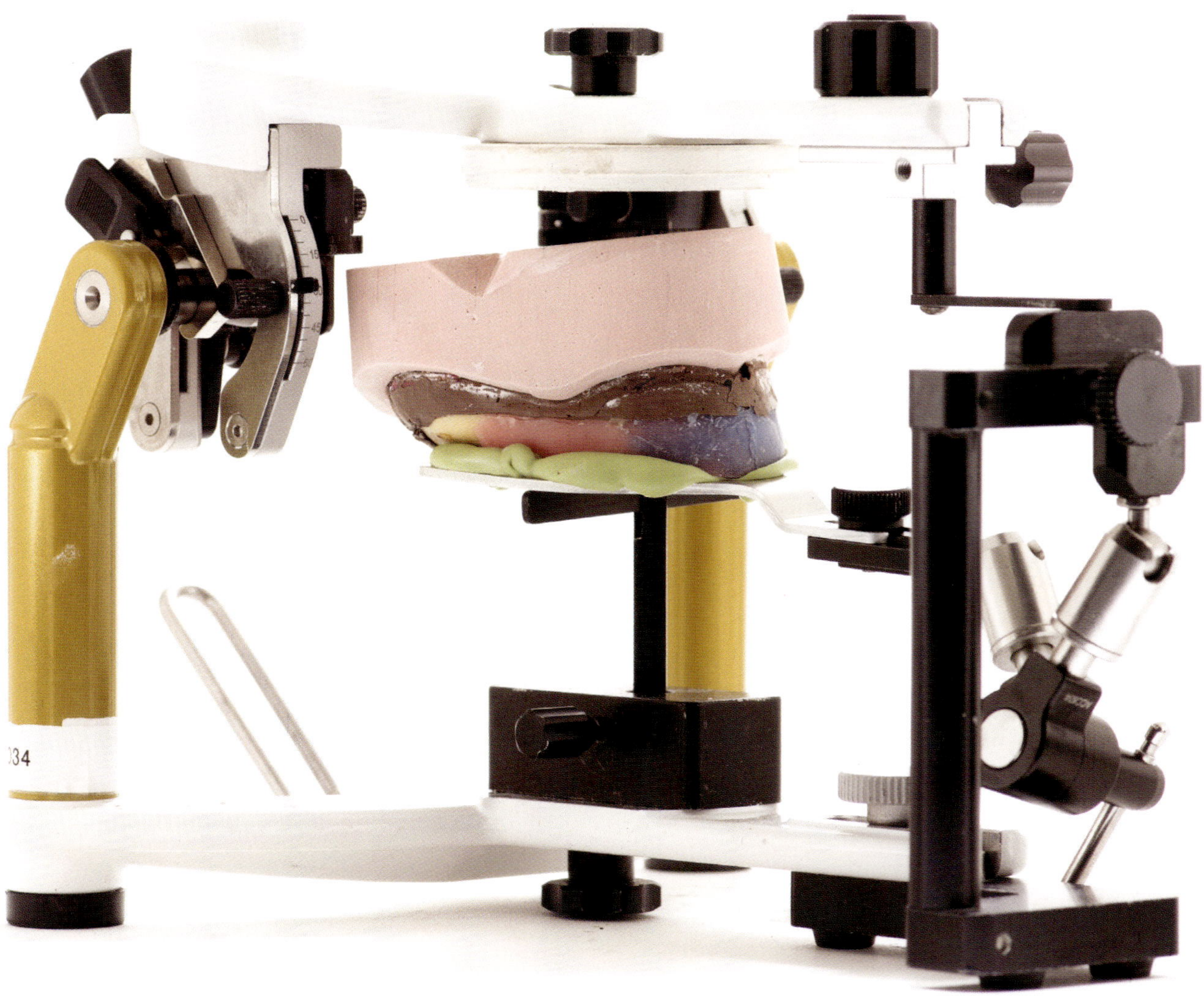

Figure 4.34 • Placement of the upper model in the articulator.

To mount the upper model in the articulator only the registration fork and related joint, through which it is connected to a support that let it positioned in the articulator, are sent to the laboratory.

The upper model is then cast, using specific low-expansion plaster.

The lower model is assembled with the occlusion bases positioned on the models [41] **(Figure 4.35)**.

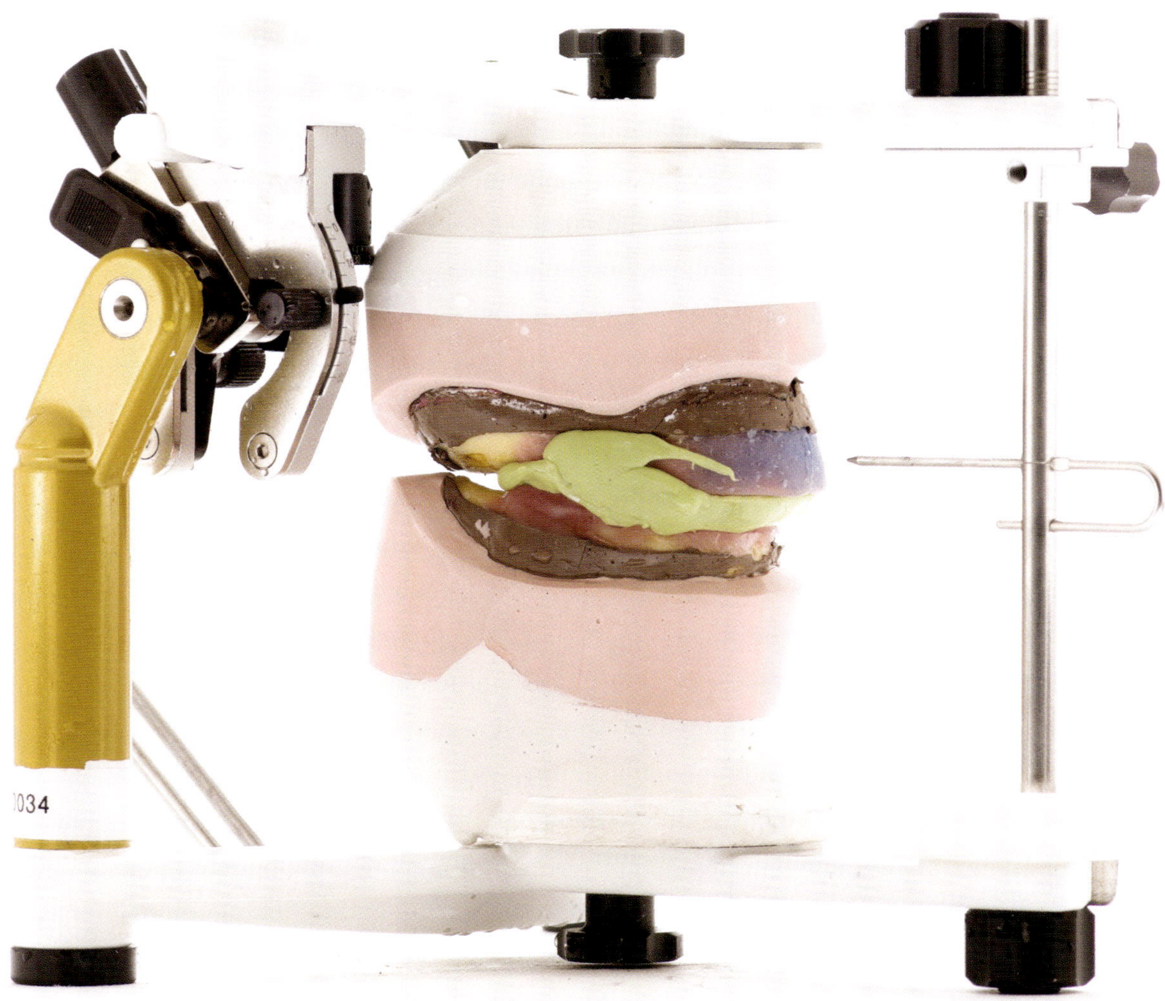

Figure 4.35 • Placement of the models in the articulator.

Making the plate for neutral zone registration

Once the models have been mounted in the articulator, the lower impression tray is removed from the model and immersed in warm water at 60° C for 5 minutes **(Figure 4.36)**.

The self-hardening resin is softened, allowing the impression tray to be removed without damaging the master model.

Any undercuts on it are highlighted and finally a plaster-resin isolating layer is applied. A resilient resin is placed in the undercuts. The self-hardening resin is prepared with the models mounted in the articulator. A part is adapted on the ridge, taking care to duplicate all the details on the model, including the borders, the remaining material is positioned in the centre of the alveolar ridge, paying attention not to lose the structure of the upper rim. The plate is finished paying attention to respect the borders. The resin rim is finished with an occlusal thickness of about 2 mm and is positioned in the centre of the ridge. The plate must be stable, rigid and retentive and must duplicate the base of the completed prosthesis [3,45,46] **(Figure 4.37)**.

After finishing the lower plate, a plaster or rigid silicone index is made in order not to lose the antero-posterior position, the length and any parameters registered on the upper rim **(Figure 4.38)**.

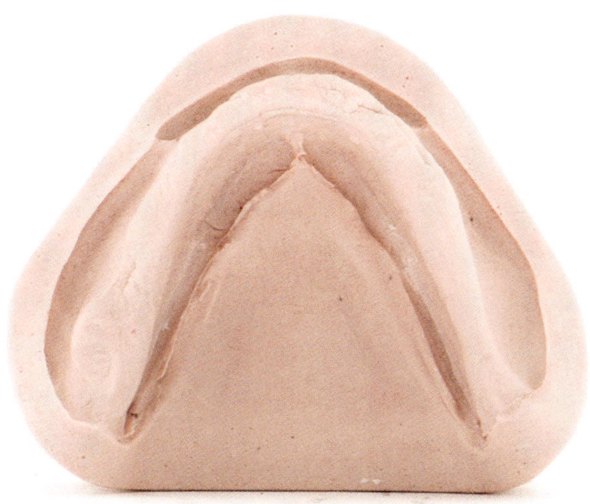

Figure 4.36 • Lower master model.

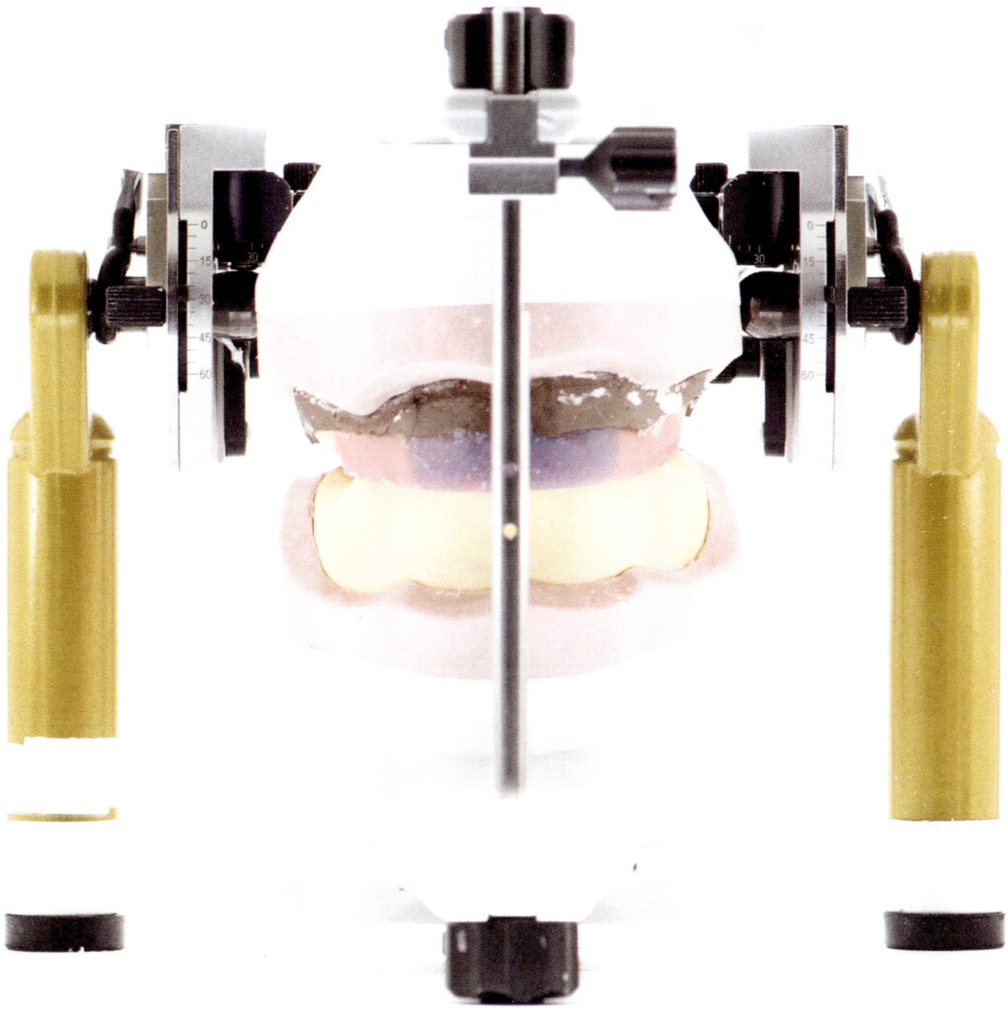

Figure 4.37 • Making the lower plate for neutral zone registration

At this point the model is immersed in lukewarm water and the upper impression tray is removed, the rugae area is discharged with wax and the insulation is placed. In this stage, the prosthetic space between the occlusal plane and the upper alveolar ridge can be checked, which in this case is particularly small. The resilient resin is placed in the undercuts, ensuring it does not end up in the fornix in a similar way to the lower model.

One waits for the resilient resin to harden then the self-hardening resin plate is made. The plate must accurately duplicate the borders, plus the palate part must have the same thickness as the definitive prosthesis.

Finally it is finished, taking care to respect borders and thicknesses, following the criteria of stability, rigidity and precision.

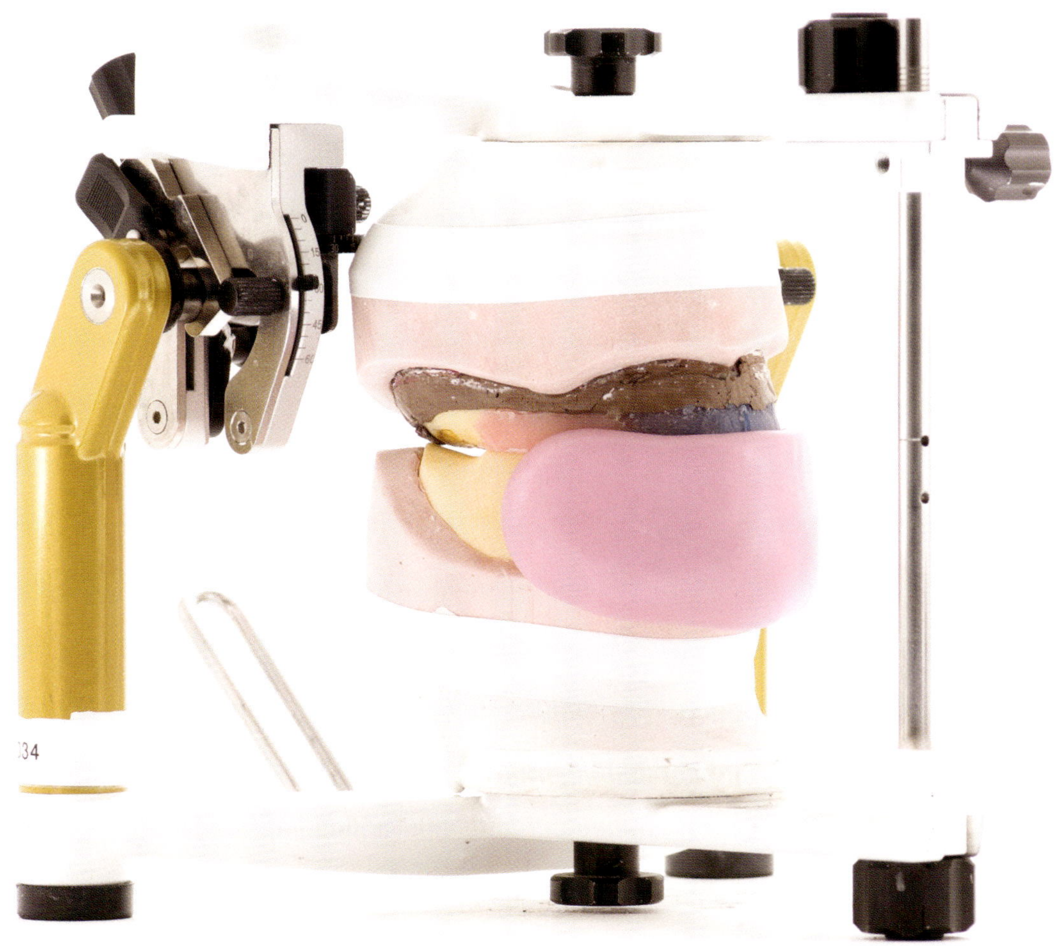

Figure 4.38 • Silicone index for maintaining the position of the upper front teeth.

Choice of the front teeth and setting

The reference lines drawn on the rims and their profile are an excellent starting point for the choice and mounting of the front teeth. Films and photographs provided by the clinician are also very useful. In natural dentition, as reported by many studies, the distance between the labial surface of the canines and the end of the first palatine fold is 10 mm, furthermore the distance between the centre of the incisive papilla and the labial surface of the central incisors is 8-10 mm. It has been observed that the tip of the canines is on a line that goes through the centre of the incisive papilla. If we start from the concept that the position of the incisive papilla and the group of palatine folds remain constant even in the course of atrophy of the alveolar ridges, the aforementioned values can be taken as a basis for mounting the artificial teeth. The anterior teeth are positioned on the plate using the index previously made on the rims **(Figure 4.39)**.

A check of the prosthetic space available for mounting the teeth can be carried out in the articulator by removing the plates one at a time **(Figure 4.40)**.

In this stage, the mounting proposed by the laboratory must be verified in the oral cavity in esthetic and phonetic terms. The dentures are therefore not yet customised on the incisal margins and any rotations are excluded to prevent them from being retouched before their validation on the patient. The upper quarter is also positioned following the orientation of the upper rim, but its final assembly must then be verified in terms of statics and occlusal relation with the lower one. Therefore, the mounting setup can be reviewed and corrected after the clinical try-in and it is therefore very useful before making the complete mounting.

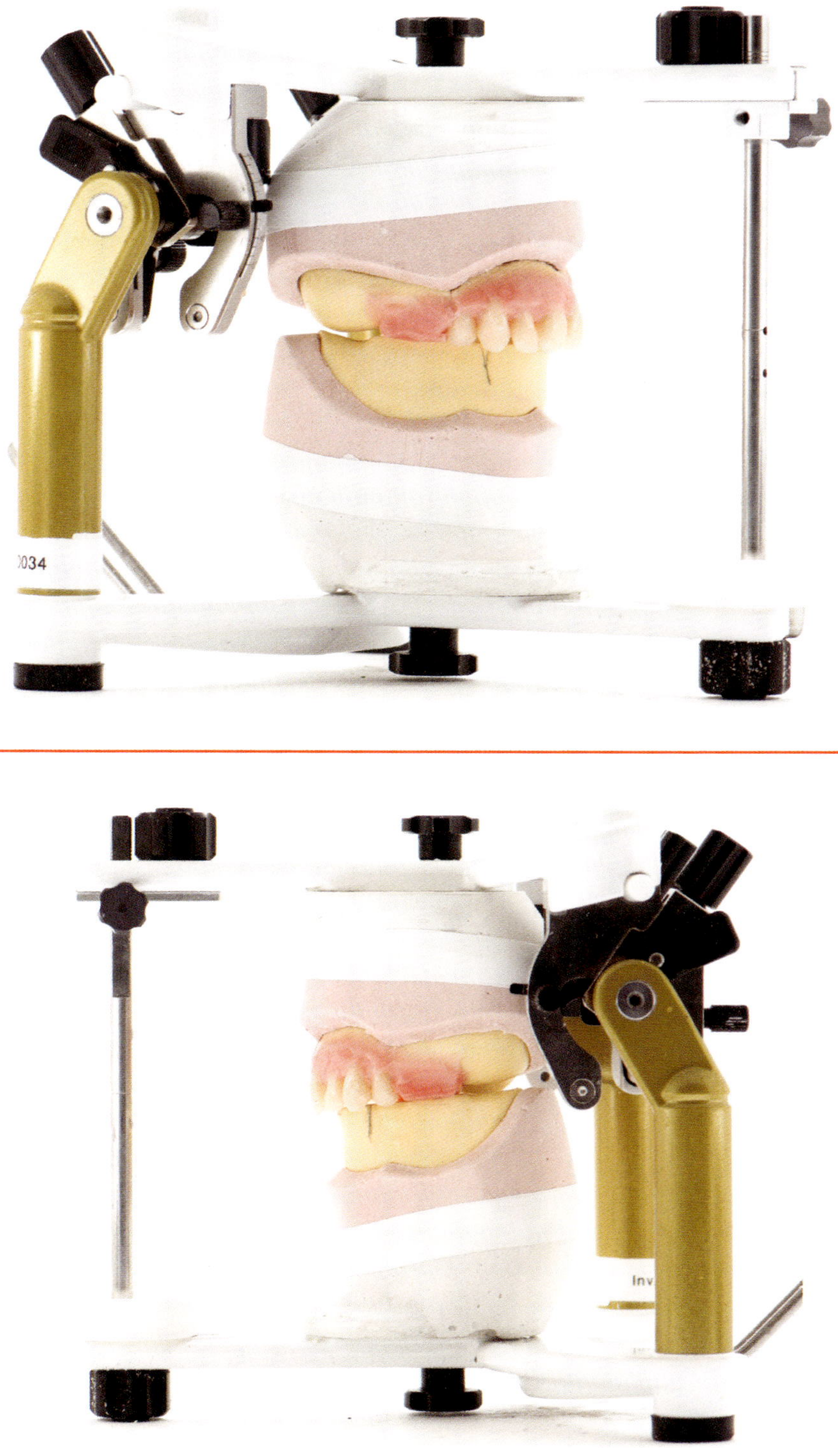

Figure 4.39 • Setting the front and upper teeth.

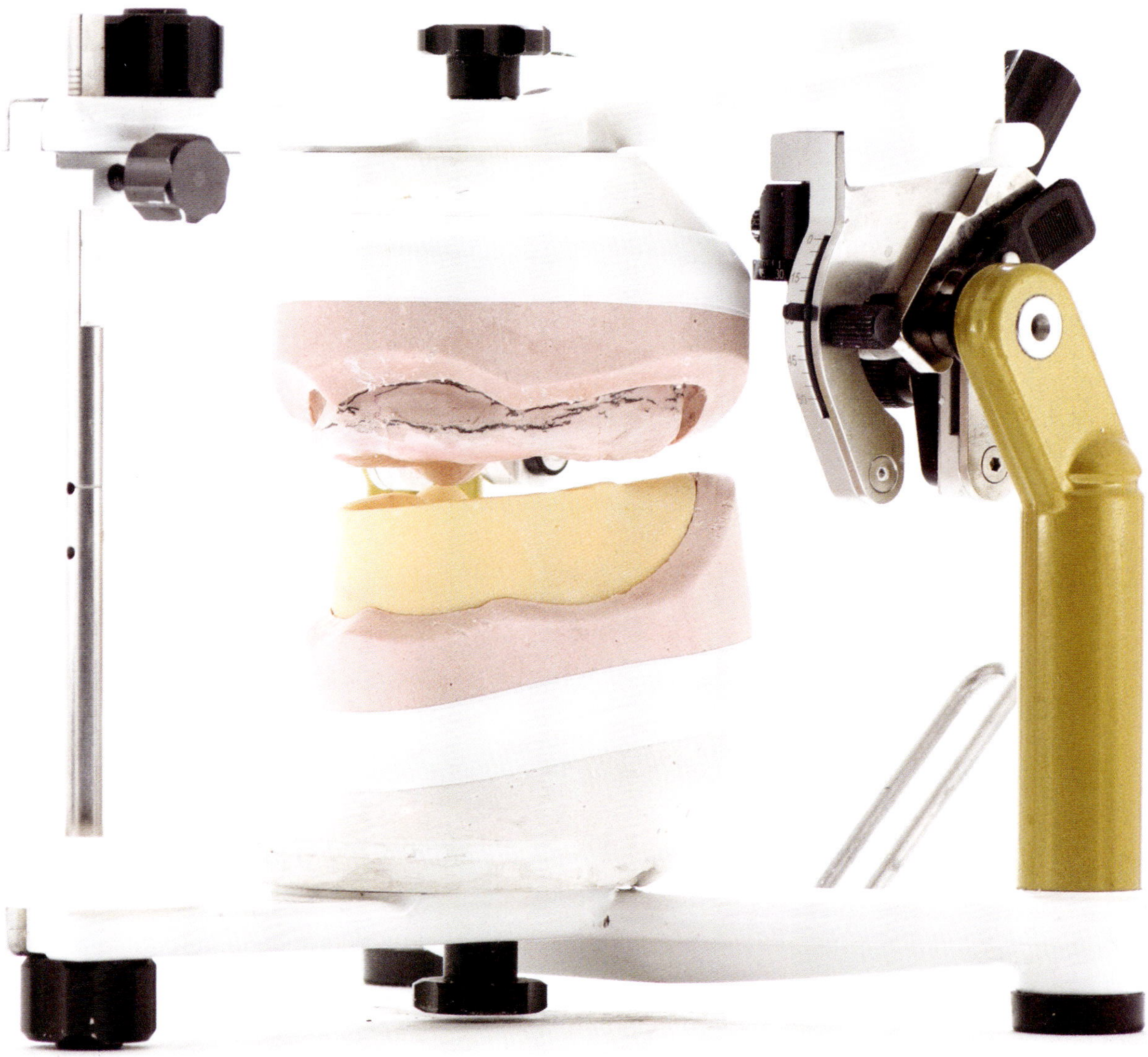

Figure 4.40 • Checking the upper prosthetic space.

Esthetic try-in and analysis of the neutral zone

In this stage it is possible to check a number of aspects before carrying out the complete mounting of the dentures.

It is possible to check the precision of the plates on the tissues, which are likely to be very close to the prosthetic bases. Obviously, in the presence of inaccurate plates or altered extensions of the bases they would need to be revised before proceeding further, by means of new registration of the impressions.

Then the esthetic, phonetic and occlusal parameters that were previously registered are analysed. First, the upper occlusal plane is considered with the Fox plane, then the chosen esthetic setup is assessed. This analysis must validate the size of the chosen dentures, the midline and their length and position with respect to the lips **(Figure 4.41)**.

By using the lower plate fabricated for the registration of the neutral zone, it is possible first of all to assess whether the chosen vertical dimension is adequate, as well as to establish whether the distribution of the prosthetic space between the upper and lower arch is satisfactory.

After making any corrections needed, the neutral zone is registered. It is defined as the virtual space taken up by the prosthesis, within which the forces generated by the lips and cheeks are in balance with those produced by the tongue. This principle is effective in order to be able to manage properly the overall dimensions of the lower prosthesis which often is subject to displacement precisely by the muscles that act in functional movements.

The registration of the neutral zone begins by making a cut in the resin rim in the anterior area of the first premolar on the right and left **(Figure 4.42)**.

The space that is thus created is filled with a material with a hardening time that is long enough to allow deformation and moulding by the muscles activated with functional movements. During this stage the patient will be asked to swallow, speak, open and close the mouth and to repeat these procedures several times, thus moulding the resin placed in the anterior space **(Figure 4.43)**.

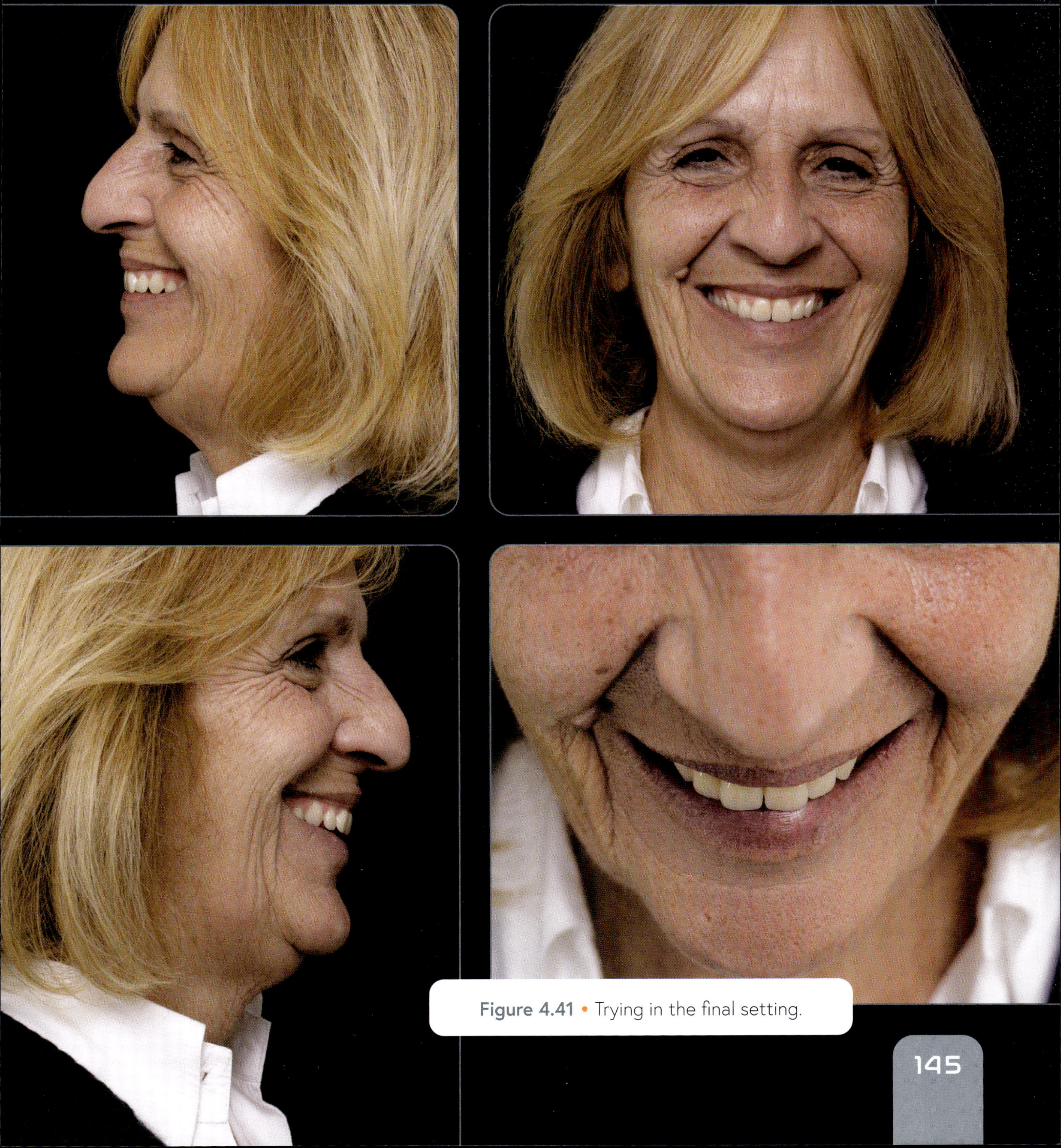

Figure 4.41 • Trying in the final setting.

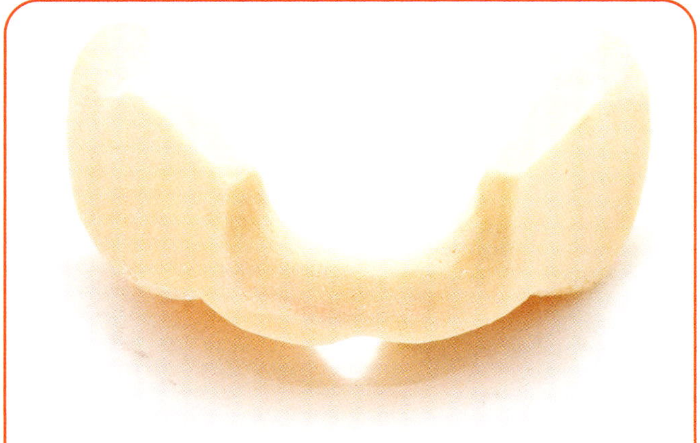

Figure 4.42 • Steps for registration of the neutral zone.

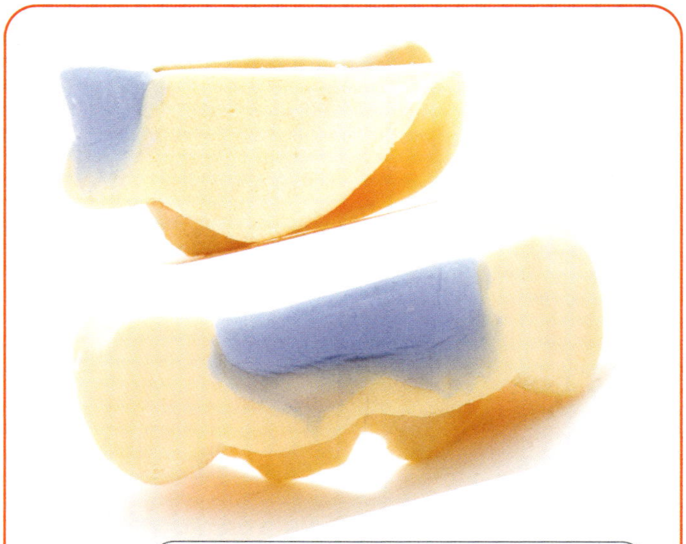

Figure 4.43 • Neutral zone, registration of the front part.

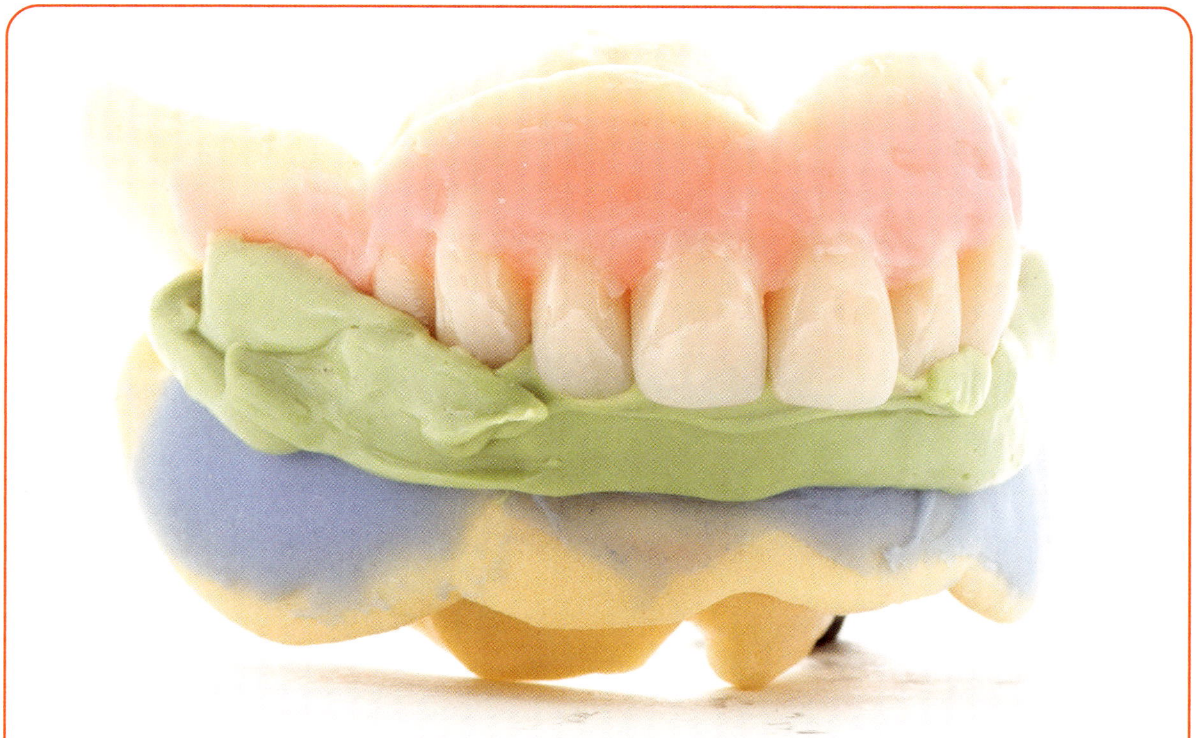

Figure 4.44 • Completed registration of the neutral zone.

After waiting for the hardening time of the material prepared for the anterior part, another quantity can be added to ensure adequate contact of the cheeks with the buccal surface of the posterior teeth. This is in order to ensure easier and more effective activity of the buccinator muscle when it retrieves the food bolus, after it has been pushed buccally by the mechanical action generated by the posterior teeth.

At the end of the registration, it is possible to make photos and videos for esthetic assessment with the laboratory and confirm the centric relation (**Figure 4.44**).

Complete setting of the teeth

Once the plates are received back from the test, the first thing to do is to check the centric relation in the articulator to ensure it is confirmed.

Then the dentures are mounted inside the registered neutral zone, starting with the first lower premolars for which the buccal cusp must be exactly in correspondence with the centre of the crest and at the same time positioned within the neutral zone. Since both these conditions must be met it is easy for the lingual part of the premolar to invade the vital space of the tongue, in this case the lingual part must therefore be reduced by transforming the tooth and making it similar to a canine. Finally, the lower fourth must be positioned slightly higher than the occlusal plane by about 1 mm.

Once the two premolars have been assembled, the lower six are chosen in order to close the anterior space between them. The incisors must have the same inclination as the neutral zone registration.

Each time the posterior teeth are set, one must take care to only remove from the customised rim the part in which the tooth will be positioned. The second premolar is mounted keeping the fossa in the centre of the ridge at the same height as the rim within the neutral zone. The first molar is positioned within the neutral zone with the fossa in the centre of the ridge; the mesial part will be placed at the height of the occlusal plane and the distal part will be slightly raised.

When positioning the upper posteriors, one starts with the first molars: from here one decides whether to perform normal occlusion or a crossbite.

In the case presented in this chapter, normal occlusion was chosen, the palatal cusp of the upper sixth was placed in occlusion in the fossa of the antagonist sixth and the palatal cusp of the second upper premolar in the fossa of the lower fifth.

Once the setting of the dentures is completed, the flanges are waxed and the gingiva is moulded, taking care not to leave residual wax on the teeth: in particular, the interdental papillae and the marginal gingiva must be defined **(Figure 4.45)**.

Final setting try-in

This appointment mainly aims at confirming the modifications that were made in light of the previous try-in **(Figure 4.46)**, where the goal is static positioning of the dentures. To perform this check, as previously explained in the similar test performed on the prosthesis the patient already has, one checks whether the load exerted causes a displacement of the prosthesis or otherwise.

In the event that one or more teeth should transmit a displacement force on the item, their positioning with respect to the centre of the ridge must be reviewed, bringing them more palatal or lingual depending on the arch considered.

At the same time, one ensures there is proper fit of the cheek with respect to the position of the dentures **(Figure 4.47)**.

The final esthetic assessments are made, making the necessary changes with regard to the position of the dentures and the abrasions to be made on them. At the end of this process it is essential to ensure the patient approves the esthetic design and that the general comfort level obtained with the try-in is satisfactory, before proceeding with finalisation. Finally, the compressibility of the tissues on the post-dam is assessed: the clinician makes a map of the compressible area, the posterior limit, under the plate, and also provides the laboratory with the resilience of the various points of the post-dam area **(Figure 4.48)**.

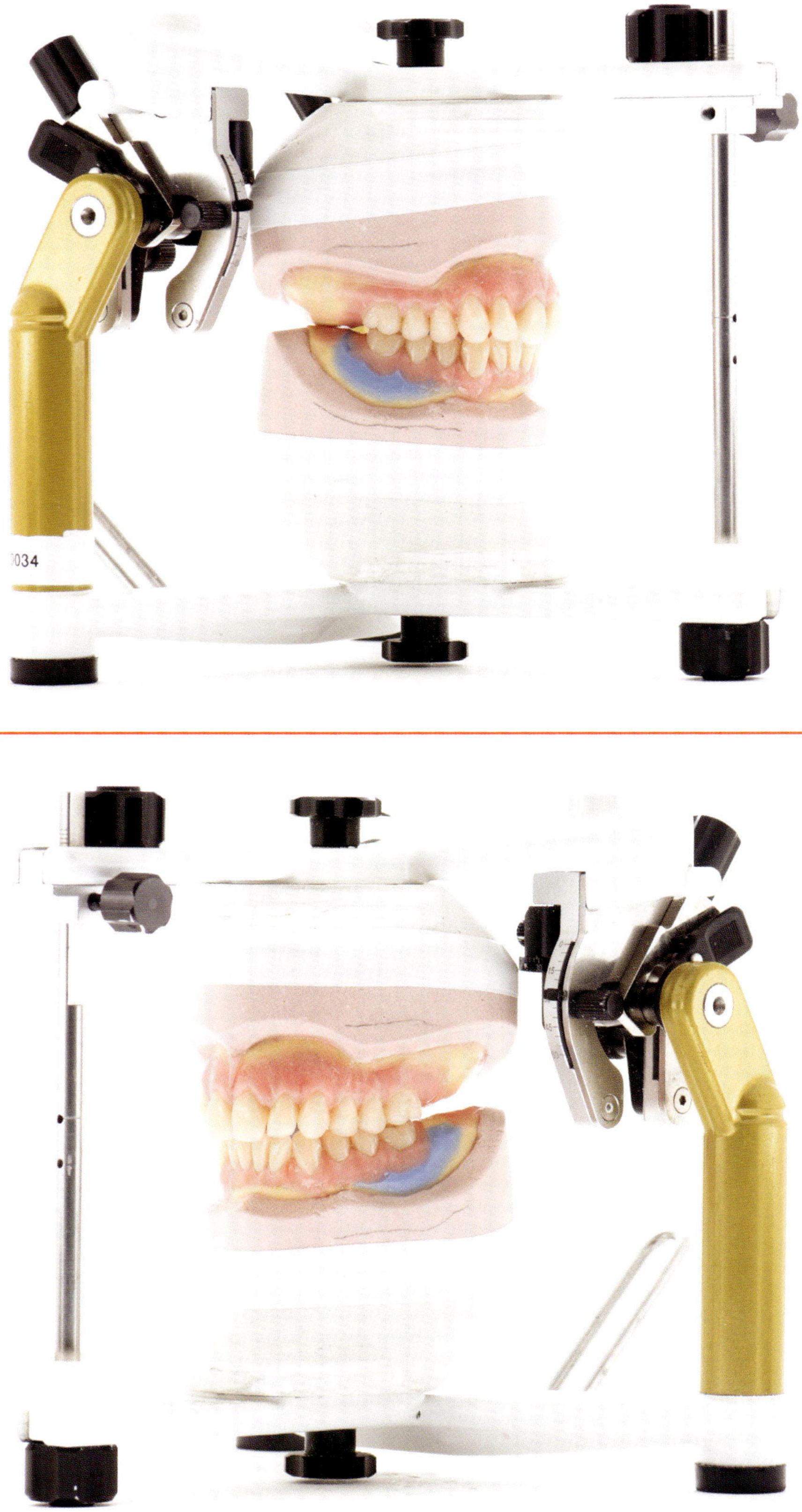

Figure 4.45 • Completed tooth setting.

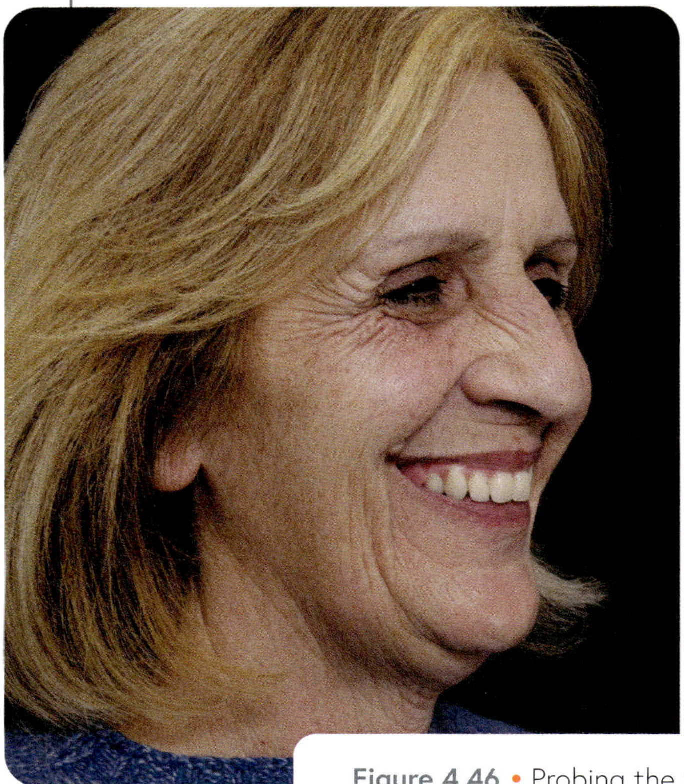

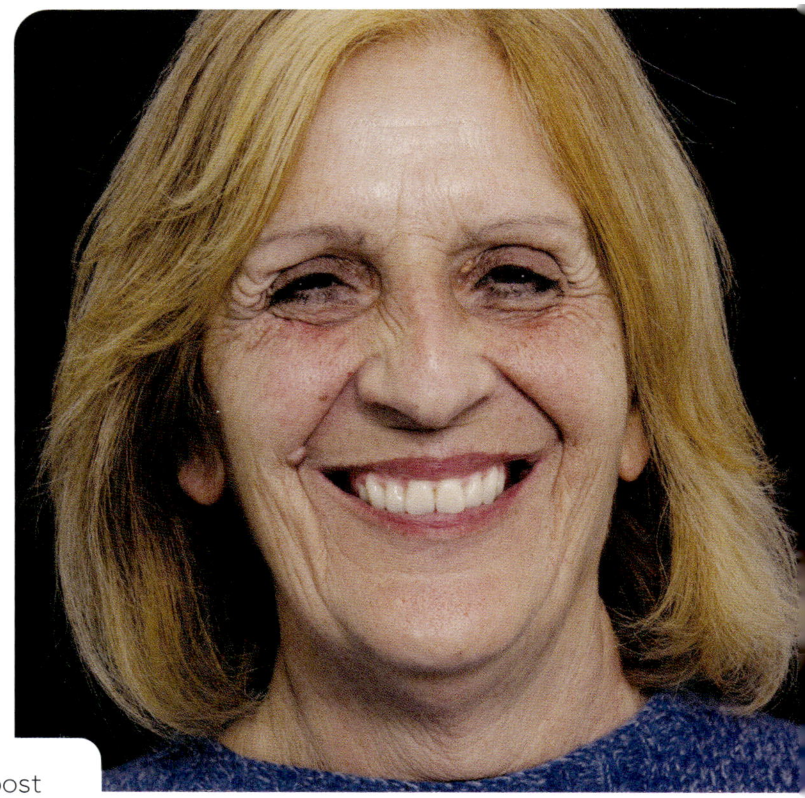

Figure 4.46 • Probing the post dam area and transferring the information on the base plate.

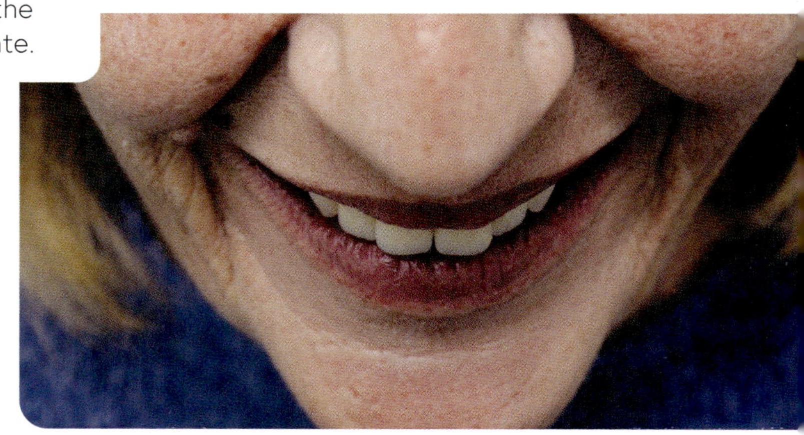

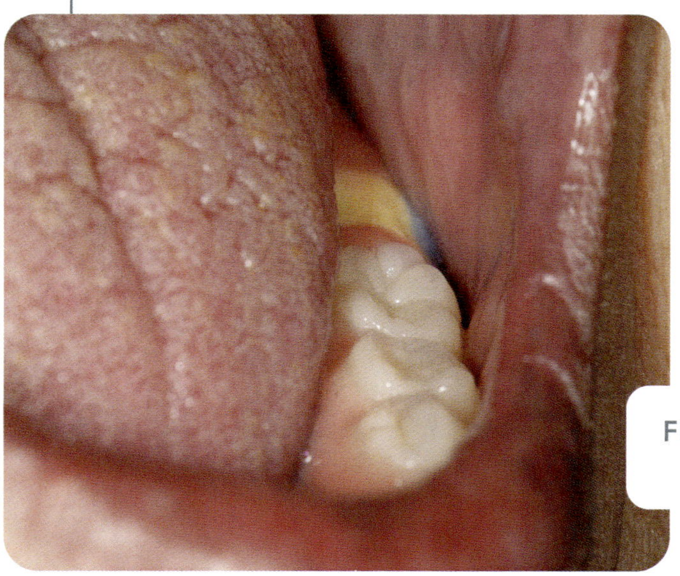

Figure 4.47 • Checking cheek fit.

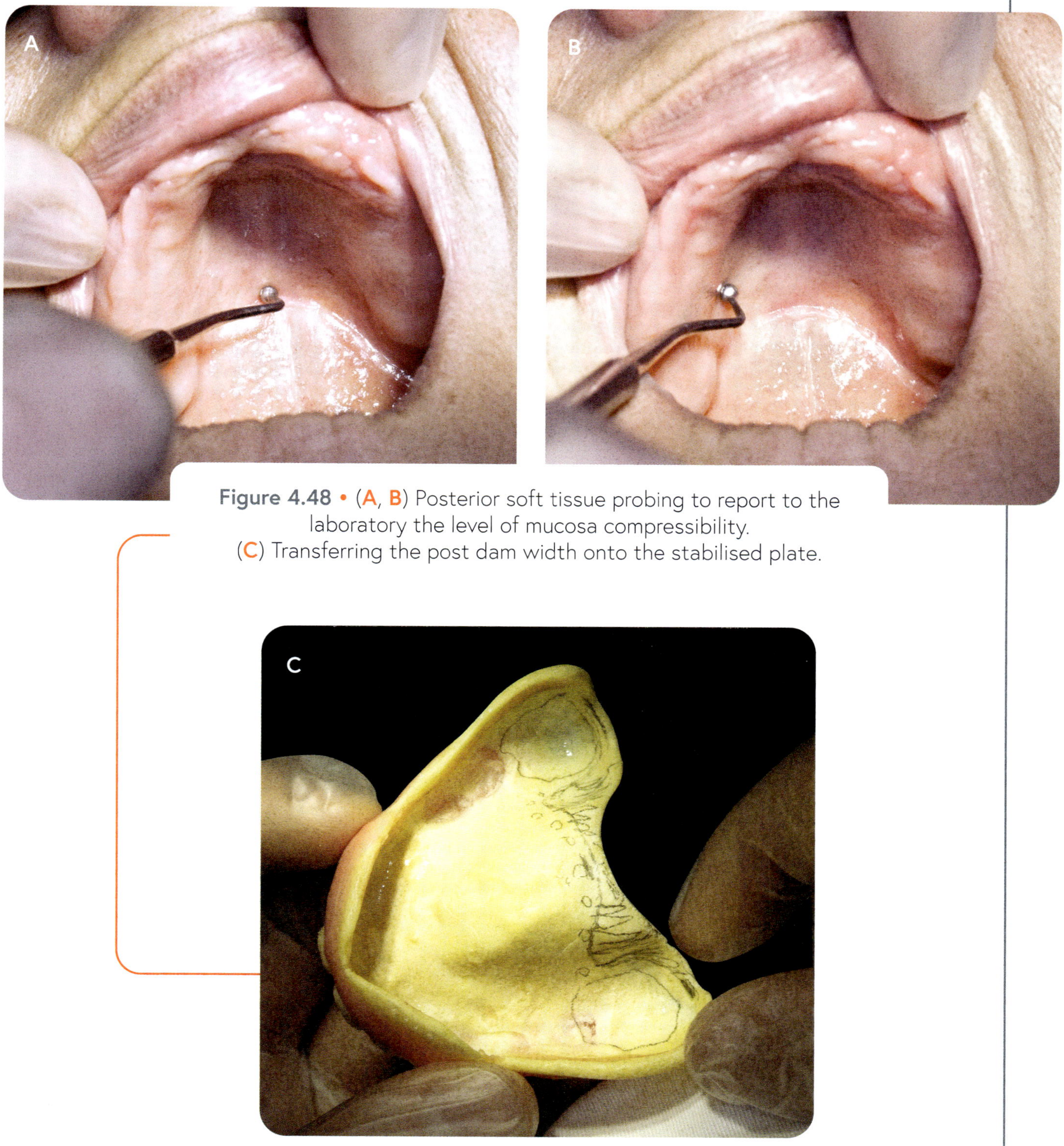

Figure 4.48 • (A, B) Posterior soft tissue probing to report to the laboratory the level of mucosa compressibility.
(C) Transferring the post dam width onto the stabilised plate.

Finalisation

The posterior limit, previously indicated, in terms of length as well as thickness due to the level of compressibility of the tissues is carved on the model with a ball burr of calibrated diameter according to the required depth. Insufficient precision of the prosthetic plate in this area results in a significant loss of retention because due to the shrinkage of the resin after curing, an actual gap is created between the master model and the support surface of the prosthesis.

Curing stage

Once the occlusal contacts have been checked again, the prostheses are locked onto the models; this operation must be carried out with the prostheses mounted in the articulator to avoid displacements. The models are immersed in cold water for about 10 minutes with the aim of saturating the plaster. Subsequently, the plaster is isolated with Vaseline, so that, once the curing stage is completed, the models can be easily removed from the flasks and mounted again in the articulator to carry out re-occlusion.

The models with the waxed prostheses must then be positioned in the flasks with level three plaster. To keep the position of the teeth stable during the resin curing stage, once the plaster of the mould is isolated, the dentures and part of the flange are covered with plaster. Finally, with closed flasks, the mould former is filled with the same plaster that is cast from above.

After this step, the flasks are placed in boiling water for about 7 minutes, in order to partially melt the wax and be able to open them, followed by washing and roughing from the remaining wax residues and a phase of isolation of the models and of the plaster on the mould and mould former.

Finally, the surface of the tooth heels is dulled to remove residual insulation and is treated with monomer, in order to improve the adhesion between dentures and palate resin **(Figure 4.49)**.

Then the resin is packed following the manufacturer's instructions. The closed flasks positioned inside a clamp are put under a hydraulic press and held for about 10 minutes at approximately 2 bars. Before releasing the pressure to remove them from the clamp, the screws of the bracket must be tightened to maintain pressure throughout the curing cycle.

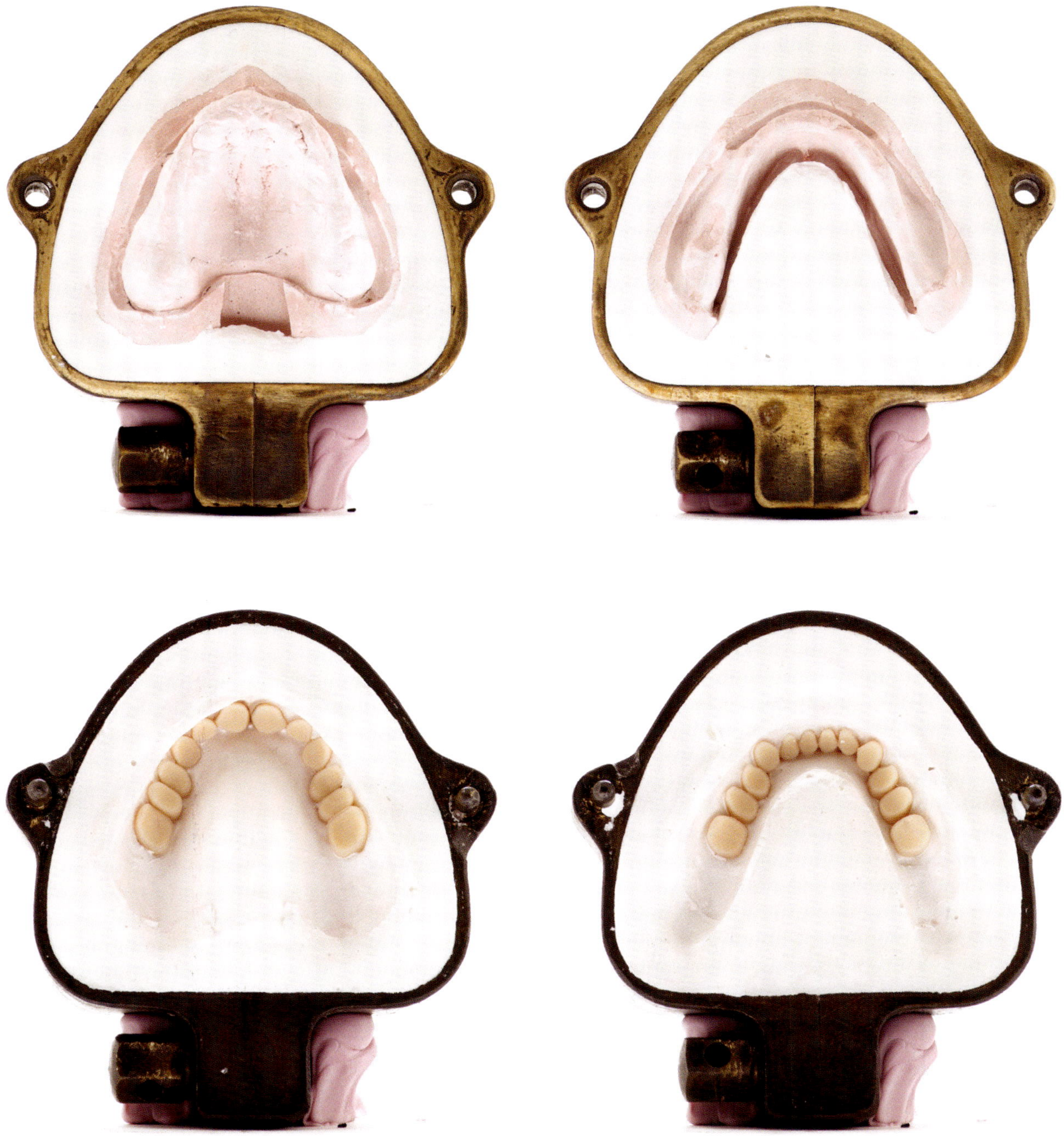

Figure 4.49 • Steps of hot curing with the conventional flask.

The clamped flasks are immersed in cold water. During the first hour, the water must reach the temperature of 70° C and keep it for the next eight hours to come to a boil (100° C) during the last half hour. When the cycle is completed, the flask is extracted and allowed to cool completely on the bench before opening it and releasing mould and counter mould polymerized protheses.

Re-occlusion

The prostheses, still placed on the models, are reassembled in the articulator to correct any occlusal discrepancies caused by curing of the resin and to achieve balanced occlusion in all mandibular movements **(Figure 4.50)**.

Balanced occlusion occurs when in mandibular movements – laterality, protrusion and retrusion – all the pairs of antagonists on both sides come into contact simultaneously.

In the protrusive movement it is preferable that in addition to the contacts of the antagonist pairs of the lateral sector, contacts are also established between the central ones.

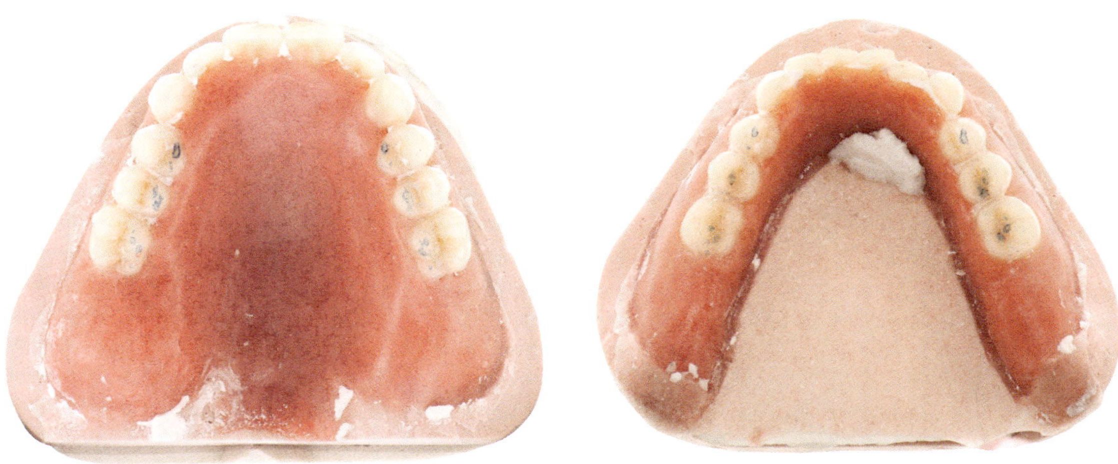

Figure 4.50 • Occlusal check after curing.

Finishing and polishing

After occlusion is restored, the prostheses are finished paying the utmost attention to the borders. They are polished only using water and pumice with the polishing wheel with low speed brushes. In addition, any plaster residues can be removed by using a sandblaster, using microbeads at 2 atm and a water sandblaster, or by immersing the prostheses in ultrasound bath with appropriate liquids.

Polishing is carried out with the brushes normally used for prophylaxis with pumice, in order not to damage the details of the gingival tissue. The rest of the prosthesis is polished with the appropriate brushes and polishing pastes (**Figure 4.51**).

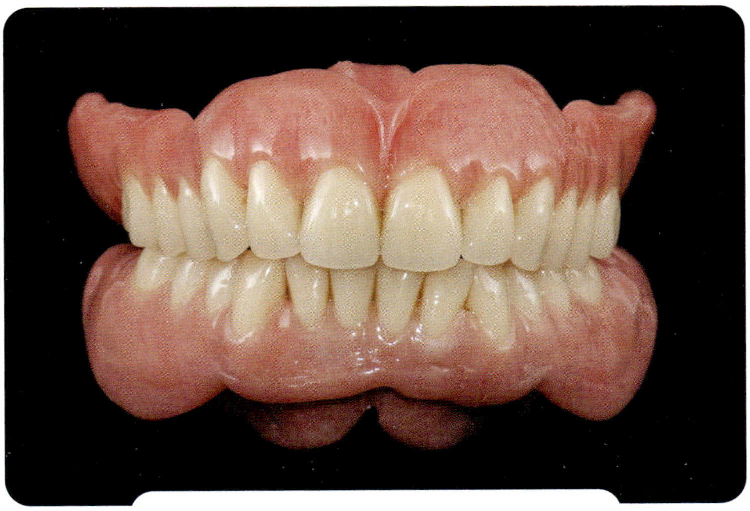

Figure 4.51 • Polished prostheses.

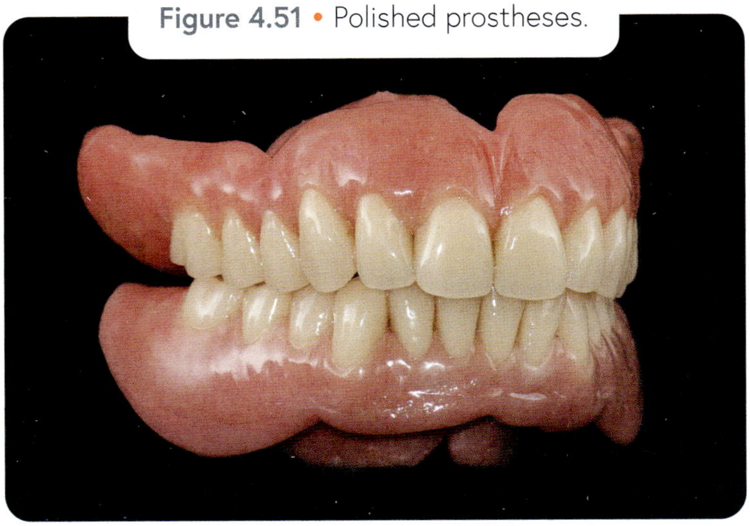

Delivery and follow-up

The appointment for delivering the prosthesis to the patient is one of the most important stages of the rehabilitation process. Small modifications can be made and some aspects can be perfected such as the fit of the prostheses to the tissues or some esthetic corrections can be made. However, should one notice occlusal problems, it might be useful to schedule re-mounting in the articulator after a few days.

The first check to be carried out regards the fit on the plates and borders. However, it should be remembered that, before performing this check, it is best to wait a few minutes so that tissue resilience is overcome and the prosthesis fits appropriately. That is why the patient is asked to bite into cotton rolls.

The check of the bases entails fitting to the tissues as well as length and thickness of the borders, subsequently an occlusal analysis can be performed **(Figure 4.52)**.

However, the actual occlusal check can be performed when the resilience of the tissues is completely overcome. The instructions on hygiene, diet and prosthesis management by the patient over the coming days are also an integral part of the delivery. Finally, the end esthetic result is assessed **(Figure 4.53)**.

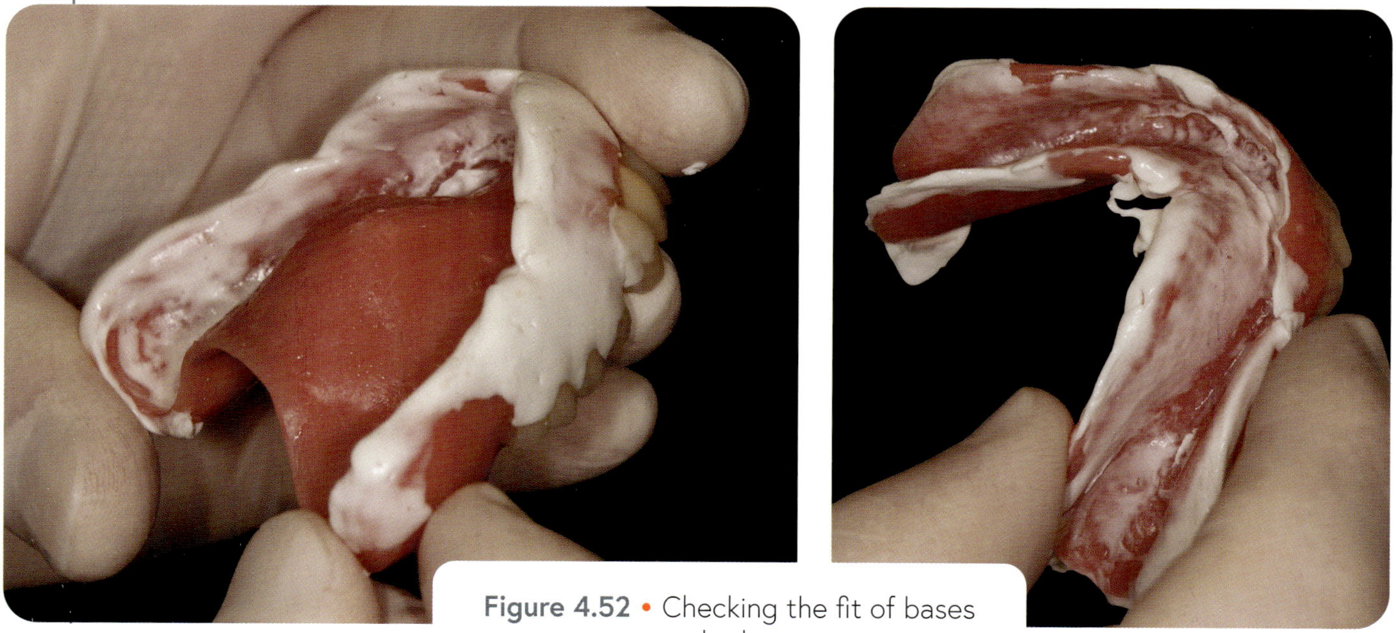

Figure 4.52 • Checking the fit of bases and edges.

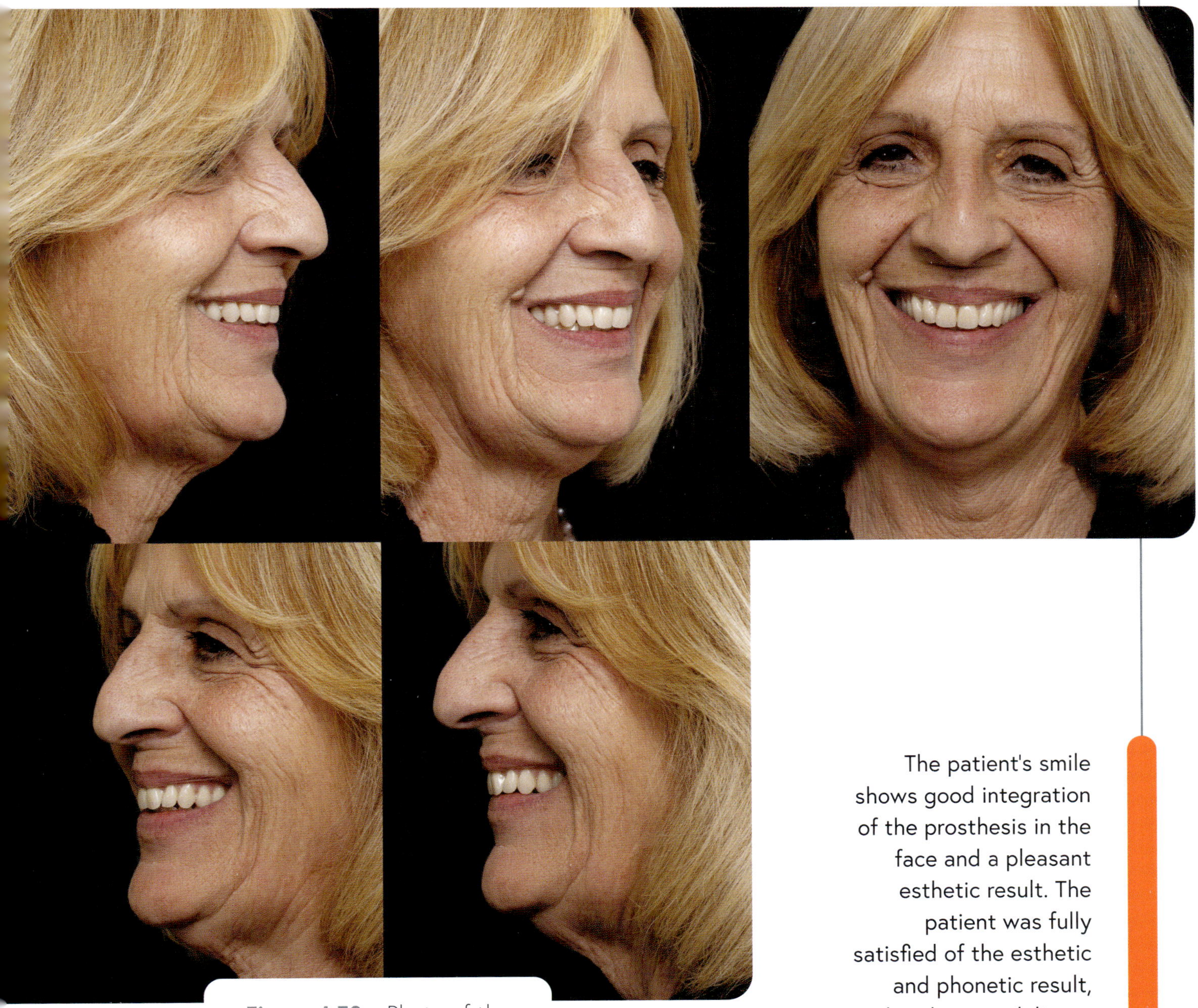

Figure 4.53 • Photo of the patient's face upon delivery.

The patient's smile shows good integration of the prosthesis in the face and a pleasant esthetic result. The patient was fully satisfied of the esthetic and phonetic result, already upon delivery. Adapting to the new prostheses was very quick also from a functional point of view.

References

1. Ogden A. *Guidelines in Prosthetic and Implant Dentistry*. Quintessence Publishing Co. Ltd; 1996. pp. 7-11.
2. Testori T, Parenti A, Perrotti G et al. *Trattamento delle edentulie totali: protocolli diagnostici e clinici*. 2014. pp. 365-85.
3. Ceruti P, Mobilio N, Bellia E et al. Simplified edentulous treatment: A multicenter randomized controlled trial to evaluate the timing and clinical outcomes of the technique. *J Prosthet Dent*. 2017;118(4):462-7.
4. ISTAT. *Il ricorso alle cure odontoiatriche*. ISTAT; 2015.
5. Ivanhoe JR, Cibirka RM, Parr GR. Treating the modern complete denture patient: A review of the literature. *J Prosthet Dent*. 2002;88(6):631-5.
6. Stewart H. bioestetica.pdf. Contemporary Esthetic;
7. Pound E. Let /S/ be your guide. *J Prosthet Dent*. 1977 Nov;38(5):482-9.
8. Burnett CA, Clifford TJ. Closest speaking space during the production of sibilant sounds and its value in establishing the vertical dimension of occlusion. *J Dent Res*. 1993;72(6):964-7.
9. Showa J. The use of phonetics in determining the vertical dimension of occlusion. *J Showa Univ Dent Soc*. 1983;2(2):139-47.
10. Davies SJ, Gray RMJ, Smith PW. Good occlusal practice in simple restorative dentistry. *Br Dent J*. 2001;191(7):365-81.
11. Kuniyal H, Katoch N, Rao PL. Occlusal plane orientor: An innovative and efficient device for occlusal plane orientation. *J Indian Prosthodont Soc*. 2012;12(2):78-80.
12. Ferrario VF, Sforza C, Serrao G, Ciusa V. A direct in vivo measurement of the three-dimensional orientation of the occlusal plane and of the sagittal discrepancy of the jaws. *Orthod Craniofacial Res*. 2000;3(1):15-22.
13. O'Callaghan MC. Using diagnostic impressions to evaluate the fit of existing removable prostheses. *J Am Dent Assoc*. 2001;132(8):1128-9.
14. Hummel SK, Wilson MA, Marker VA, Nunn ME. Quality of removable partial dentures worn by the adult U.S. population. *J Prosthet Dent*. 2002;88(1):37-43.
15. Sabir S, Regragui A, Merzouk N. Maintaining occlusal stability by selecting the most appropriate occlusal scheme in complete removable prosthesis. *Jpn Dent Sci Rev*. 2019;55(1):145-50.
16. Troendle GR, Troendle KB. Polyvinyl siloxane as a disclosing medium. *J Prosthet Dent*. 1992;68(6):983-4.
17. Shetty MS, Shenoy KK. Techniqu es for evaluating the fit of removable and fixed prosthesis. *ISRN Dent*. 2011;2011(4):1-4.
18. Chan CA. A review of the clinical significance of the occlusal plane. its variation and effect of head posture. *Int Coll CranioMandib Orthop Anthol*. 2007;1-63.
19. Desjardins RP. The tongue as it relates to complete dentures. *J Am Dent Assoc*. 1974;88(4):814-22.
20. To P, Complete O, Dentures R, Boyle H a. Practical to occlusion complete. 1951;
21. Niedermeier W, Huber M, Fischer D et al. Significance of saliva for the denture-wearing population. *Gerodontology*. 2000;17(2):104-18.
22. Niedermeier WHW, Krämer R. Salivary secretion and denture retention. *J Prosthet Dent*. 1992;67(2):211-6.
23. Acharya S, Lohe V, Bhowate R. Evaluation and comparison of alveolar bone loss of maxilla and mandible in completely edentulous patients on digital panoramic radiographs. *J Oral Med Oral Surgery, Oral Pathol Oral Radiol*. 2016;2(3):112.
24. Jivraj S, Chee W, Corrado P. Treatment planning of the edentulous maxilla. *Br Dent J*. 2006;201(5):261-79.
25. Passamonti G, Vergnano A. Atlante di protesi totale. CIDES ODONTO, Torino 1978.
26. Fernandes A, Dua N, Herekar M. Corrective primary impression technique. *Open Dent J*. 2010;4(1):27-8.
27. Golden WG, Driscoll CF. *Making the preliminary impression*. Wiley-Blackwell; 2020. pp. 5-15
28. Vrespa D, Ferretti G, Augusti G. I materiali di impronta. *Il Dentista Moderno*. 2014;30-44.
29. Jone A, Jain AR. Clinical demonstration of border molding using various materials: a review. *J Pharm Res*. 2018;12(2):185-9.
30. Solomon EGR. Single stage silicone border molded closed mouth impression technique – Part II. *J Indian Prosthodont Soc*. 2011;11(3):183-8.
31. Daou EE. The elastomers for complete denture impression: A review of the literature. *Saudi Dent J*. 2010;22(4):153-60.

32. Carlsson GE, Örtorp A, Omar R. What is the evidence base for the efficacies of different complete denture impression procedures? A critical review. *J Dent.* 2013;41(1):17-23.
33. Golden WG, Driscoll CF. *Treating the complete denture patient.* Wiley-Blackwell; 2020. pp. 17-23.
34. Smith PW, Richmond R, McCord JF. The design and use of special trays in prosthodontics: Guidelines to improve clinical effectiveness. *Br Dent J.* 1999;187(8):423-6.
35. Kresnoadi U, Rostiny R. Closed mouth method with dynamic and muco compressive impression on upper and lower jaw flat ridges for aid full denture retention. *Dent J (Majalah Kedokt Gigi).* 2007;40(4):193.
36. Plates FB. *Base plates and occlusion rims. Treating the Complete Denture Patient.* Wiley-Blackwell; 2020. pp. 51-56.
37. Abbas H, Bulad K. Complete denture achievement in three visits. 2016;5-7.
38. Inamdar AHMA, Dange SP, Mahale KM, Khalikar SA. A device for occlusal plane determination. *J Indian Prosthodont Soc.* 2019;19:93-6.
39. Turrell AJW. Clinical assessment of vertical dimension. *J Prosthet Dent.* 2006;96(2):79-83.
40. Freitas de Souza R, Marra J, Carolina Pero A, Antonio Compagnoni M. Effect of denture fabrication and wear on closest speaking space and interocclusal distance during deglutition. *J Prosthet Dent.* 2007;97(6):381-8.
41. Marin DOM, Leite ARP, De Oliveira Junior NM et al. Reestablishment of occlusal vertical dimension in complete denture wearing in two stages. *Case Rep Dent.* 2015;2015:762914.
42. Driscoll J. Changing vertical dimension: a solution or problem? *Sth Hosp.* 1973;41(3):15-6.
43. McGee GF. Use of facial measurements in determining vertical dimension. *J Am Dent Assoc.* 1947;35(5):342-50.
44. Al-Ahmar AO, Lynch CD, Locke M, Youngson CC. Quality of master impressions and related materials for fabrication of complete dentures in the UK. *J Oral Rehabil.* 2008;35(2):111-5.
45. Porwal A, Sasaki K. Current status of the neutral zone: A literature review. *J Prosthet Dent.* 2013;109(2):129-34.
46. Beresin VE, Schiesser FJ. The neutral zone in complete denture. *Educ Forum.* 1969;33(3):342.

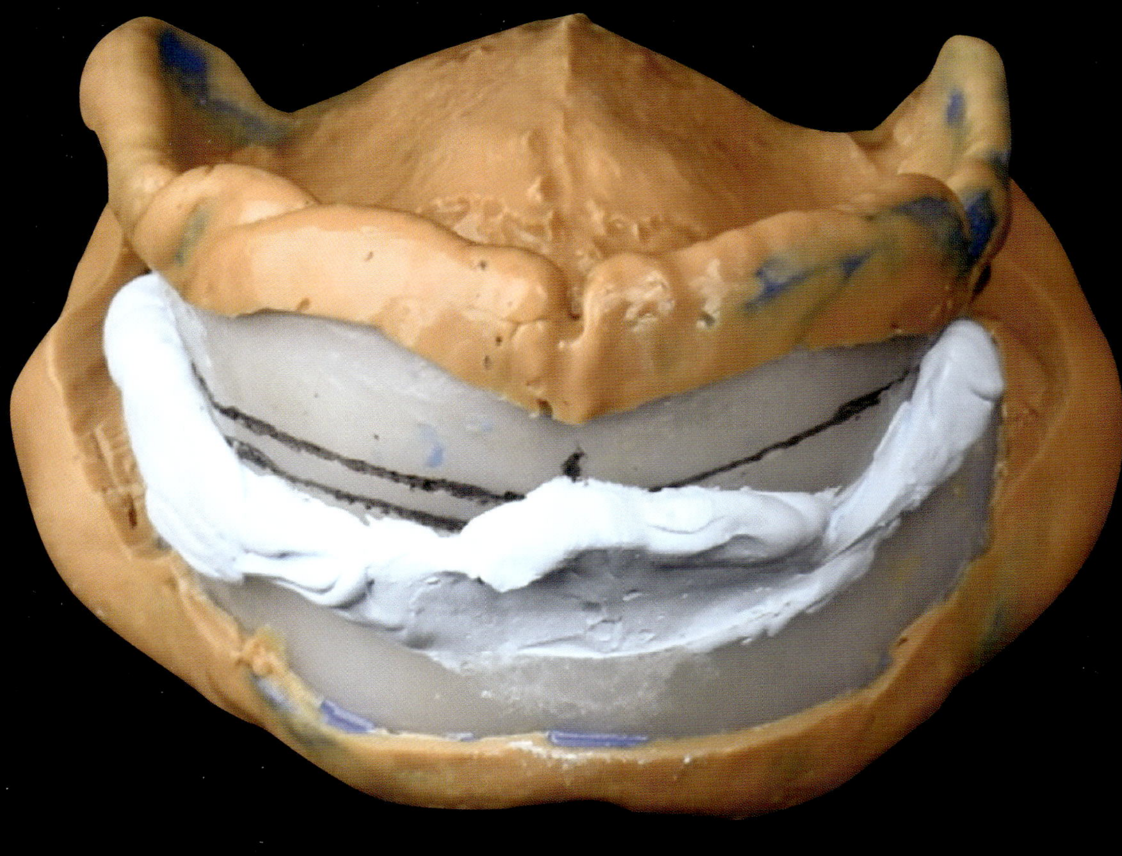

CHAPTER 5

P. VENEZIA, P. LACASELLA

Digital Denture: CAD/CAM protocols in total prosthesis

CAD/CAM technologies (Computer Aided Design/Computer Aided Manufacturing) have been adopted in dentistry starting from the early 1980s. Their use has especially concerned dental laboratories and has made it possible to significantly reduce their production lead times [1]. CAD/CAM procedures have become an indispensable factor in prosthetics. In the past, however, attention focused mainly on fixed restorations and the idea to make full dentures with CAD/CAM procedures did not seem very realistic until a few years ago [2,3].

In recent years, digital workflows have been proposed for the design and production of removable partial prostheses, although there is still a lack of long-term data to validate the clinical applicability of these processes [4-7].

Within digital workflows in dentistry, fabrication of total prostheses is the last to have been described. Historically, the first published experimental papers date back to the mid 1990s [8].

The protocol used by the Author entails use in the laboratory of a five-axis milling machine, a bench scanner and CAD software (3Shape); for the finalisation of the prosthetic rehabilitation with upper and lower removable total prosthesis, four clinical stages are required, with three laboratory stages in between.

Clinical stage 1

The following steps are carried out during the first clinical stage, illustrated below in the chapter:

- taking the primary impressions;
- registration of the preliminary occlusion vertical dimension (OVD) and of the intermaxillary relations;
- registration of Camper's plane and of the bipupillary line.

Primary impressions

The case presented in the chapter refers to the rehabilitation of a patient fully edentulous for about two years **(Figure 5.1)**. For the primary impression, an elastomer from the polyvinyl-siloxane family and the double impression technique were used, with materials of varying viscosities (Virtual®, Ivoclar Vivadent, Schaan Liechtenstein).

The trade impression tray was treated with specific adhesive (Virtual® Tray Adhesive, Ivoclar Vivadent). The base paste and the catalyst were mixed manually in equal quantities (Virtual® Putty Regular Set) and the impression of the upper arch was taken **(Figure 5.2)**. Areas of excessive compression were discharged with a micromotor handpiece at low speed and using a tungsten carbide burr (Imperial no. 500.104.198.110.023).

The impression procedure was completed thanks to the use of low viscosity silicone (Virtual® Light Body Regular Set, Ivoclar Vivadent), complying with the setting and hardening times indicated by the manufacturer. The same procedure was adopted for the impression of the lower edentulous arch **(Figure 5.3)**.

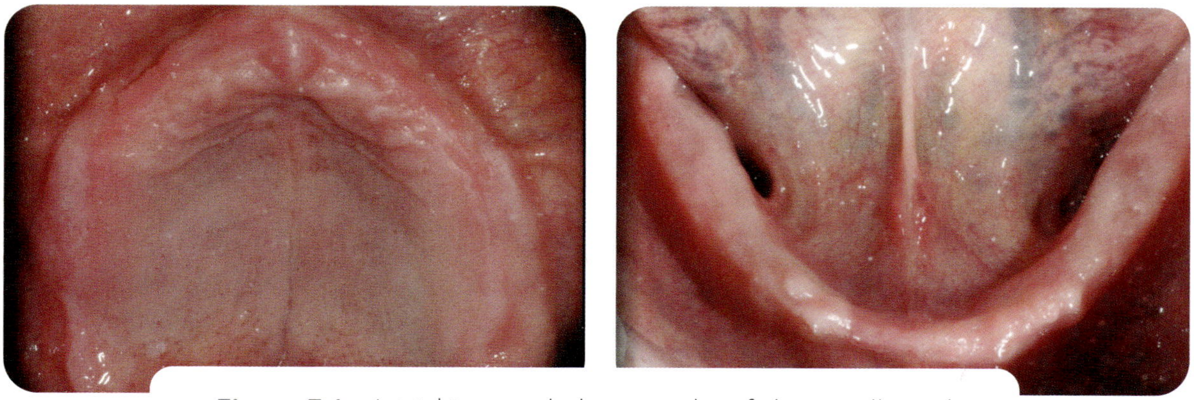

Figure 5.1 • Initial intraoral photographs of the maxilla and mandible of the patient's edentulous condition.

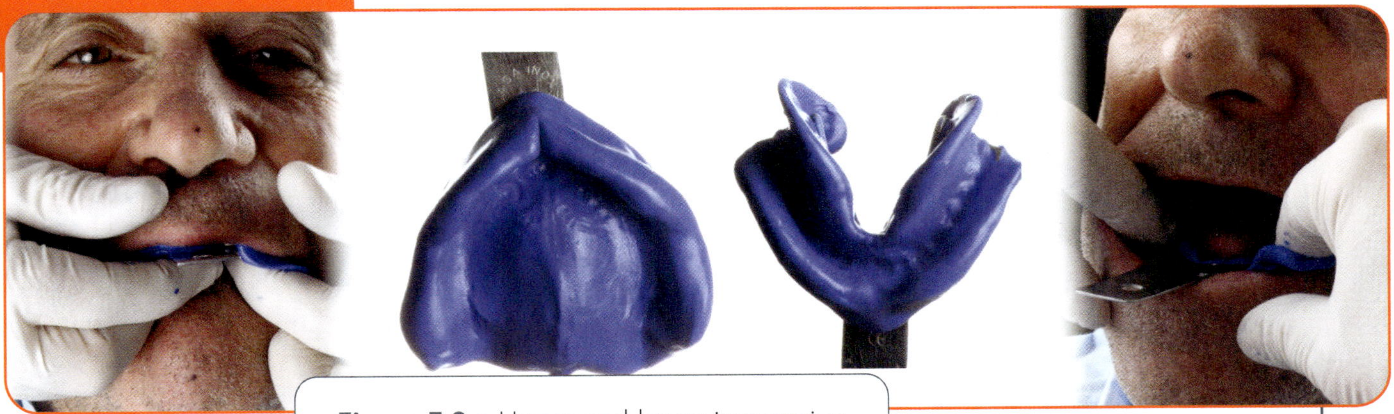

Figure 5.2 • Upper and lower impression with silicone putty.

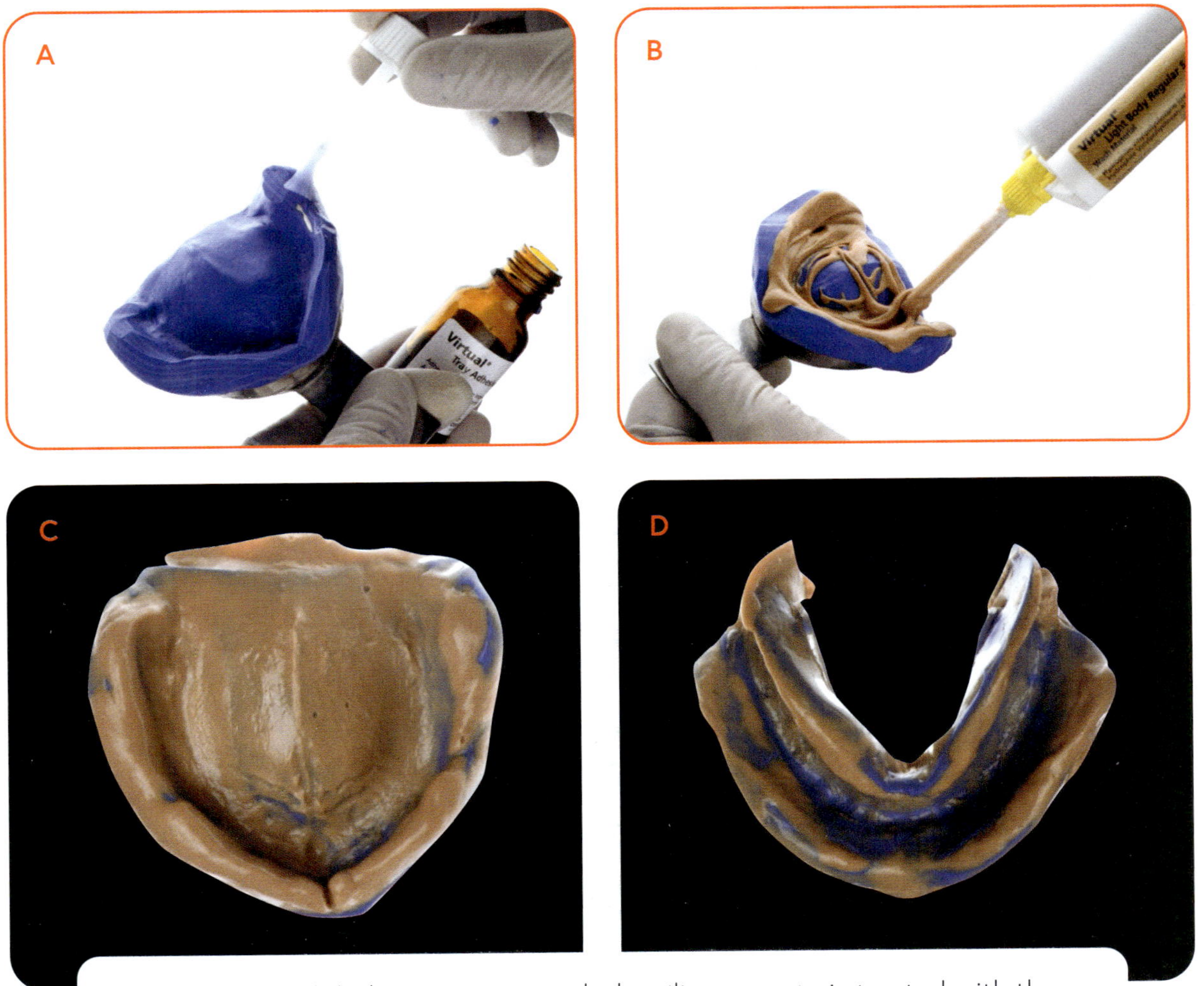

Figure 5.3 • (**A**) The impression with the silicone paste is treated with the adhesive (Virtual® Tray Adhesive, Ivoclar Vivadent, Schaan Liechtenstein). (**B**) The low viscosity silicone (Virtual® Light Body Regular Set, Ivoclar Vivadent, Schaan Liechtenstein) is placed on the surface of the previous impression to be able to record the anatomical details. (**C**) The upper arch impression is taken. (**D**) The lower arch impression is taken.

Registration of the preliminary OVD and of the intermaxillary relations in the sagittal direction

The next step concerned registration of a "preliminary" OVD.

Two landmark points were marked on the skin and their distance was measured in the jaw rest position.

This value corresponds to the occlusal Free Way Space (FWS) which on average ranges between 3 and 5 mm, although this measurement varies from person to person. The preliminary occlusion vertical dimension was estimated as 3 mm lower than that previously registered in rest position.

The Centric Tray instrument was used to measure the intermaxillary relations (Ivoclar Vivadent). This device consists of a plastic support with standard stabilisers of the impression material and movable fins that can be adapted in relation to the dimensions of the arches to be registered. The displacement of the impression material is prevented also by a retention edge. A vestibular shield allows the labial support required for the patient's esthetic and functional rehabilitation to be assessed. The material used for the registration was Virtual® Putty Regular Set (Ivoclar Vivadent) **(Figure 5.4)**.

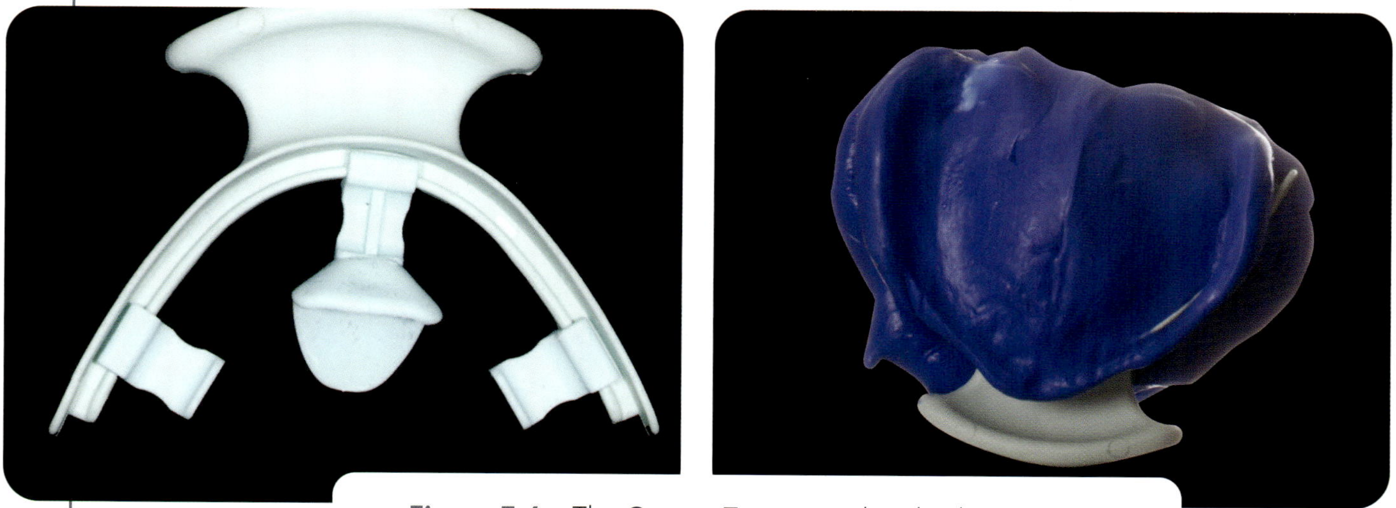

Figure 5.4 • The Centric Tray is used with silicone putty (Virtual® Putty Regular Set, Ivoclar Vivadent, Schaan Liechtenstein) to be able to register the intermaxillary relations.

The patient was guided to close at an OVD 3 mm shorter than the resting vertical dimension measured previously (**Figure 5.5**).

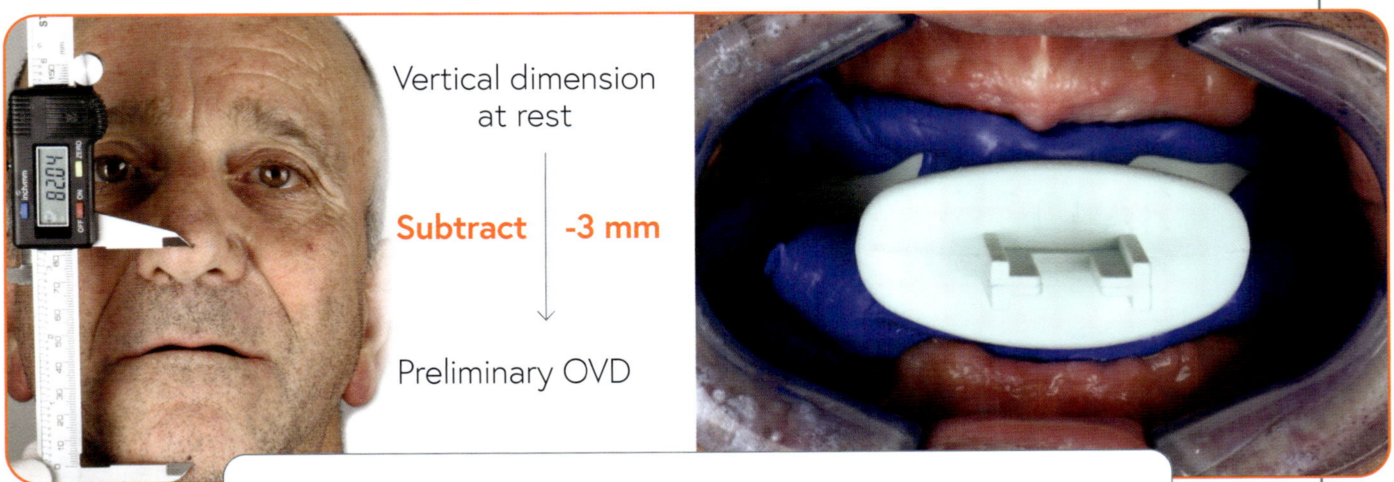

Figure 5.5 • Two fixed anatomical points are registered on the skin and their distance at rest is calculated. The patient is then guided to preliminary OVD closure 3 mm less than the measurement taken previously.

Registration of Camper's plane and of the bipupillary line

After the impression material hardened, the UTS CAD (Ivoclar Vivadent), an instrument very similar to the Fox plane, was attached to the Centric Tray. This device is extremely light and sturdy because it is made of carbon fibre (**Figure 5.6**).

The side arms of the UTS CAD must be set parallel to the Camper's Plane (CP). When their position is correct, the CP fixing screw can be tightened (**Figure 5.7**).

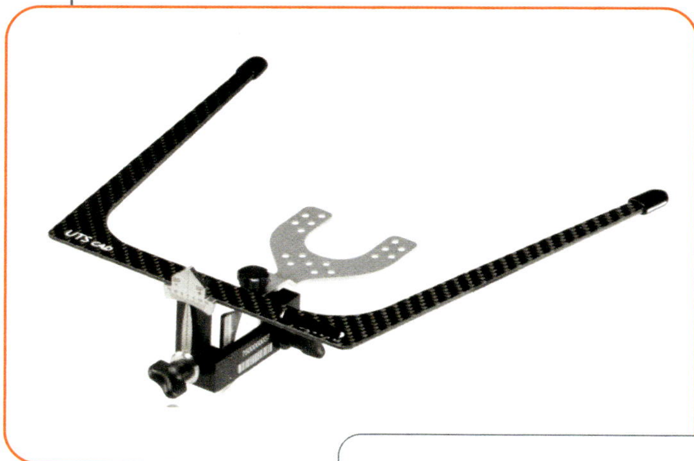

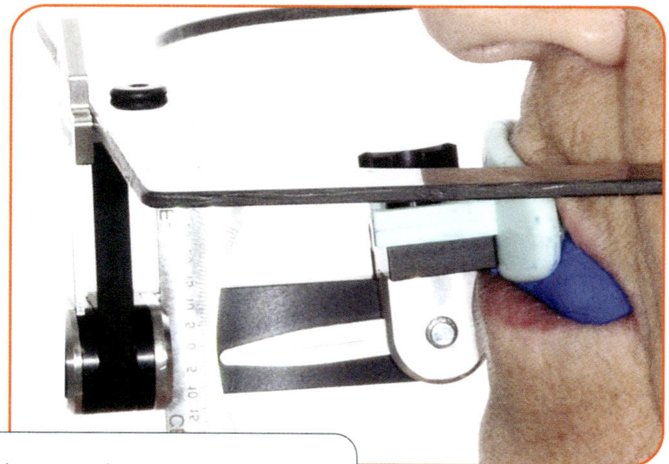

Figure 5.6 • UTS CAD (Ivoclar Vivadent), instrument to measure the Camper plane.

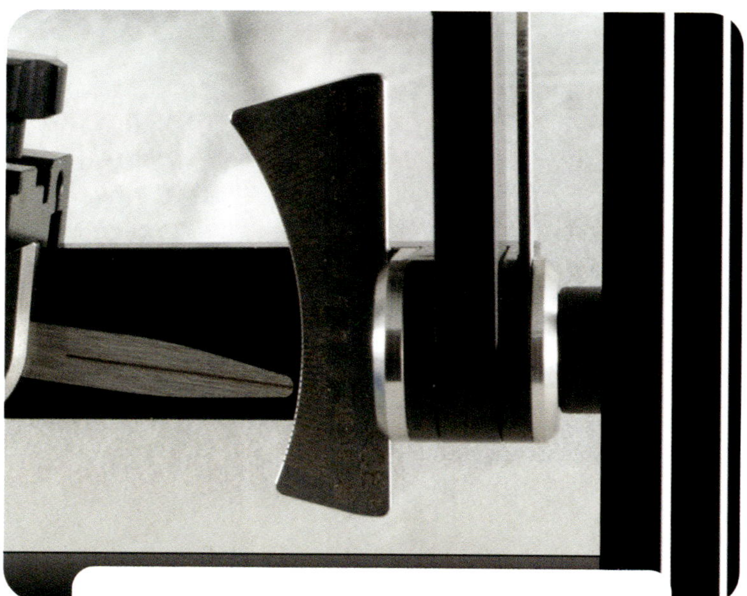

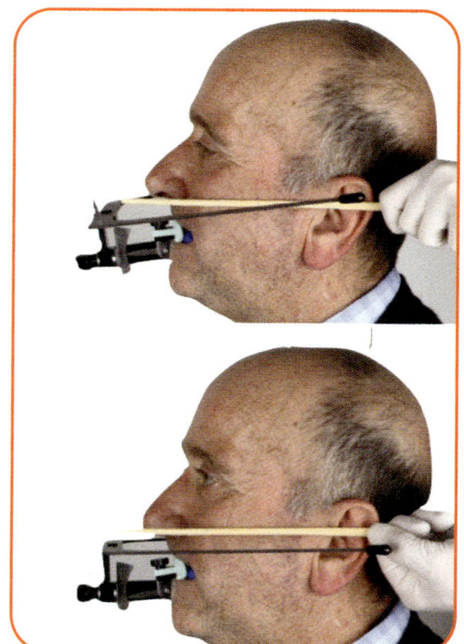

Figure 5.7 • The Camper plane is registered by locking its fixing screw.

Then the front arm of the bow is adjusted so it is parallel to the bipupillary line (BL). After adjusting, the joint can be fixed with the BL screw **(Figure 5.8)**. The measured CP/BL angular discrepancies (in excess or in defect) are communicated to the laboratory and can be transferred within the prosthesis design software in order to produce the correct spatial orientation of the virtual models **(Figure 5.9)**.

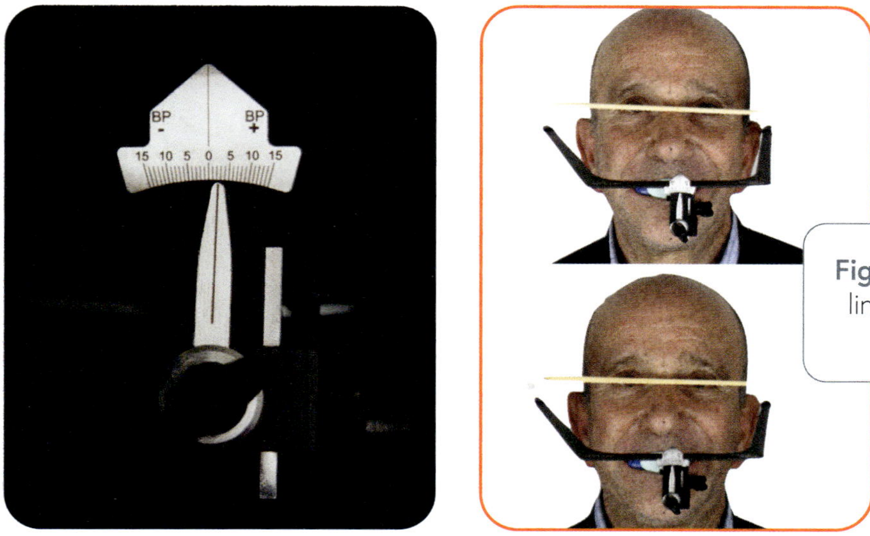

Figure 5.8 • The bipupillary line is registered by fixing the screw.

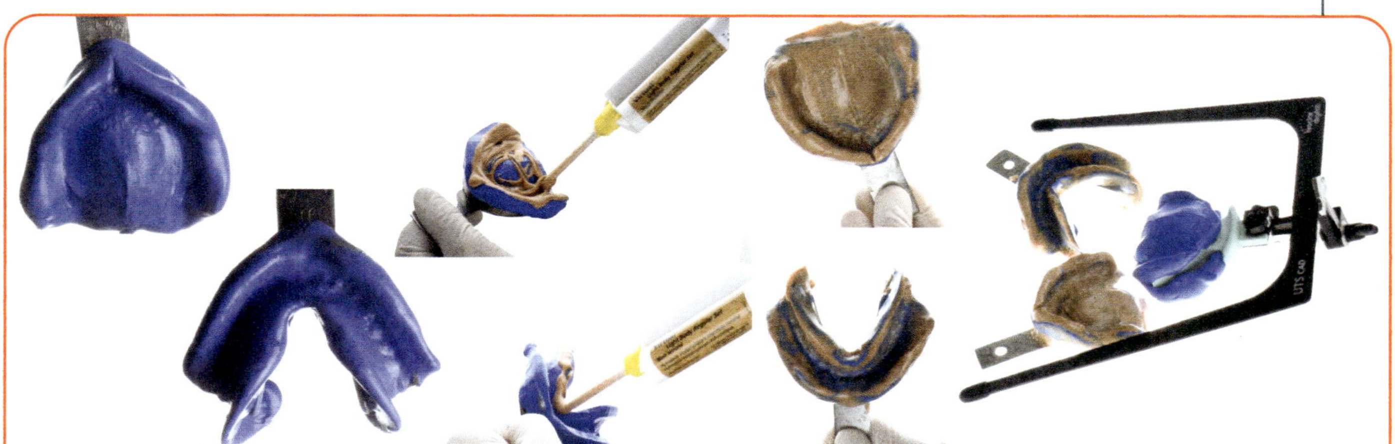

Figure 5.9 • Summary of the first clinical stage. Taking the upper and lower impressions. The preliminary impressions and the information collected with UTS CAD are sent to the laboratory.

Laboratory stage 1

The laboratory receives from the office the impressions, the Centric Tray with the occlusal registrations and the angular corrections to be applied thanks to the analysis with UTS CAD.

The program used is Denture Digital Design (3Shape, Copenhagen Denmark); with this instrument, both the surfaces of the Centric Tray are scanned and the UTS CAD angular compensation data are entered into the software (**Figures 5.10** and **5.11**).

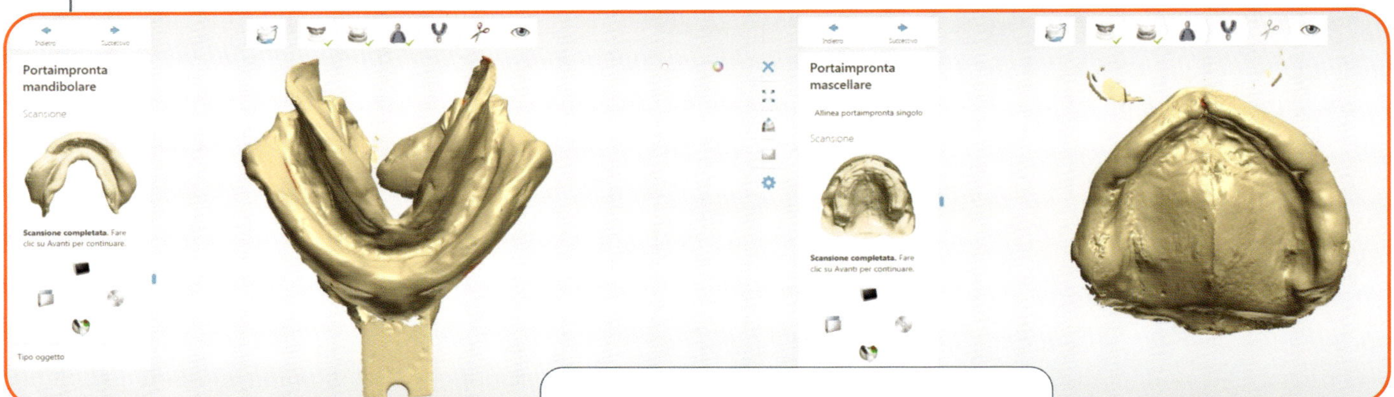

Figure 5.10 • The impressions are scanned at the laboratory.

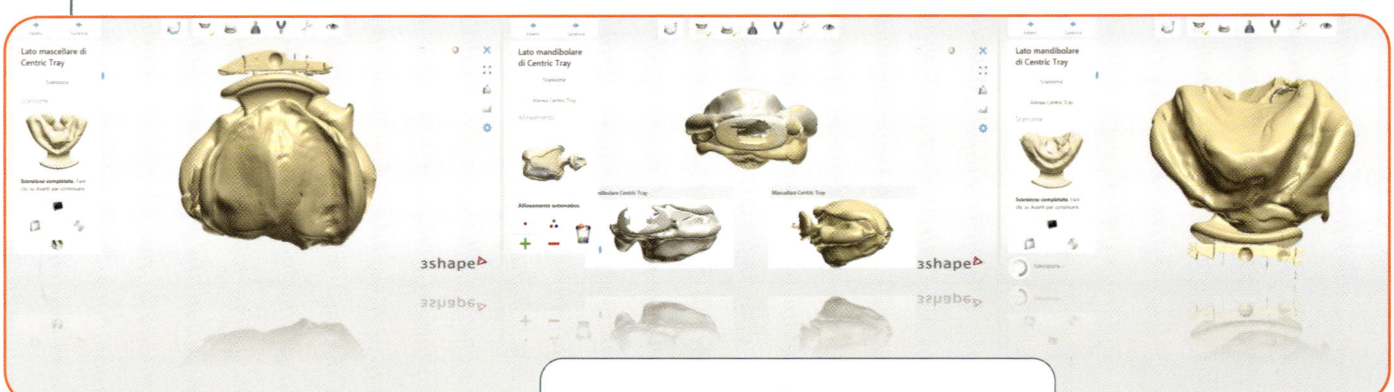

Figure 5.11 • The Centric Tray is scanned at the laboratory.

The data are analysed by the computer by matching the scans and setting up the two virtual models of the edentulous arches according to that registered clinically **(Figure 5.12)**.

The CAD designer analyses the edentulous ridges indicating in the software the precise landmark points, assesses the occlusal plane in relation to that recorded with UTS CAD and the extent of the undercuts on the maxilla and mandible, and identifies the extent of the registration plate to be milled, to be used in the next step **(Figure 5.13)**.

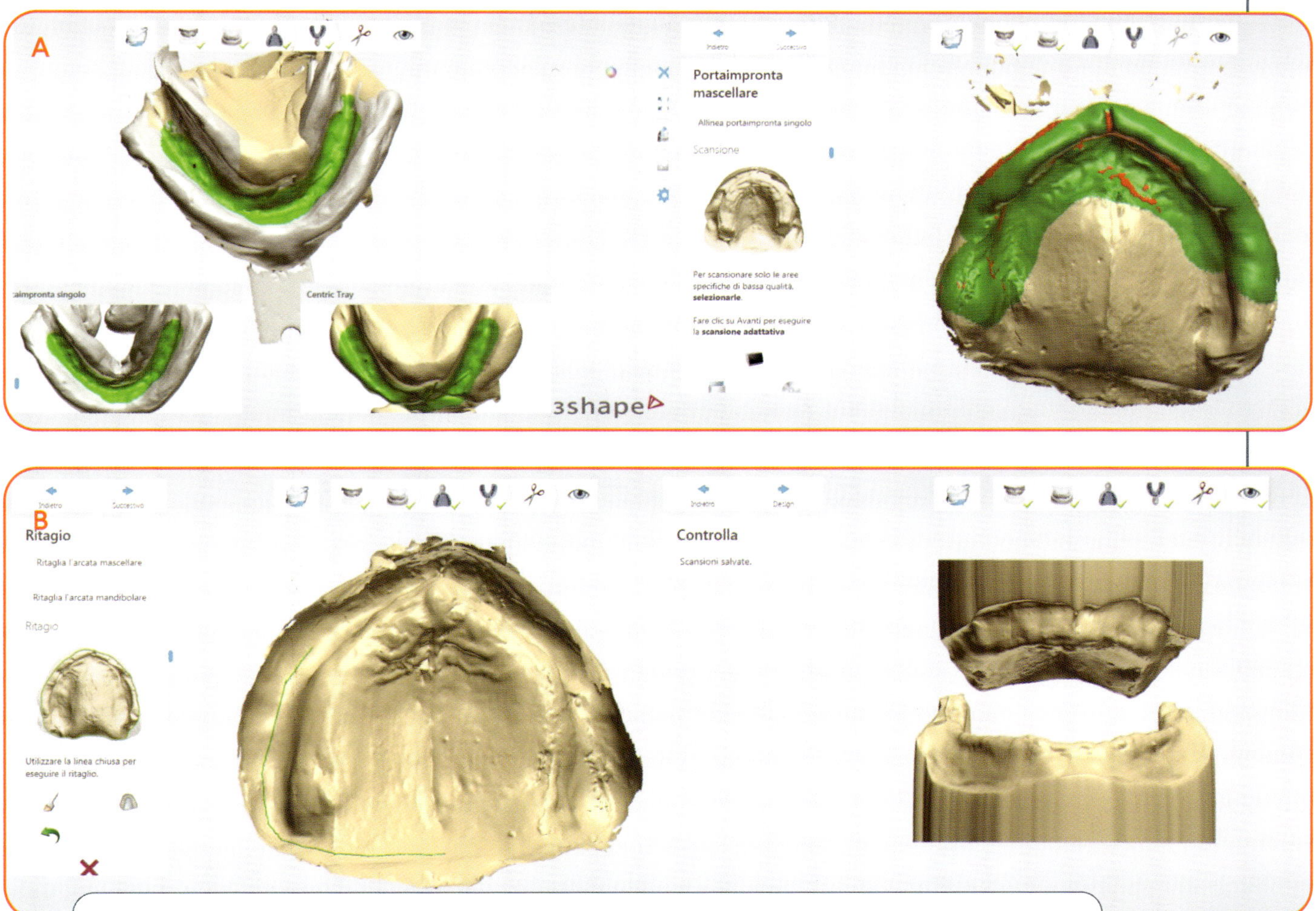

Figure 5.12 • (**A**) The software pairs the information related to the Centric Tray with that of the impressions. (**B**) The software relates the upper virtual model to the lower one according to the preliminary OVD registered clinically with the Centric Tray.

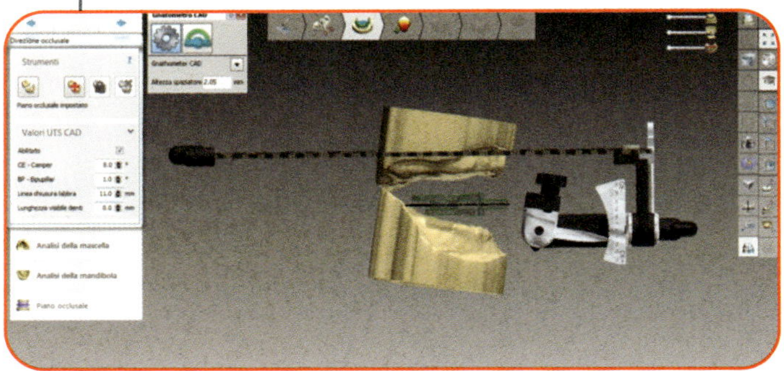

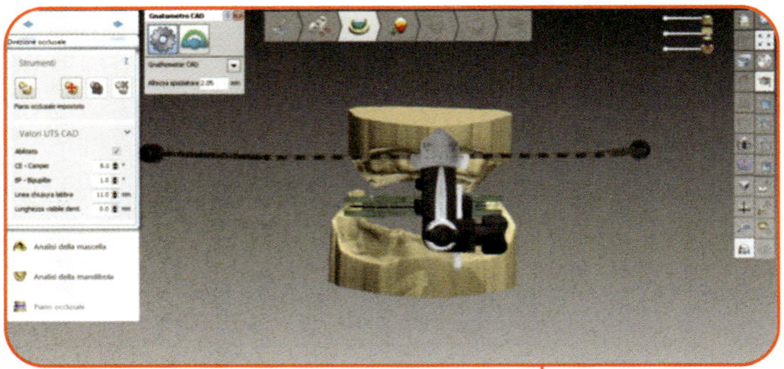

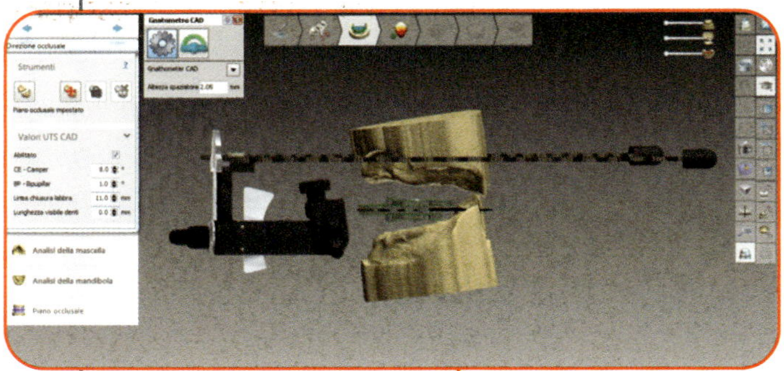

Figure 5.13 • The CAD adjusts the virtual models according to the angular values of Camper plane and bipupillary line registered clinically with UTS CAD. The occlusal plane is also defined.

The base plate design is sent to the machine that will mill round PMMA discs (polymethyl-methacrylate) **(Figure 5.14)**.

Once finished, the plates are sent to the dentist's office **(Figure 5.15)**.

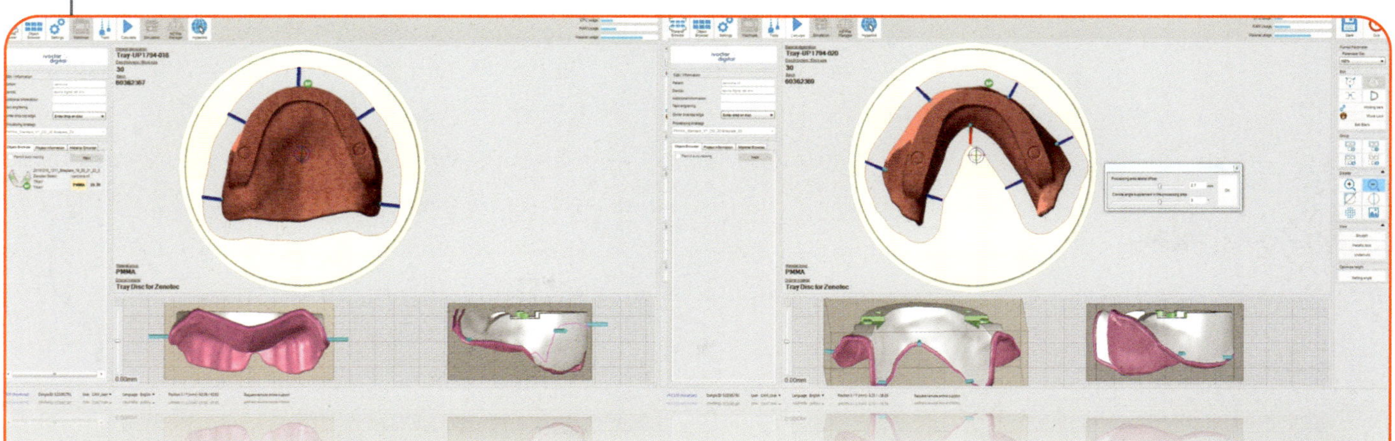

Figure 5.14 • The material of choice is PMMA.

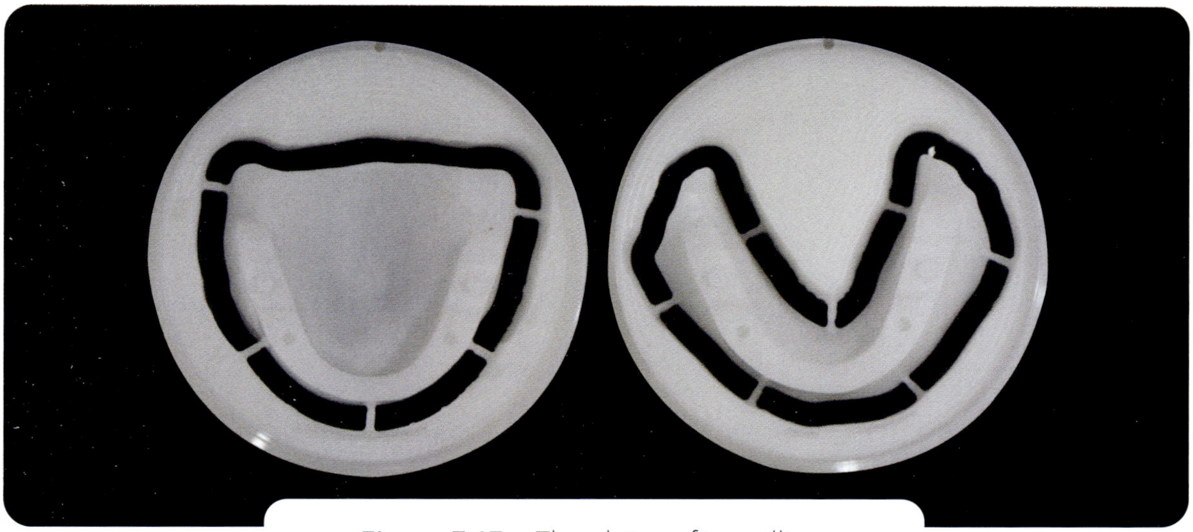

Figure 5.15 • The plates after milling.

A gothic arch system is to be seated within the resin base plate, the Gnathometer CAD (Ivoclar Vivadent) (**Figures 5.16** and **5.17**).

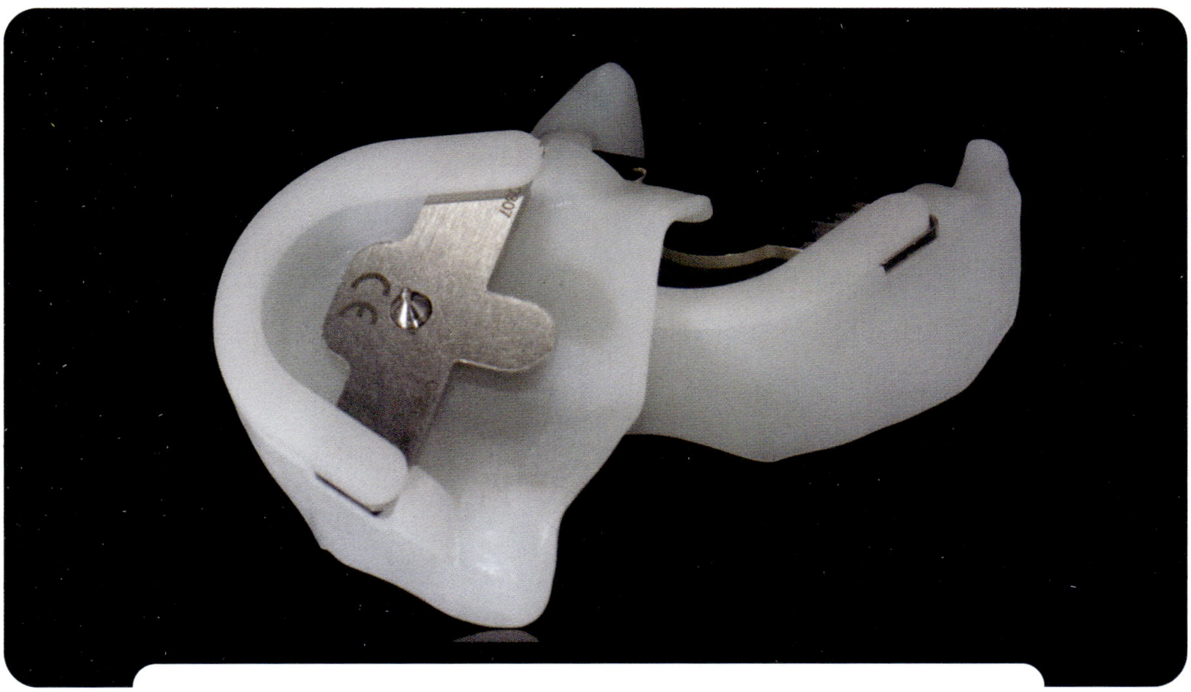

Figure 5.16 • The plate contains a housing for the Gnathometer CAD system (Ivoclar Vivadent, Schaan Liechtenstein).

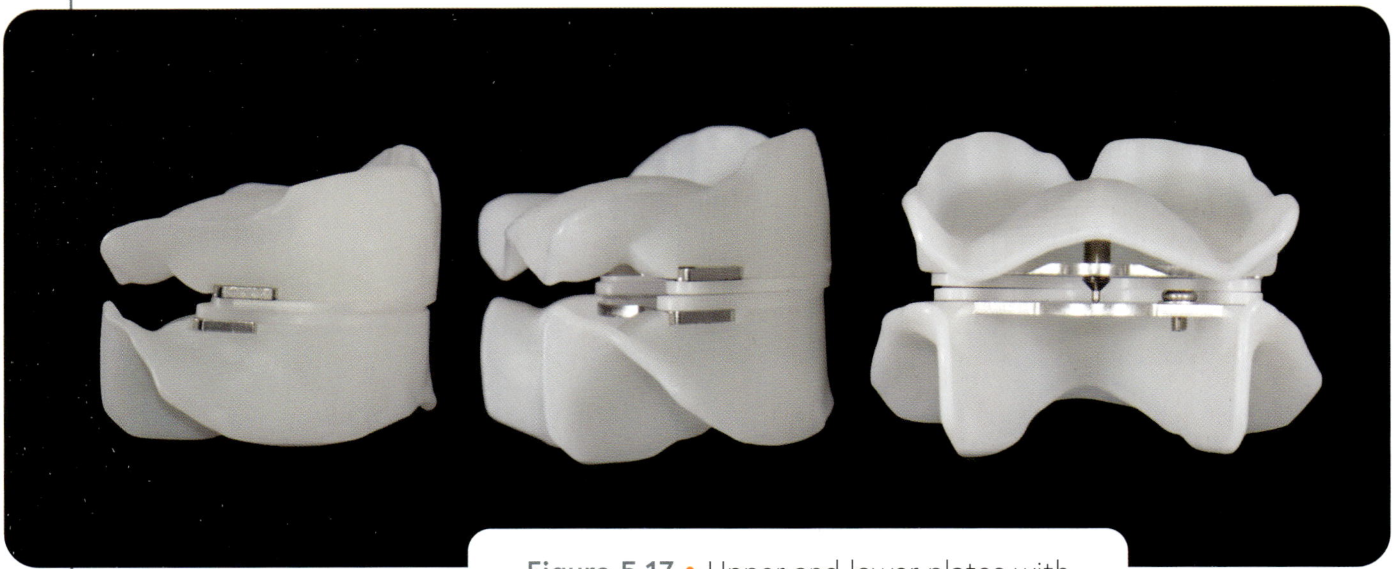

Figure 5.17 • Upper and lower plates with occlusal registration device inserted.

Clinical stage 2

During the second clinical stage, the following steps are performed (to be illustrated in detail below):

- assessment of the base plates to identify any pressure points;
- checking the proper setup of the occlusal plane;
- definition of the plate borders;
- application of the adhesive on the plate;
- taking the precision impression;
- registration of the intermaxillary relations.

The base plates are tried on and any pressure points are detected with a silicone paste (Pressure Spot Indicator, Coltene) (**Figure 5.18**).

The proper alignment of the occlusal plane is checked with the plates inserted intraorally with respect to the Camper plane and the bipupillary line, both joints of the UTS CAD are locked at 0° and a specific fork is clenched, attached to the instrument (**Figure 5.19**).

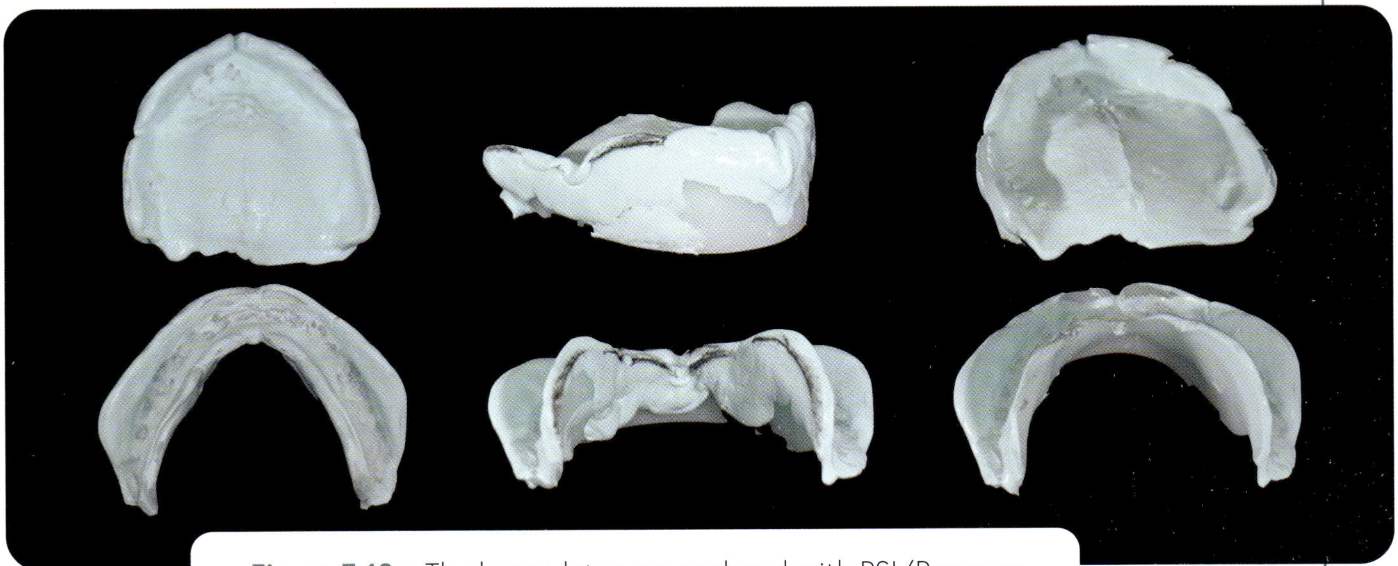

Figure 5.18 • The base plates are analysed with PSI (Pressure Spot Indicator – Coltene) to identify points of excessive pressure.

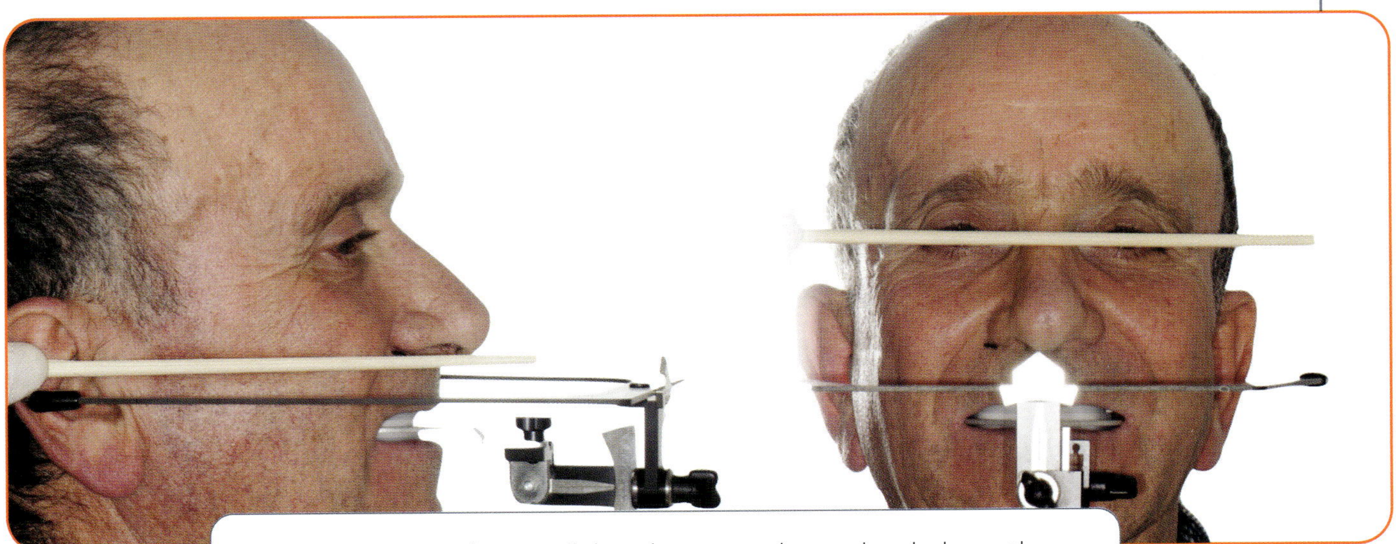

Figure 5.19 • The parallelism between the occlusal plane, the Camper plane and the bipupillary line is verified by locking the UTS CAD joints at 0°.

The borders are defined by using a silicone material by addition (Virtual® Light Body, Ivoclar Vivadent) which is placed on the border of the upper plate. Once the plate is positioned in the oral cavity, the muscle fascias are activated actively and passively.

After the impression material has set, the possible areas of impression tray over-extension are assessed again and the excess material is removed in order to eliminate raised steps in the impression. The same procedure is performed for functionalisation of the lower plate borders.

The adhesive is then spread on the plate and, after the solvent has evaporated, the impression material is placed within the plate (Virtual® Light Body, Ivoclar Vivadent), the patient is asked to bring the plates in contact then the measurement is performed according to the "closed mouth" technique **(Figure 5.20)**.

After the impression material has set, the plates are removed **(Figure 5.21)**. The Gnathometer CAD gothic arch system (Ivoclar Vivadent) is then seated within the base plates to perform registration of the intermaxillary relations.

The Gnathometer CAD (Ivoclar Vivadent) is a device for intraoral registration with support pins for individual assessment of the centric relation position of edentulous patients. The principle of the intraoral support pin method is based on the idea of the three-point support of both mandibular joints and the registration pin, which is positioned in the centre of the lower jaw [9,10].

The plate with the tracing pin is fixed in the appropriate housing of the upper plate **(Figure 5.22)**.

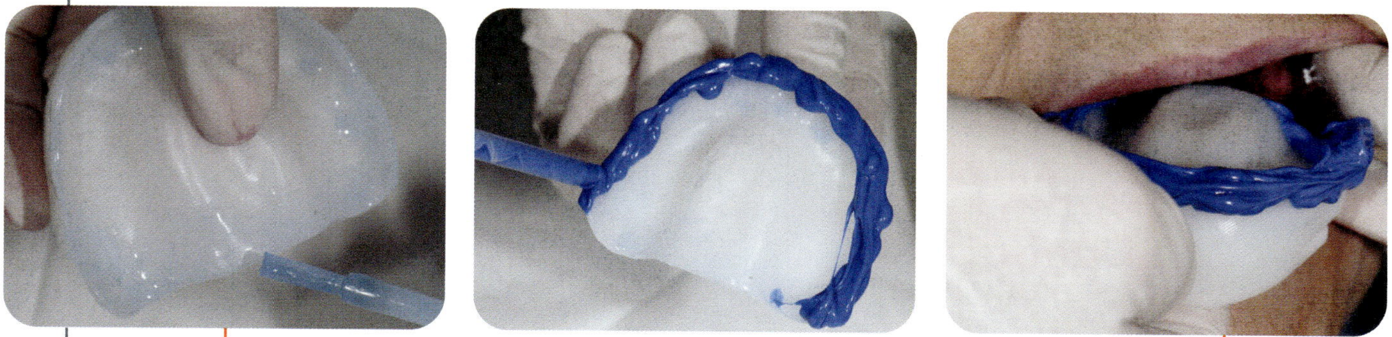

Figure 5.20 • Functional edging is carried out to measure the muscle activity.

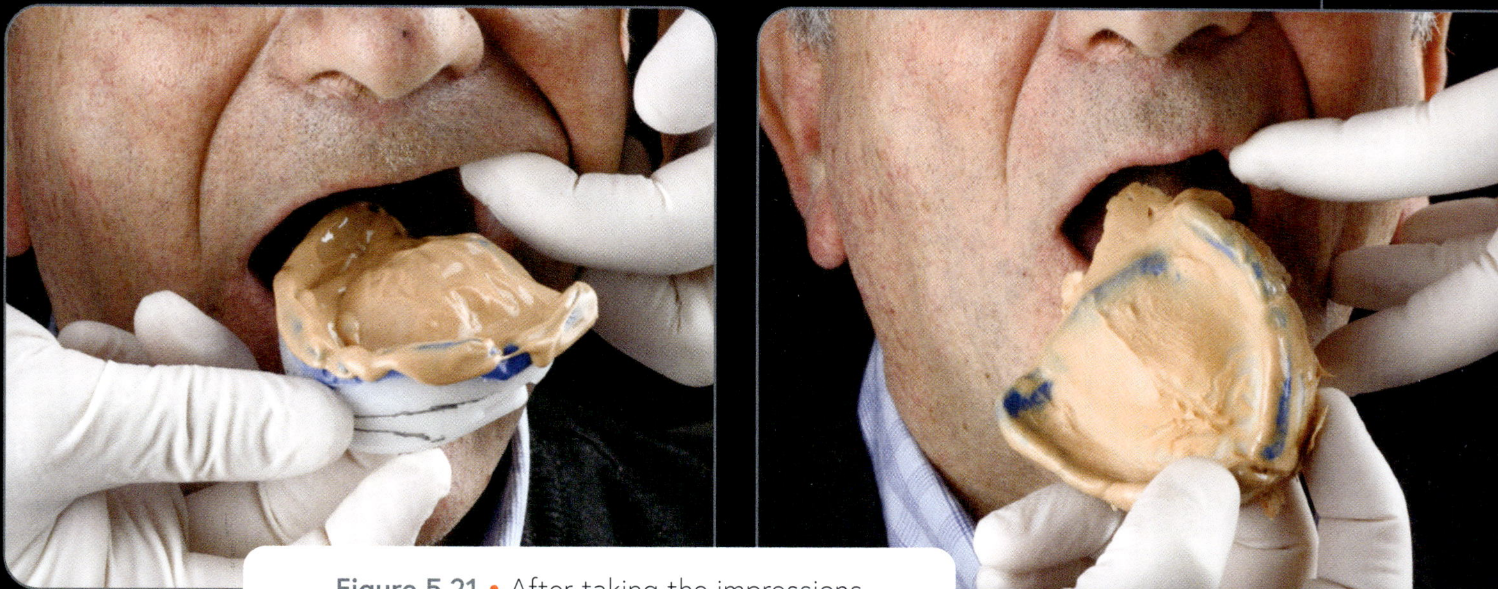

Figure 5.21 • After taking the impressions (with closed mouth), the plates are removed.

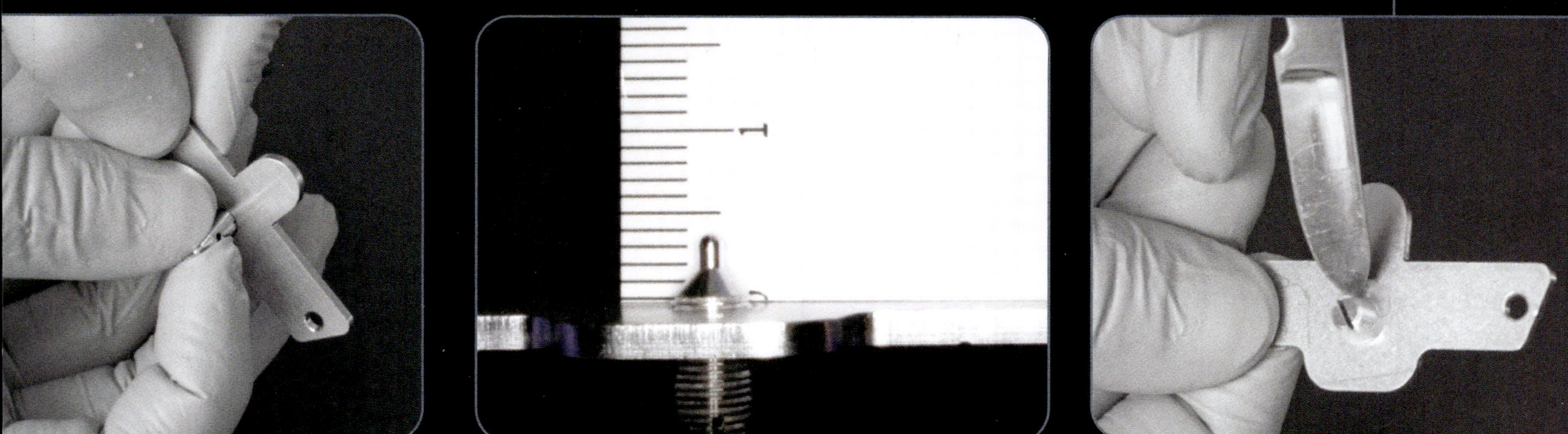

Figure 5.22 • The plate with the tracing pin is set at 4 mm and blocked with a drop of wax.

The vertical dimension is defined thanks to esthetic and phonetic assessments. A suitable dye (wax pencil, marker pen) is applied to the registration plate, which is housed in the lower plate, and the patient is asked to perform the retrusion, protrusion and left and right lateral movements **(Figure 5.23)**. The support pin will draw the typical gothic arch pattern on the stained registration plate, highlighting its travel. The neuromuscular centre must match the apex of the gothic arch. A fixing plate is used to lock the registered centric position and the hole of the tracing tip of the fixing plate is then oriented on the tip of the gothic arch, then the plate is locked with the fixing screw **(Figure 5.24)**.

The patient is then asked to close his/her mouth carefully and you check whether the tracing tip of the pin is in the hole of the fixing plate and whether the fixed registration of the gothic arch is correct. The entire intermaxillary registration is attached three-dimensionally with occlusal registration silicone (CAD Bite, Ivoclar Vivadent, material that can be scanned in the laboratory) applied directly between the registration plates **(Figure 5.25)**

The esthetic references (midline, canine position, smile line, maximum and minimum dental display) can be transferred to the laboratory by marking them on the base plates with a permanent marker. The entire fixed registration is then sent to the laboratory **(Figure 5.26)**.

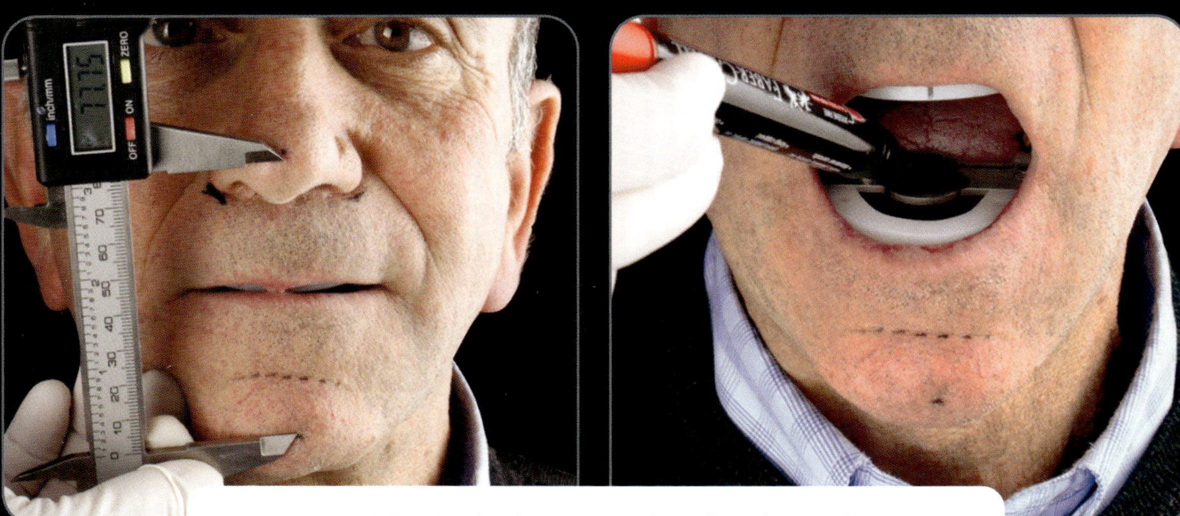

Figure 5.23 • Both plates are placed in the oral cavity. The patient's esthetics and phonetics are evaluated to check the vertical dimension.

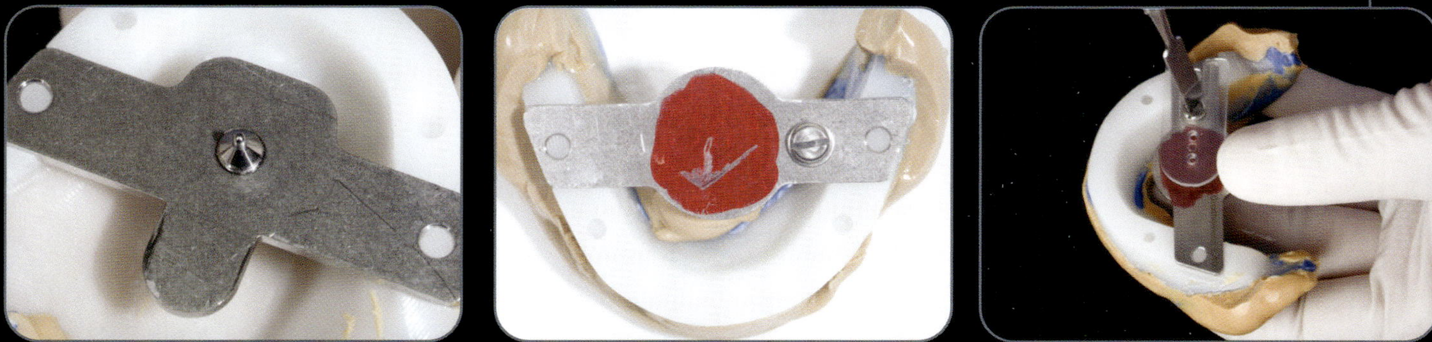

Figure 5.24 • The registered centric position is locked with the fixing screw.

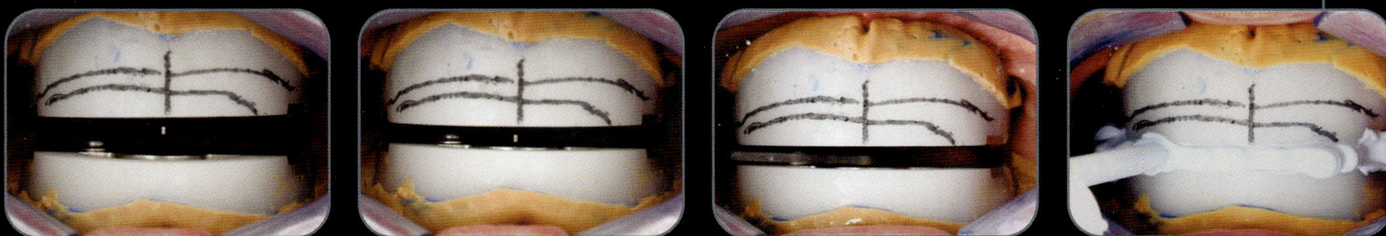

Figure 5.25 • The intermaxillary relation is registered with the aid of the Gnathometer CAD (Ivoclar Vivadent). A scannable occlusal registration silicone is used to fix the entire registration.

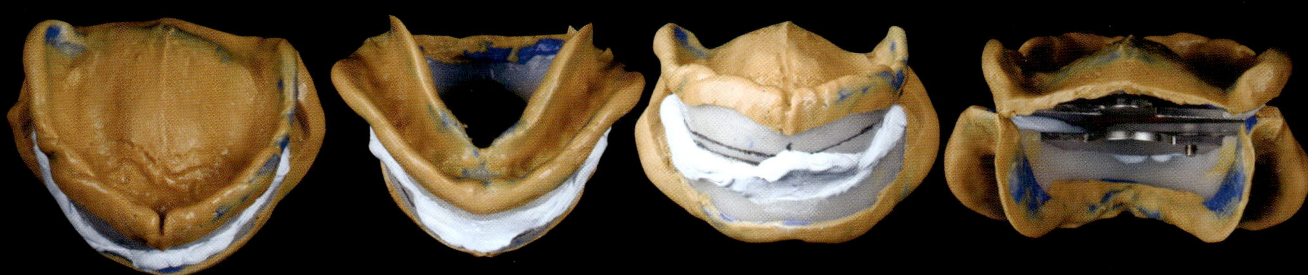

Figure 5.26 • Final registration.

Laboratory stage 2

By using a specific scanning support, the registration can be placed into the laboratory scanner for digitisation (**Figures 5.27** and **5.28**).

The edentulous arches are adjusted in space in the virtual articulator thanks to the registration performed with UTS CAD and in the intermaxillary relations checked with the Gnathometer CAD (Ivoclar Vivadent) (**Figure 5.29**).

The anatomical landmark points, which can be wholly superimposed to those of the analogue technique, are identified on the virtual models. These are required to mount both the anterior and posterior dentures, also assessing the information collected in the previous clinical step (**Figure 5.30**).

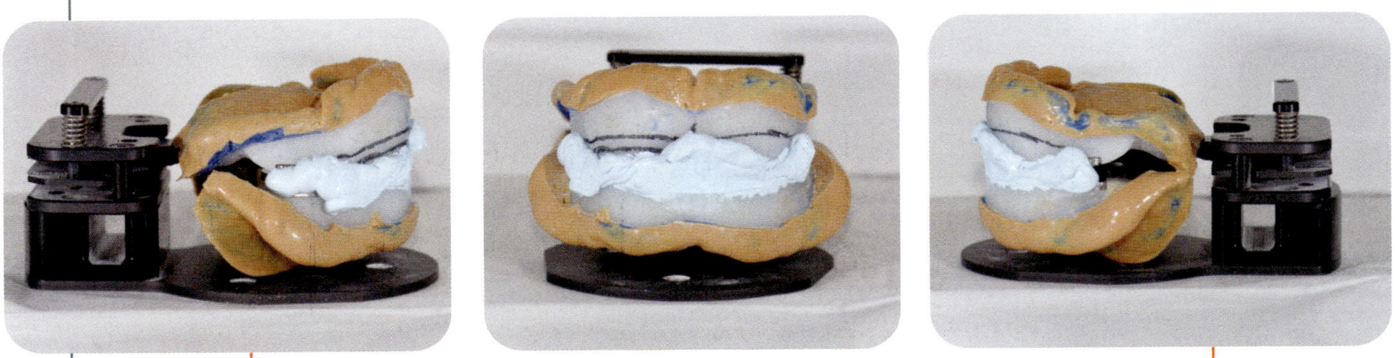

Figure 5.27 • In the laboratory, the final registration is placed on a scanning support.

All the materials used to take the impressions and also the material to attach the plates after completing the occlusal registration must enable convenient scanning by the laboratory scanners. In laboratory scanners that use laser technology, an unsuitable impression material would not be adequately scannable and would need to be treated with opacifying powder.
The most recent bench scanners with structured light no longer require opacifying procedures.

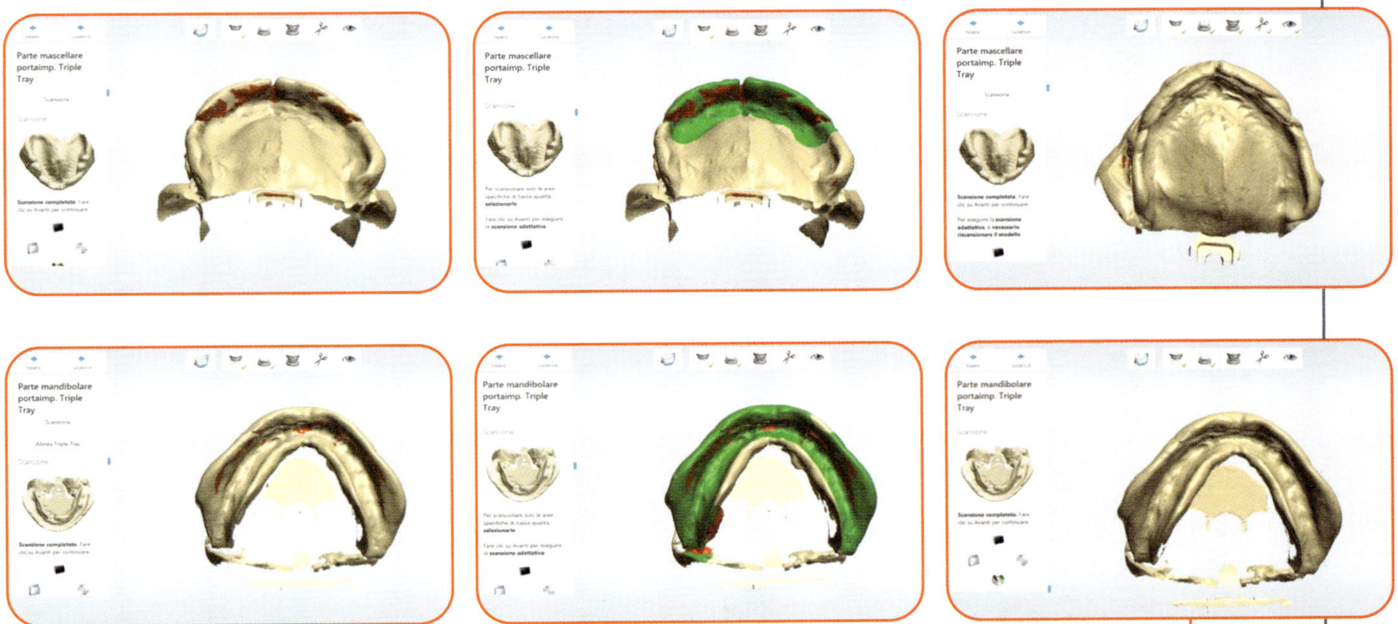

Figure 5.28 • Digitisation of the final data.

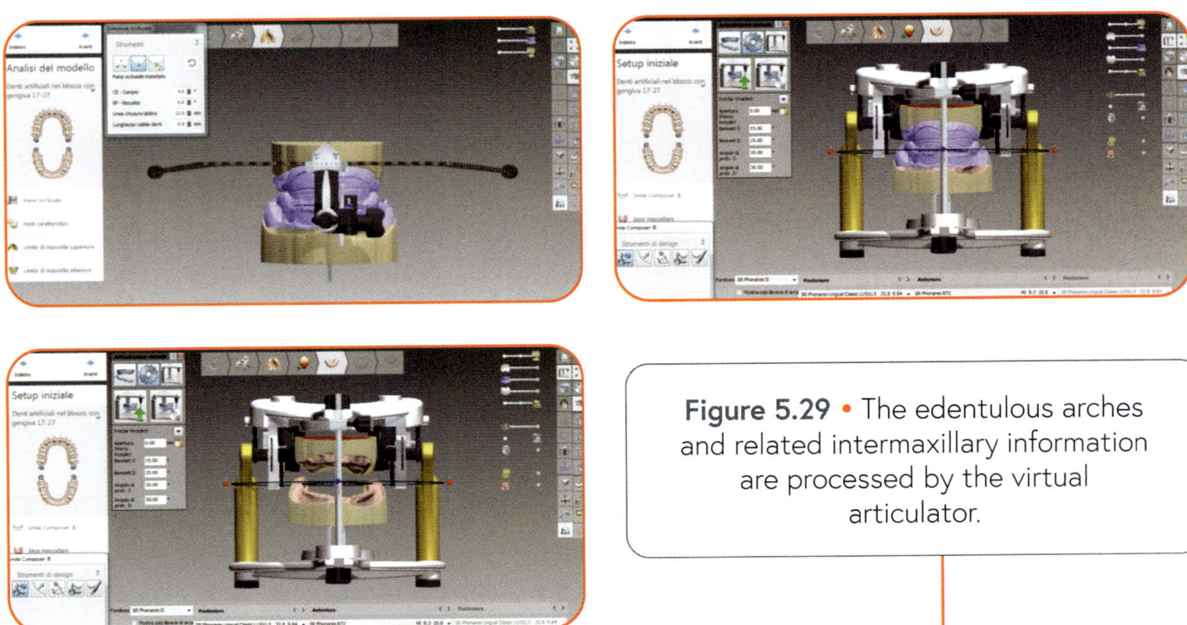

Figure 5.29 • The edentulous arches and related intermaxillary information are processed by the virtual articulator.

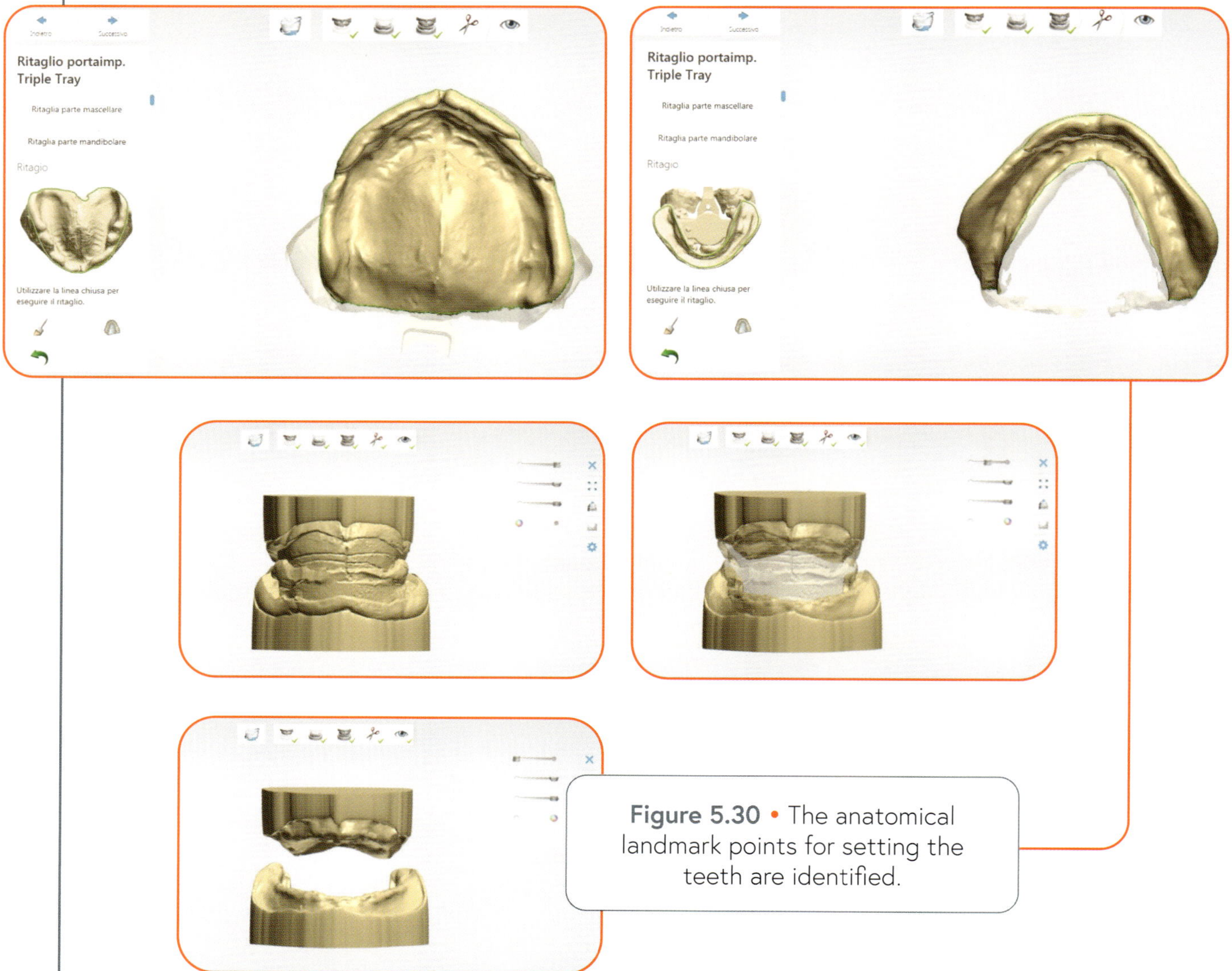

Figure 5.30 • The anatomical landmark points for setting the teeth are identified.

The dental shape is selected from the virtual library and the software proposes the mounting **(Figure 5.31)**.

The latest updates of these design programs offer wide design discretion to the dental-technician: it is now possible to rehabilitate even one of the two arches, move or delete the individual teeth without causing movement of the other teeth **(Figure 5.32)**.

The proposed occlusal diagram is bilaterally balanced occlusion **(Figure 5.33)**. The design file is then sent to the miller that produces the PMMA prototypes of the final prosthesis **(Figure 5.34)**.

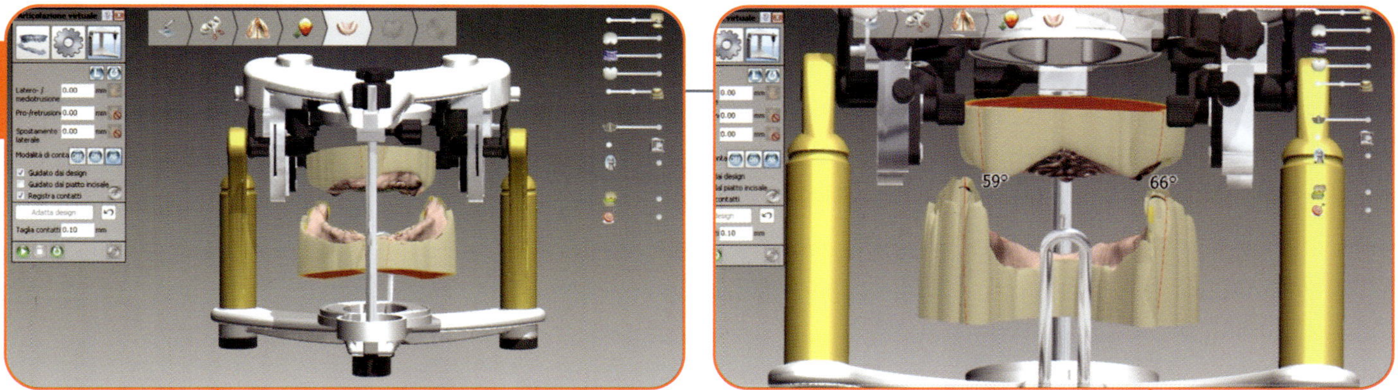

Figure 5.31 • The software makes it possible to customise the design of the prosthesis.

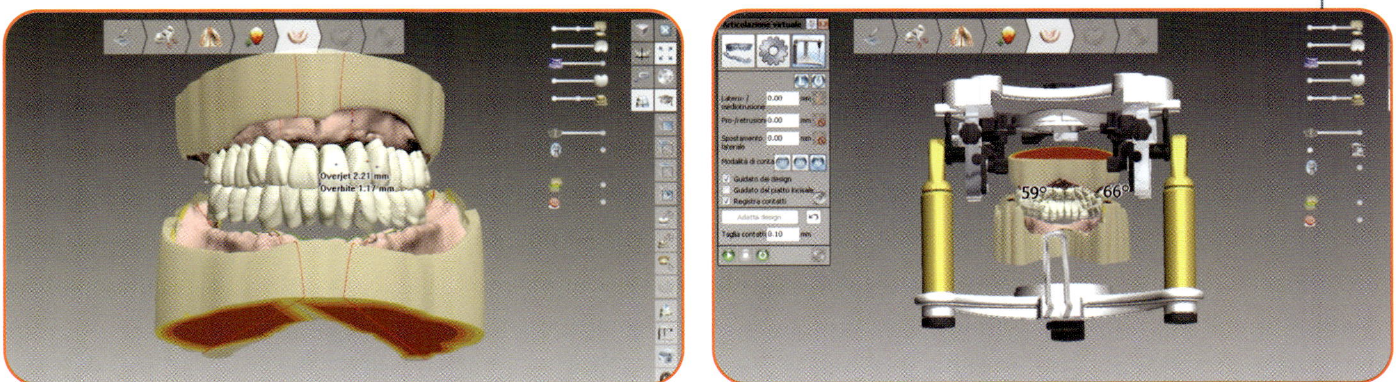

Figure 5.32 • The artificial teeth are selected and inserted.

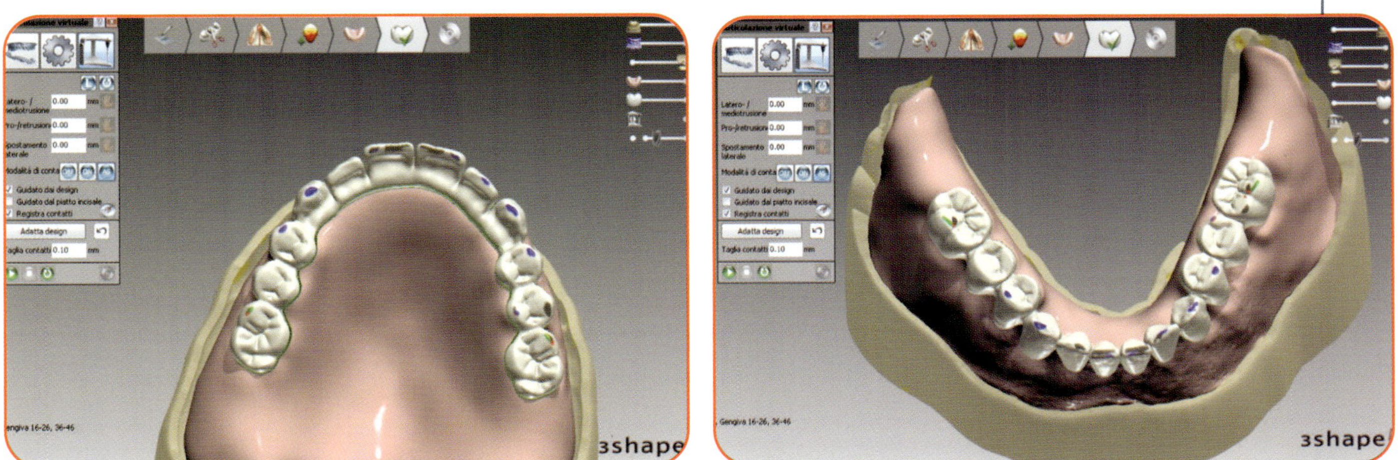

Figure 5.33 • The occlusal scheme is optimised.

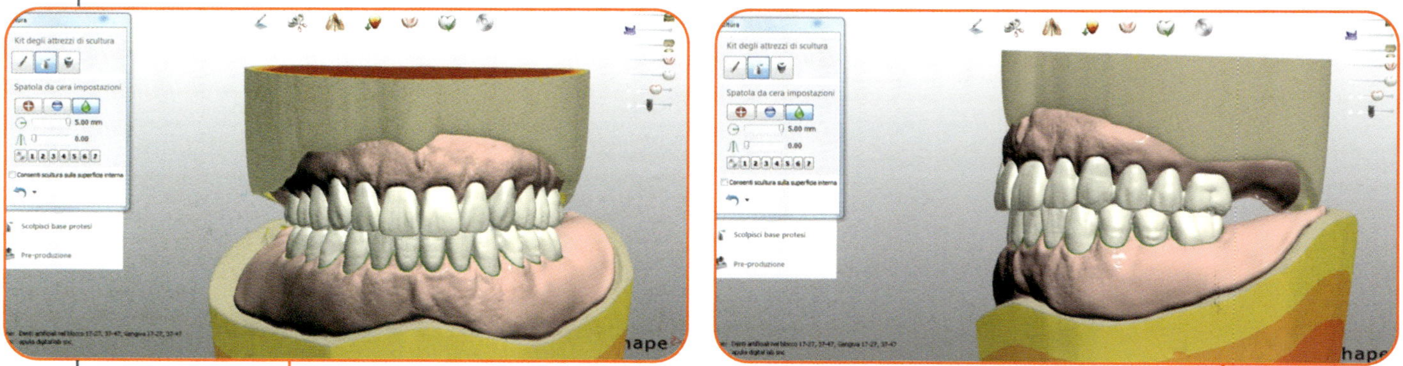

Figure 5.34 • The prosthesis is designed and is ready for milling.

Clinical stage 3

The third clinical stage is optional, but strongly recommended.

During this appointment, occlusion, esthetics, phonetics and prosthesis fit are checked. If these parameters are satisfactory, the design is validated **(Figure 5.35)**.

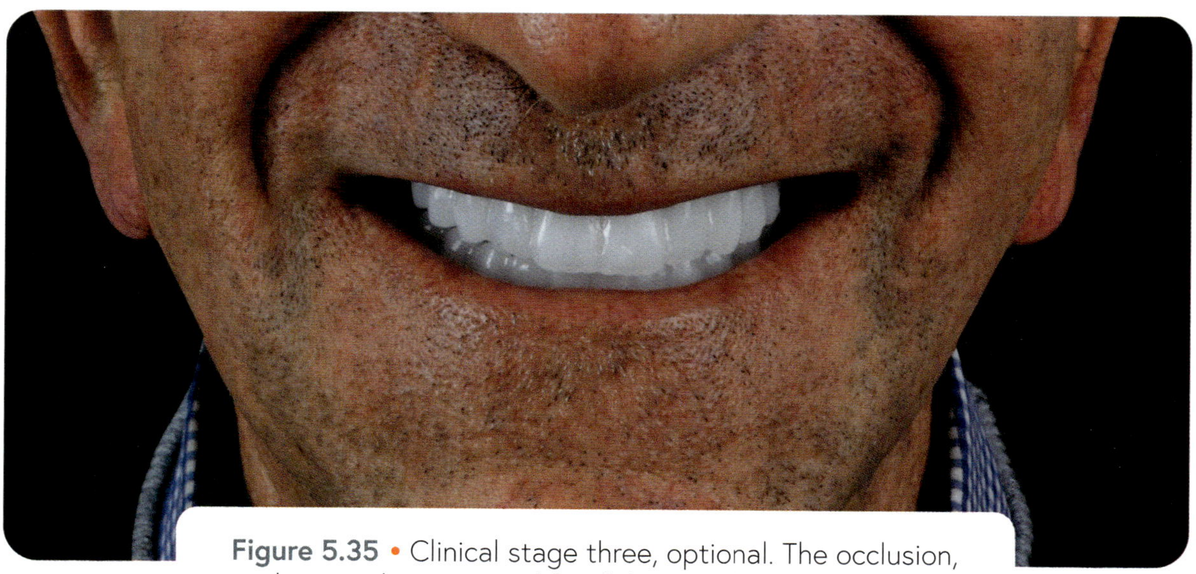

Figure 5.35 • Clinical stage three, optional. The occlusion, esthetics, phonetics and fit of the prosthesis are checked thanks to a milled PMMA prototype.

Laboratory stage 3

Four steps are required to complete the full prosthesis. The first two consist in milling the extrados pf the prosthesis starting from a pink PMMA disc. The sockets that will contain the artificial teeth are milled **(Figure 5.36)**.

The entire arch is milled from a disc in the chosen colour. Multilayer resin blocks are available on the market, which ensure excellent esthetic results.

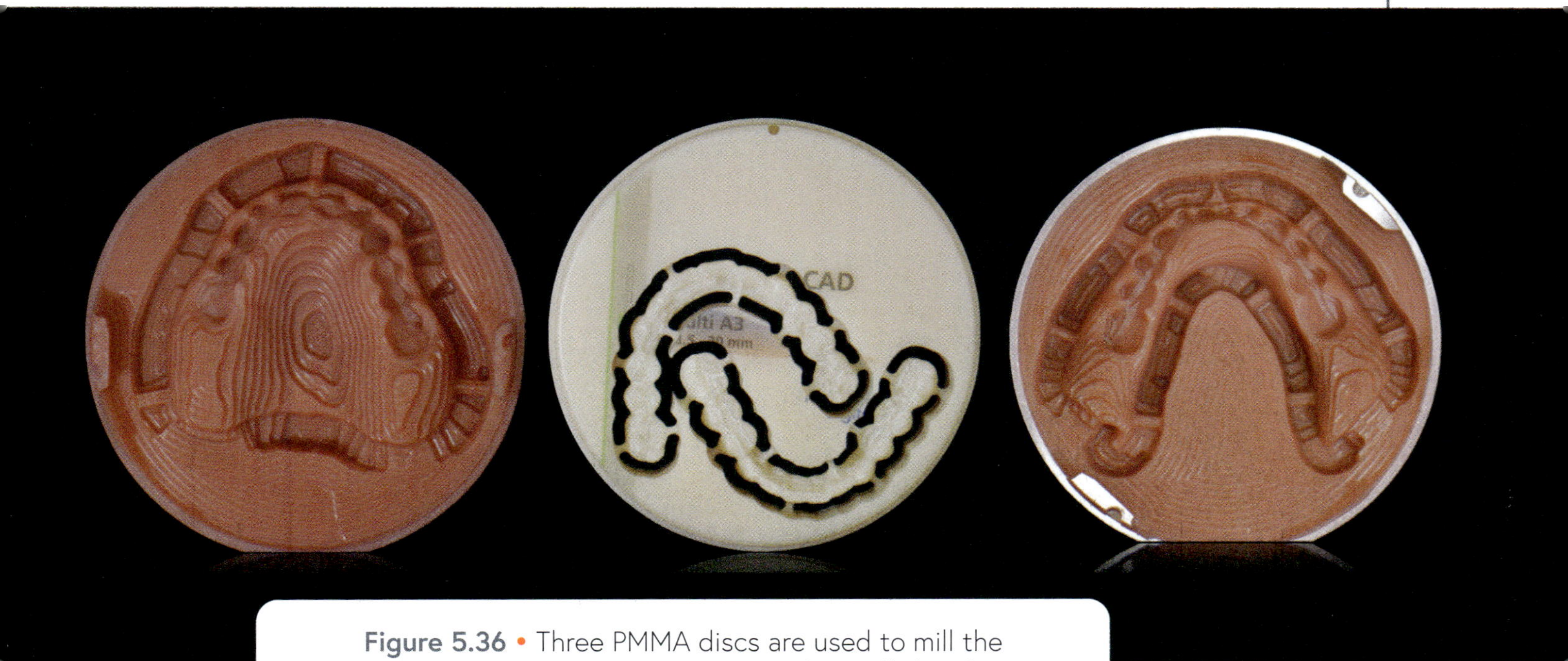

Figure 5.36 • Three PMMA discs are used to mill the prostheses: the two pink ones are used to mill the plates, while the white one is used to mill the artificial teeth.

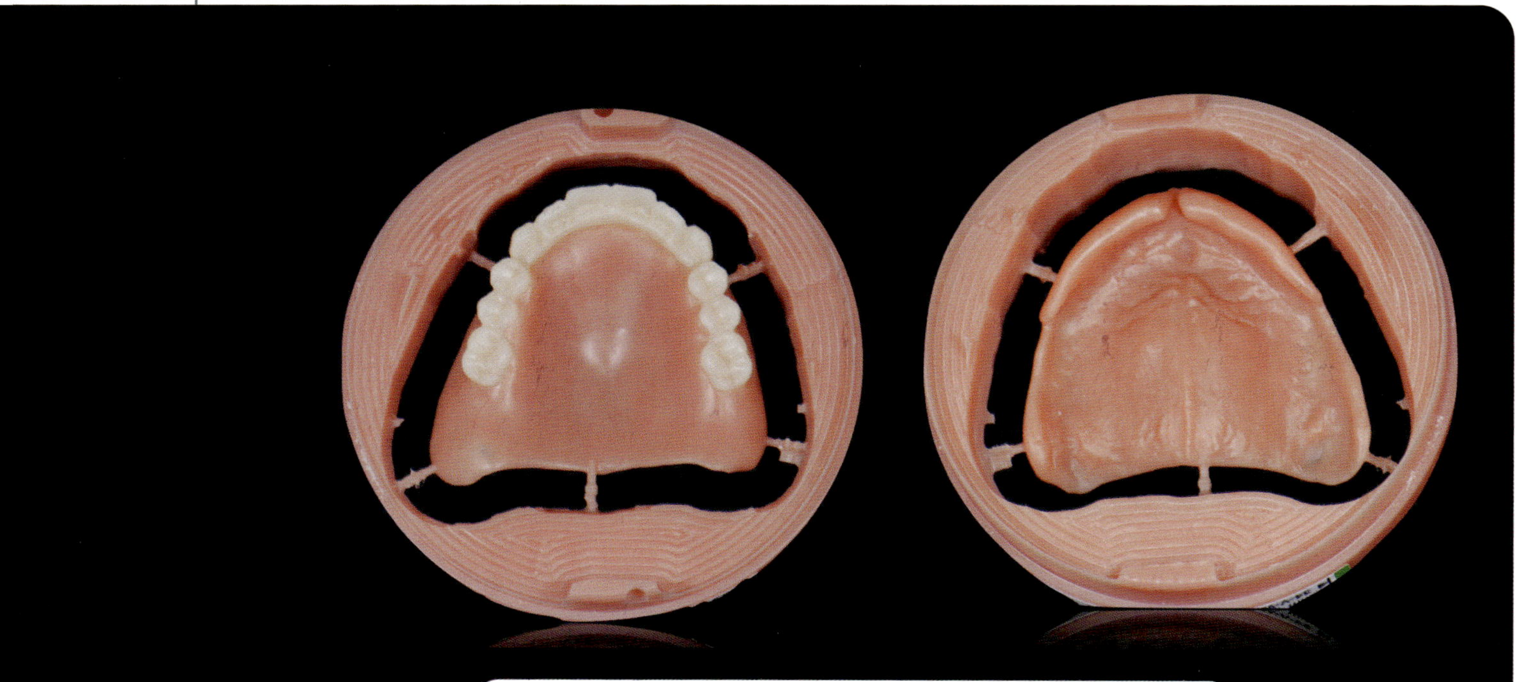

Figure 5.37 • The teeth are set into the milled sockets with specific primer and bonding.

The third step entails gluing the artificial teeth within the sockets. A specific primer and bonding are used (**Figure 5.37**).

When the adhesion procedure of the trade teeth to the prosthetic base has been completed, the disc is put back into the milling machine to mill the intrados.

Intrados of the prosthesis in accordance with the virtual design

In the fourth step, the machine corrects even the small discrepancies of the occlusal surface of the prosthesis with respect to the final design.

The machine also finishes the prostheses which can therefore be removed from the milling disc.

Clinical stage 4

During this appointment, the prostheses are delivered to the patient. The occlusion, stability, phonetics and esthetics are checked again.

Strict compliance with the protocol ensures the CAD design perfectly matches the CAM fabrication **(Figure 5.38)**.

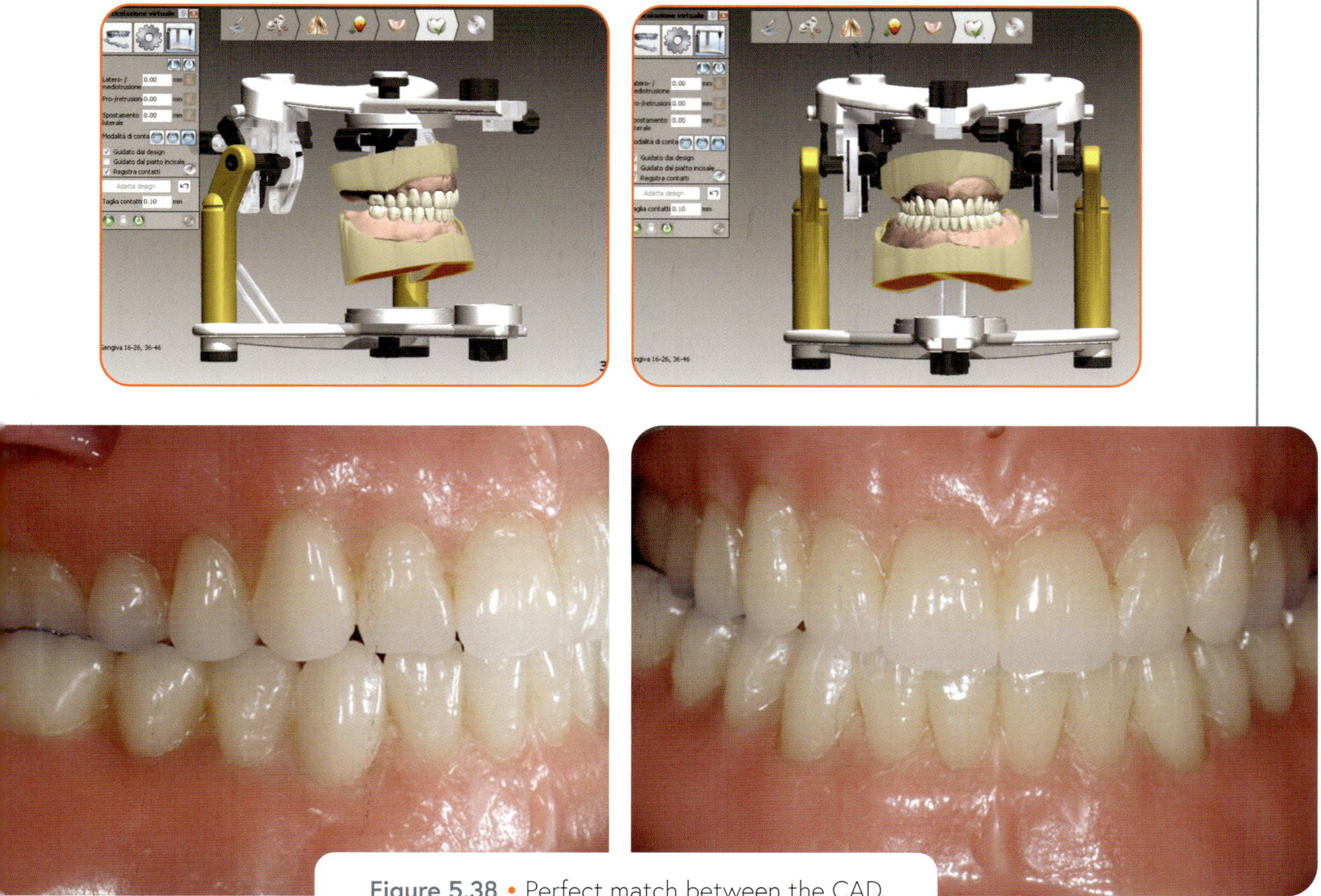

Figure 5.38 • Perfect match between the CAD design and the CAM fabrication is observed.

The checks during delivery of the total digital prostheses and subsequent adjustments are obviously identical to those performed for conventional prostheses (**Figure 5.39**). When the patient is in a hybrid situation, with residual individual teeth or implants with attachments, the matrices can be incorporated intraorally using the conventional techniques.

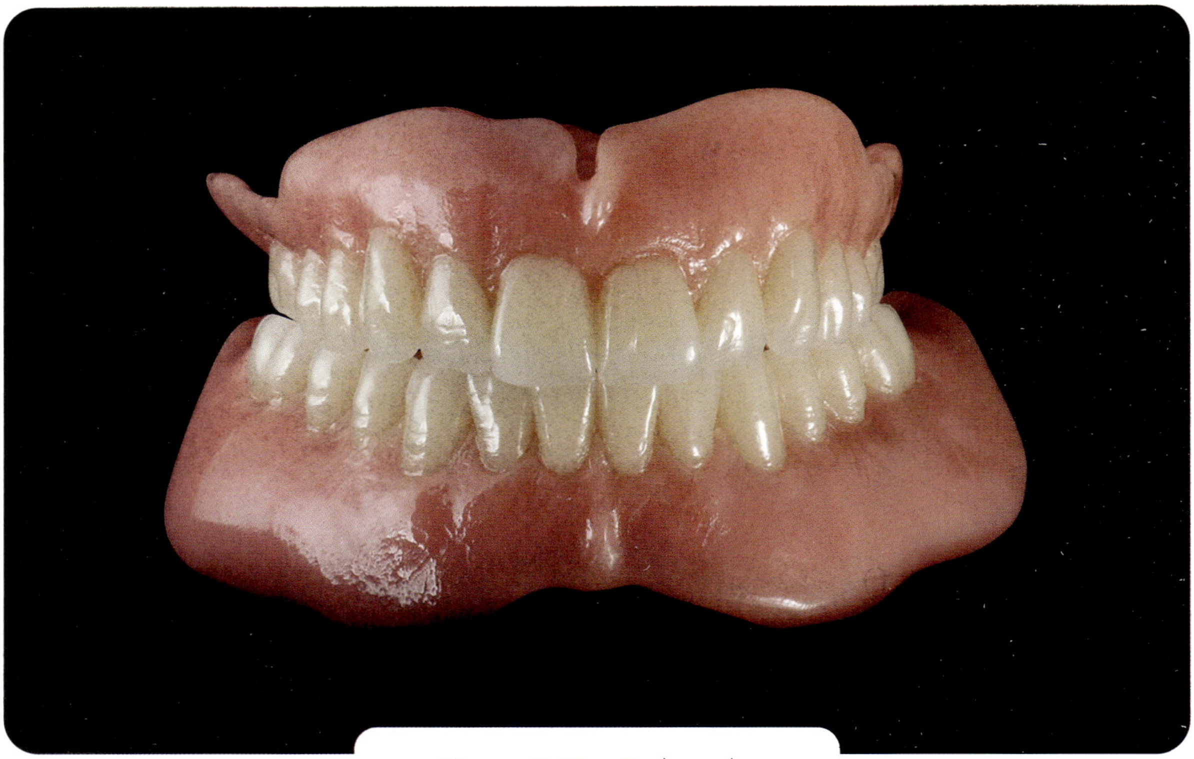

Figure 5.39 • End result.

Conclusions

Recent studies [2,11] have ascertained that the CAD/CAM fabrication process is the most accurate among the workflows used for the production of full dentures.

The combined use of the scanning technology and the CAD/CAM procedures makes it possible to significantly reduce the working times of the clinician and dental technician. Virtual modelling (CAD) and milling of the prosthesis (CAM) from a resin disc make it possible to avoid the time-consuming procedures for placing in the flask and packing. As there is no curing shrinkage, the fit of the prosthesis is accurate.

Other advantages are the lower number of appointments required to complete the therapy and, consequently, the benefits for elderly patients who find it difficult to get to the dentist's office [3].

A huge advantage is the fact that the digital design of the full prosthesis can be superimposed in some software to the DICOM files of three-dimensional radiology. This option enables accurate prosthetically guided design of implant placement in the implant treatment of edentulous patients (Chapter 7).

Further developments will be discussed in Chapter 7 related to perspectives in complete prostheses.

References

1. Steinmassl PA, Klaunzer F, Steinmassl O et al. Evaluation of currently available CAD/CAM denture systems. *Int J Prosthodont.* 207;30(2):116-22.
2. Goodacre CJ, Garbacea A, Naylor WP et al. CAD/CAM fabricated complete dentures: Concepts and clinical methods of obtaining required morphological data. *J Prosthet Dent.* 2012;107(1):34-46.
3. Bidra AS, Taylor TD, Agar JR. Computer-aided technology for fabricating complete dentures: Systematic review of historical background, current status, and future perspectives. *J Prosthet Dent.* 2013;109(6):361-6.
4. Mendes TA, Marques D, Lopes LP, Caramês J. Total digital workflow in the fabrication of a partial removable dental prostheses: A case report. *SAGE Open Med Case Reports.* 2019;7:2050313X1987113.
5. Oh SL, Hack G, Gurman S, Idzik-Starr C. Provisional removable prosthesis fabricated from a digital impression. *Decis Dent.* 2020;6(1):22-24.
6. Al-Haj Husain N, Özcan M, Schimmel M, Abou-Ayash S. A digital cast-free clinical workflow for oral rehabilitation with removable partial dentures: A dental technique. *J Prosthet Dent.* 2020; 123(5):680-5.
7. Lo Russo L, Salamini A. Removable complete digital dentures: A workflow that integrates open technologies. *J Prosthet Dent.* 2018;119(5):727-32.
8. Maeda Y, Minoura M, Tsutsumi S et al. A CAD/CAM system for removable denture. Part I: Fabrication of complete dentures. *Int J Prosthodont.* 1994;7(1):17-21.
9. McGrane HF. Five basic principles of the McGrane full denture procedure. *J Fla State Dent Soc.* 1949;20(11):5-8.
10. Gysi A. *The problem of articulation.* Philadelphia: S.S. White Dental Manufacturing Co; 1910. pp. 1-19, 148-169, 269-283.
11. Infante L, Yilmaz B, McGlumphy E, Finger I. Fabricating complete dentures with CAD/CAM technology. *J Prosthet Dent.* 2014;111(5):351-5.

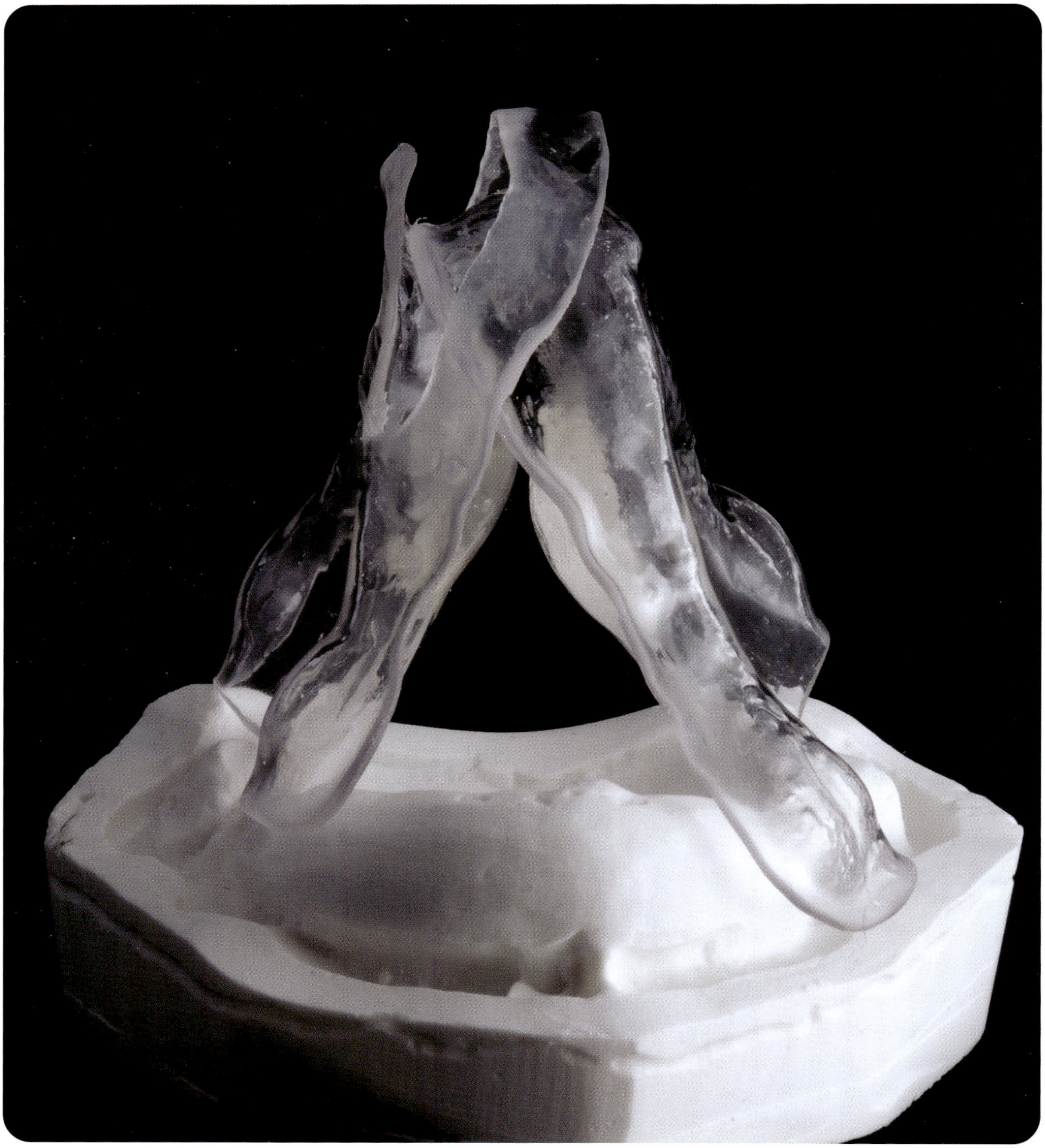

CHAPTER 6

P. VENEZIA, P. LACASELLA, R. CAVALCANTI, S. D'AMATO

Immediate denture in hopeless dentition patients

Immediate prosthesis: analogue flow

P. Venezia, P. Lacasella, R. Cavalcanti

Removable complete prostheses play an ever more significant role in modern dentistry. The introduction of new materials such as, for example, artificial teeth, resins, composites for the characterisation of dentures and flanges allows functional and esthetic excellence to be achieved, essential when dealing with patients with very high expectations.

The rehabilitation route with removable prosthesis is even more important in patients who must undergo a complex implant-prosthetic treatment. The ideal position of the teeth registered with phonation, occlusion and esthetics [1-5] is tested and subsequently replicated in the prosthesis on implants.

If the patient has not lost all their teeth, but has terminal dentition, the protocols for fabricating the complete prosthesis must be modified. In these cases, the retrieval of prosthetic coordinates such as the vertical dimension and the registration of the intermaxillary relations and that of the centric relation are hindered by the presence of residual teeth, often with high mobility and in an unsuitable position due to malposition and/or extrusion.

Even taking primary or panoramic impressions may be especially difficult or painful for the patient. The protocol for this type of patient has been used in the case illustrated in this chapter.

The patient treated is a 54-year-old woman suffering from severe periodontitis in terminal dentition. The patient complains of considerable mobility of the residual upper teeth, high difficulty in chewing [6], considerable instability of the lower prosthesis which should be stabilised by two spherical root attachments and, finally, considerable discomfort linked to the esthetics of the face with negative implications from a psychological point of view.

The first stage of the therapy focused on studying the prosthetic case: photographic and radiographic surveys were carried out and panoramic alginate impressions were taken for the upper as well as lower arch (**Figures 6.1** and **6.2**).

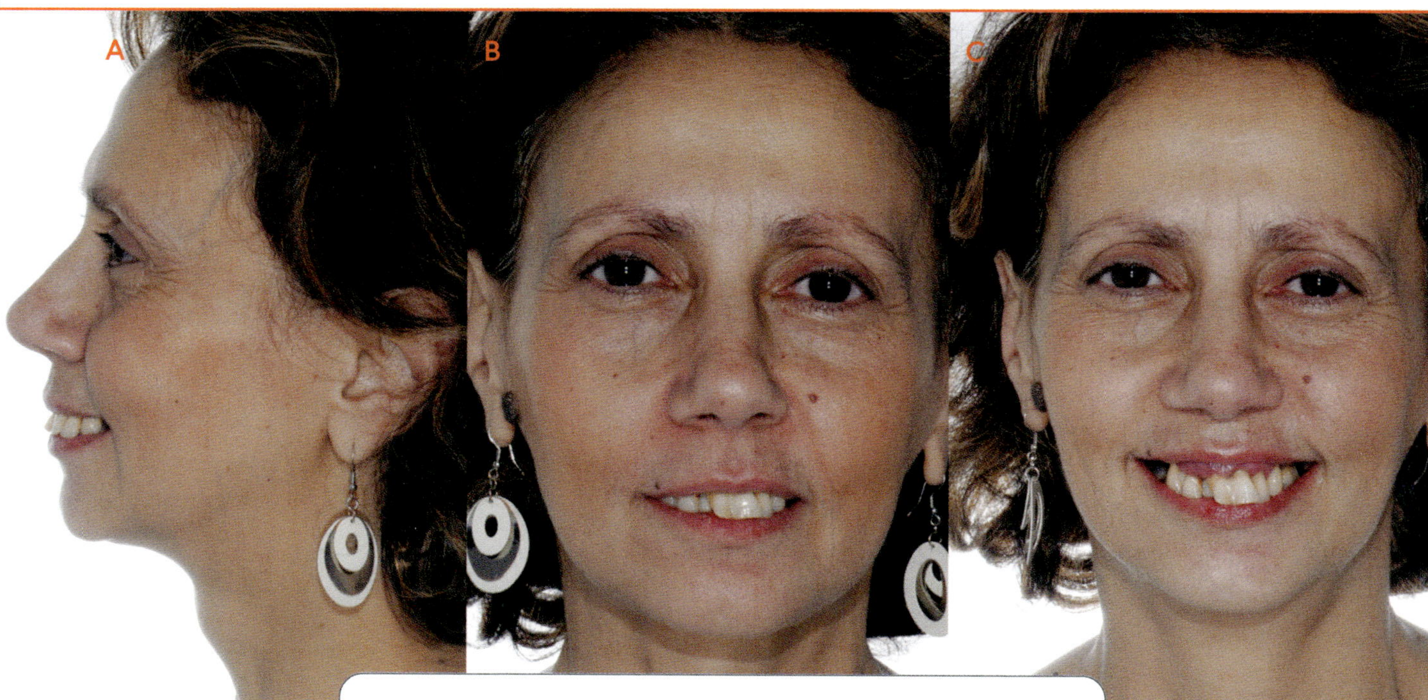

Figure 6.1 • Profile (**A**); dental display at rest (**B**) and maximum smile display (**C**).

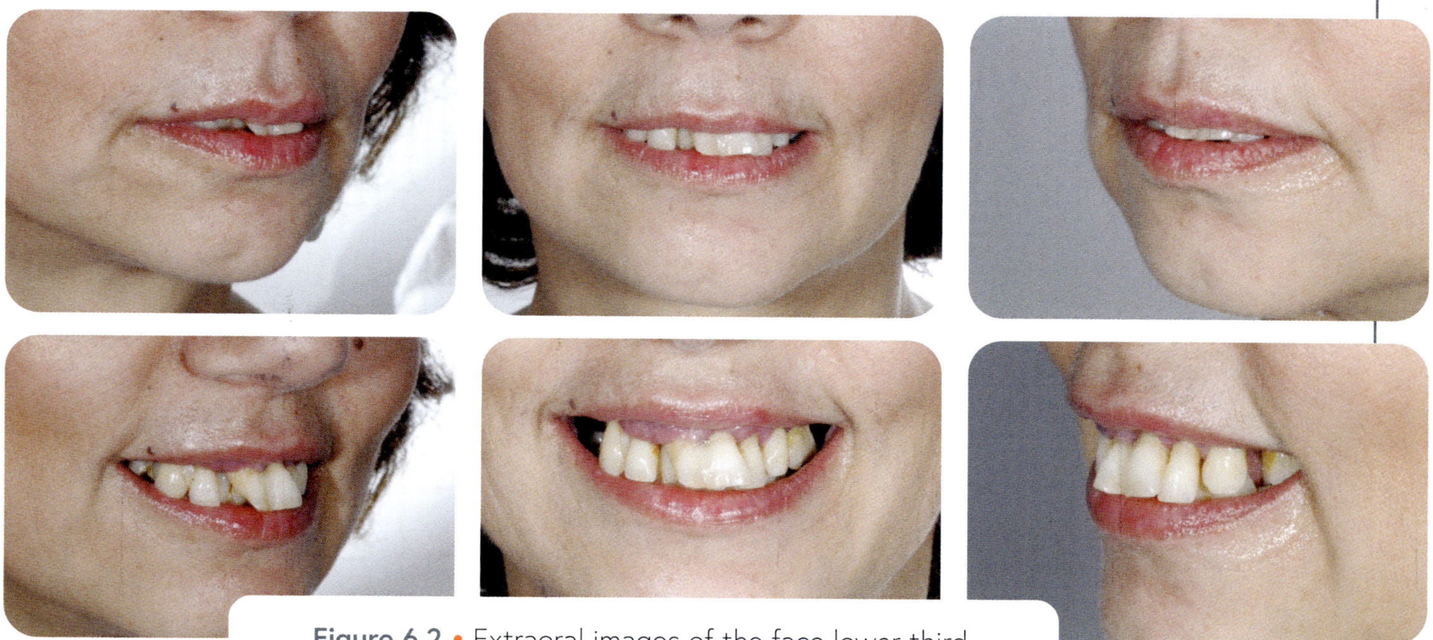

Figure 6.2 • Extraoral images of the face lower third.

Special attention was paid to the esthetic analysis and specifically, to the facial, dento-labial and phonetic analysis. Parallelism between the bipupillary and commissural lines in the frontal plane was evaluated **(Figure 6.3)**, as well as the relation between the E-Line (Esthetic line) [7] **(Figure 6.4)** and the lips on the sagittal plane. Advanced periodontal disease caused the loss of correspondence between the facial midline and the upper dental line, which appears off-centre and significantly slanted **(Figure 6.5)**.

The dento-labial analysis showed a 7 mm resting dental display **(Figure 6.6)**, with vestibularisation of the incisal ridge of the upper frontal teeth, which lost any normal relation with the lower lip, either in dynamic or static position, during phonation. The smile line is very high **(Figure 6.7)** because the extrusion of the front teeth has led to coronal migration of the soft tissues. The smile and labial corridors are wide.

The phonetic analysis confirmed the loss of vertical dimension and the existence of a wider than average FWS.

The extrusion of the upper front teeth causes the entire dental display to be taken up when uttering the phoneme /i/ [8-17] **(Figure 6.8)**.

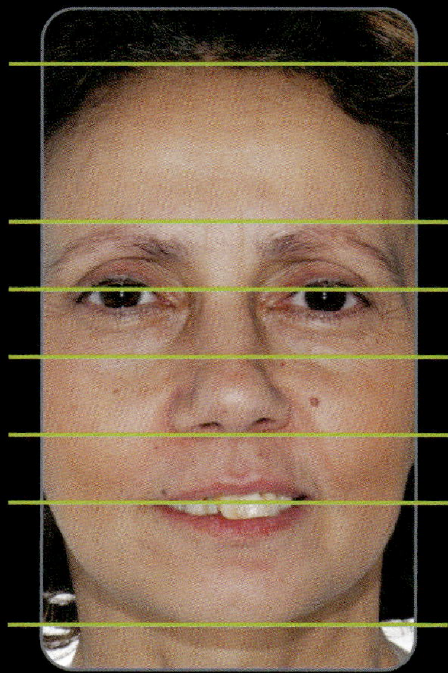

Figure 6.3 • Horizontal reference lines.

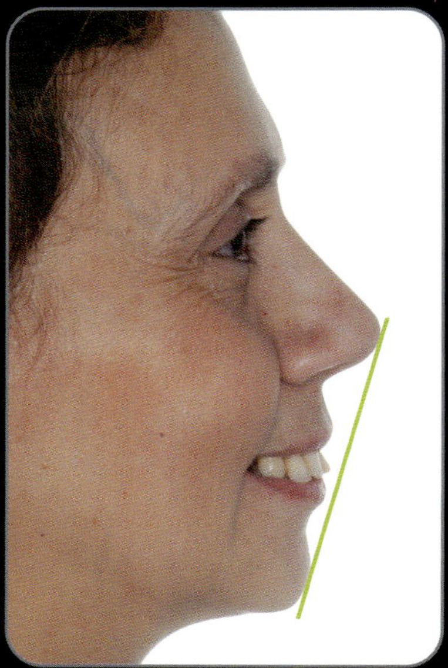

Figure 6.4 • Relation between lips and E-line.

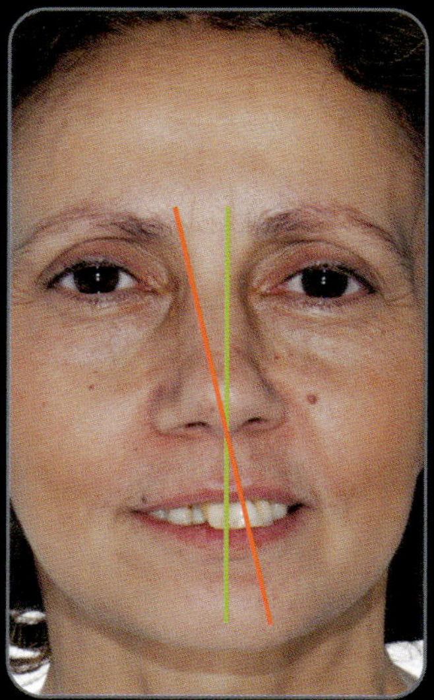

Figure 6.5 • Discrepancy between dental and facial midline.

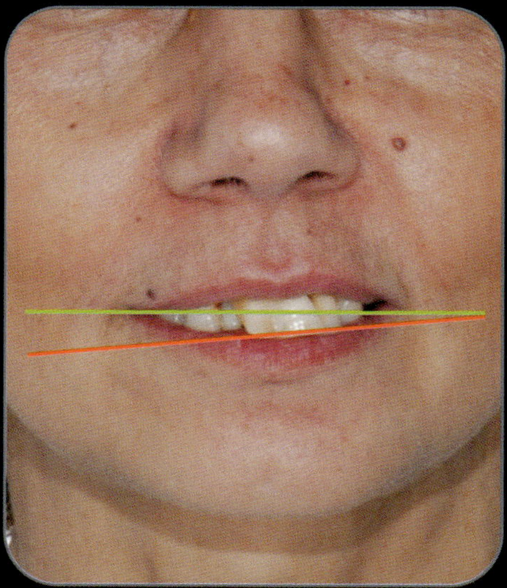

Figure 6.6 • Inconsistency between commissural and incisal line.

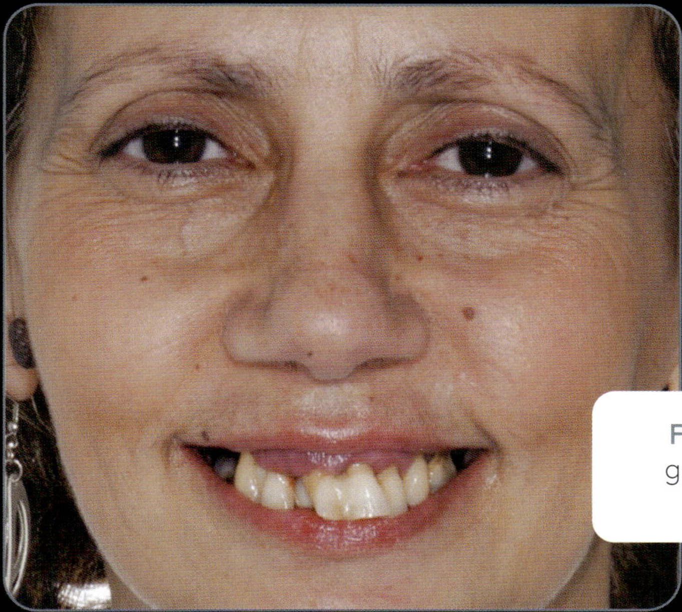

Figure 6.7 • The patient's gummy smile linked to the extrusion of the teeth.

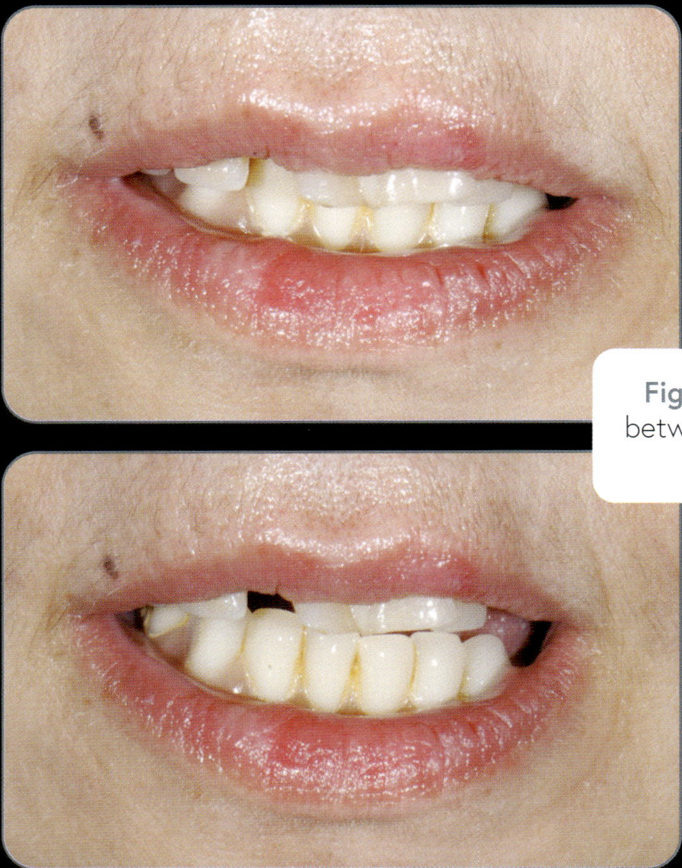

Figure 6.8 • Incorrect relations between teeth and lips during the phonetic tests.

The poor prognosis of all the residual teeth has led to the need to schedule their extraction with immediate delivery of a rehabilitation with removable prostheses.

Panoramic alginate impressions of both the upper and lower arch were taken and subsequently developed in the laboratory.

An individual self-curing resin impression tray was made on the models obtained **(Figure 6.9)**; following its functionalisation, it was used to take a precision impression.

With regard to the upper arch, different impression materials were used: polyether (Impregum™, 3M ESPE) to take the impression of the dentate area and zinc oxide-eugenol

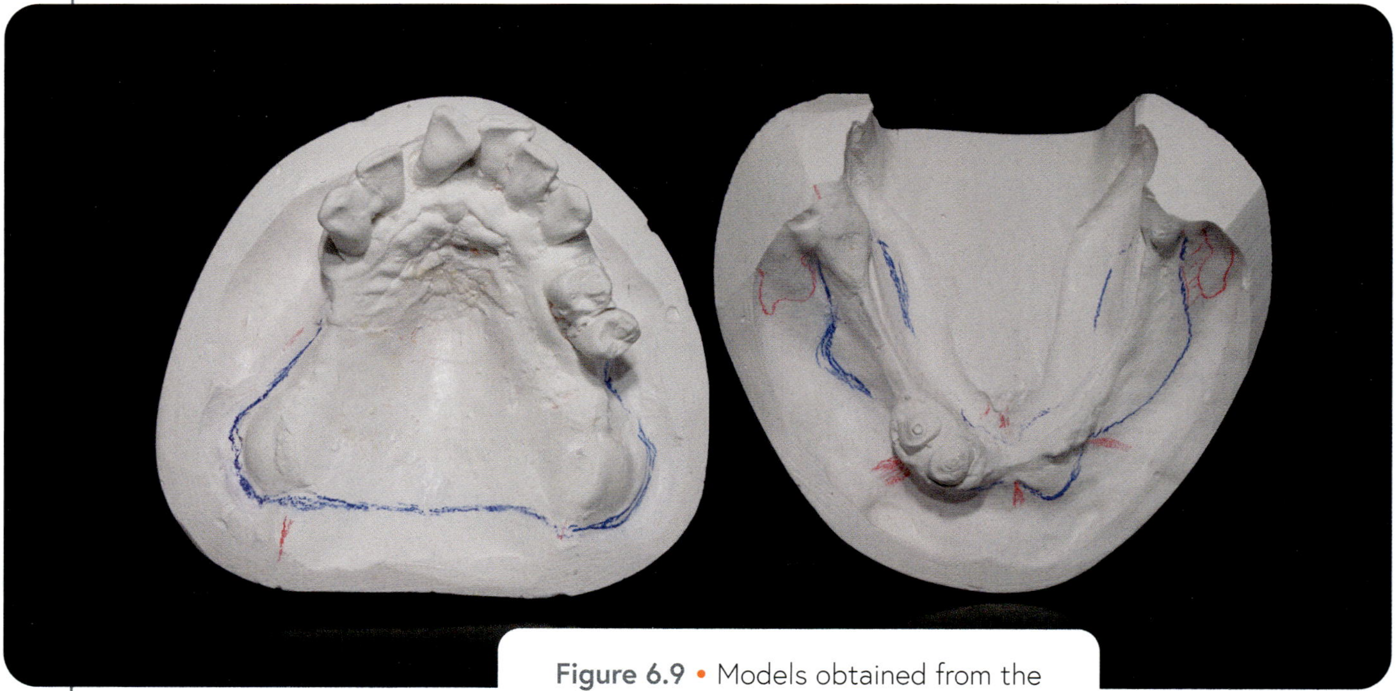

Figure 6.9 • Models obtained from the "panoramic" primary impressions.

paste (SSWhite, Kerr Dental, Canton Ticino Switzerland) for the edentulous one **(Figure 6.10)**.

The lower impression was made in polyether, after treatment with specific adhesive of the tray. The master models obtained **(Figure 6.11)** were used to make the wax rims for occlusal registration on self-curing resin plates. In the subsequent clinical

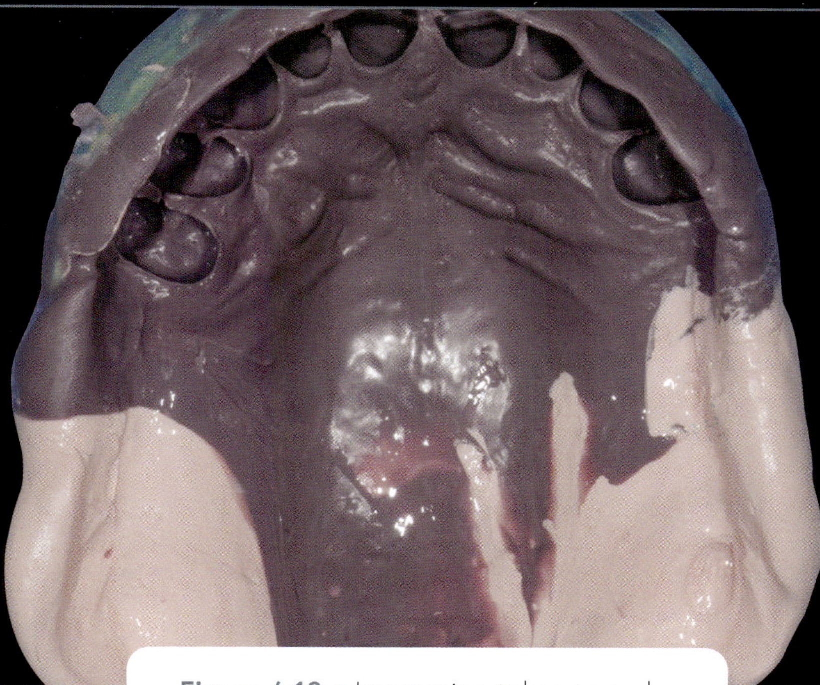

Figure 6.10 • Impression taken to make the master model.

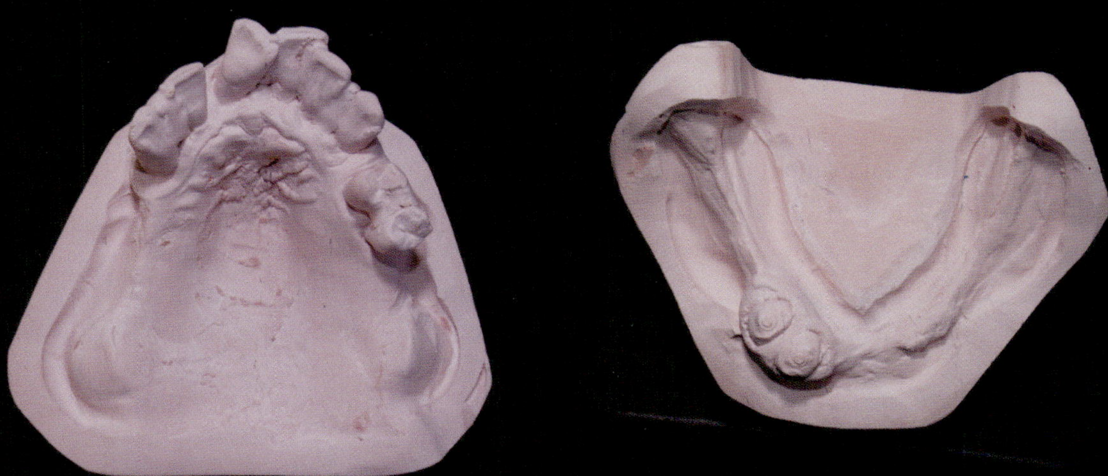

Figure 6.11 • Master models.

stage, the plates were used for the registration of the intermaxillary relations (**Figure 6.12**).

In the same session, the facebow was taken, which made it possible to mount the master models in the articulator at semi-individual values (**Figure 6.13**) [18].

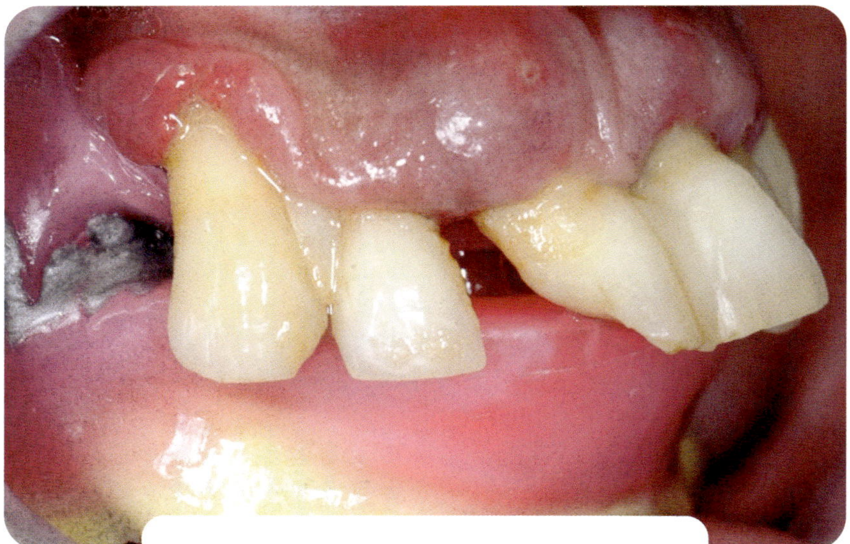

Figure 6.12 • Registration of the intermaxillary relations.

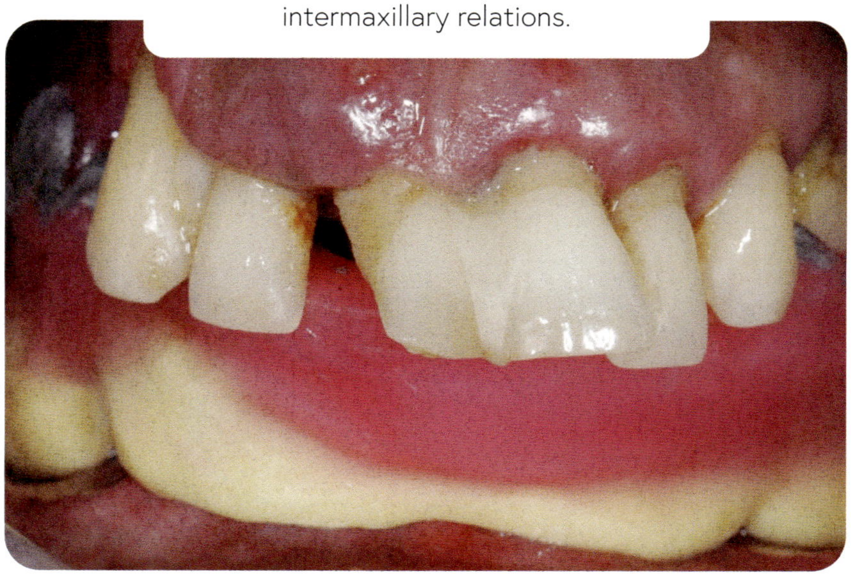

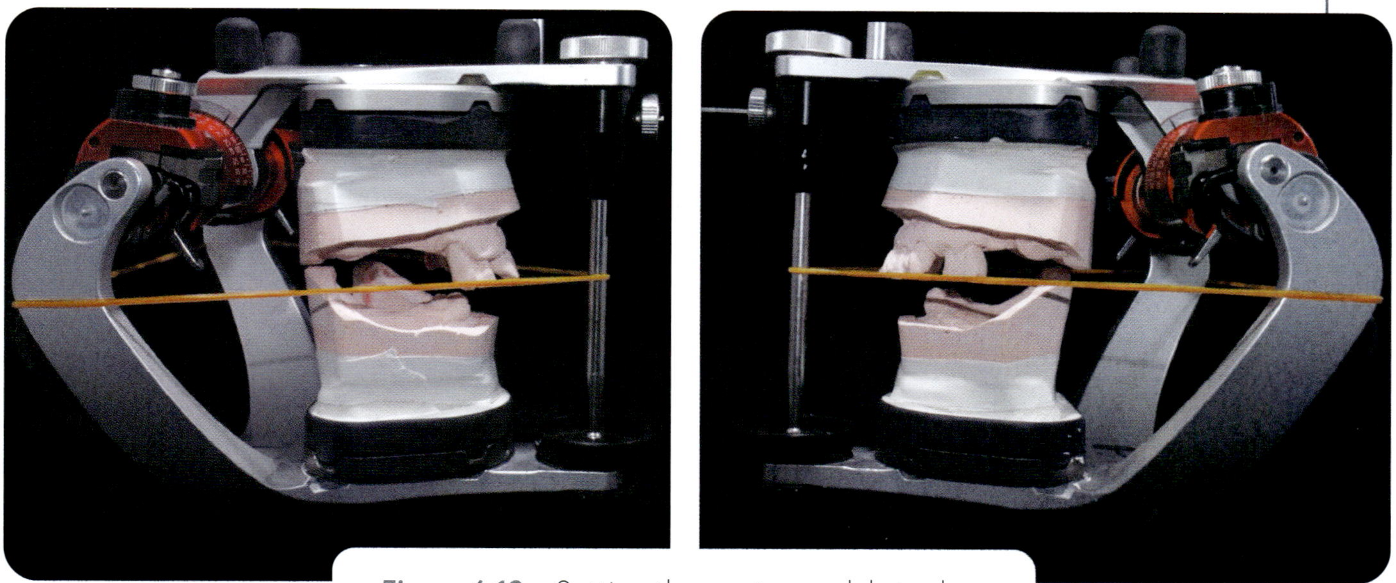

Figure 6.13 • Setting the master models in class three articulator (semi-adjustable).

The analysis of the models took into account the initial esthetic evaluations (**Figure 6.14**): the front teeth were shortened as per clinical indication to establish a dental display at rest of 3-5 mm (**Figure 6.15**). The position of the central upper incisors on the horizontal plane was set up at about 10 mm from the incisive papilla. (**Figures 6.16** and **6.17**).

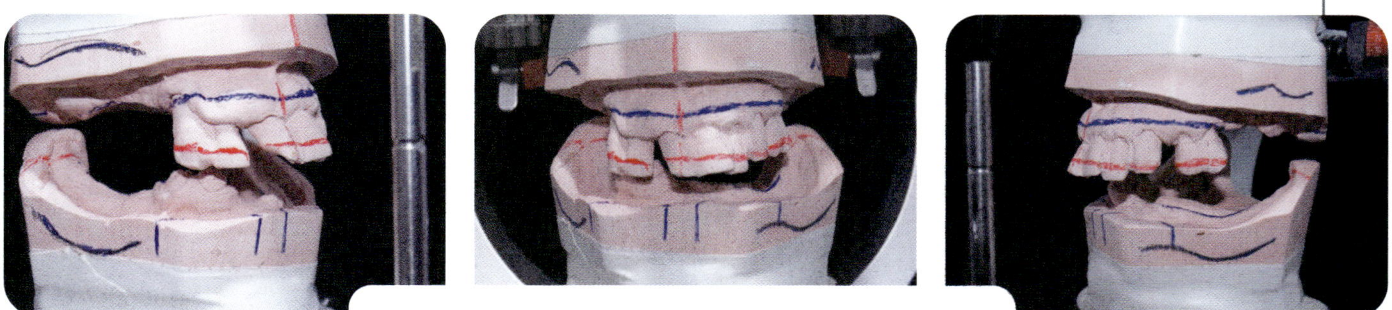

Figure 6.14 • The initial esthetic evaluations are transferred to the plaster models.

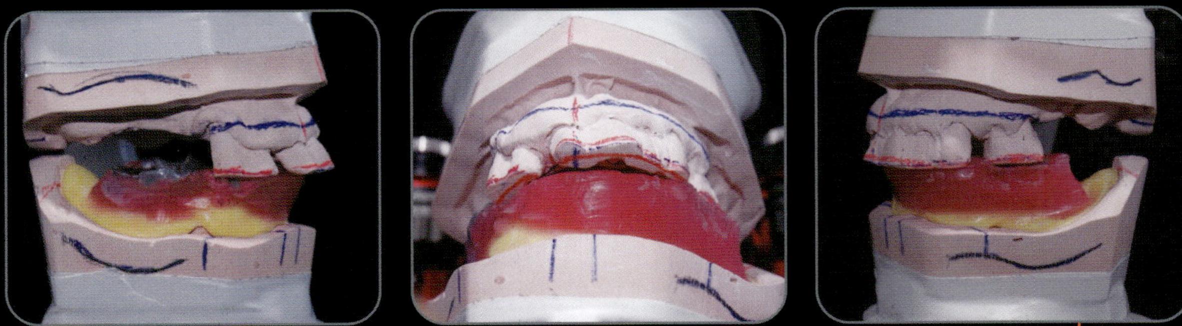

Figure 6.15 • The length of the dentures has been reduced on the model in order to have a dental display at the end of the therapy of about 3 mm.

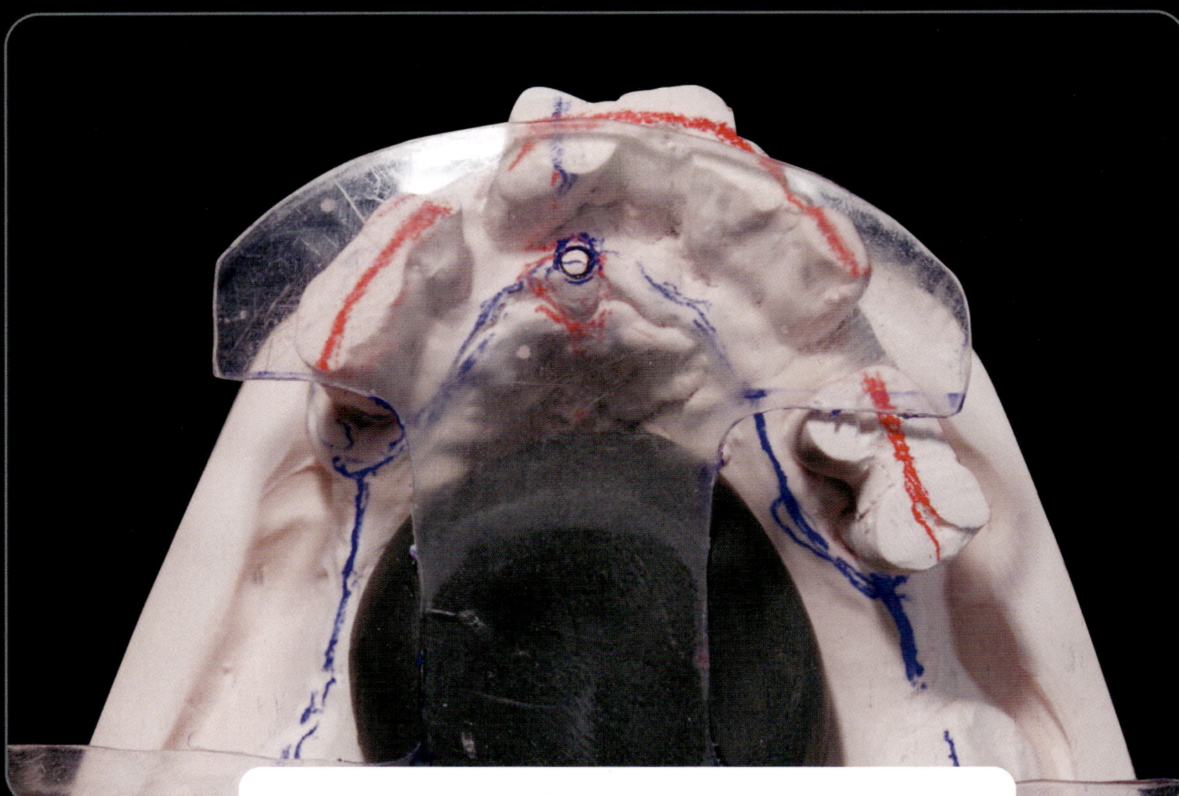

Figure 6.16 • On the horizontal plane, the upper incisors were placed 10 mm from the incisive papilla.

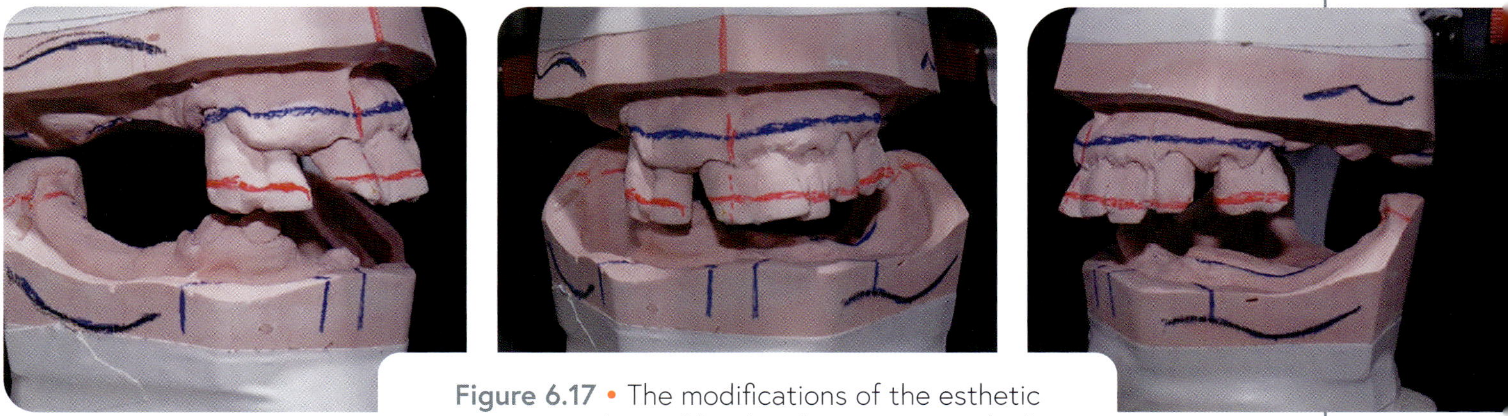

Figure 6.17 • The modifications of the esthetic parameters indicated by the clinician are applied on the master models.

The residual teeth were then removed from the plaster model taking care not to remove the gingival papillae in such a way as to avoid excessive compression by the prosthesis on the surgical wound. The set-up was prepared according to a combined occlusal scheme: the semi-anatomic upper teeth were set, i.e. with cusps at 18°, and the non-anatomical lower teeth with cusps at 0° [19] (Ivoclar Vivadent, Schaan Liechtenstein).

Furthermore, a 12 mm overjet was designed. An overbite was not planned to avoid interference in protrusive movements: muscle de-conditioning was achieved thanks to the combined occlusal scheme in a similar way as that carried out by the bite-plane in the case of a fixed prosthesis.

The immediate prostheses were finalised and subsequently finished in accordance with the procedures described in Chapter 4 (**Figures 6.18-6.22**).

The esthetic and functional assessments pointed to the need to plan osteotomy in the premaxilla region. To this end, two guides were prepared: a fenestrated plate and a plate that replicated the impression surface of the immediate prosthesis (**Figures 6.23** and **6.24**).

The first guide was used in the surgical stage to evaluate the amount of hard and soft tissues to be removed, the second to assess the possibility of passive seating of the post-extraction prosthesis in the absence of compressions and before performing the surgical wound suture.

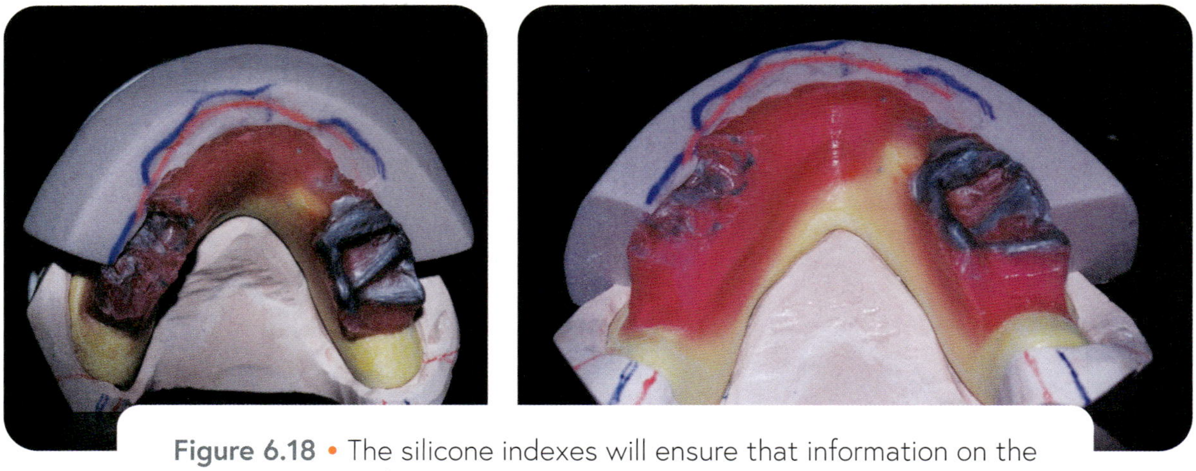

Figure 6.18 • The silicone indexes will ensure that information on the original position of the patient's teeth is not lost once the plaster teeth are removed from the master model.

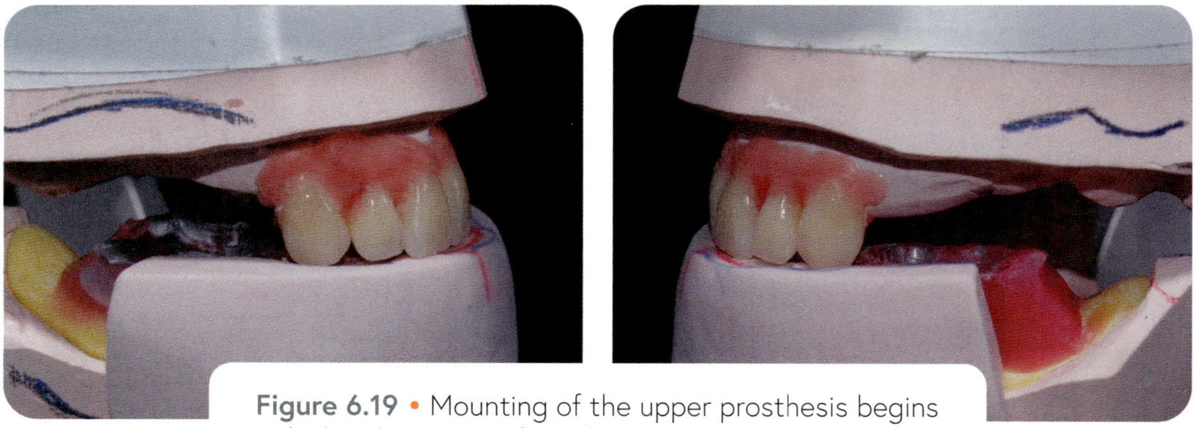

Figure 6.19 • Mounting of the upper prosthesis begins with the placement of the front group of artificial teeth.

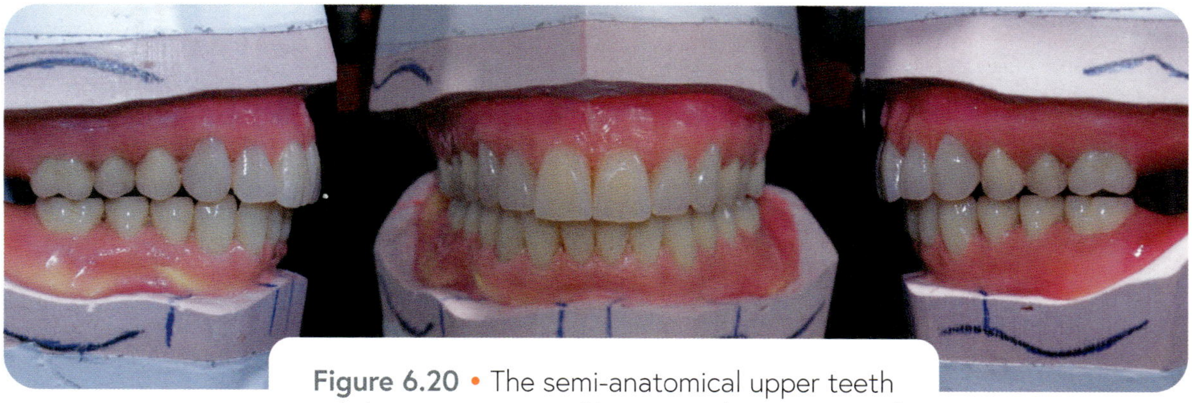

Figure 6.20 • The semi-anatomical upper teeth and the non anatomical lower teeth are mounted.

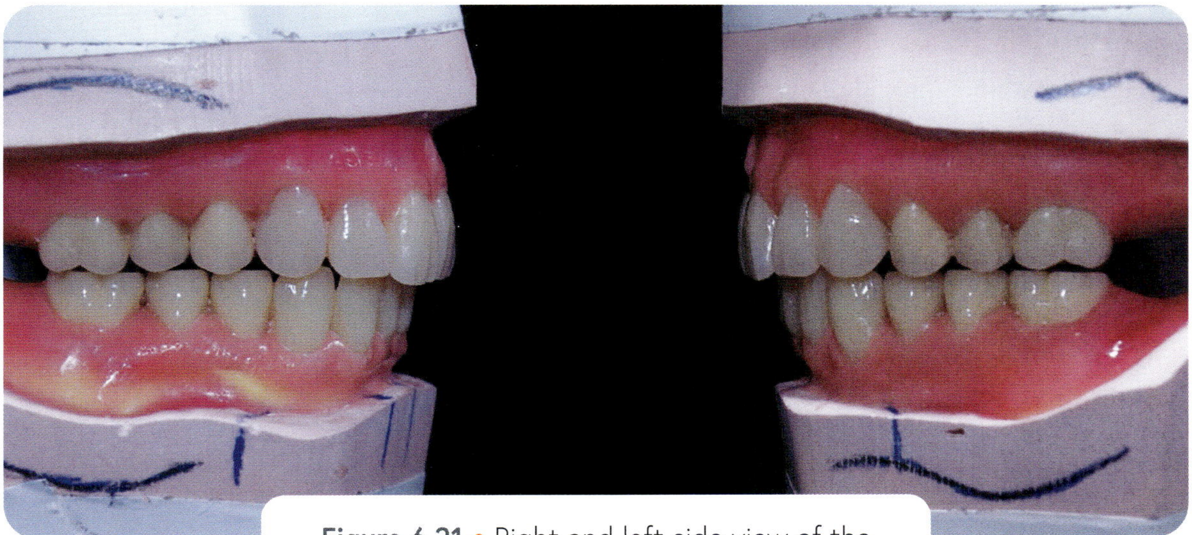

Figure 6.21 • Right and left side view of the finalised prosthesis.

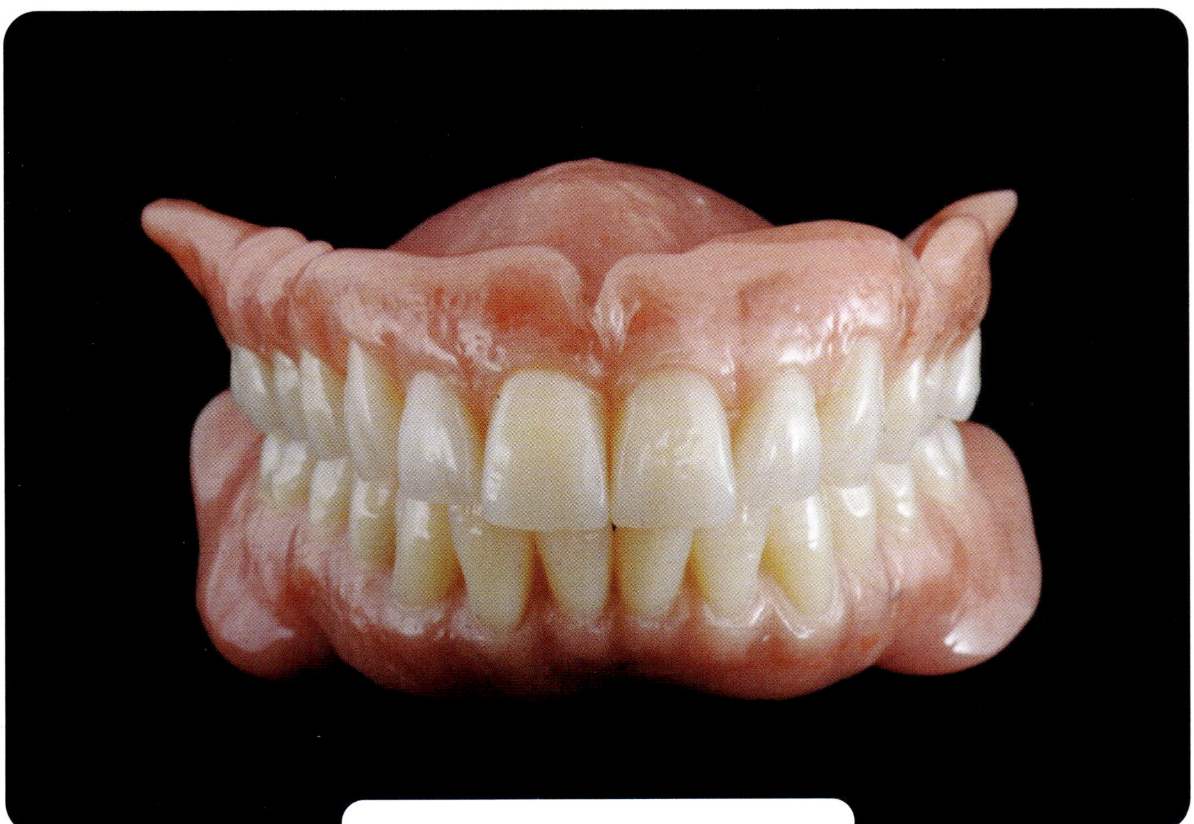

Figure 6.22 • Completed prosthesis.

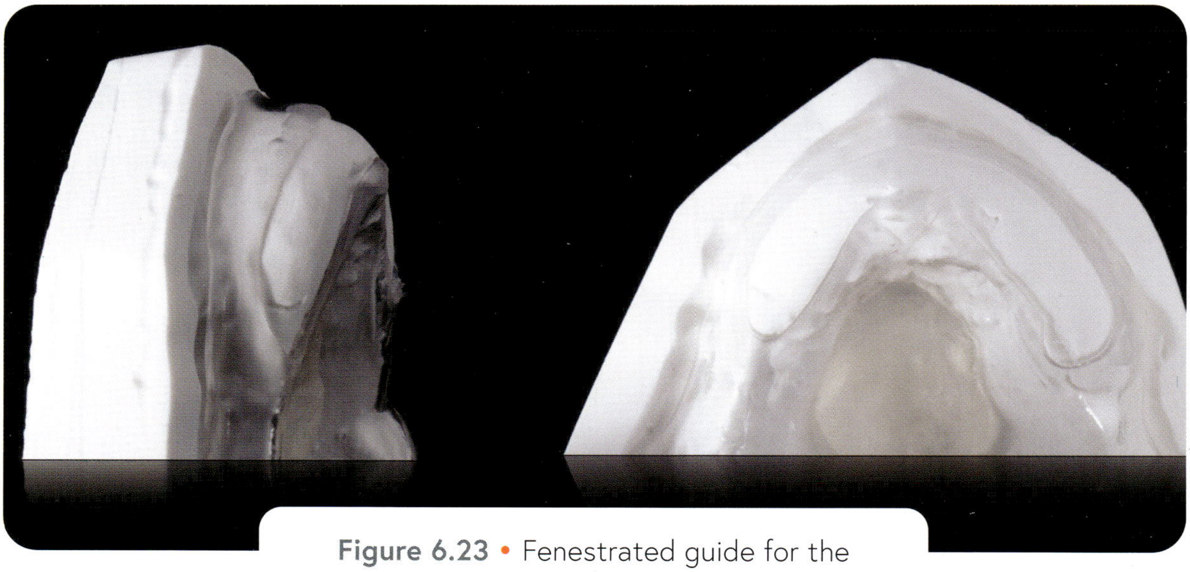

Figure 6.23 • Fenestrated guide for the surgical stage.

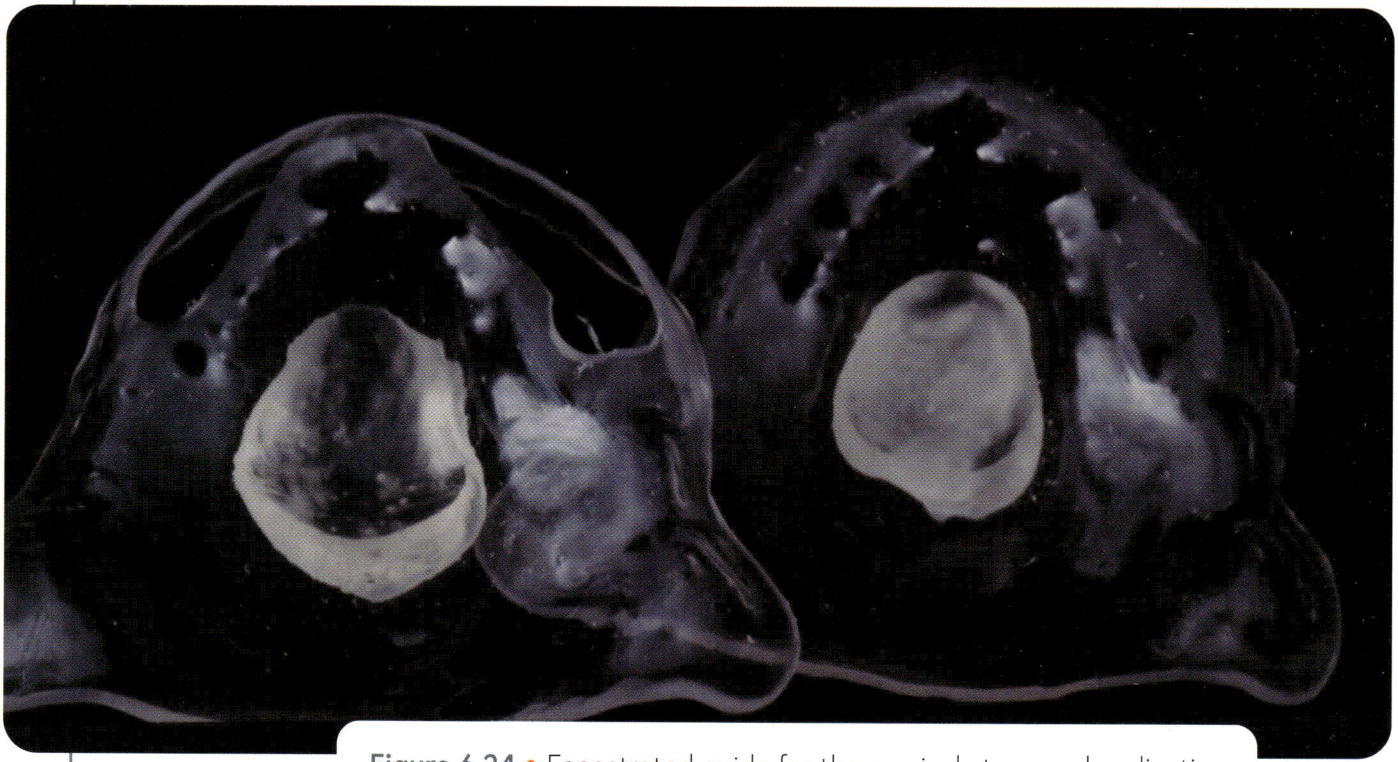

Figure 6.24 • Fenestrated guide for the surgical stage and replicative guide of the impression surface of the immediate prosthesis.

All the teeth and root residues were then extracted, the ridges were regularised in accordance with the indications of the surgical guide **(Figure 6.25)** and the absence of compression areas was ascertained by means of the transparent replica of the impression surface of the prosthesis **(Figures 6.26-6.28)**. The sutures were made and the prosthesis was delivered.

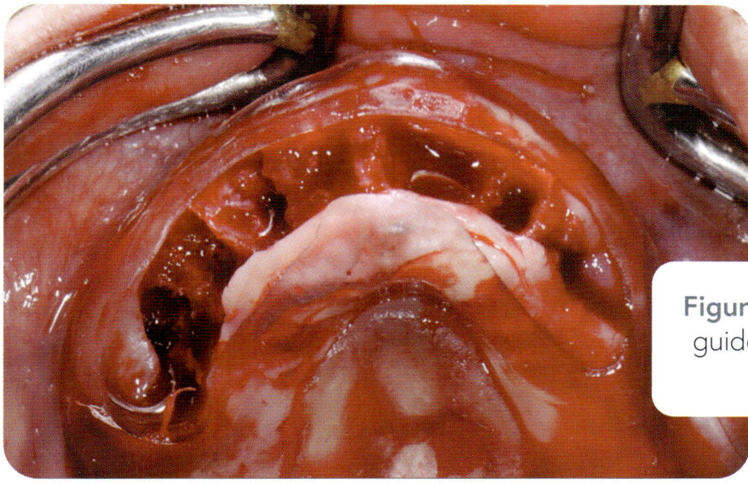

Figure 6.25 • The fenestrated surgical guide is inserted following extraction of the residual teeth.

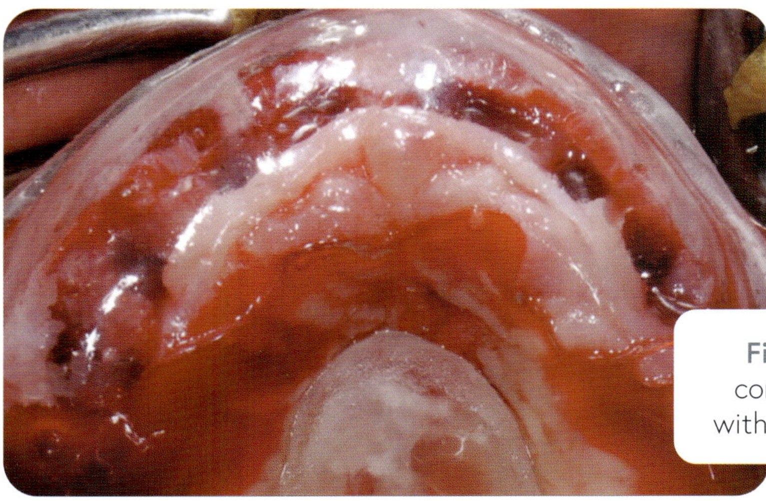

Figure 6.26 • The absence of compression areas is confirmed with the second transparent plate.

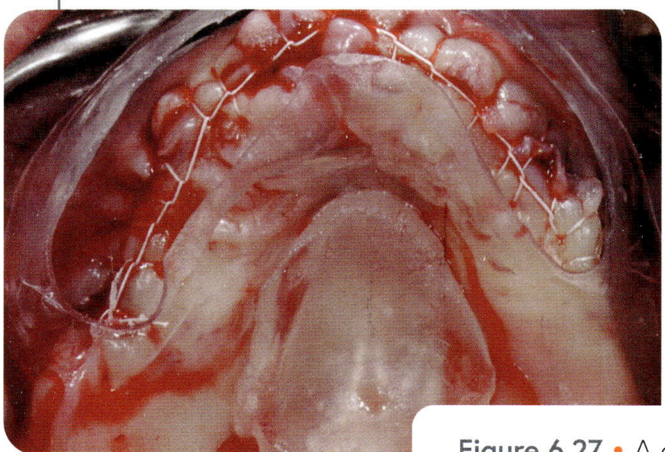

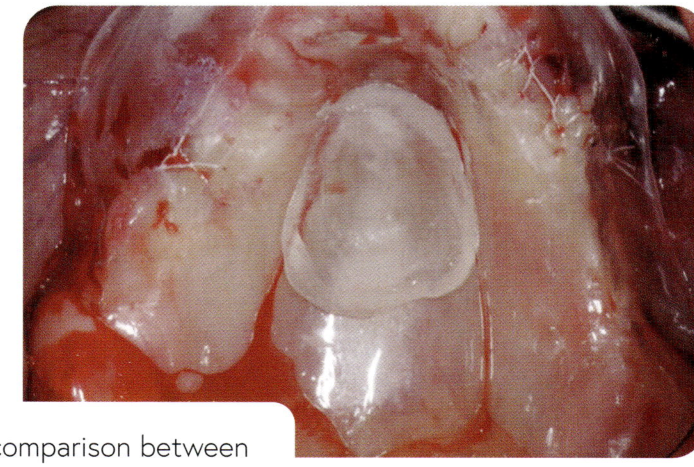

Figure 6.27 • A comparison between the two guides.

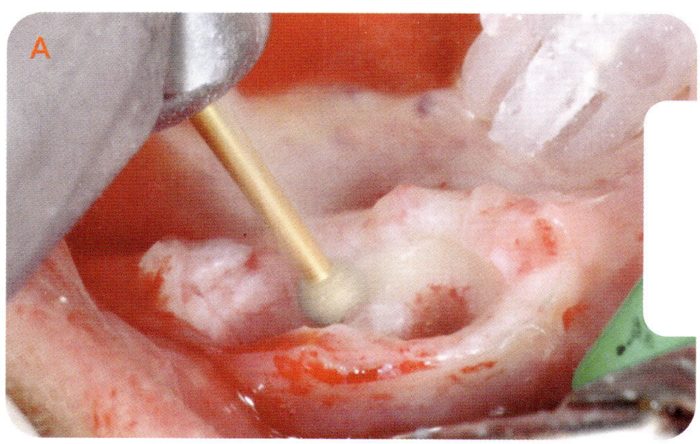

Figure 6.28 • (**A**) An osteotomy is performed to regularise the bone and to enable better prosthetic fit. (**B**) Guide to check the sufficient osteotomy in the lower arch.

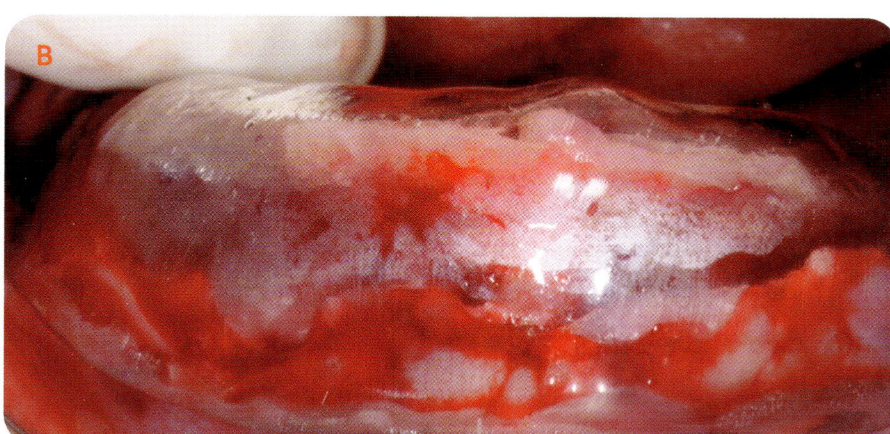

The rehabilitation seemed adequate from the esthetic point of view as well as in terms of occlusal relations and tissue support (**Figures 6.29** and **6.30**).

This assessment was confirmed at the time of the follow-up visit to remove the sutures: the phonetic tests showed the esthetic and functional adequacy of the prosthetic design. The tissues continued healing in an optimal manner (**Figure 6.31**).

The patient was checked approximately every 2 weeks and, as envisaged, a slight mandible post-rotation was observed, which gradually stabilised.

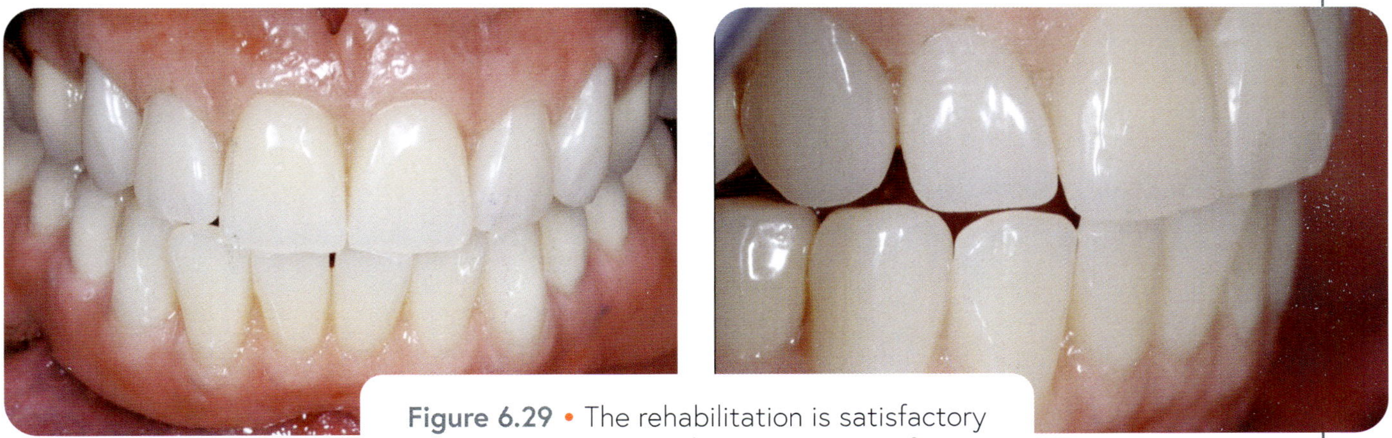

Figure 6.29 • The rehabilitation is satisfactory from the esthetic and functional point of view.

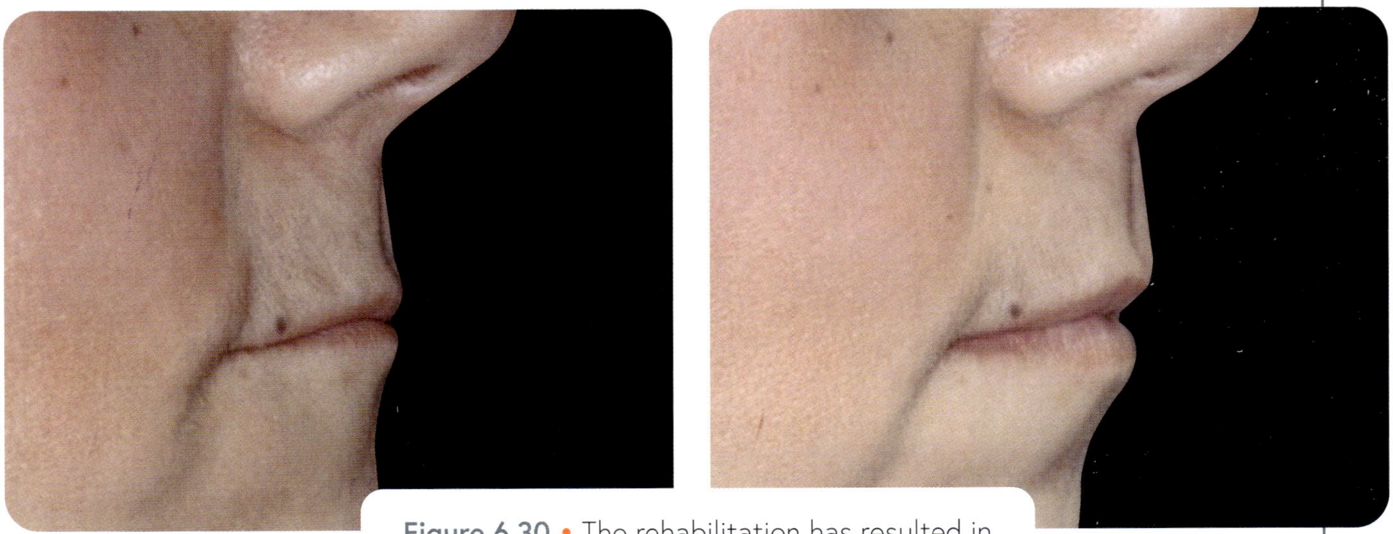

Figure 6.30 • The rehabilitation has resulted in good support of the perioral tissues.

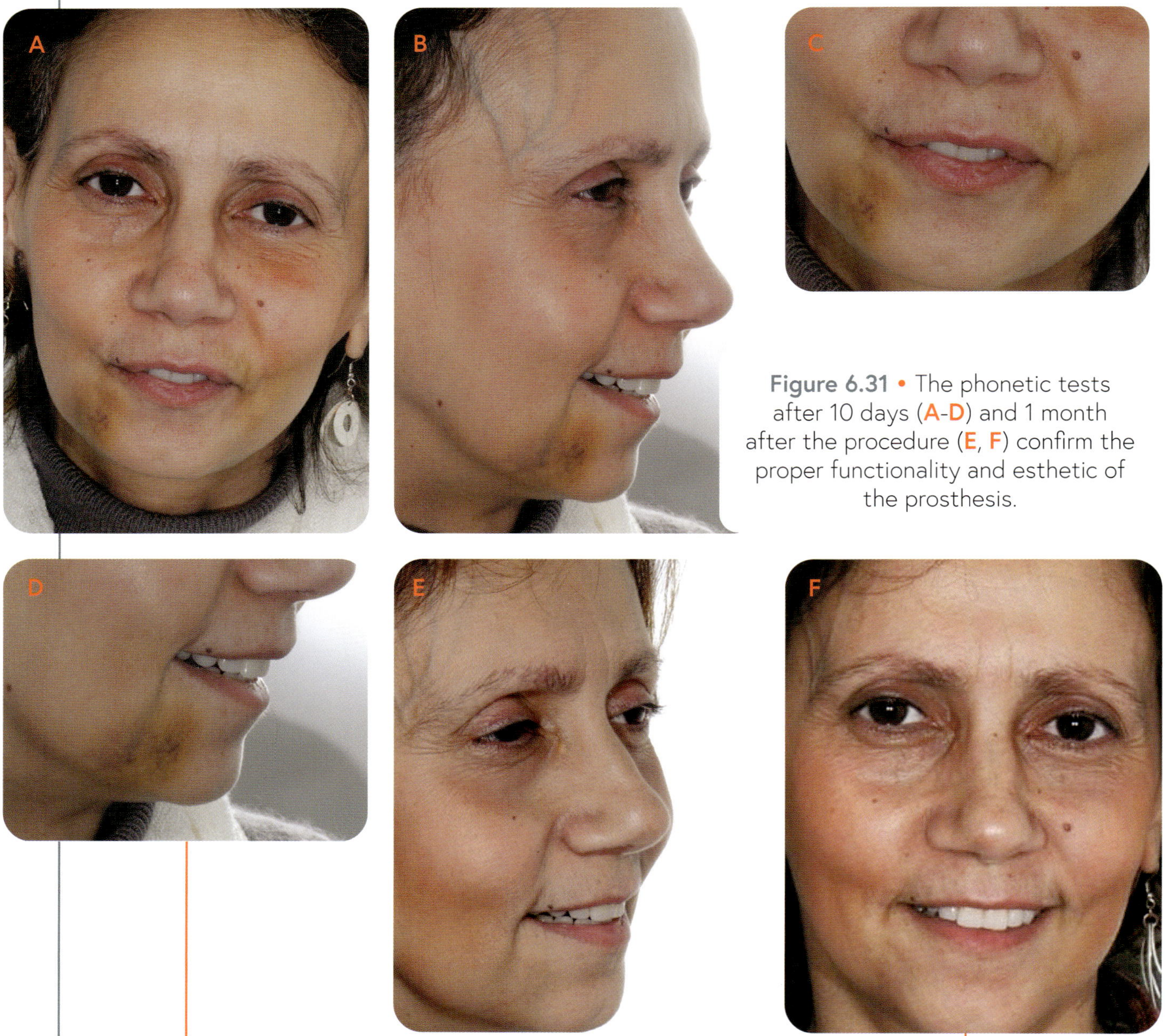

Figure 6.31 • The phonetic tests after 10 days (**A**-**D**) and 1 month after the procedure (**E**, **F**) confirm the proper functionality and esthetic of the prosthesis.

After one month, the prostheses were treated with a tissue conditioner, and after a further three-month period, they were rebased in the laboratory.

Four months after the extractions, the soft tissues showed perfect healing and occlusion proved to be stable and repeatable **(Figure 6.32)**.

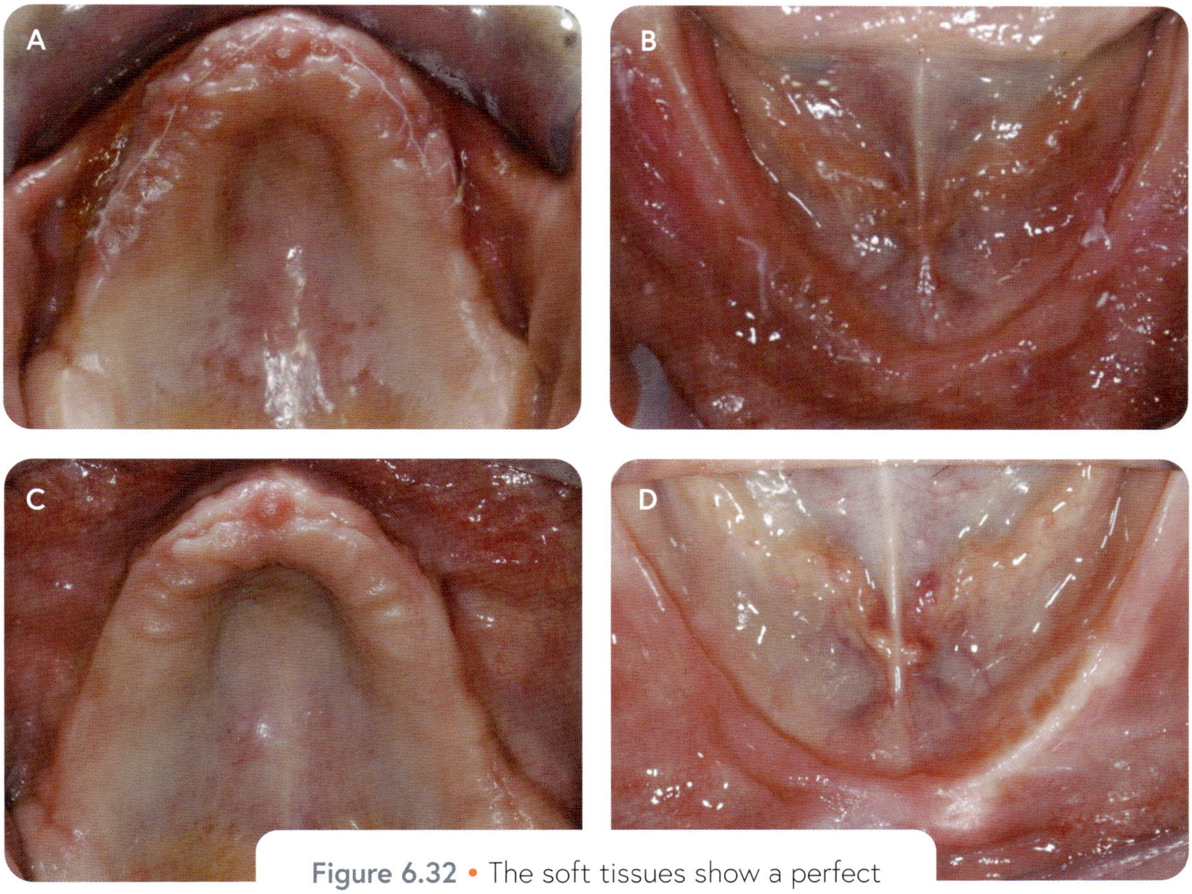

Figure 6.32 • The soft tissues show a perfect healing process at the 10-day follow-up (A,B) and after 4 months (C,D).

However, the perioral tissues underwent re-adaptation to the extent of preventing the teeth from being displayed in a resting condition (Figure 6.33).

That is why the facebow was taken again and the prostheses were therefore set again in the articulator and modified in relation to the new functional and esthetic evaluations [20,21] (Figure 6.34).

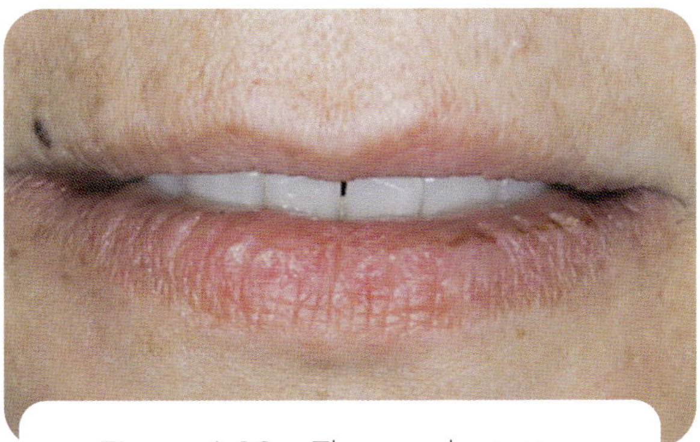

Figure 6.33 • The re-adaptation of the perioral tissues does not enable proper display of the upper teeth in the resting position.

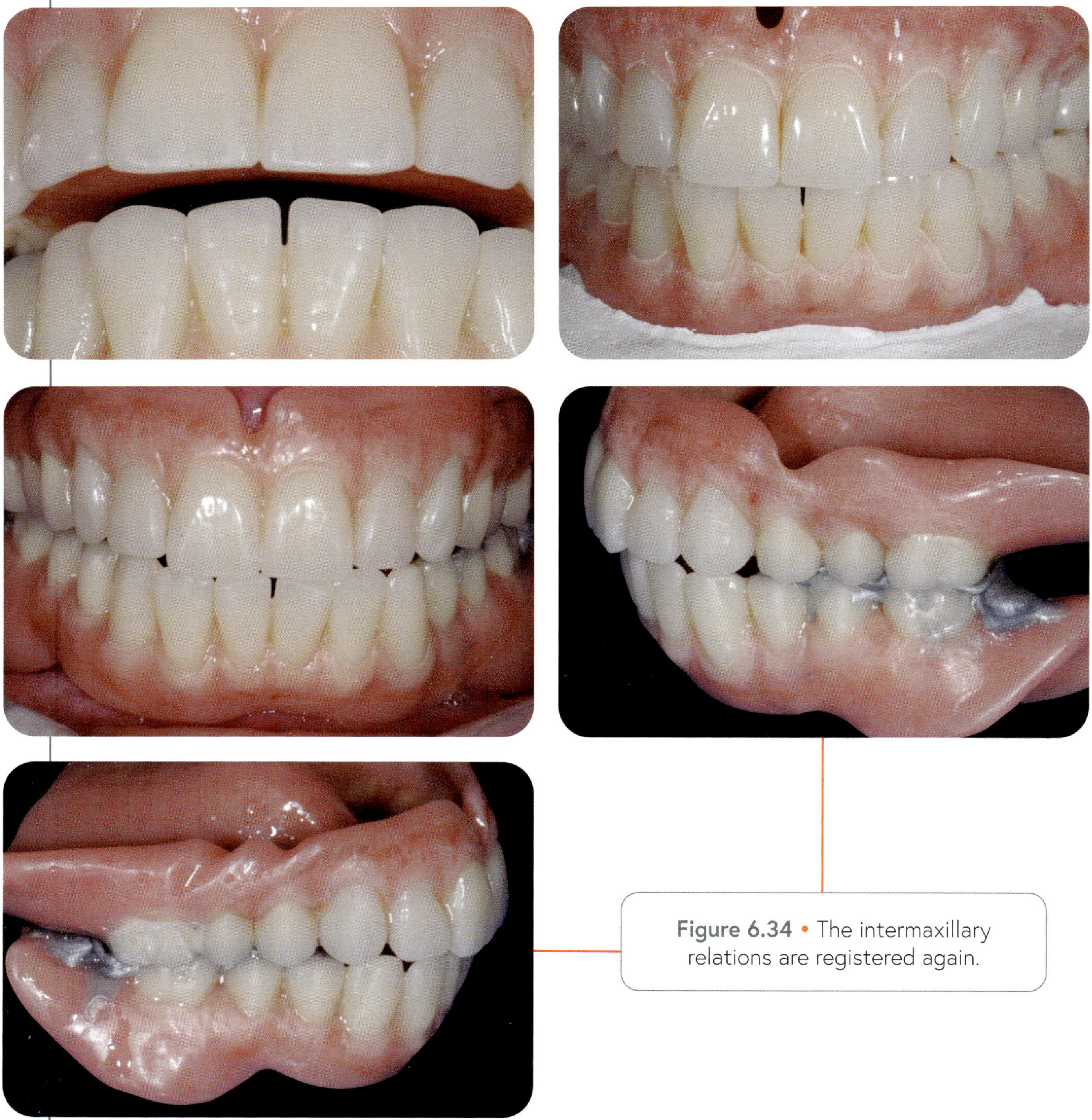

Figure 6.34 • The intermaxillary relations are registered again.

After another two months, occlusal stability, esthetics and phonetics were checked (**Figure 6.35**).

The patient's prostheses were duplicated in a self-curing resin (polymethyl-methacrylate) according to the procedures that will be described in Chapter 7. The replicas were used to perform cross-mounting in complete prosthesis: the acrylic teeth were replaced by trade ones (Phonares® II, Ivoclar Viva-dent) without losing any of the already tested parameters: shape, position and occlusion (**Figures 6.36** and **6.37**).

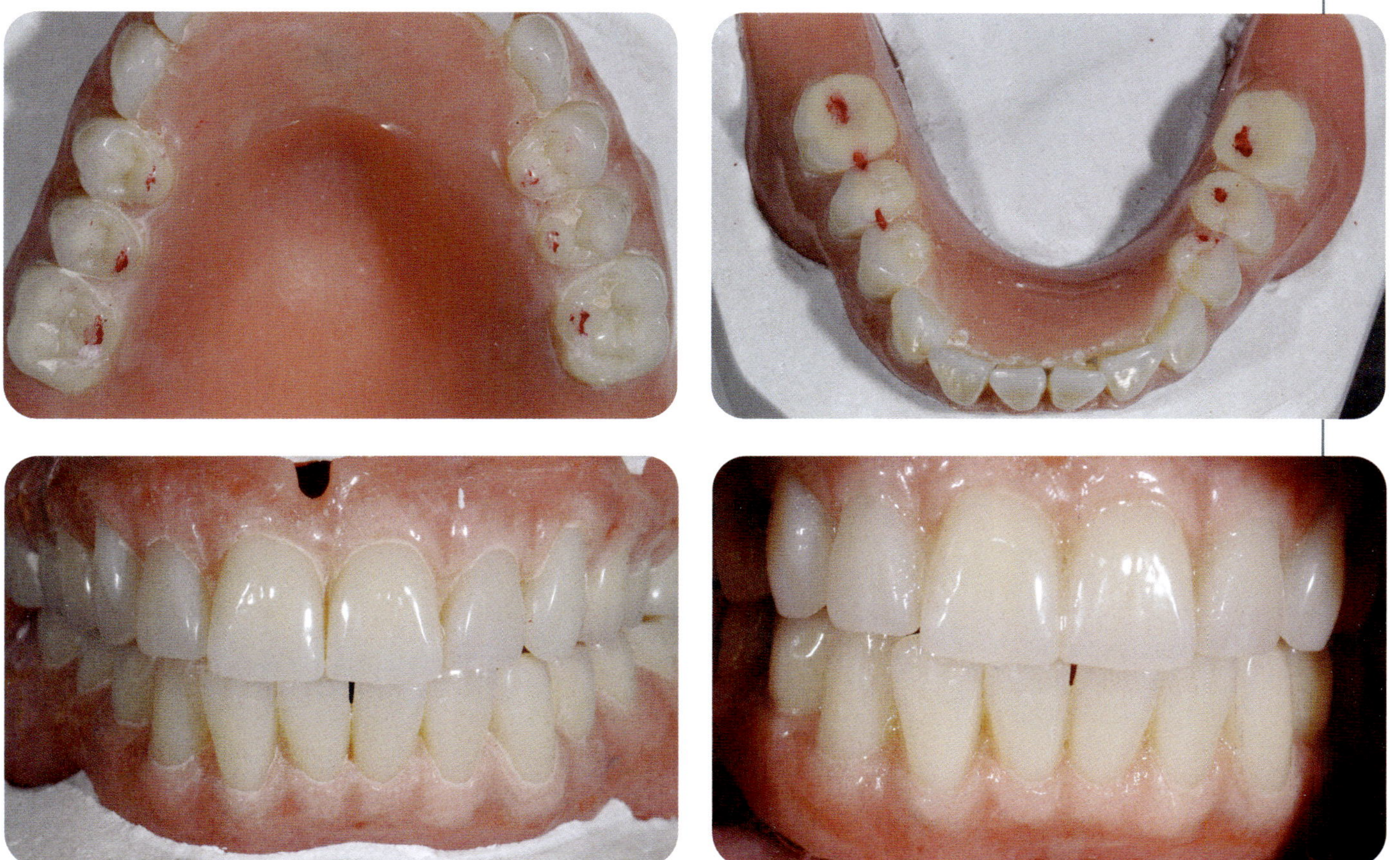

Figure 6.35 • Occlusal contacts after setting the posterior teeth again.

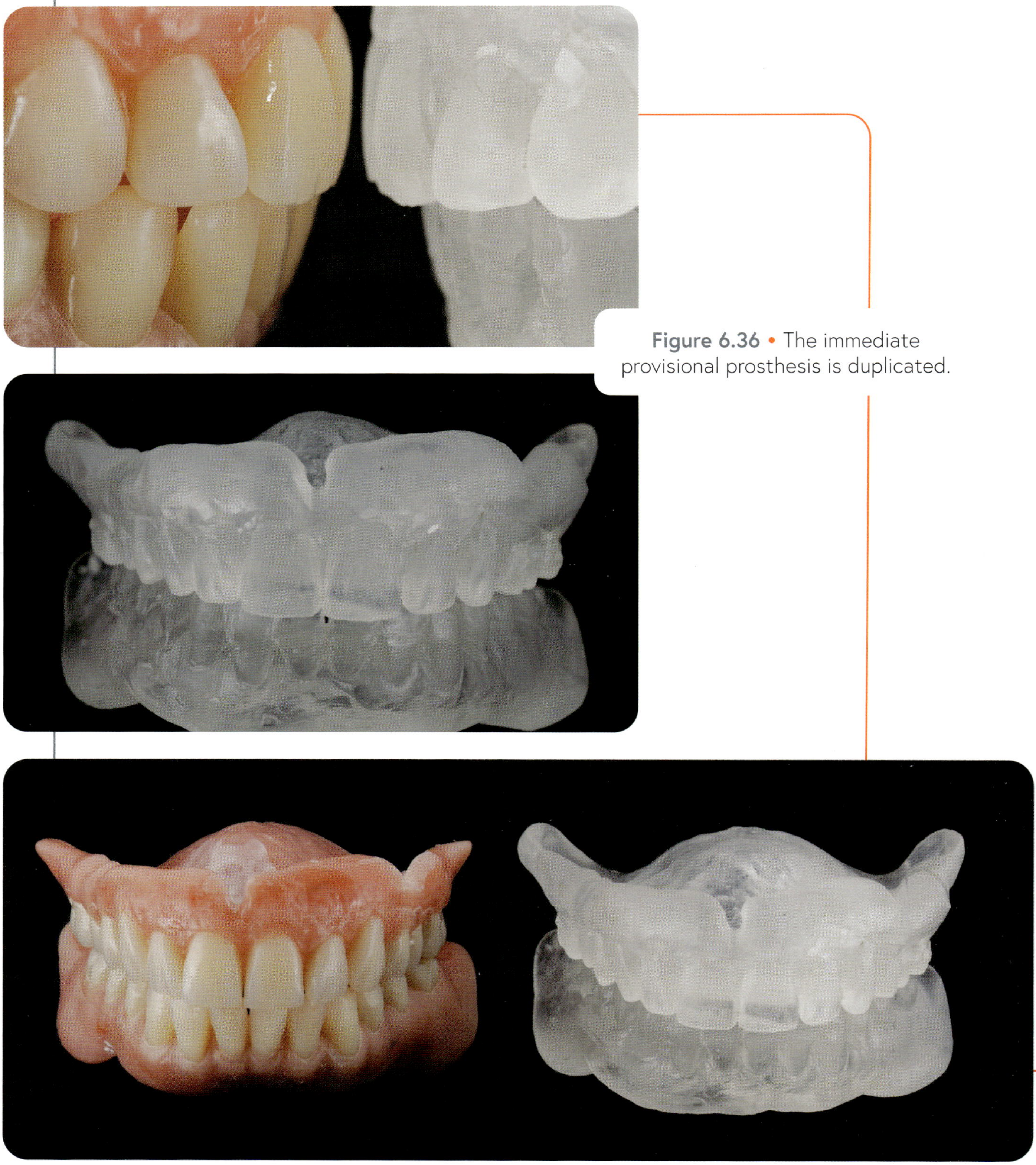

Figure 6.36 • The immediate provisional prosthesis is duplicated.

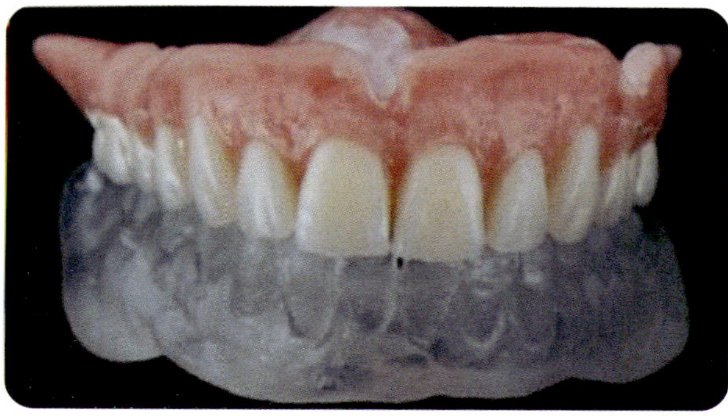

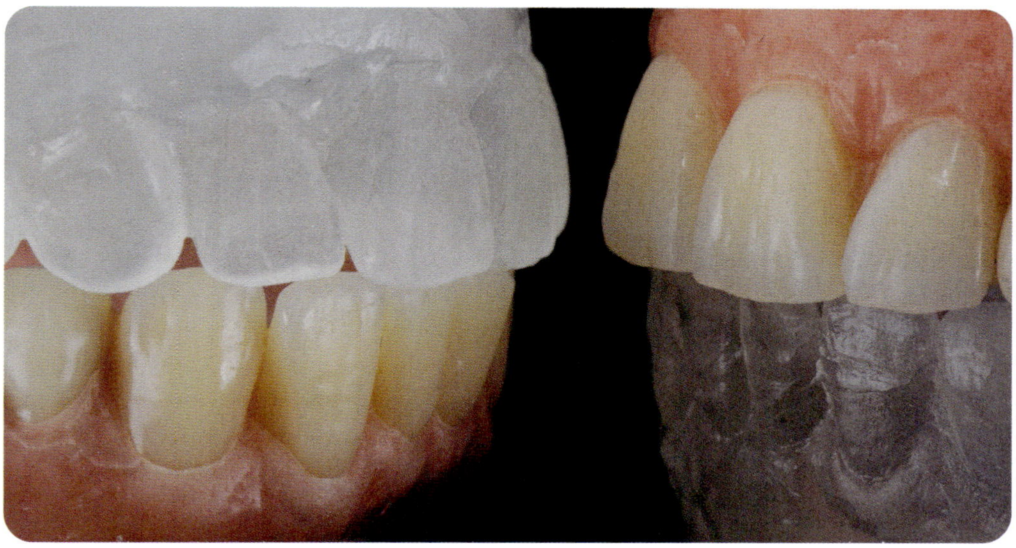

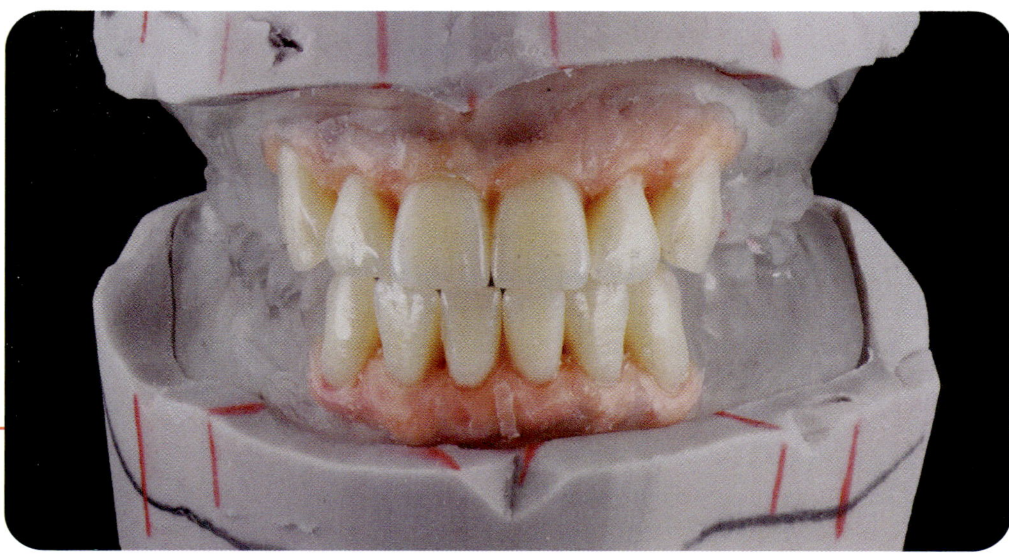

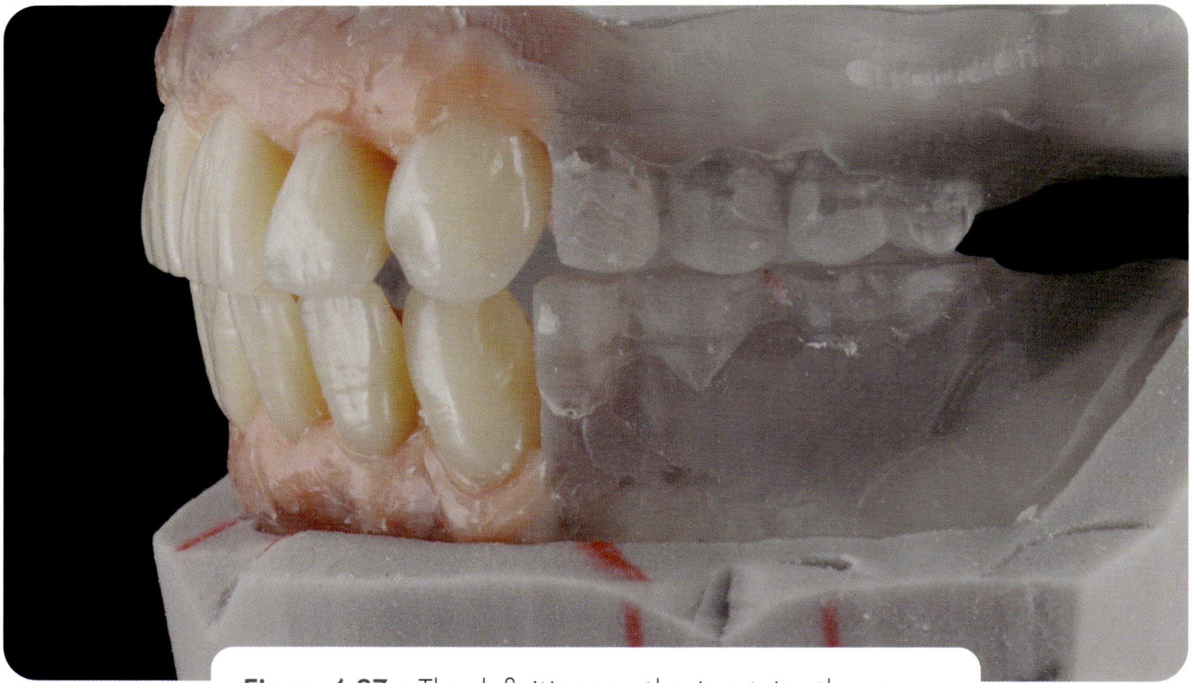

Figure 6.37 • The definitive prosthesis retains the parameters already confirmed with the provisional prosthesis.

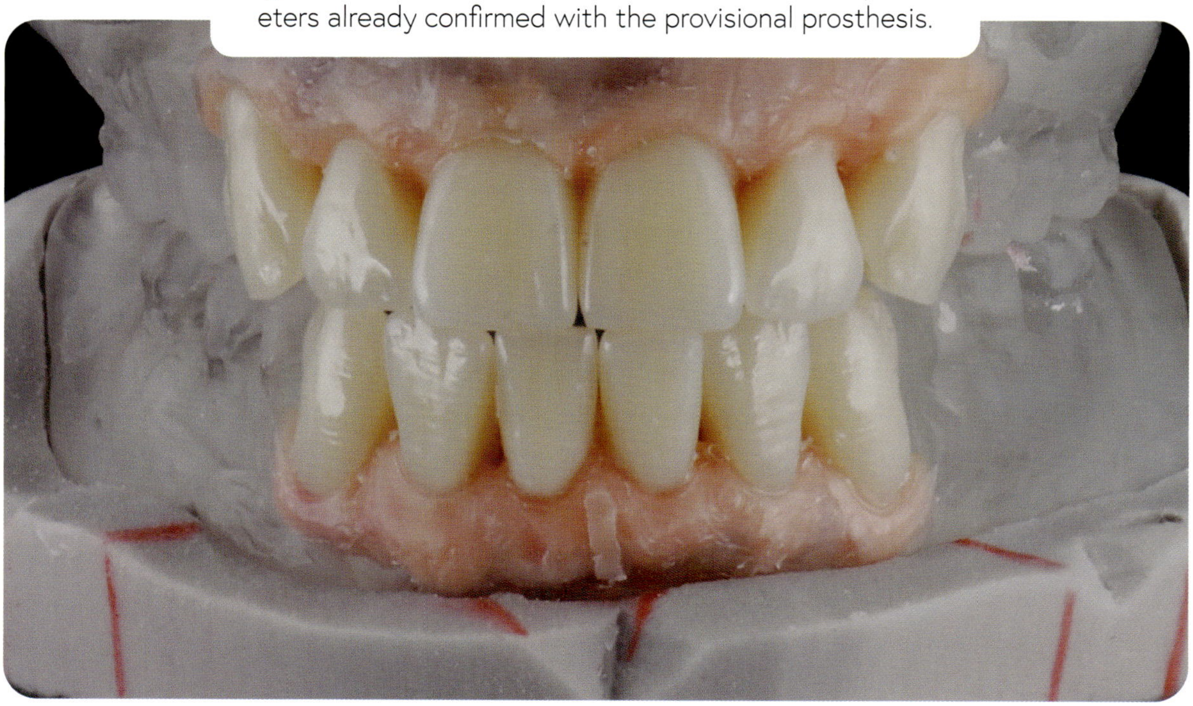

An esthetic test was then performed of the upper and lower six (**Figure 6.38**). The prostheses were finalised and delivered without any occlusal touch-up and with the utmost satisfaction of the patient (**Figure 6.39**).

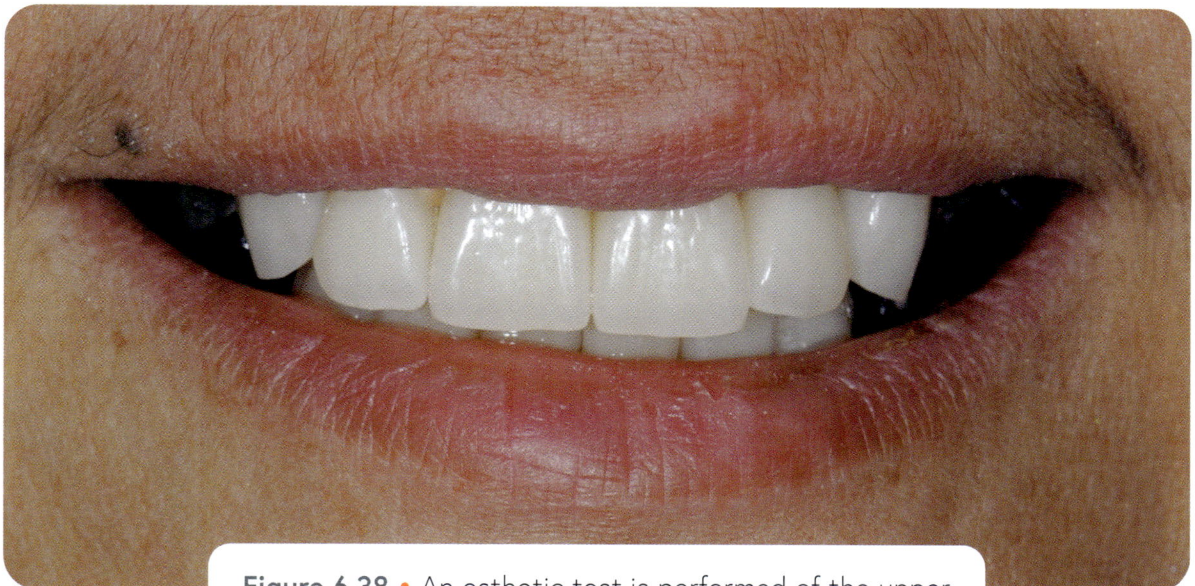

Figure 6.38 • An esthetic test is performed of the upper and lower six.

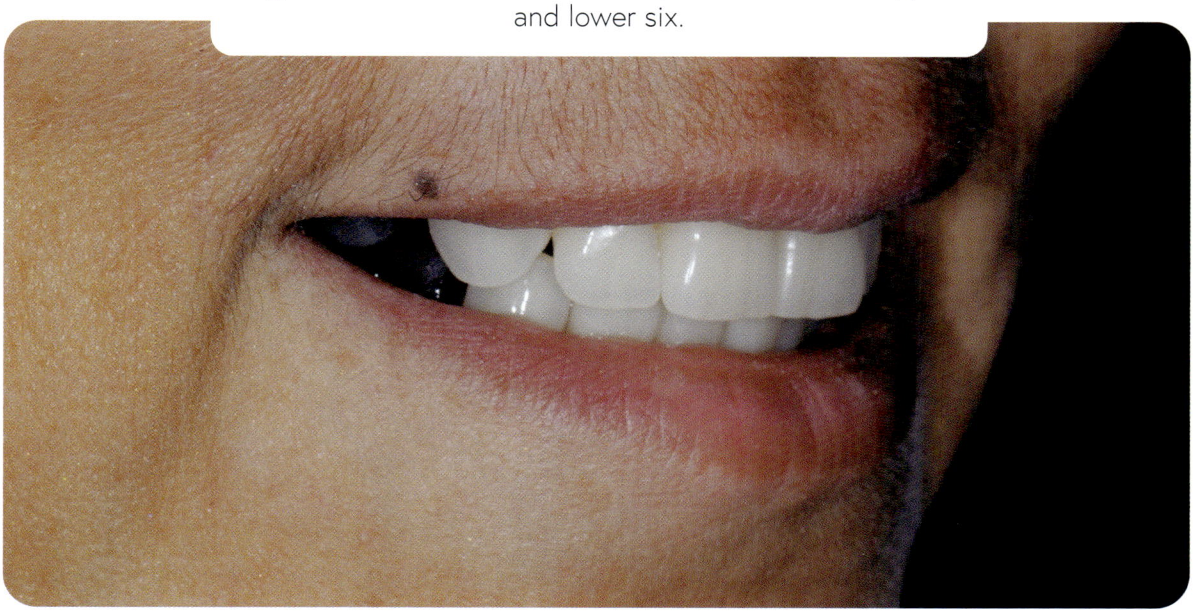

Continues

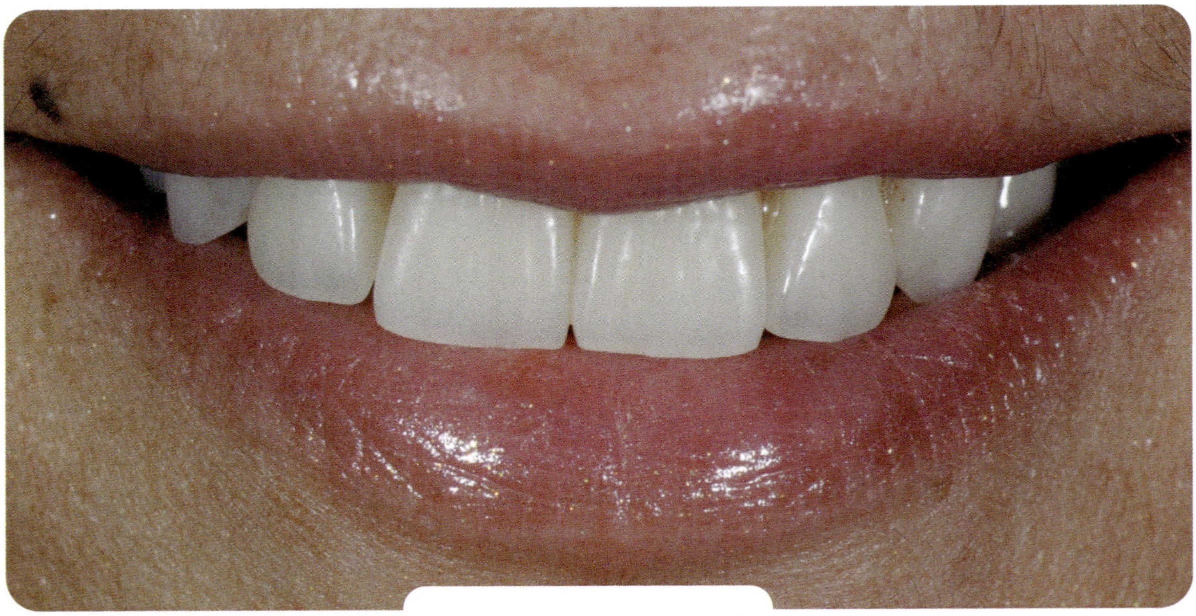

Figure 6.38 • *Continued*

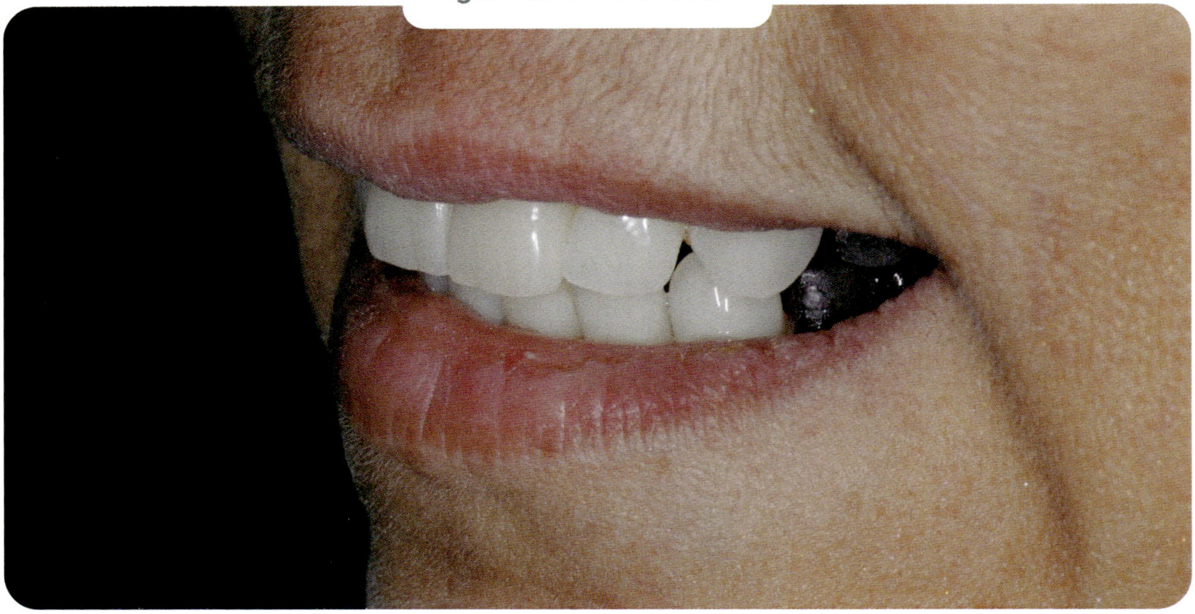

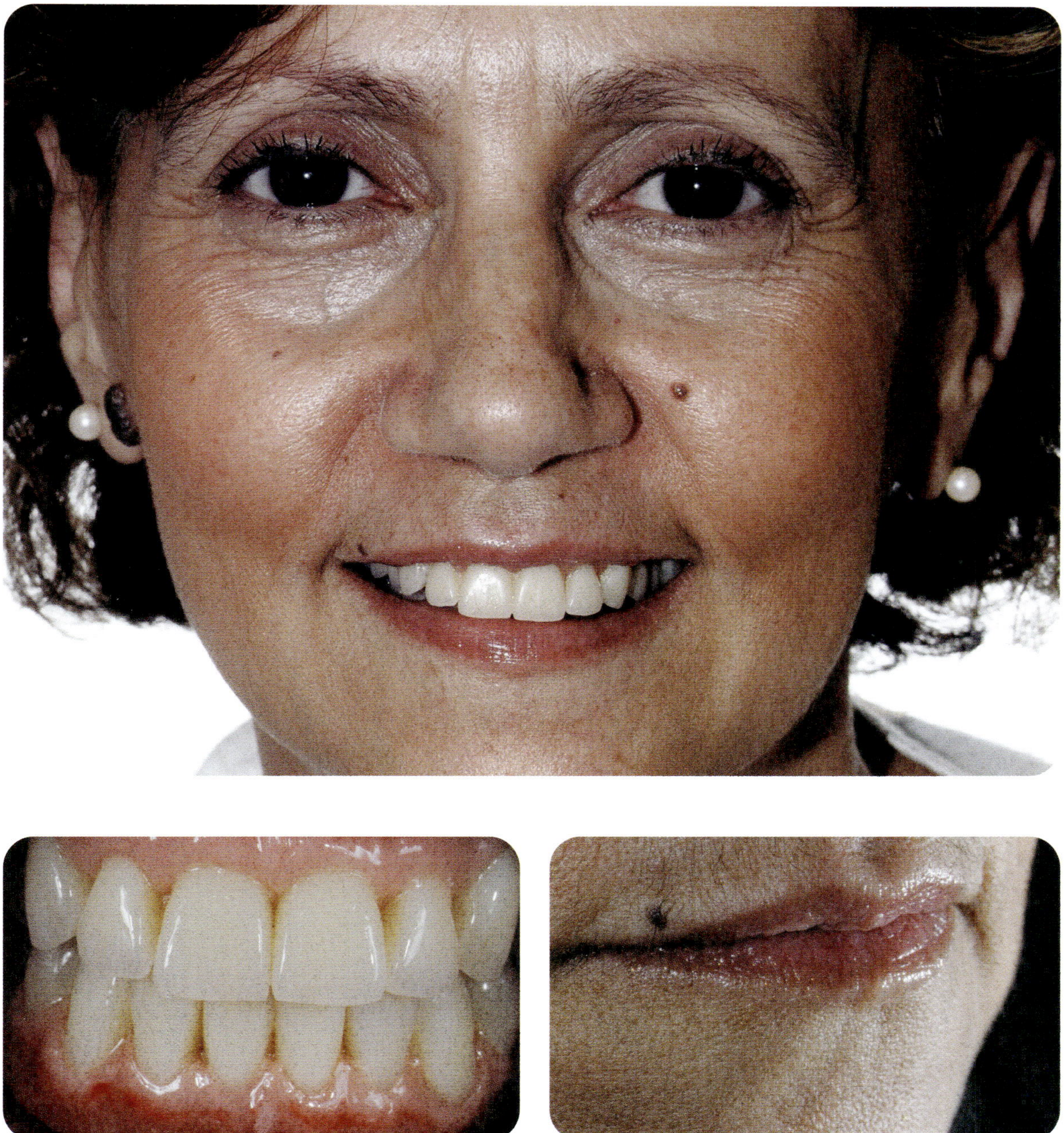

Figure 6.39 • The prosthesis is delivered without making any changes.

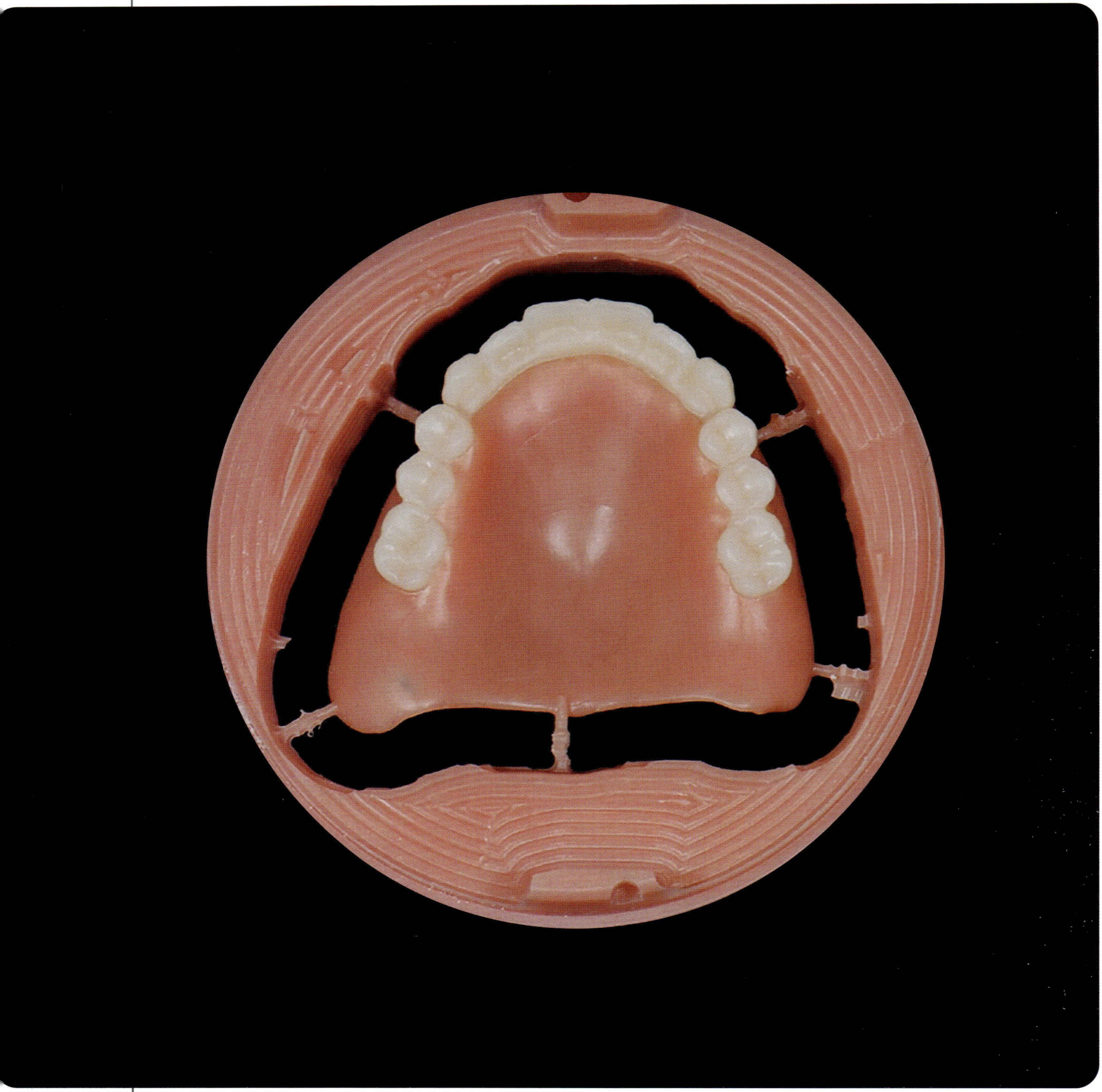

Immediate digital prosthesis

P. Venezia, P. Lacasella, S. D'amato

Fabrication of an immediate complete prosthesis according to analogue workflows may pose several critical issues.

Patients with terminal dentition have common characteristics: they have a decrease in the lower face height, anterior and superior sliding of the mandible, fanning, extreme mobility and migration of residual teeth, presence of diastemas and significant undercuts due to recessions as well as dental migration.

The procedures described in Chapters 4 and 5 for the design of full dentures are therefore even more complicated.

Any step required for obtaining the prosthetic coordinates (impressions, intermaxillary registrations, esthetic and phonetic assessments) is considerably difficult. All the testing procedures of the prosthetic design, which in cases of total edentulism are carried out before delivery of the prosthesis (esthetic assessments of the upper and lower frontal teeth, stability tests, phonetic tests), are however impossible to perform as the prostheses will be delivered immediately after extraction of the residual teeth.

The technical difficulty is often compounded by the discomfort and pain that may be caused to the patient.

The advantages of performing immediate prostheses are:

- preservation and restoration of the facial esthetics;
- preservation of the masticatory and phonation functions;
- preservation or restoration of the vertical dimension;
- preservation of the alveolar bone volumes;
- protection of the surgical wound;
- containing the increase in tongue volume in the lower arch.

The conventional methods used for making this type of prosthesis have not changed in the last 50 years and require a number of clinical stages and long laboratory procedures.

A number of articles have been published in the literature describing the fabrication of immediate total prostheses and which have the advantage of optimising the finalisation time of the prosthetic procedure with considerable patient satisfaction [22-25].

These studies report that the use of digital flows in complete prostheses can reduce the number of appointments, enables a greater fit of the prosthesis than all other production procedures and, obviously, allows for easy duplication of the final prosthesis [25-30].

The protocols for the production of immediate full dentures with digital flows are very similar to those already described in Chapter 5.

The steps for the production of an immediate full denture with CAD-CAM procedures are as follows:

1. esthetic and functional assessment of the case;
2. performance of the photographic status;
3. performance of the digital impressions of the arches and registration of the inter-maxillary relations;
4. extraction of the residual teeth on the virtual models;
5. designing the prosthetic rehabilitation;
6. milling the plate (PMMA – polymethyl-methacrylate – pink) and the artificial teeth (PMMA);
7. procedures for gluing the artificial teeth to the plate;
8. finishing;
9. extraction of the residual teeth and delivery.

Essentially, just two clinical appointments are required and one laboratory step only to finalise the rehabilitation with immediate full prosthesis.

Clinical stage 1

After carrying out the esthetic analysis of the case, also including the phonetic assessments, the photographic status is performed which will be sent to the laboratory to allow the dental technician to make the analyses relating to facial and dental esthetics **(Figures 6.40-6.42)**.

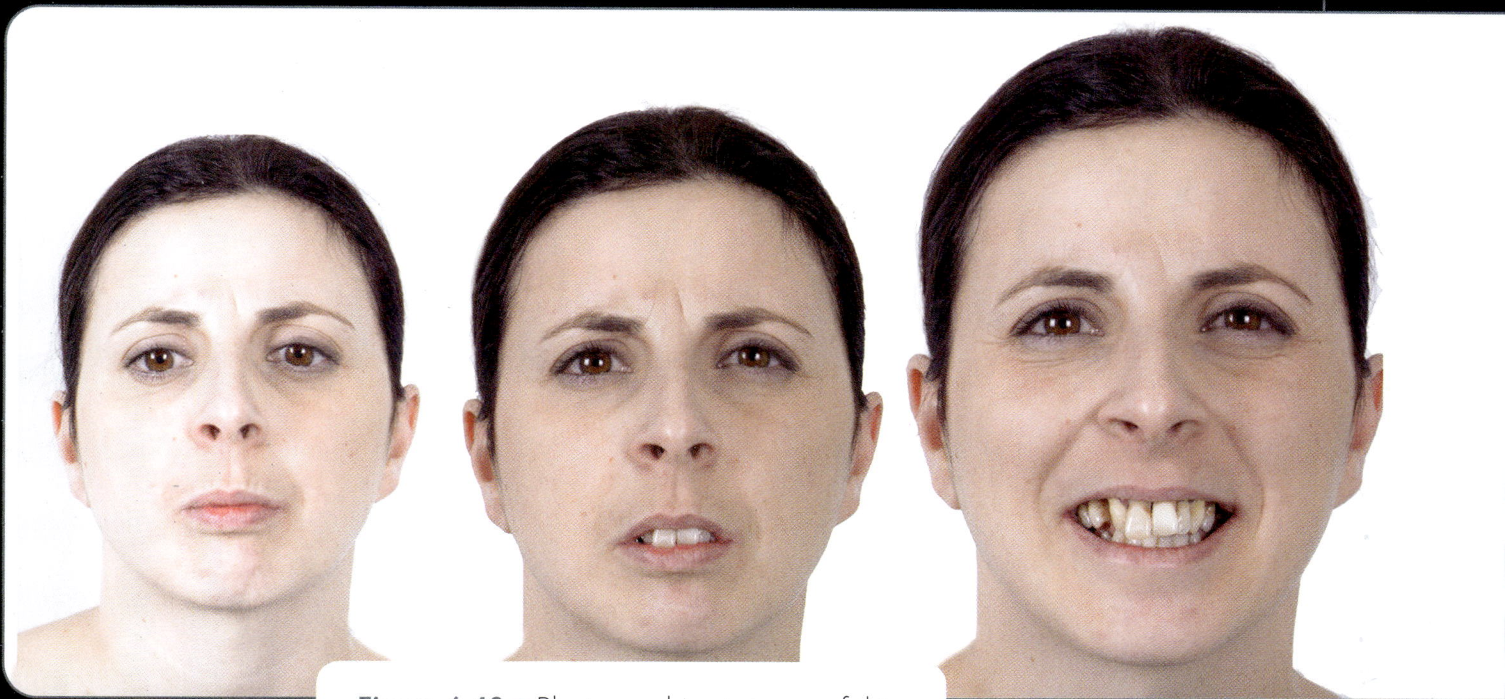

Figure 6.40 • Photographic status useful to assess the three stages of the smile.

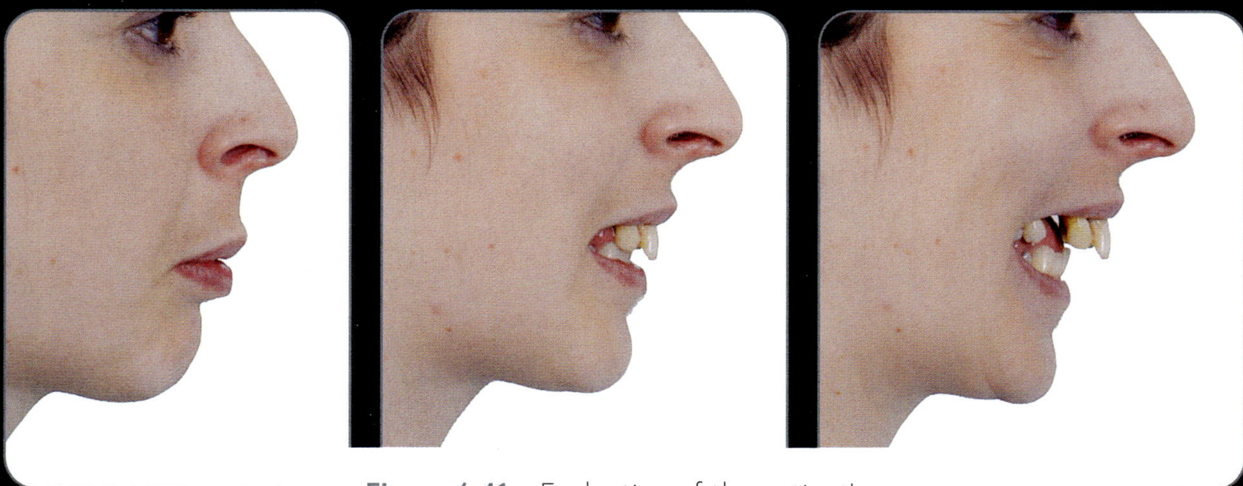

Figure 6.41 • Evaluation of the patient's profile and her dental display.

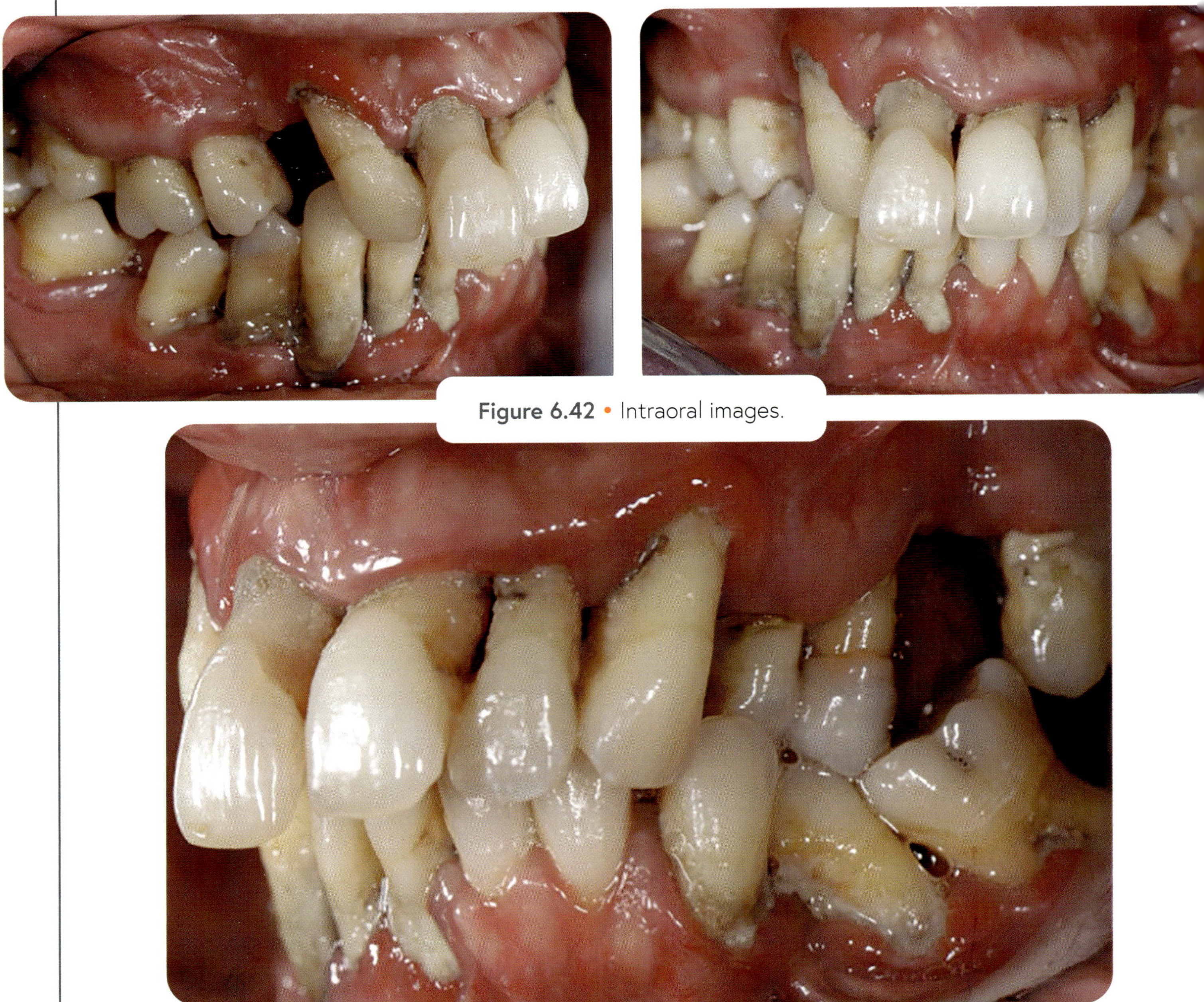

Figure 6.42 • Intraoral images.

In these patients, the impressions can be taken with intraoral scanners (I.O.S.) (see Chapter 3). This technology makes it possible to eliminate the patient discomfort described above **(Figures 6.43** and **6.44)**.

The scanner can be used to register dental display at rest and support of the perioral tissues **(Figure 6.45)**.

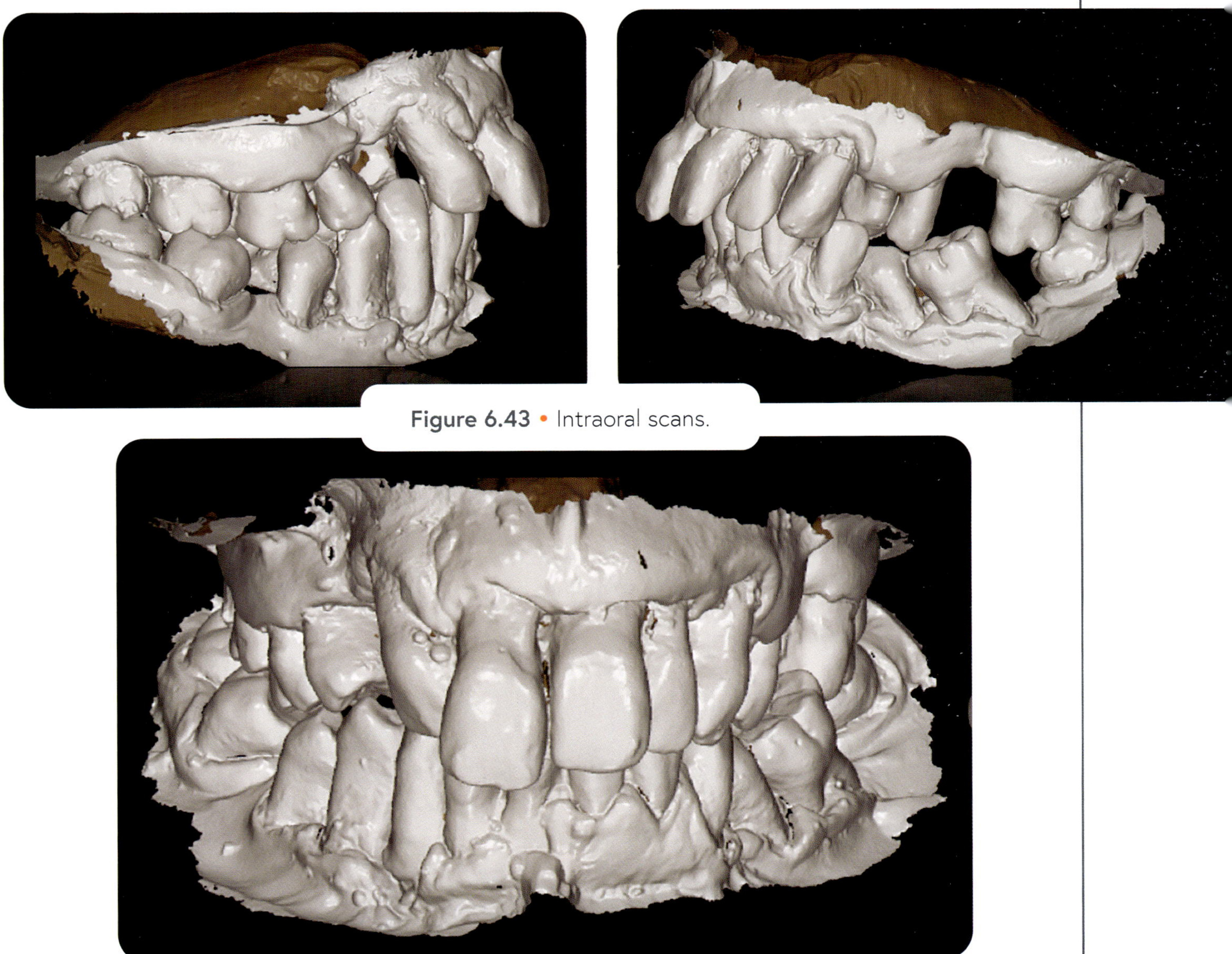

Figure 6.43 • Intraoral scans.

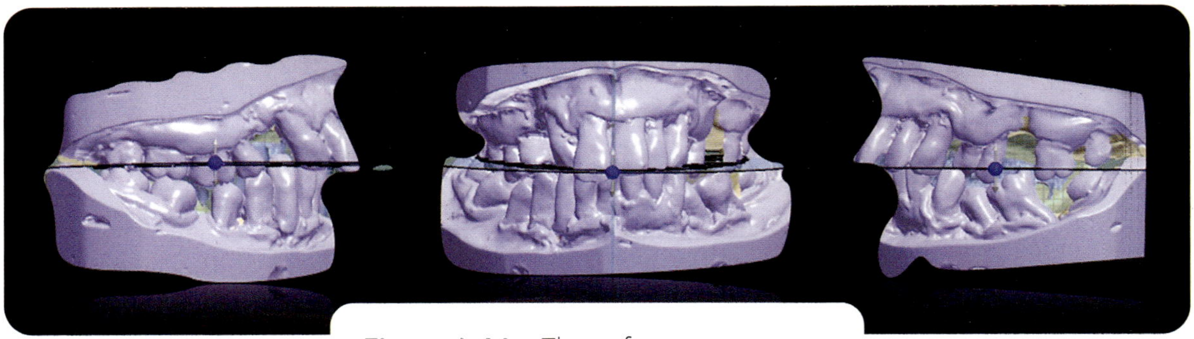

Figure 6.44 • The software processes and optimises the impression.

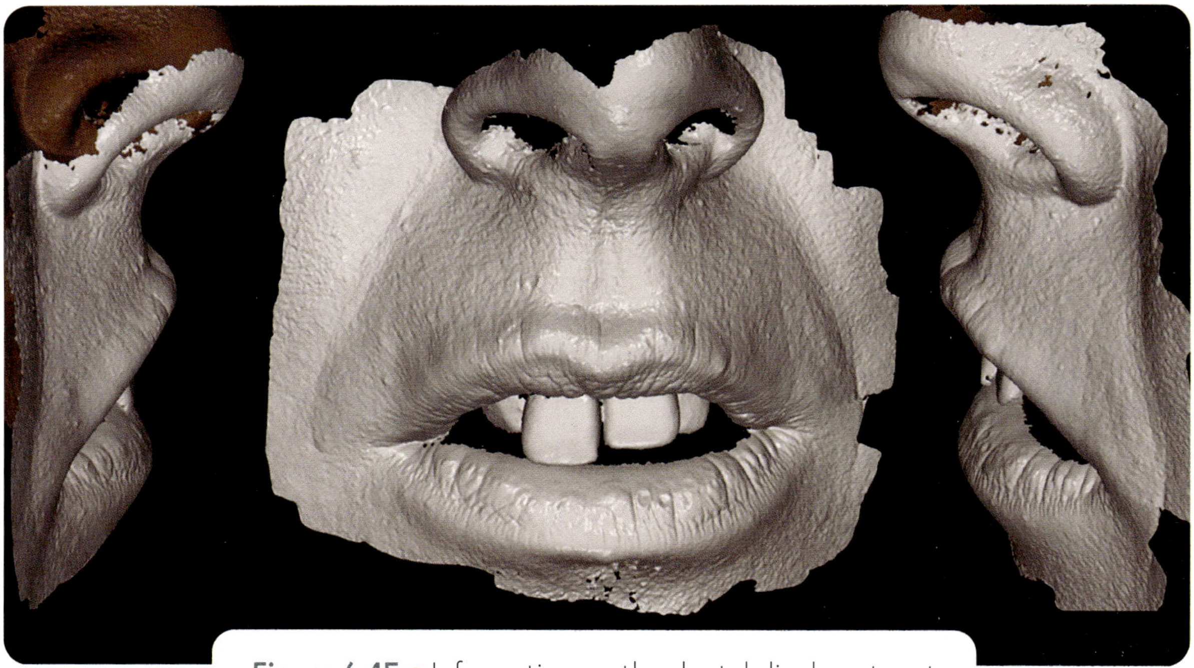

Figure 6.45 • Information on the dental display at rest and on the perioral tissues is recorded.

However, it is possible to take panoramic alginate impressions that can be developed to create models that will later be scanned and imported into a digital environment **(Figures 6.46** and **6.47)**.

Once the models have been digitised, the patient's 2D image can be superimposed on the 3D model in virtual environment **(Figure 6.48)**.

There is the option of superposing the previous files to the perioral tissue scan **(Figure 6.49)**.

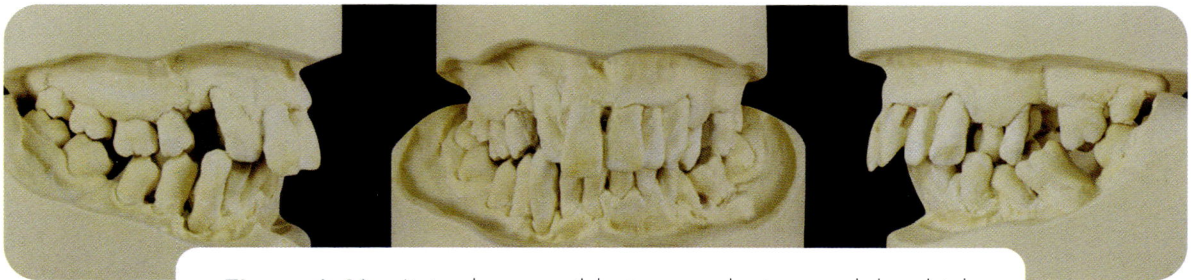

Figure 6.46 • It is also possible to use plaster models which may be scanned and imported into the virtual environment.

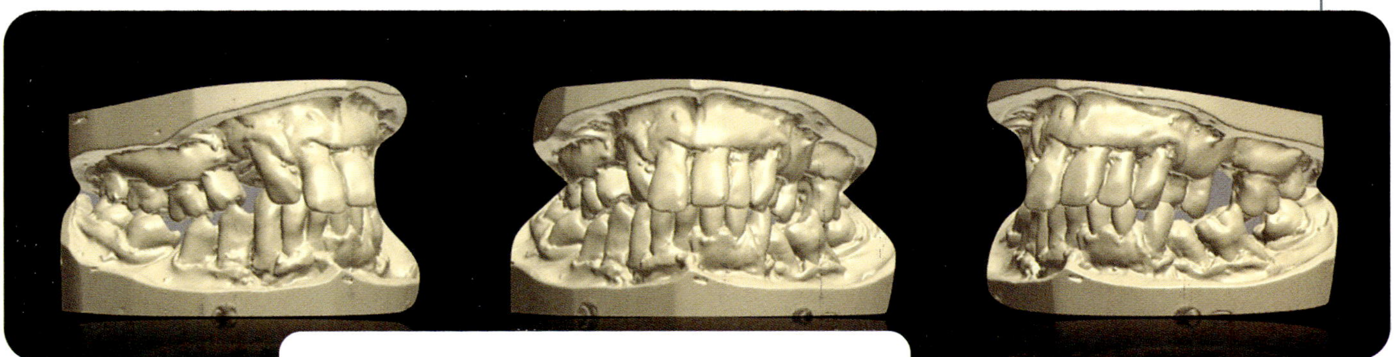

Figure 6.47 • The digitised plaster models.

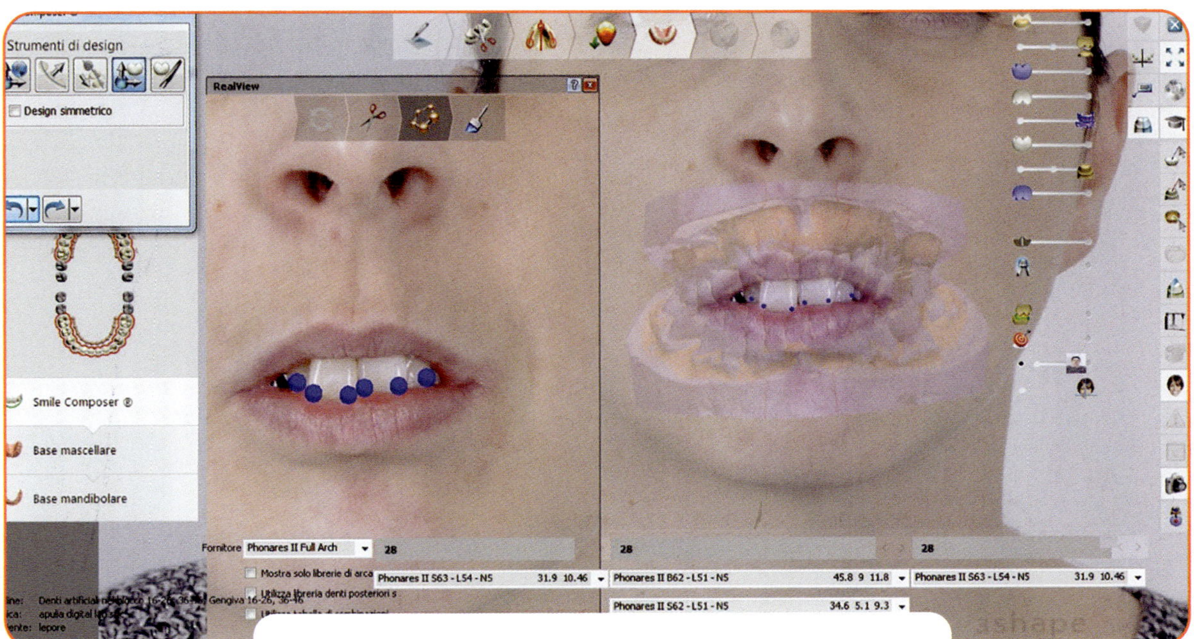

Figure 6.48 • The 2D images previously registered and the 3D model are superimposed

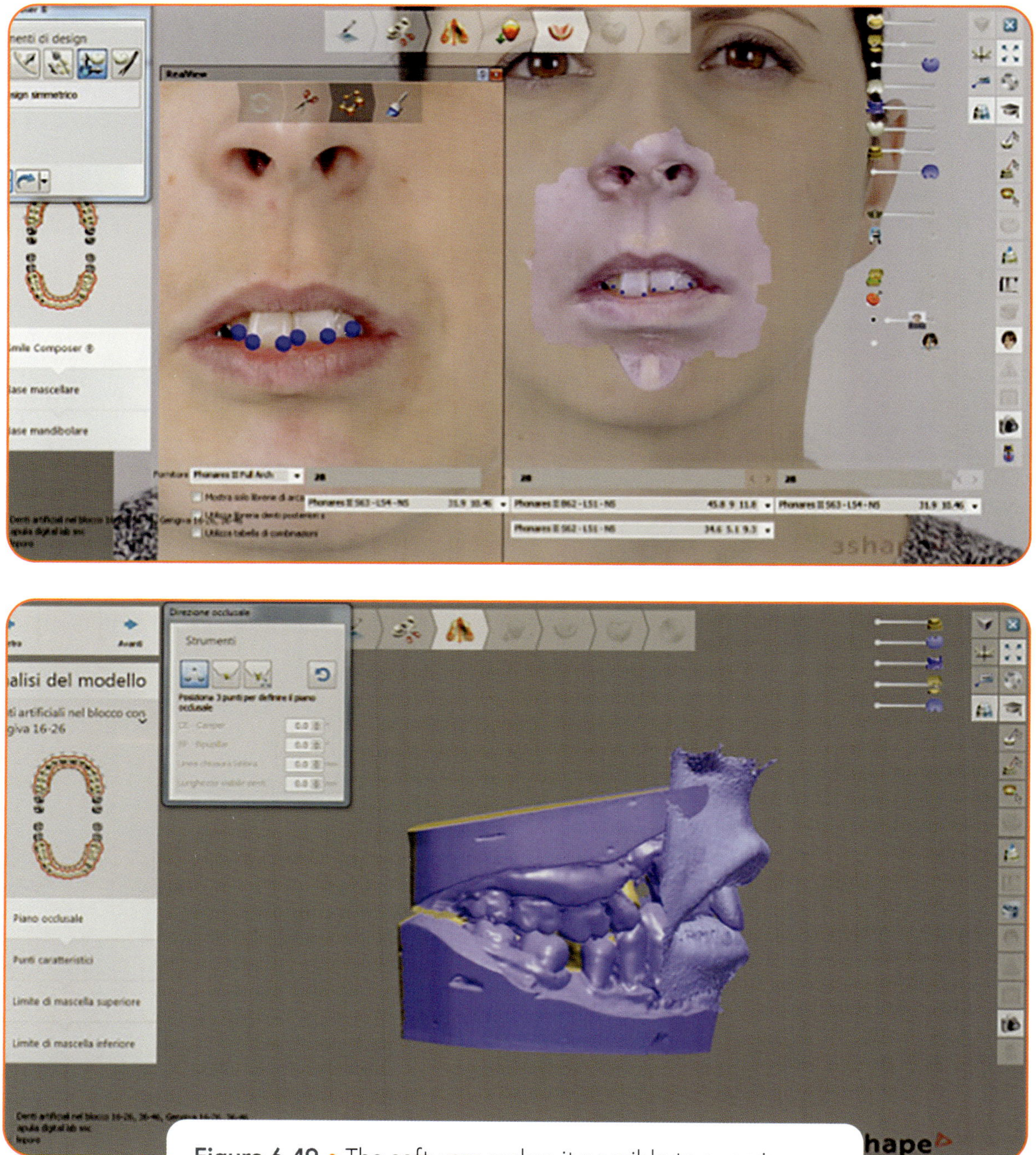

Figure 6.49 • The software makes it possible to superimpose the scan of the perioral tissues to the virtual 3D model.

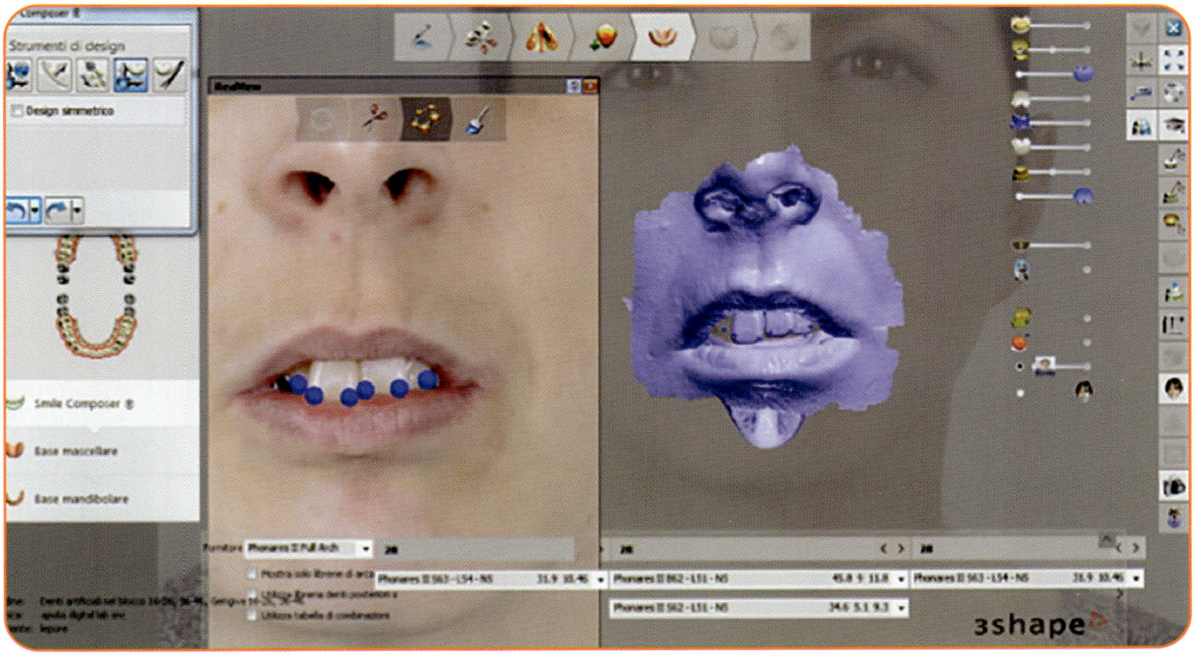
Strumenti di design
Design simmetrico
Smile Composer ®
Base mascellare
Base mandibolare
3shape

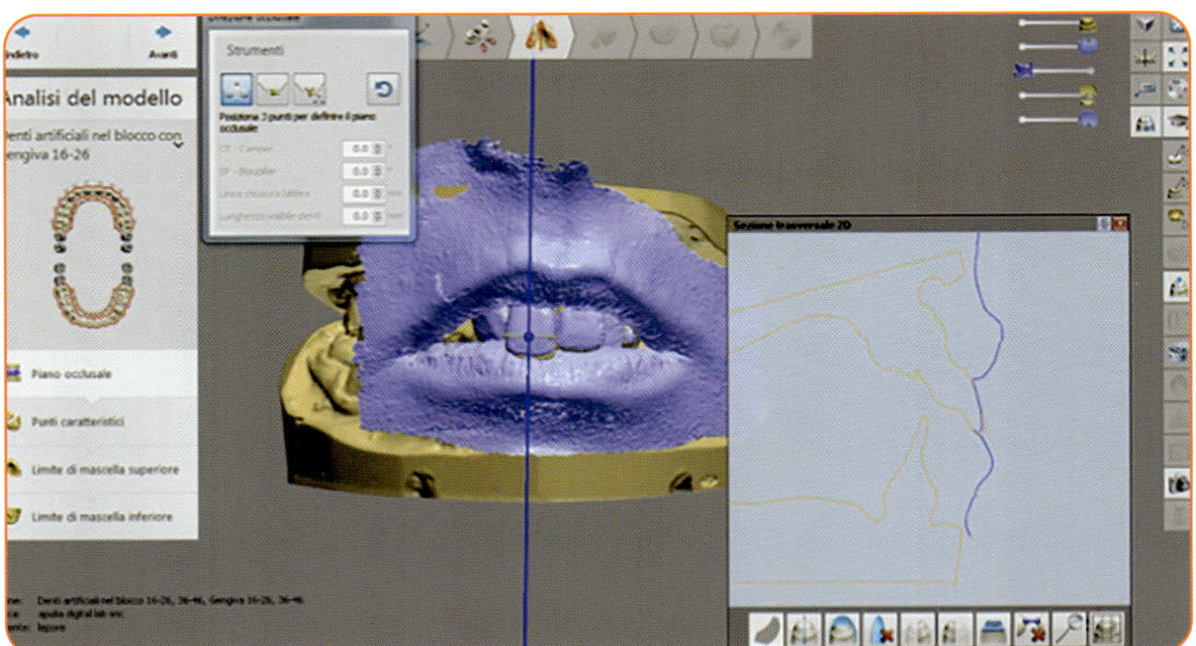
Avanti
Analisi del modello
Strumenti
Piano occlusale
Punti caratteristici
Limite di mascella superiore
Limite di mascella inferiore
Sezione trasversale 2D

The relations between lips and teeth are analysed in section and it is possible to decide what the three-dimensionally correct position of the upper central incisors should be in the space **(Figure 6.50)**.

The software makes it possible to perform a virtual extraction of the teeth concerned before the real one **(Figure 6.51)** and the CAD operator will take care to space the

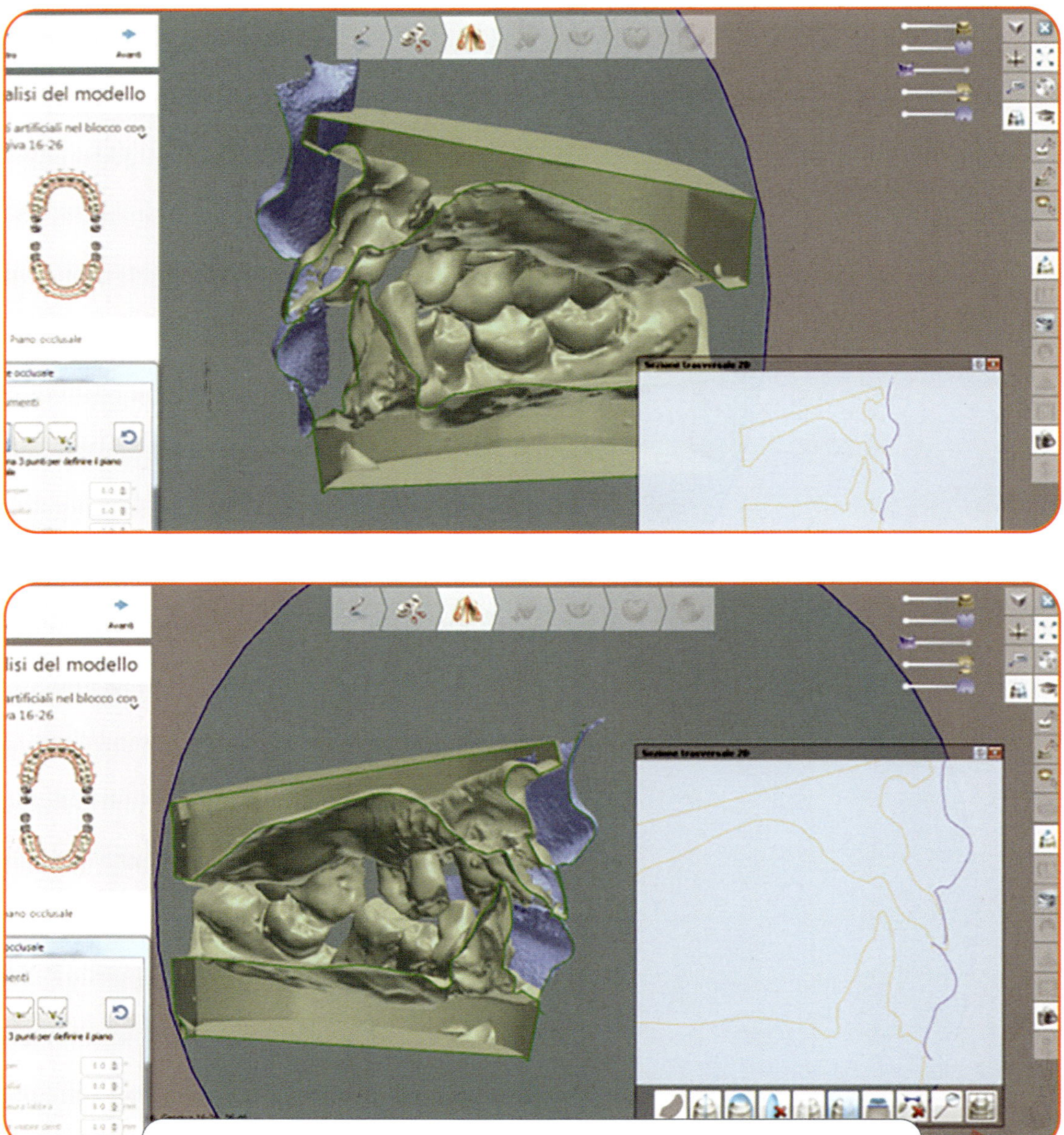

Figure 6.50 • Analysis of the relation between lips and teeth.

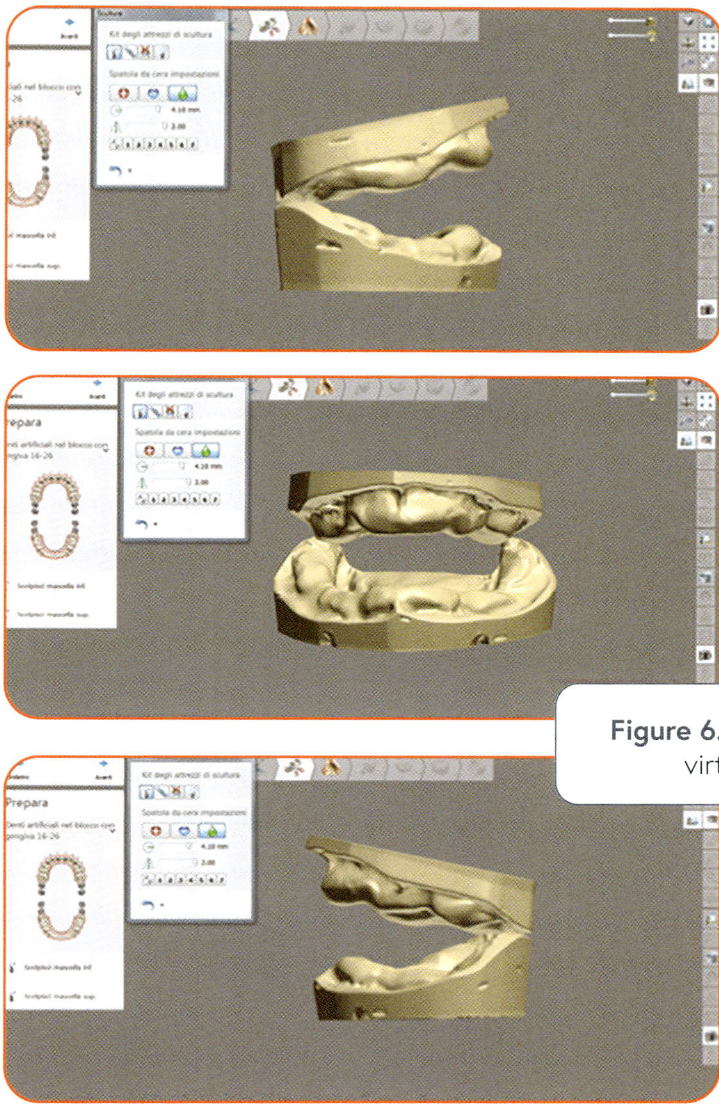

Figure 6.51 • Intermaxillary relations after virtual extraction of the teeth.

model in the areas of the extractions in order to avoid compression by the impression surface of the immediate prosthesis on the surgical wound **(Figure 6.52)**.

The models will be later analysed. The software will read the presence and extent of the undercuts **(Figure 6.53)**.

Based on the identified anatomical findings **(Figure 6.54)**, the software will propose a setup that can be customised by the dental technician (see Chapter 5) **(Figure 6.55)**.

Occlusal optimisation will be performed thanks to a virtual articulator that will make it possible to remove any interference **(Figures 6.56 and 6.57)**.

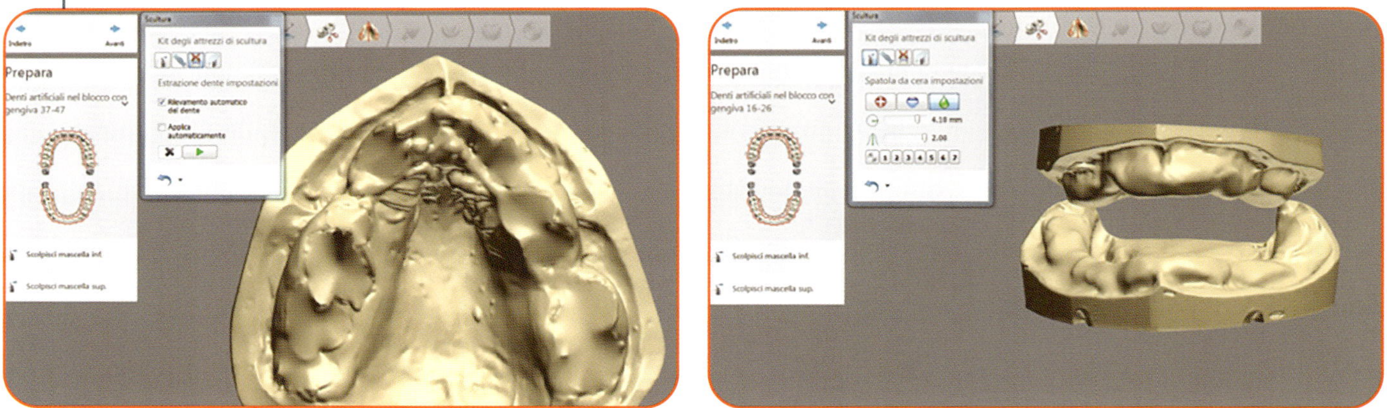

Figure 6.52 • Finishing the virtual models after the extractions.

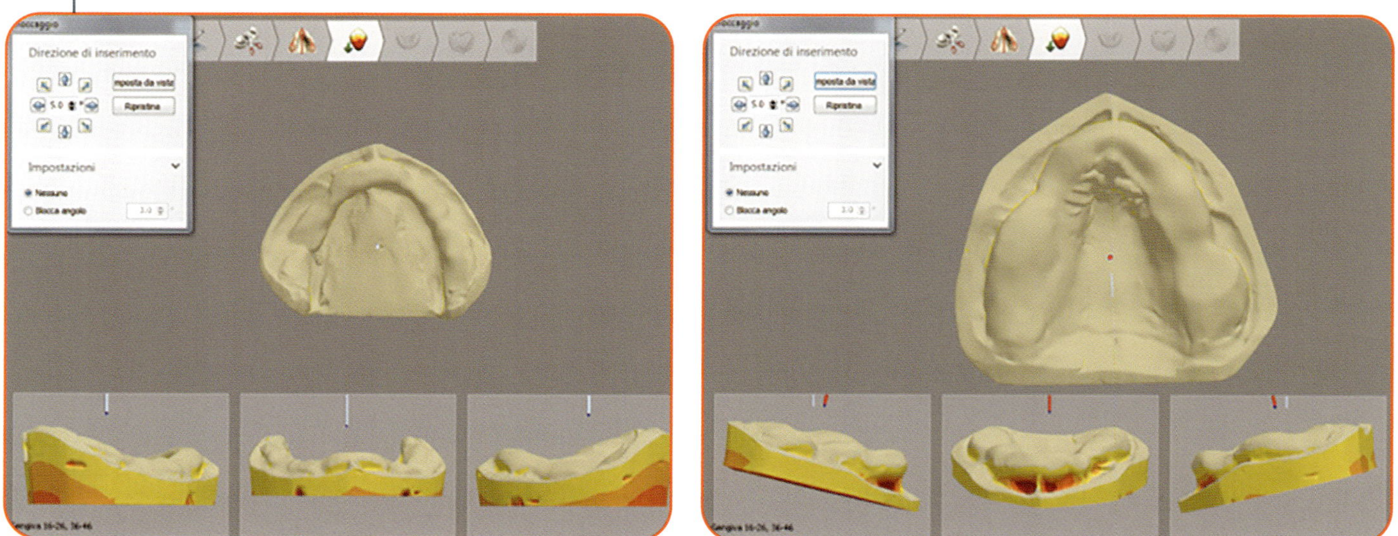

Figure 6.53 • Checking for the presence and extent of undercuts.

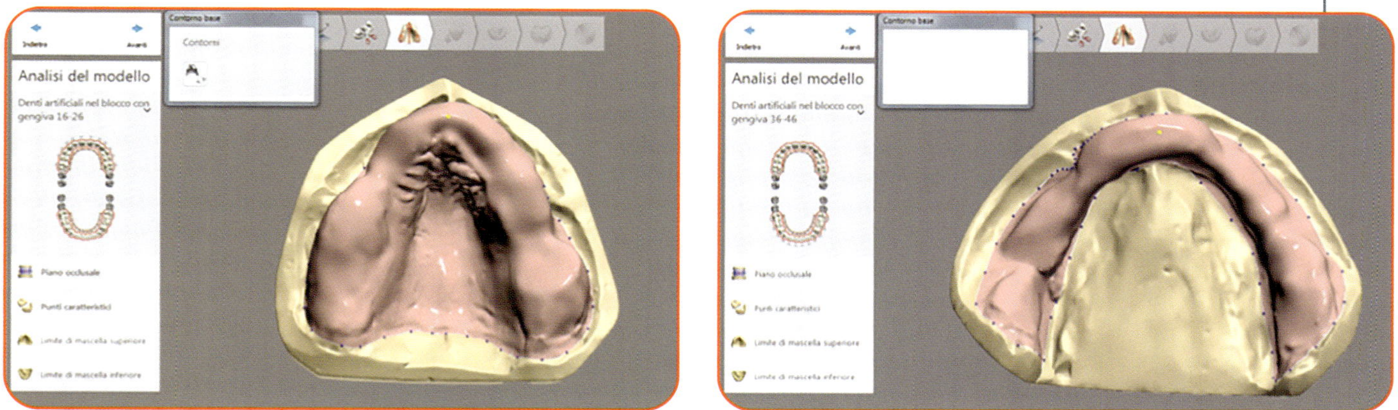

Figure 6.54 • Analysis of the anatomical structures that will ensure stability and retention of the immediate prosthesis.

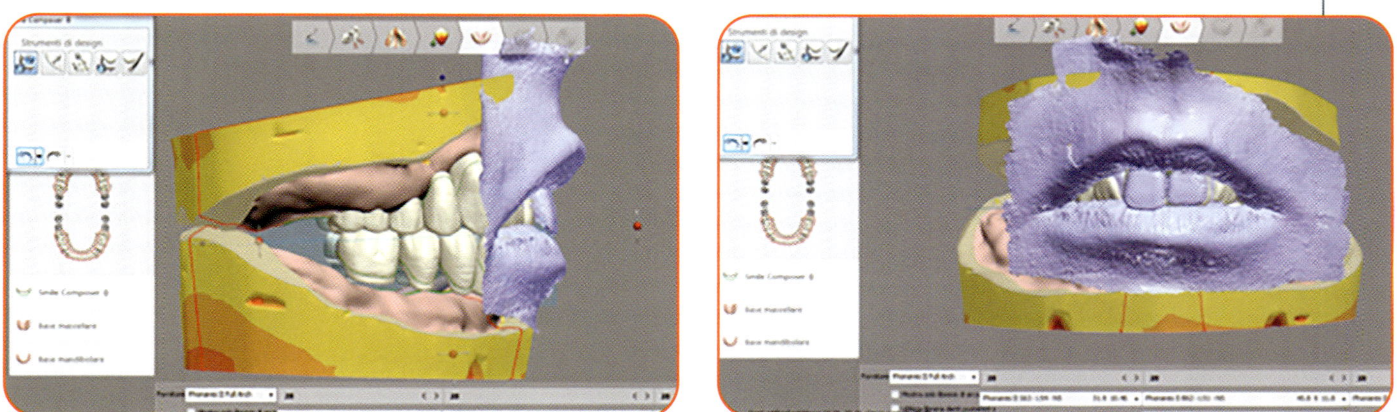

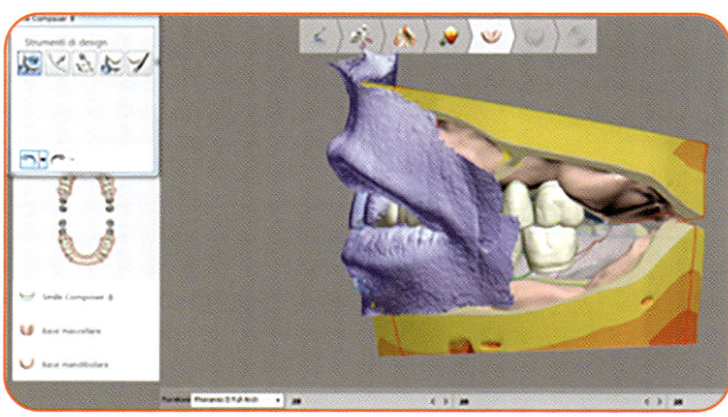

Figure 6.55 • Rehabilitation design in compliance with the esthetic and functional parameters.

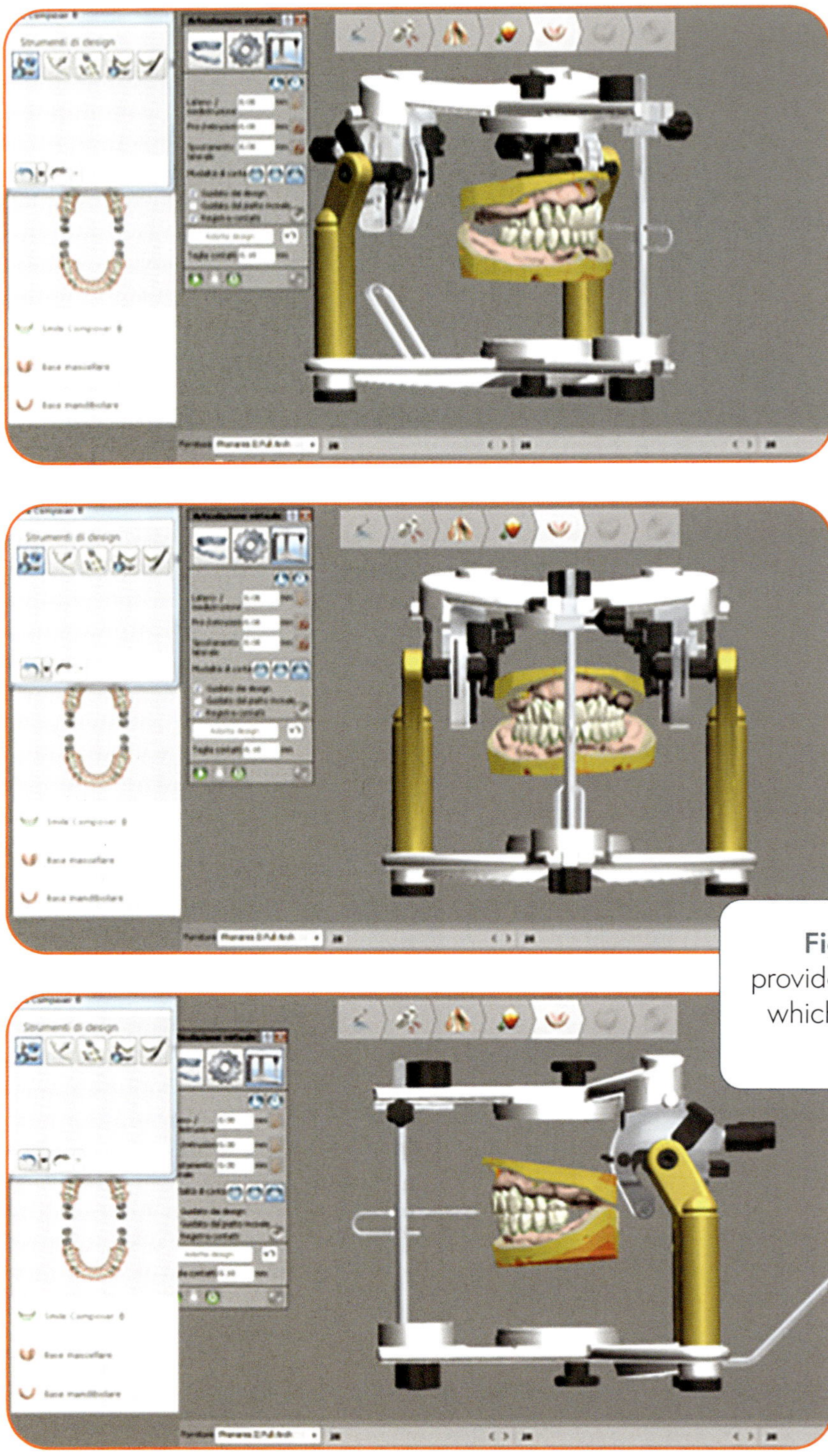

Figure 6.56 • The software provides the setup in the articulator, which can then be customised by the dental technician.

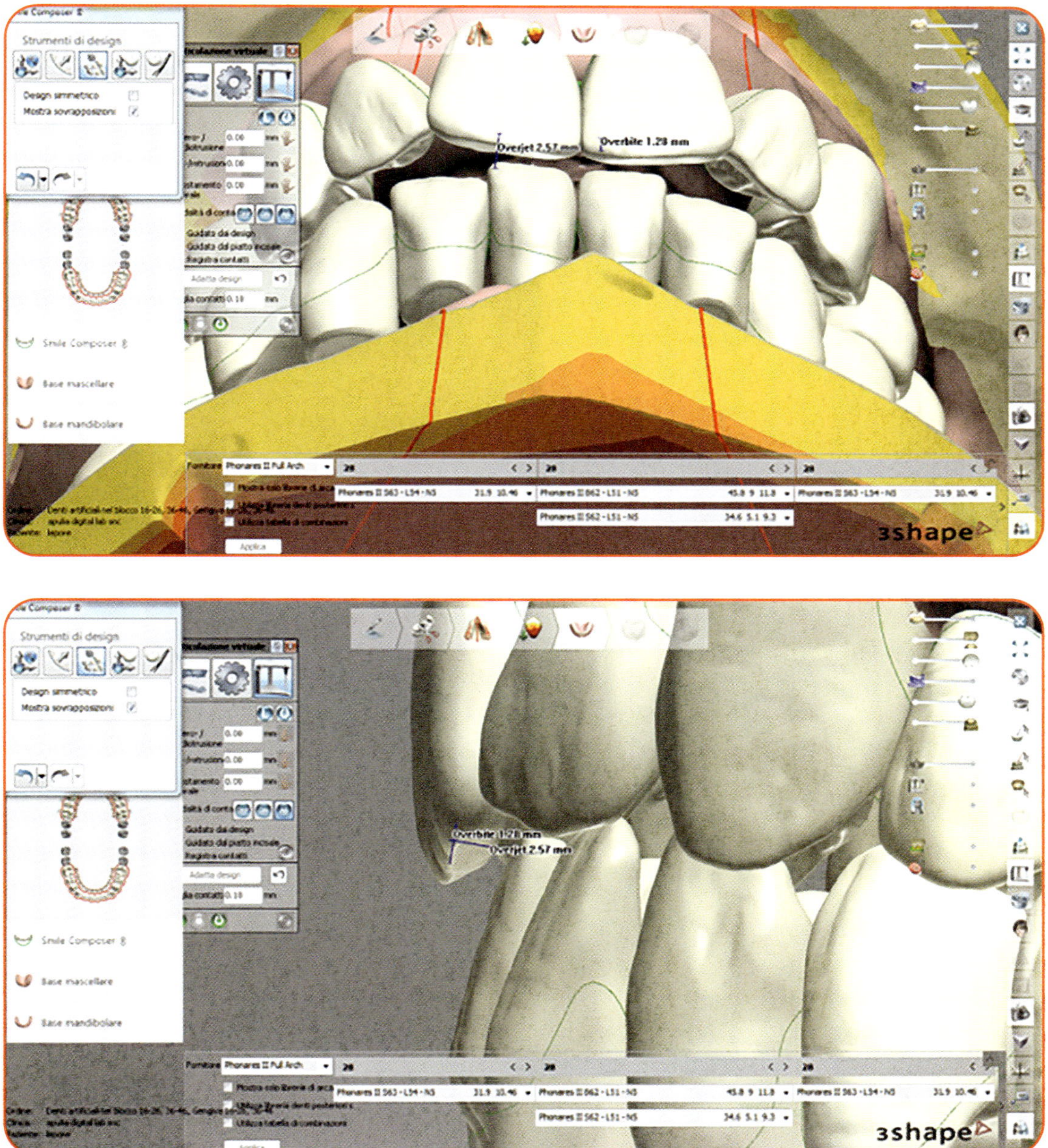

Figure 6.57 • The occlusal contacts are optimised in the virtual articulator.

The overlap between prosthetic design and perioral tissues will allow the end result to be previewed in the 2D image **(Figure 6.58)**.

The CAD design **(Figure 6.59)** is transferred to CAM **(Figure 6.60)**.

The first milling procedure concerns the extrados **(Figures 6.61** and **6.62)**.

The next step concerns the production of the artificial teeth.

The CAM design relating to the occlusal surfaces of the prostheses is transferred to the milling machine which will fabricate an entire arch of artificial teeth starting from a block of compact resin (PMMA) **(Figures 6.63** and **6.64)**.

The pink resin plate and the arch of artificial teeth are set and joined using a specific adhesive system **(Figures 6.65-6.68)**.

The item is placed in the machine again for milling the intrados and for finishing **(Figures 6.69-6.71)**.

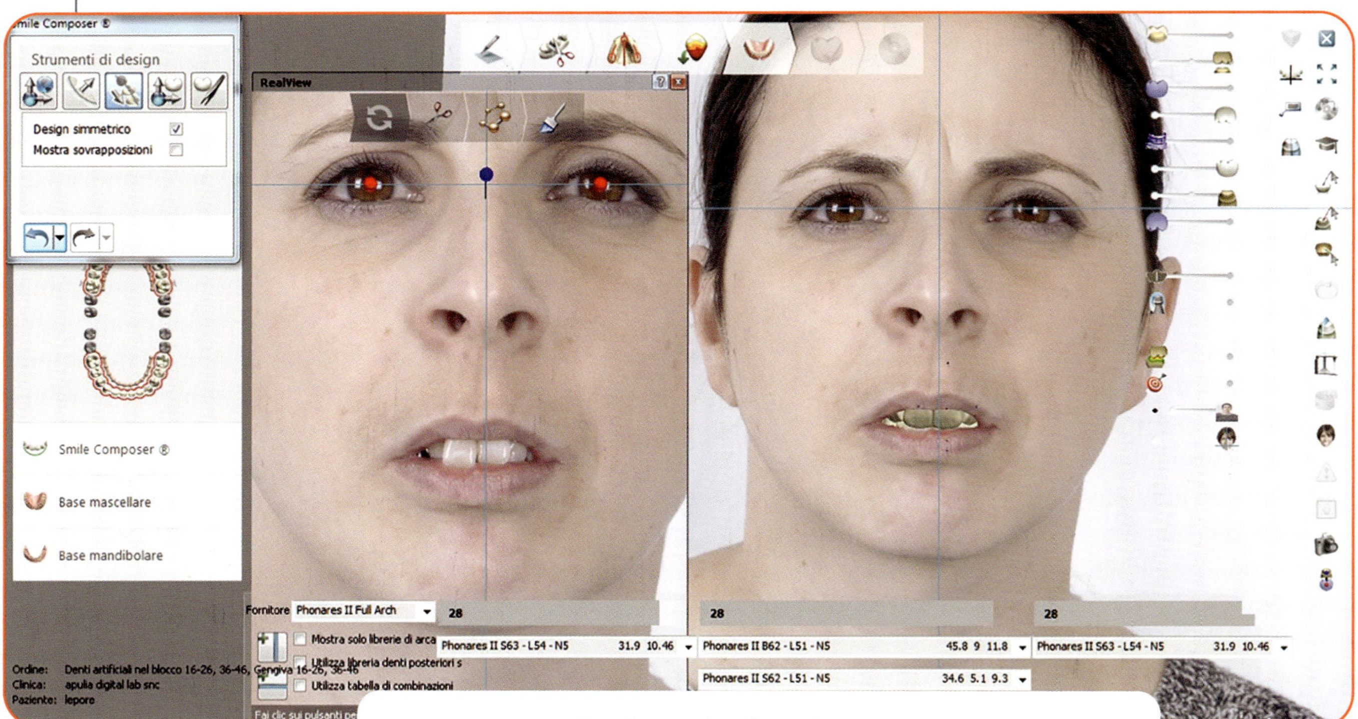

Figure 6.58 • Thanks to the fact that the 3D design can be superimposed on the 2D image documents, it is possible to obtain a preview of the end result.

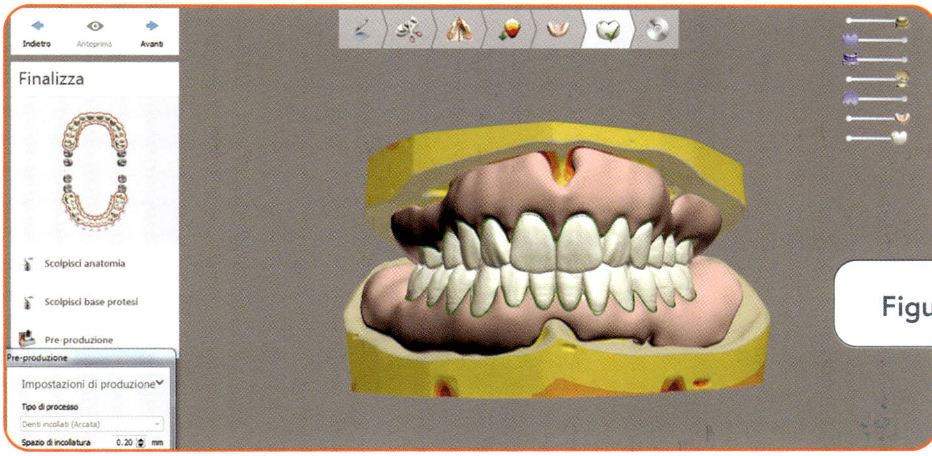

Figure 6.59 • CAD design.

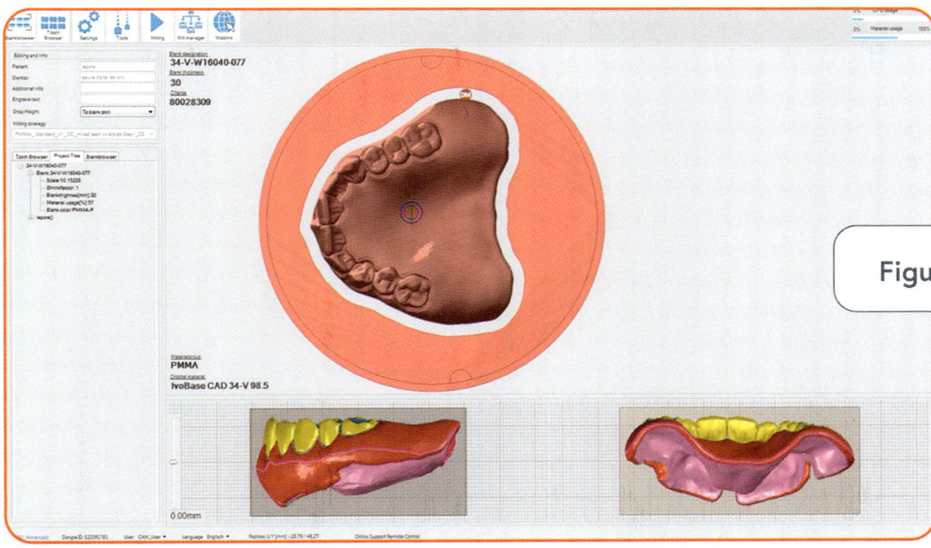

Figure 6.60 • CAM design.

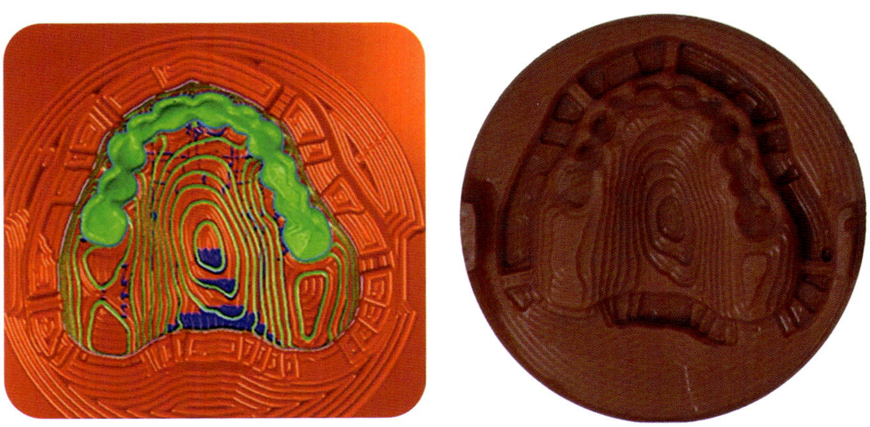

Figure 6.61 • Design and milling of the upper extrados.

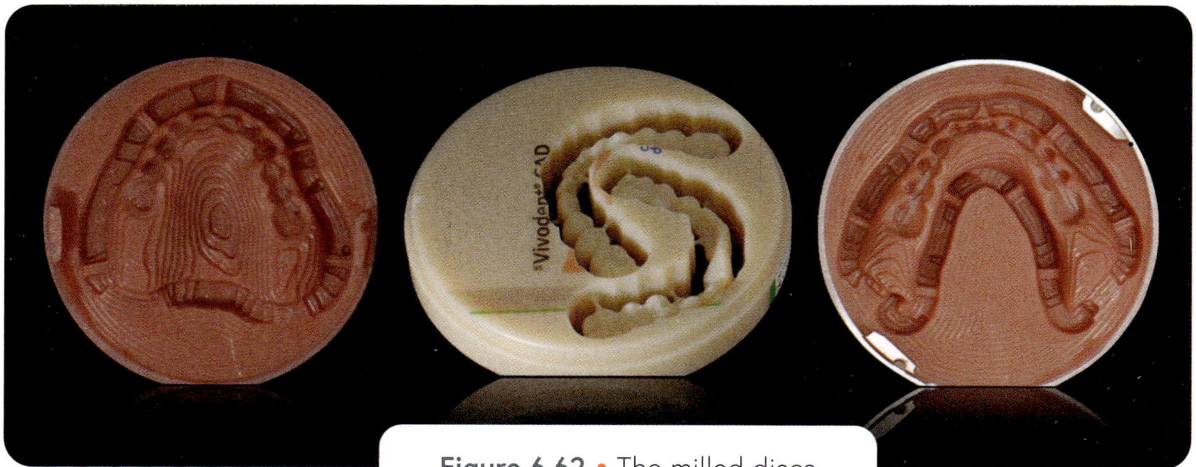

Figure 6.62 • The milled discs of the extrados and artificial teeth.

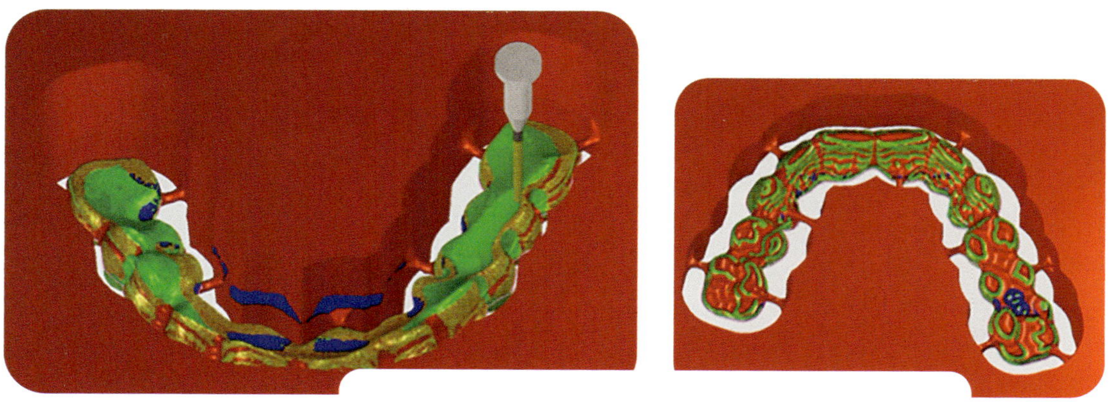

Figure 6.63 • Design of the artificial teeth.

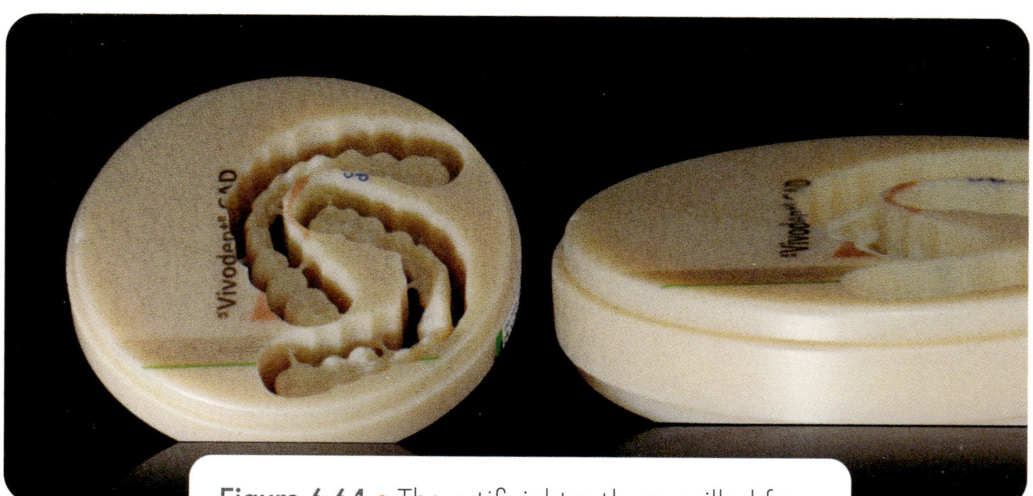

Figure 6.64 • The artificial teeth are milled from a disc of the colour chosen in the initial stage.

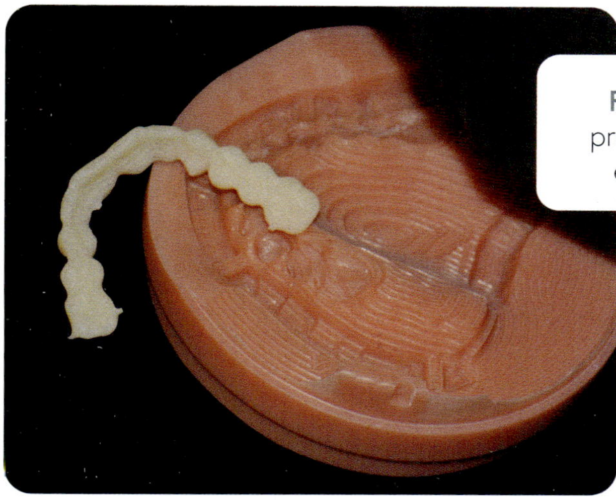

Figure 6.65 • Completion of the milling procedure of the artificial teeth and of the extrados of the total upper prosthesis.

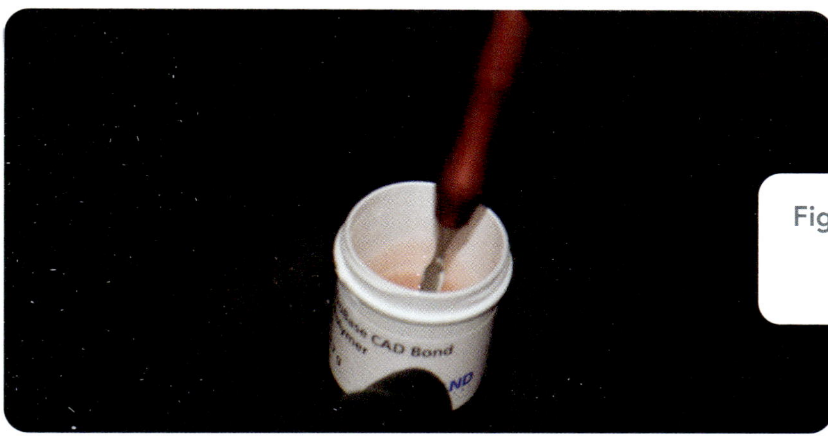

Figure 6.66 • Adhesive used in the adhesion procedures of the artificial teeth.

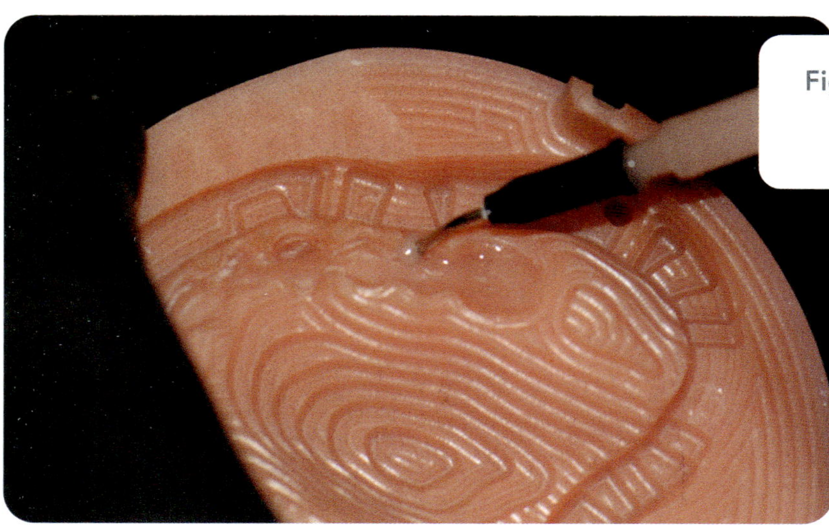

Figure 6.67 • Placement of the adhesive inside the sockets.

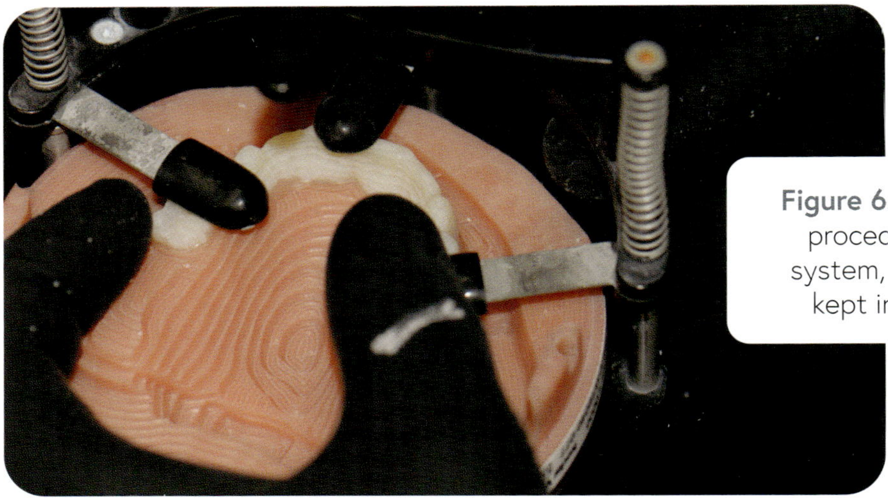

Figure 6.68 • During the curing procedures of the adhesive system, the artificial teeth are kept in place by a support.

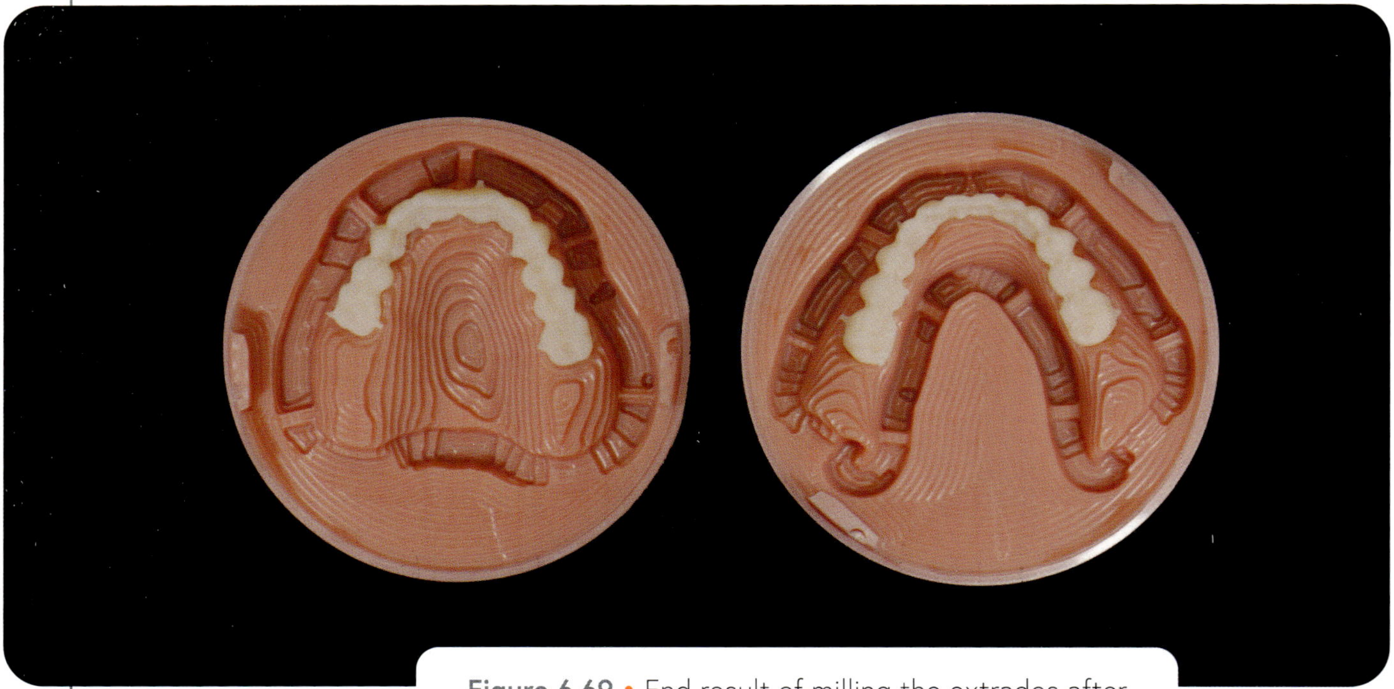

Figure 6.69 • End result of milling the extrados after placement of the artificial teeth.

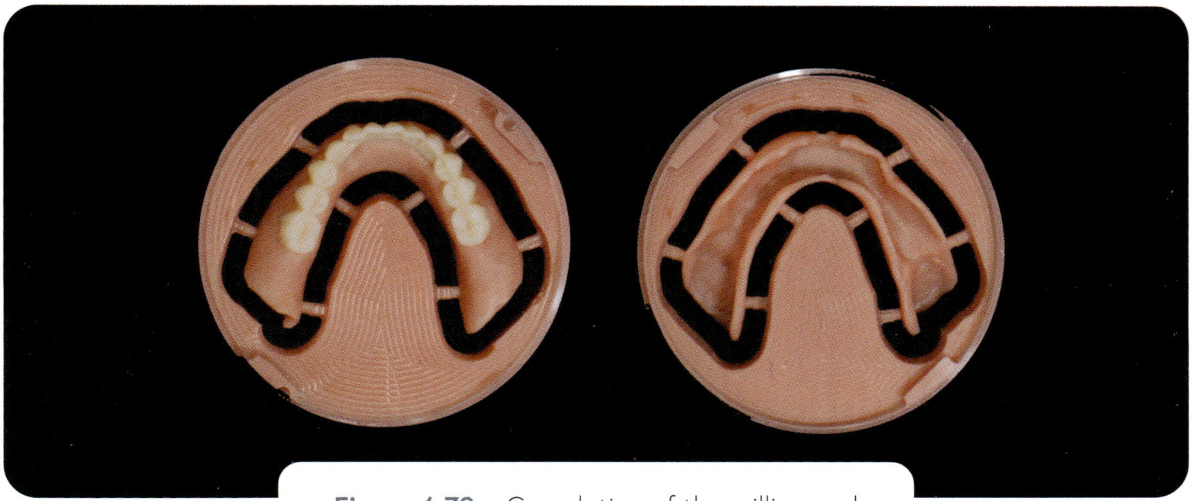

Figure 6.70 • Completion of the milling and finishing procedures of the complete prosthesis.

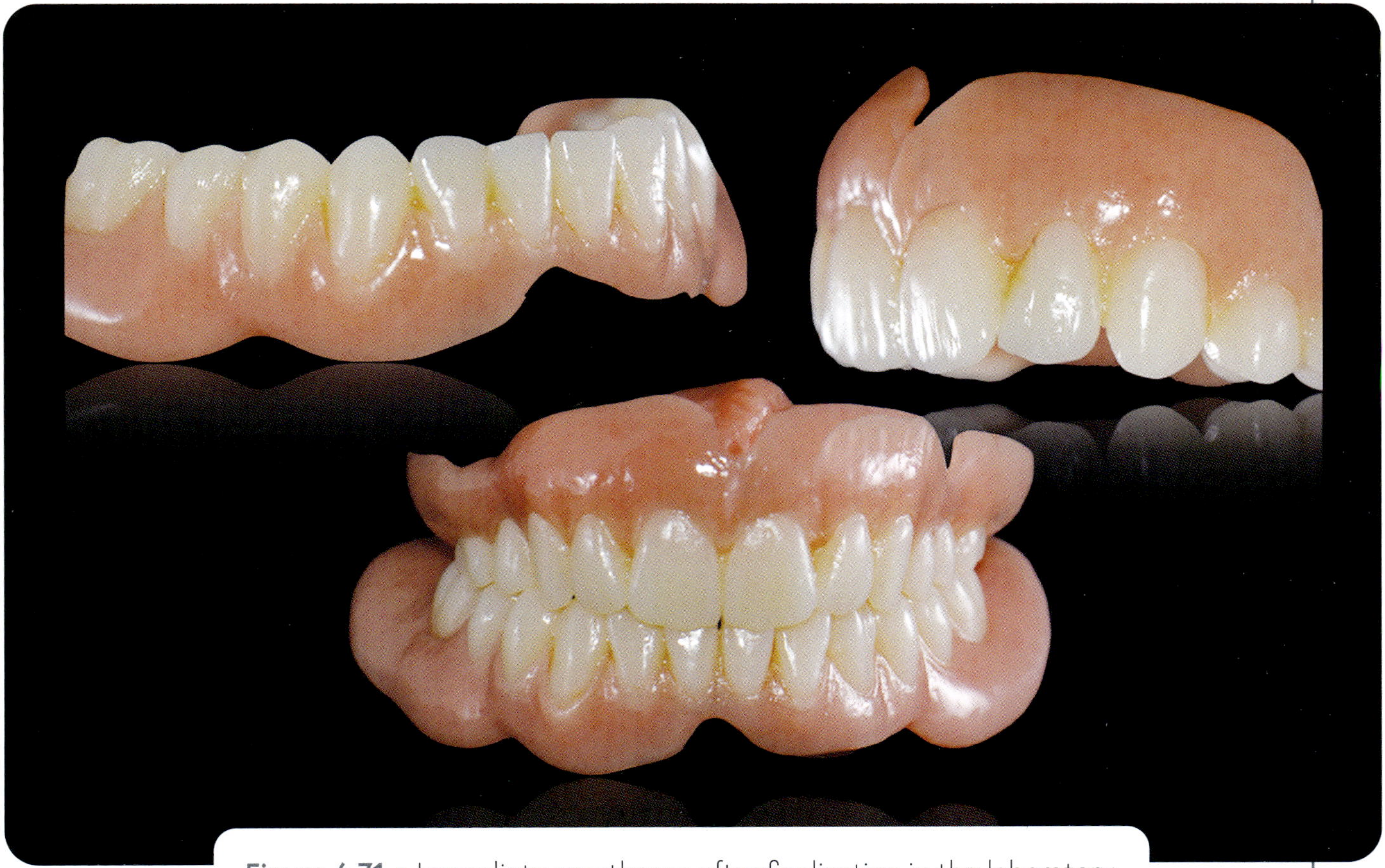

Figure 6.71 • Immediate prostheses after finalisation in the laboratory.

Clinical stage 2

During the second appointment, the patient undergoes all the extractions of both the upper and lower arch **(Figure 6.72)**. The digital flow has ensured the perfect match between the CAD design and the finalisation of the prosthetic case **(Figure 6.73)**.

Using these flows allows the case to be finalised rapidly, with considerable satisfaction by the patient with a change in the intraoral part, as well as perioral **(Figures 6.74** and **6.75)**.

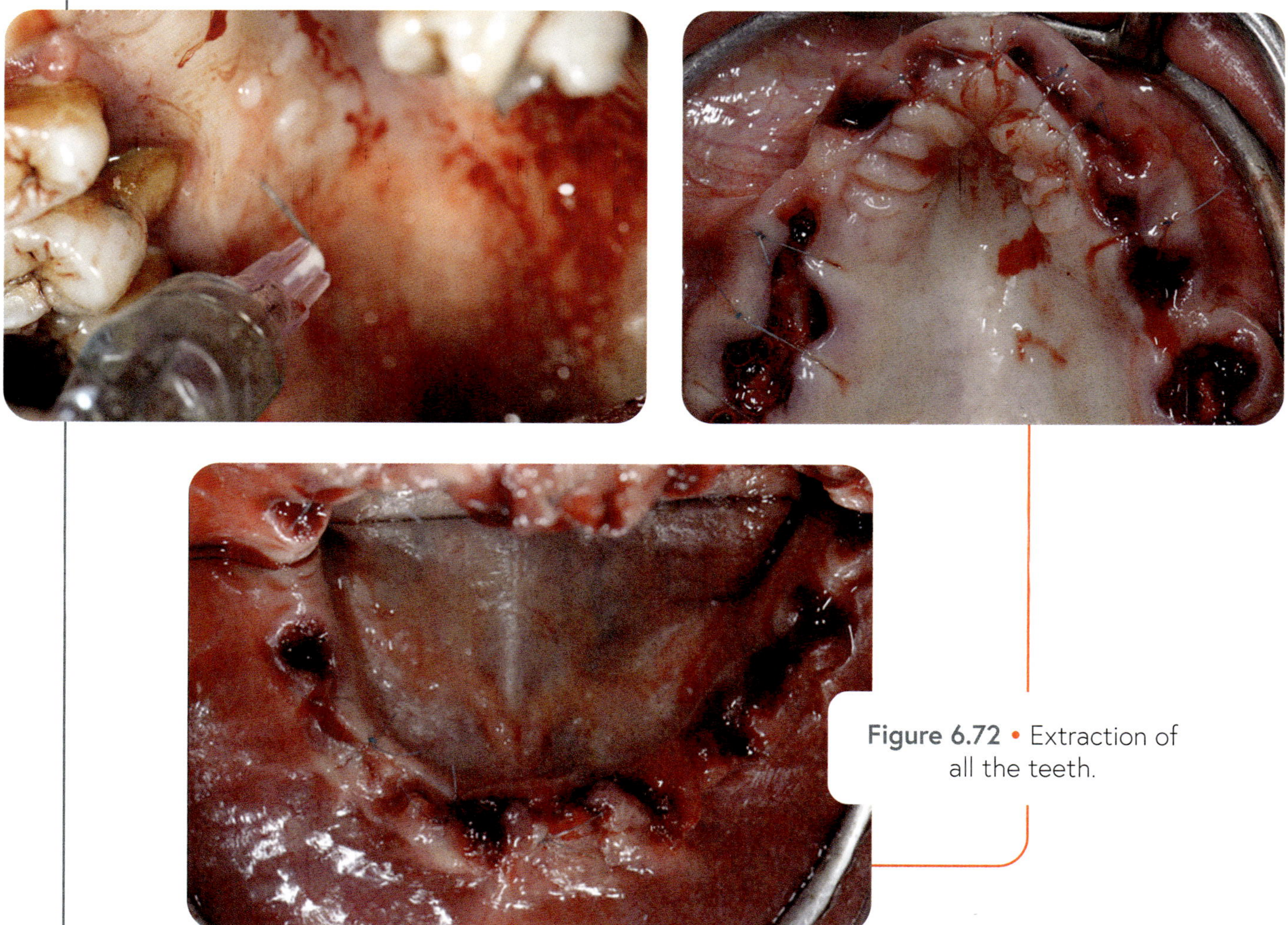

Figure 6.72 • Extraction of all the teeth.

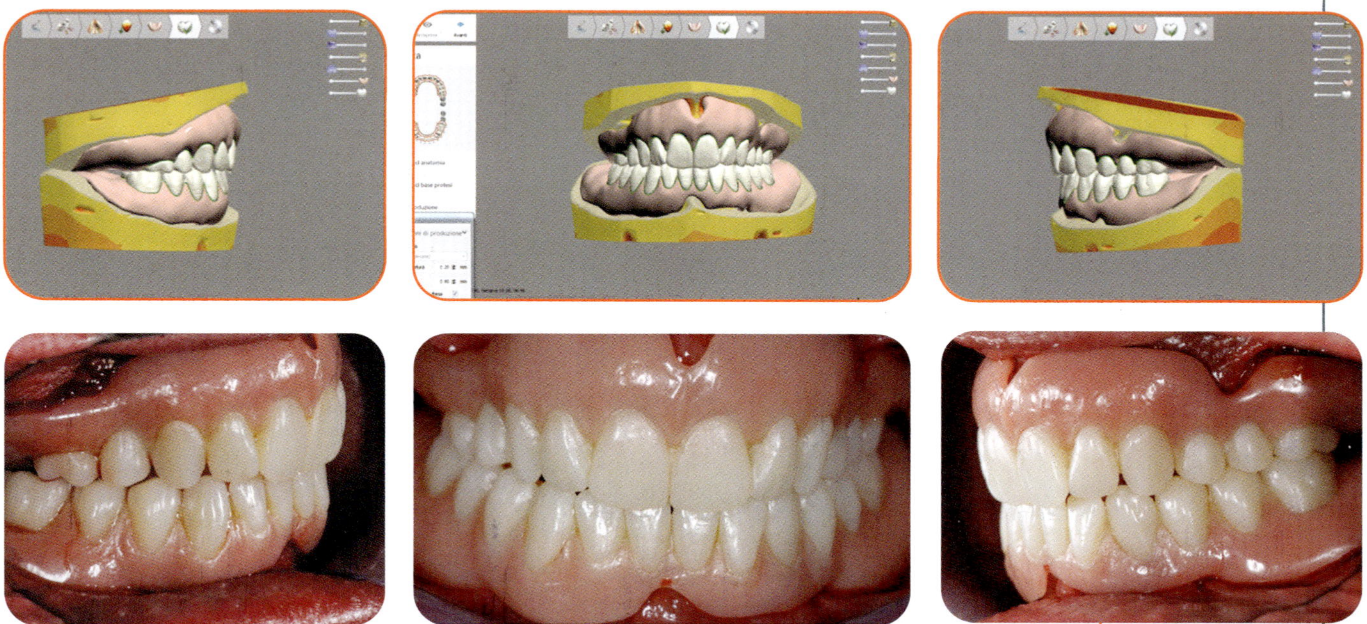

Figure 6.73 • Perfect consistency between the CAD design and the end prosthetic result.

In the treatment of patients with terminal dentition, the Authors prefer using a digital local anesthesia system, with controlled anesthetic release. This allows the surgical procedures to be performed without causing the perioral tissues to be blocked. The relation of the immediate prosthesis rehabilitation to the lips can therefore be assessed immediately.

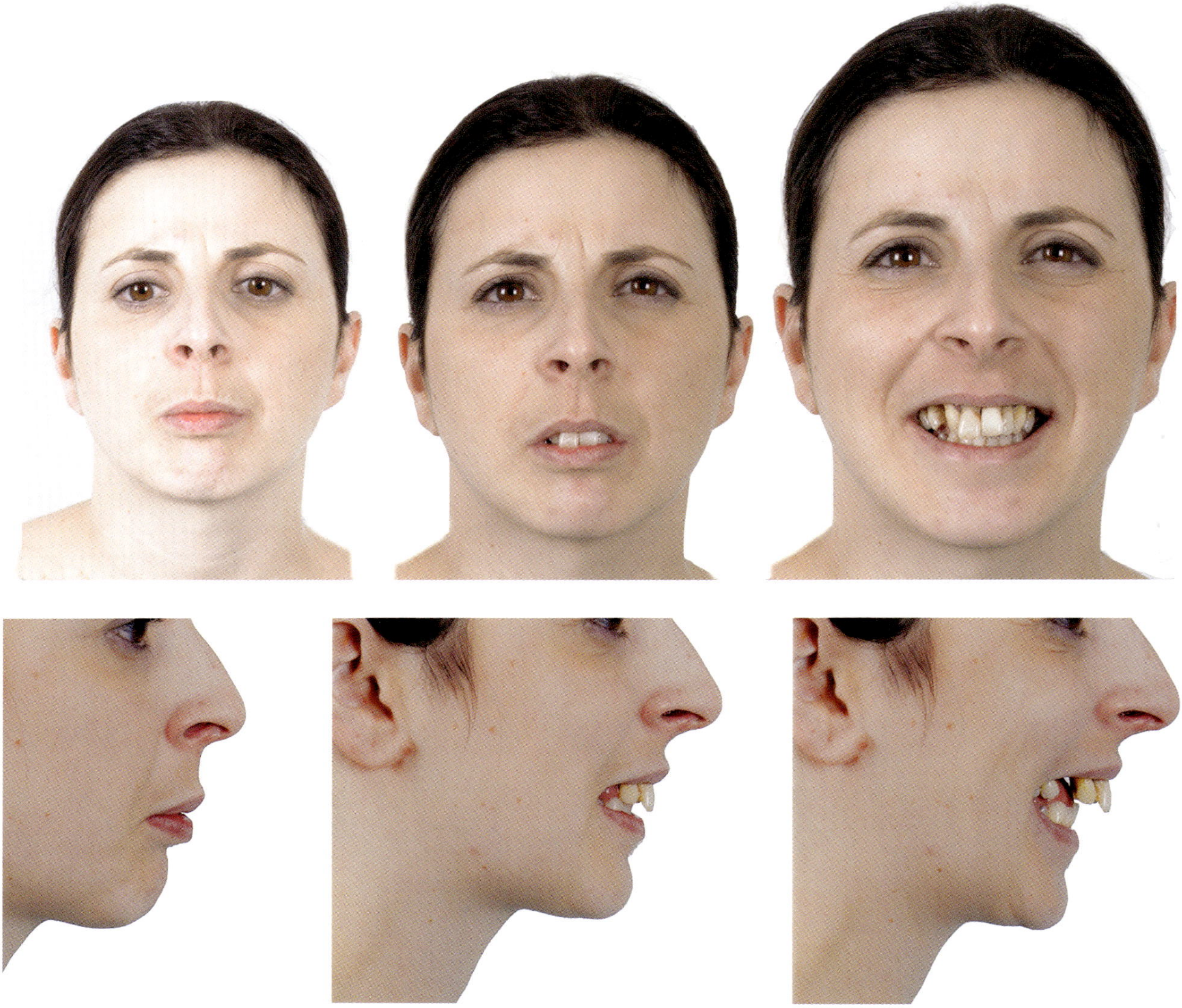

Figure 6.74 • Front and side view before the treatment.

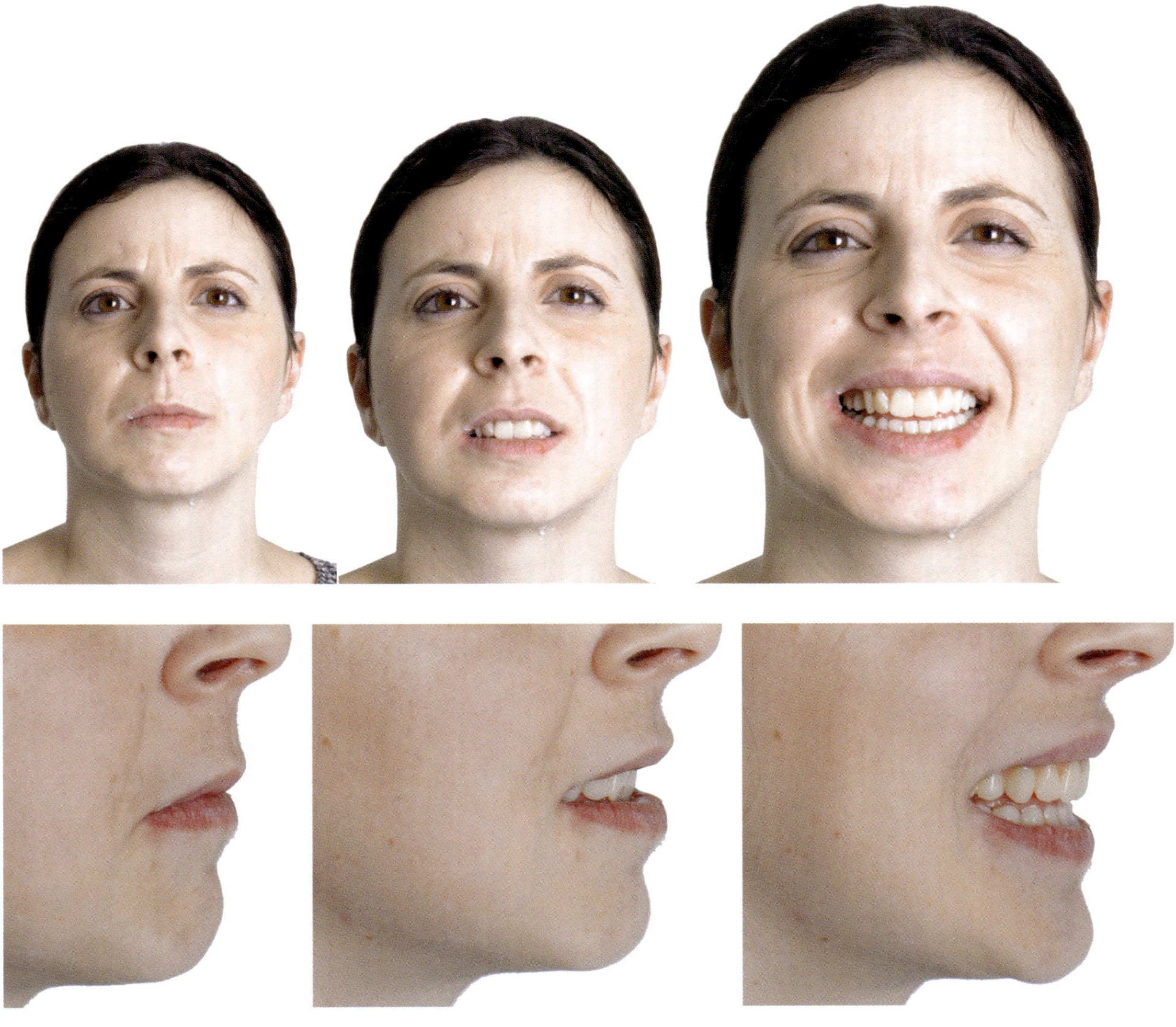

Figure 6.75 • Front and side view after the treatment.

References

1. Pound E. Esthetic dentures and their phonetic values. *J Prosthet Dent*. 1951;1(1-2):98-111.
2. Garnick J, Ramfjord S. Rest position: An electromyographic and clinical investigation. *J Prosthet Dent*. 1962;12(5):895-911.
3. Mansour RM, Reynik RJ. In vivo occlusal forces and moments: I. forces measured in terminal hinge position and associated moments. *J Dent Res*. 1975;54(1):114-20.
4. Rugh JD, Drago CJ, Barghi N. Comparison of electromyographic and phonetic measurements of vertical rest position. *J Dent Res*. 1979;58:316.
5. Pound E. Applying the vertical dimension of speech to restorative procedures. In: Lefkovitz W (ed). In: *Proceedings of the Second International Prosthodontic Congress*. St. Louis: Mosby; 1979.
6. Boos RH. Intermaxillary relation established by biting power. *J Am Dent Assoc*. 1940;27(8):1192-9.
7. Ricketts RM. Esthetics, environment, and the law of lip relation. *Am J Orthod*. 1968;54(4):272-89.
8. Pleasure MA. Correct vertical dimension and freeway space. *J Am Dent Assoc*. 1951;43(2):160-3.
9. Landa JS. The free-way space and its significance in the rehabilitation of the masticatory apparatus. *J Prosthet Dent*. 1952;2(6):756-79.
10. Mehringer E. The use of speech patterns as an aid in prosthodontic reconstruction. *J Prosthet Dent*. 1963;13(5):825-36.
11. Fenn HRB, MacGregor AR. *Fenn, Liddelow, and Gimsons' clinical dental prosthetics*. 3rd ed. London; Boston: Wright; 1989.
12. Chiche G, Pinault A. *Esthetics of anterior fixed prosthodontics*. Chicago: Quintessence; 1994. p. 13-32.
13. Burnett CA. Mandibular incisor position for English consonant sounds. *Int J Prosthodont*. 1999;12 (3):264-71.
14. Vig RG, Brundo GC. The kinetics of anterior tooth display. *J Prosthet Dent*. 1978;39(5):502-4.
15. Gibbs CH, Messerman T, Reswick JB, Derda HJ. Functional movements of the mandible. *J Prosthet Dent*. 1971;26(6):604-20.
16. Arnett WG, Bergman RT. Facial keys to orthodontic diagnosis and treatment planning. Part I. *Am J Orthod Dentofac Orthop*. 1993;103(4):299-312.
17. Strub JR, Blatz MB, Turp JC. Gingival and dental esthetics: mimicking mother. *Nature*. 2001;38:55-76.
18. Passamonti G, Vergnano A. *Atlante di protesi totale*. Torino: Editrice Cides Odonto; 1978.
19. Dawson P. Determining the determinants of occlusion. *Int J Periodontics Restor Dent*. 1983;3(6):8-21.
20. Pound E. *Personalized denture procedures*: Dentists' Manual. Denar Corporation; 1973. p. 112.
21. Robison SC. Physiological placement of artificial anterior teeth. *J Can Dent Assoc*. 1969;35(5):260-6.
22. Zarb G, Hobkirk J, Eckert S, Jacob R. *Prosthodontic treatment for edentulous patients*. 13th ed. St. Louis: Mosby/Elsevier; 2012. p. 464.
23. Souza BV, Faria AD, Ferreira S et al. Root-supported overdentures associated with temporary immediate prostheses - a case report. *Oral Health Dent Manag*. 2014;13(2):159-63.
24. Caputi S, Murmura G, Ricci L et al. Immediate denture fabrication: a clinical report. *Ann Stomatol* (Roma). 2013;4(3-4):273-7.
25. Woloch MM. Nontraumatic immediate complete denture placement: a clinical report. *J Prosthet Dent*. 1998;80(4):391-3.
26. Gilboa I, Cardash HS. An alternative approach to the immediate overdenture. *J Prosthodont*. 2009;18(1):71-5.
27. Goodacre CJ, Garbacea A, Naylor WP et al. CAD/CAM fabricated complete dentures: Concepts and clinical methods of obtaining required morphological data. *J Prosthet Dent*. 2012;107(1):34-46.
28. Infante L, Yilmaz B, McGlumphy E, Finger I. Fabricating complete dentures with CAD/CAM technology. *J Prosthet Dent*. 2014;111(5):351-5.

29. Kattadiyil M, Goodacre CJ, Baba NZ. CAD/CAM complete dentures: a review of two commercial fabrication systems. *J Calif Dent Assoc.* 2013;41(6):407-16.

30. Kattadiyil MT, Jekki R, Goodacre CJ, Baba NZ. Comparison of treatment outcomes in digital and conventional complete removable dental prosthesis fabrications in a predoctoral setting Presented at the Academy of Prosthodontics annual meeting, Kursaal, Berne, Switzerland, May 2014. *J Prosthet Dent.* 2015;114(6):818-25.

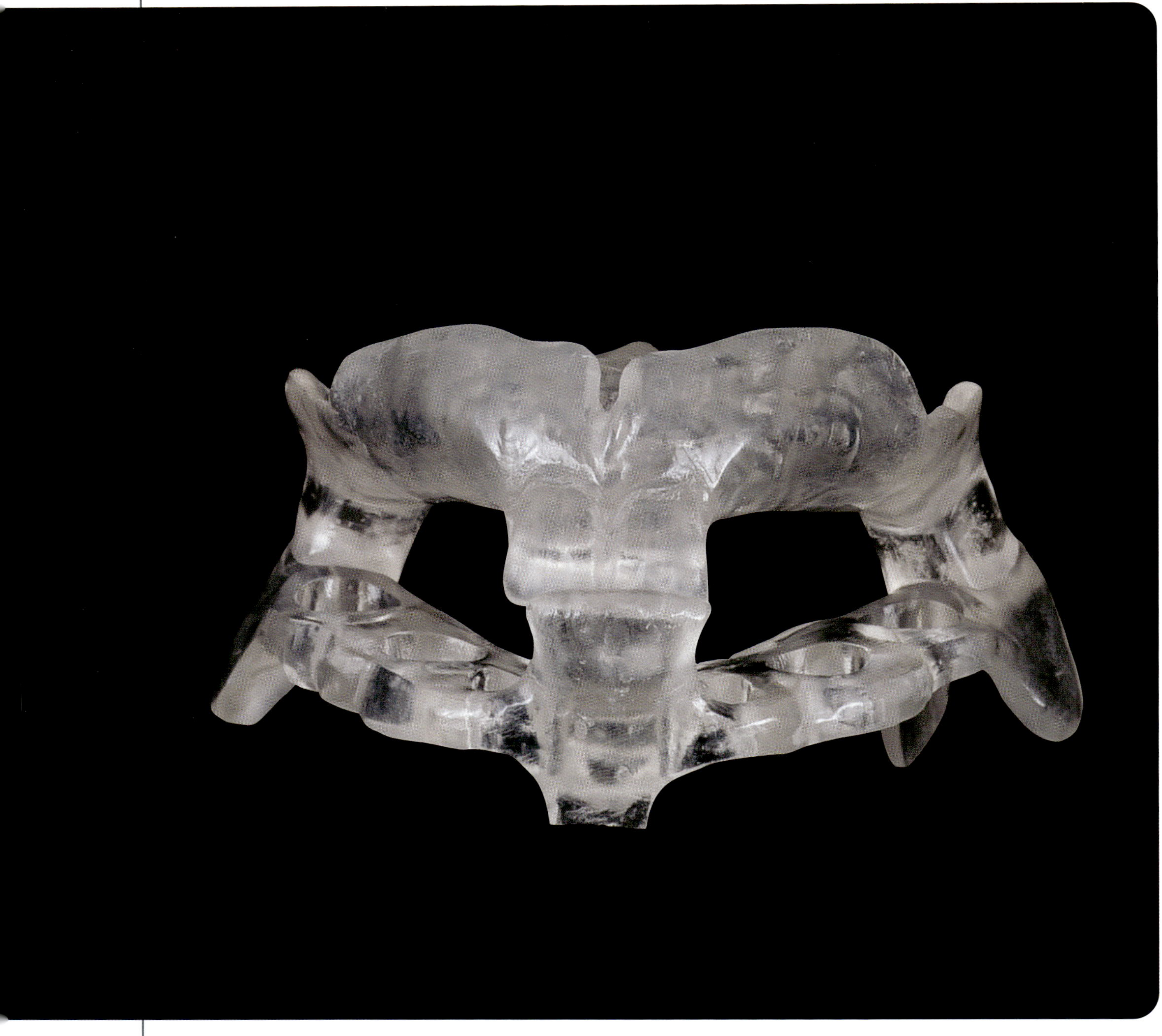

CHAPTER 7

P. VENEZIA, P. LACASELLA, R. CAVALCANTI

B.A.R.I. Technique: a new approach to immediate loading

In prosthetics, all complex rehabilitations must call for a re-organisational approach. In these cases, the occlusal, phonetic and esthetic information available at the time of the initial data collection cannot be replicated in the final rehabilitation (see Chapter 2).

In these patients, edentulous for a long time or with terminal dentition, it is essential to:

- obtain the new prosthetic coordinates (occlusion vertical dimension, position of the incisal crest of the upper anterior teeth, proper sagittal cranial-mandibular relations);
- test the soundness of the prosthetic design with a provisional prosthesis, and make any changes accordingly;
- replicate all the information from the provisional rehabilitation into the definitive one.

A variety of techniques have been developed to transfer the information from the fixed provisional prostheses on teeth or on implants to the definitive restorations.

The B.A.R.I. (Boosted Advanced Rehabilitation on Implants) Technique makes it possible to turn the patient's removable prosthesis, already tested and functionalised, into a hybrid prosthesis on implants, thus maintaining all the information relating to function, esthetics and phonetics.

In recent years, the immediate loading procedure has become increasingly popular and consists of delivering a fixed restoration in occlusal function within 48 hours of implant placement [1,2]. This technique has been developed and initially used for the edentulous lower arches [3], where the quality and quantity of bone are more favourable and the likelihood of achieving primary implant stability is high [4].

Immediate loading in the lower arch can be considered a well documented and scientifically validated approach. In the edentulous upper arch, the results of immediate loading are promising, but further studies are required to validate definitively these procedures [2].

Various protocols have been proposed in order to rehabilitate patients with immediate loading, in order to reduce treatment time frames and deliver fixed prostheses to them in one day [5-9]. The development of implant design and surfaces, as well as surgical approaches has made it possible to considerably decrease treatment time frames. Very often, the treatment of totally edentulous patients with immediate loading procedures might be difficult to achieve as the whole diagnostic stage would be lost. In most cases, the totally edentulous patient, in terminal dentition or rehabilitated with old removable prostheses, shows alterations in the mandibular position (anterior and superior sliding), alterations in the vertical dimension, inadequate occlusal relations, altered esthetics and phonetics [10].

In these cases, it is essential to rehabilitate the patient with new removable prostheses that ensure conditions of stability and occlusal repeatability and optimised function and esthetics. At this point, the treatment can be finalised quickly and predictably by making use of the information from the complete prosthesis. Any implant planning, as will be seen, can also be really simplified by the possibility of the new software to reliably superimpose the prosthetic design on three-dimensional radiology images [11-13].

Analogue flow

The first part of the technique entails duplication of the full prostheses already tested by the patient (see Chapter 5).

The prostheses are impressed with laboratory silicone (Zeta Labor, 85 shore Zhermack, Italy).

The impression surface is impressed first **(Figure 7.1)**, creating a model on which pivots used for repositioning are made, after the material has set.

Two wax cylinders are placed at the level of the tubers, on the upper prosthesis, and at the level of the trigones, on the lower one, distal to the distal teeth, which will allow the casting channels of the flask to be obtained **(Figure 7.2)**.

After performing the isolation of both the silicone model and the prosthesis, the occlusion surface and the polished surface are impressed, always with the same material **(Figure 7.3)**.

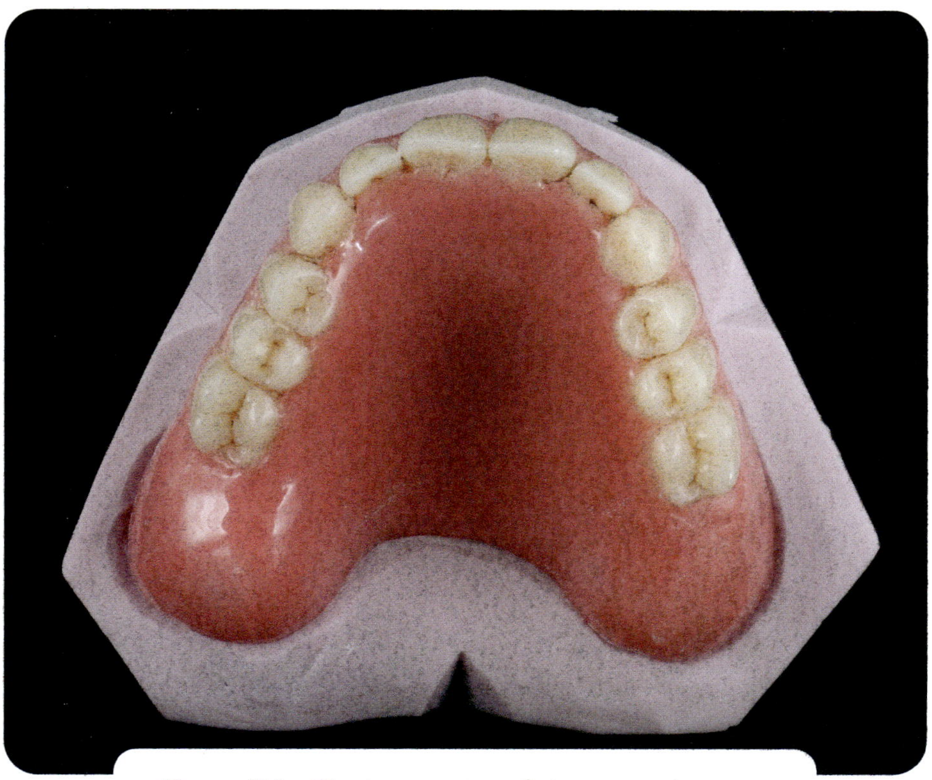

Figure 7.1 • The impression of the patient's upper prosthesis is added with silicone.

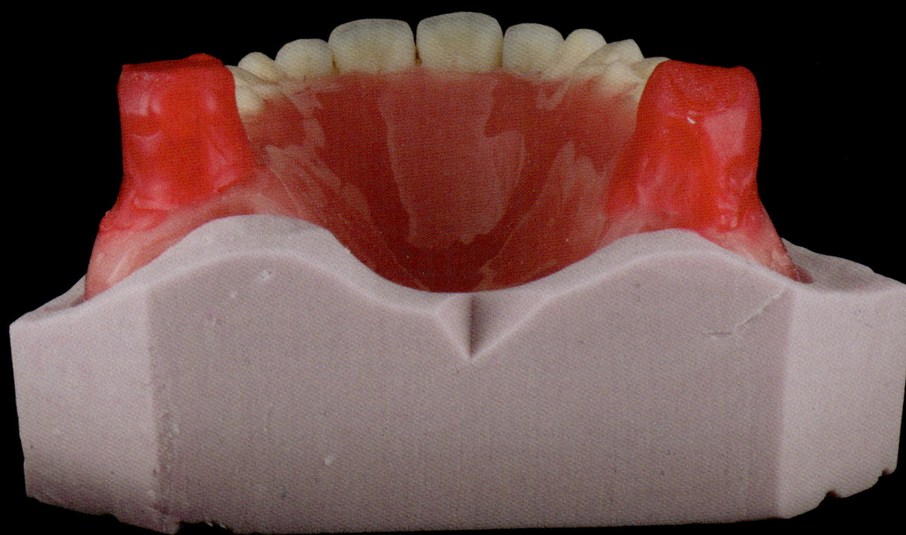

Figure 7.2 • Red wax cylinders are placed in the distal area to the molars of the upper prosthesis.

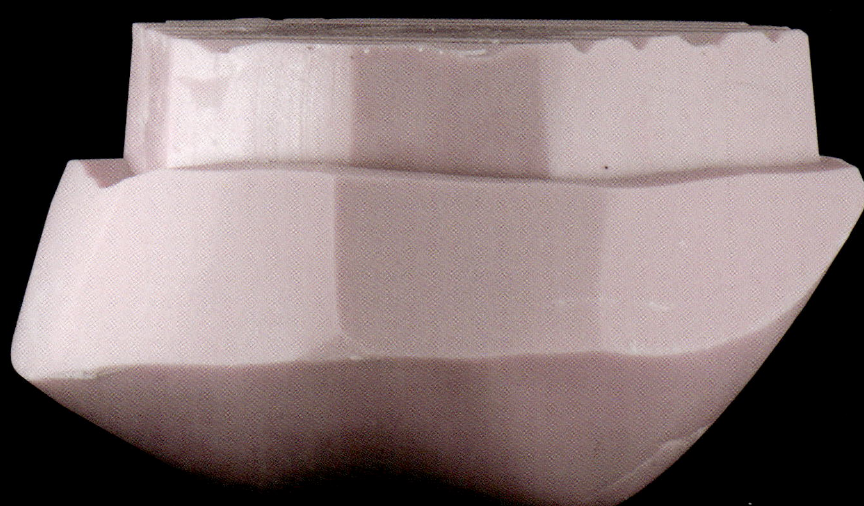

Figure 7.3 • A mould former is made of the occlusal part and of the polished surface of the prosthesis.

After vulcanisation of the material in a pressure pot at 2.2 bar **(Figure 7.4)**, the flask is opened, the prosthesis is removed and moulds and formers are obtained which will allow the prosthesis to be duplicated **(Figures 7.5** and **7.6)**.

To avoid the formation of air bubbles and inaccuracies, the fluid resin is injected through one of the two channels left free by the wax, which will be able to enter the cavity left free by the prosthesis, fill it and come out of the contralateral opening **(Figure 7.7)**.

The duplicates of the prostheses are finished, polished **(Figure 7.8)** and subsequently boxed with wax **(Figure 7.9)**.

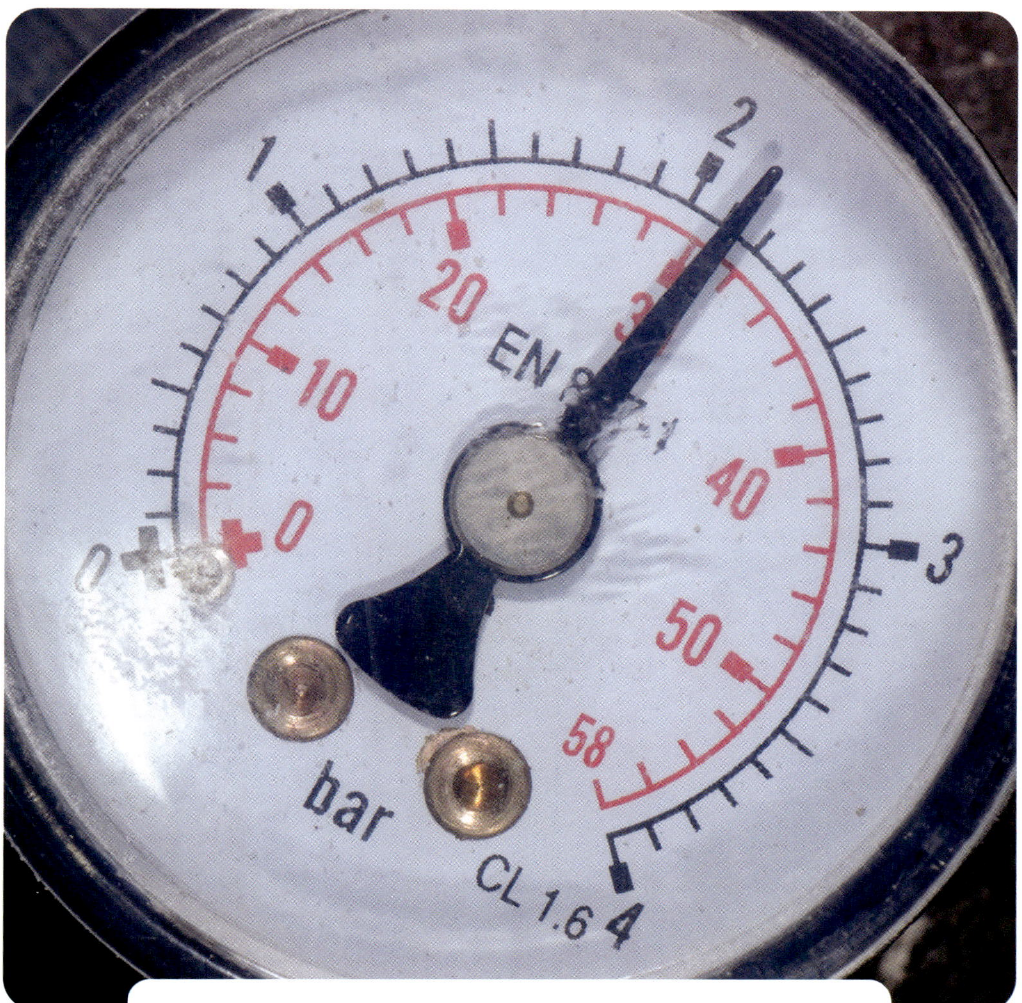

Figure 7.4 • The pressure pot is set at 2 bar.

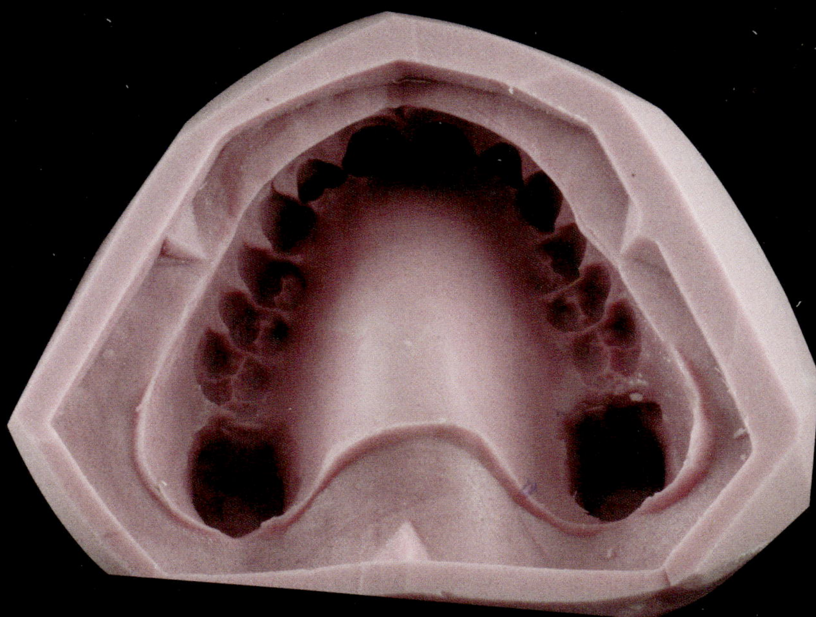

Figure 7.5 • Mould former of the upper prosthesis after opening the silicone flask.

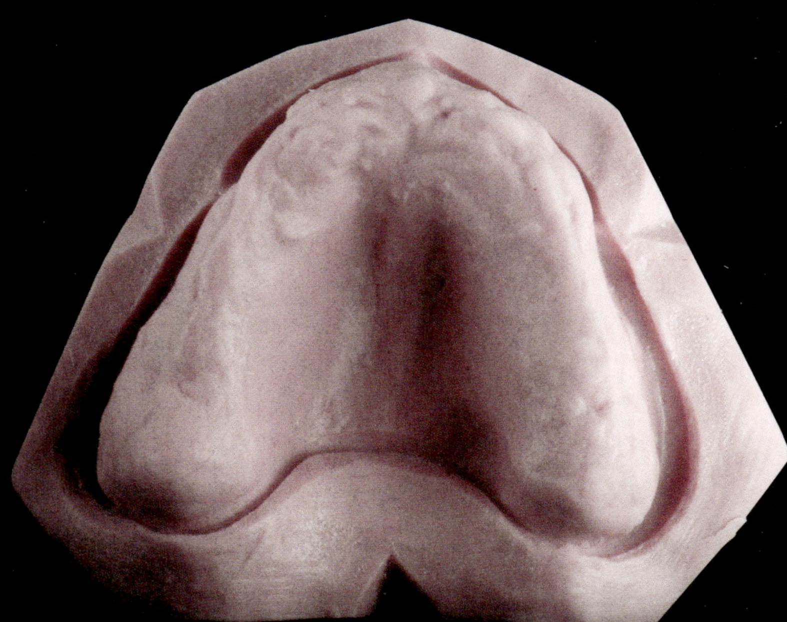

Figure 7.6 • Mould of the upper prosthesis after opening the flask and removing the pre-existing prosthesis.

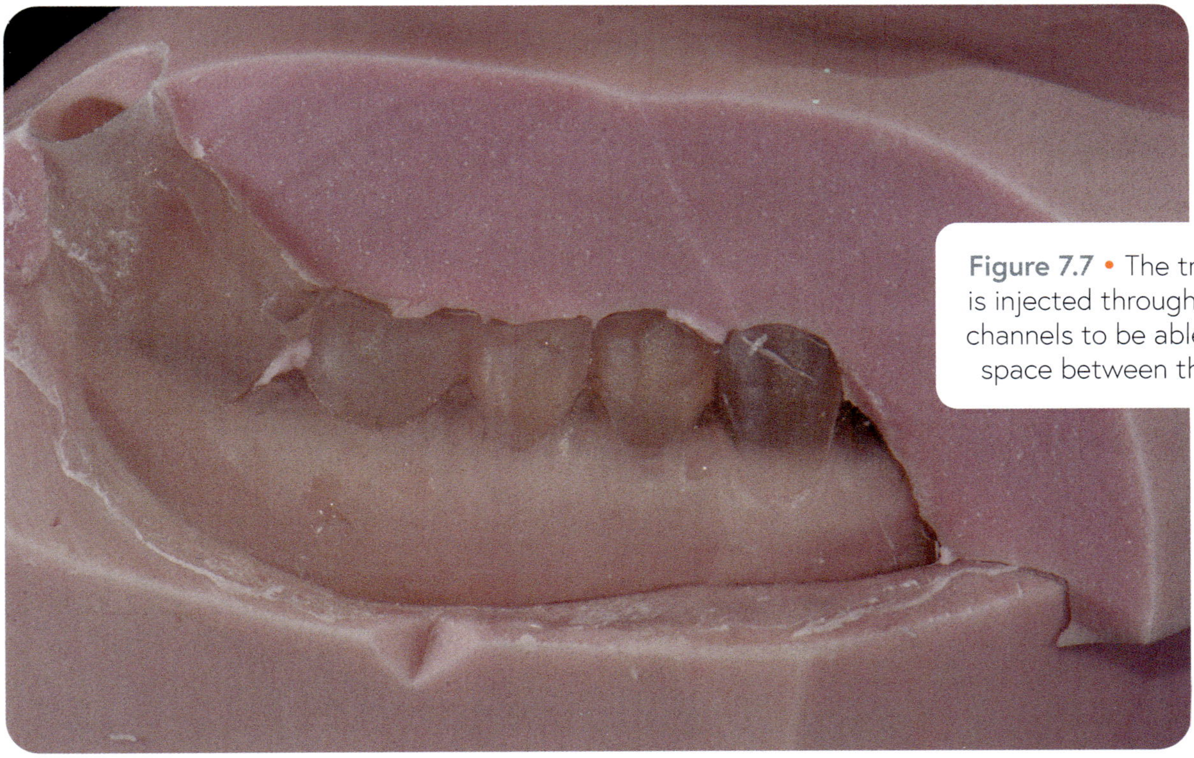

Figure 7.7 • The transparent resin is injected through one of the two channels to be able to take up the space between the two moulds.

Figure 7.8 • The duplicates in transparent PMMA of the upper and lower prostheses after finishing and polishing.

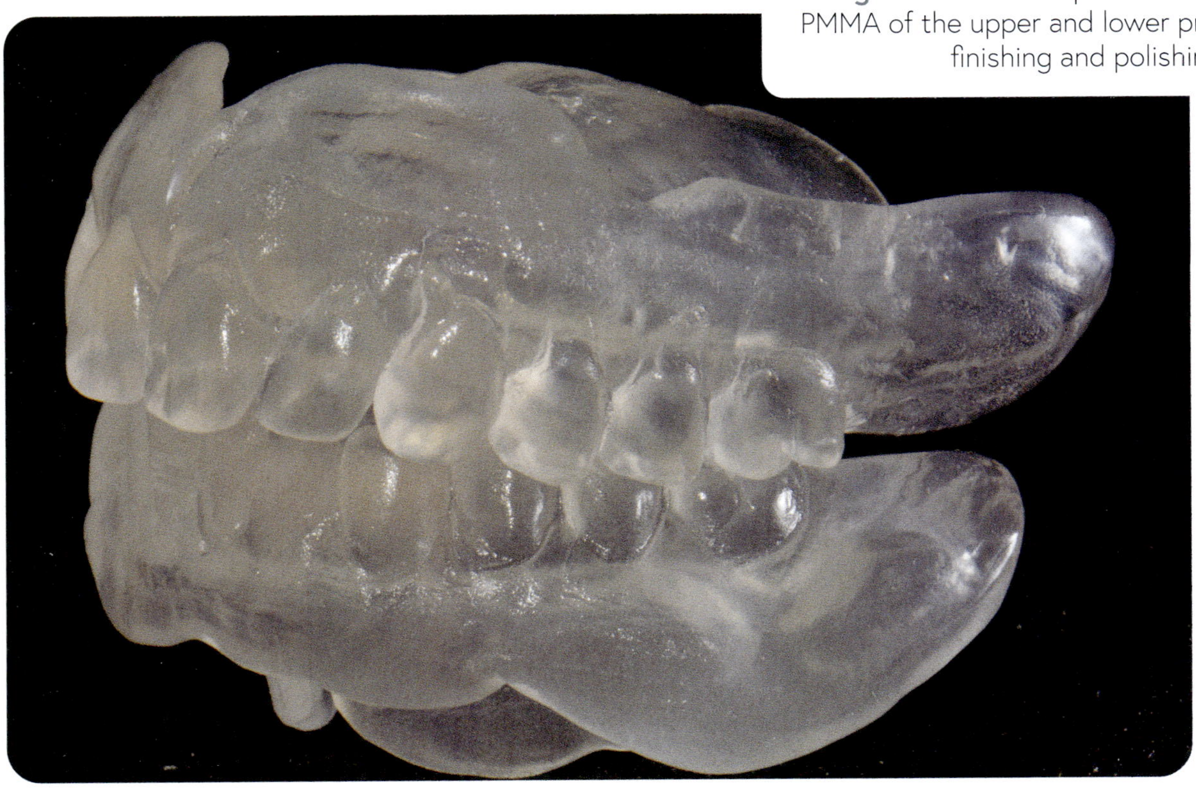

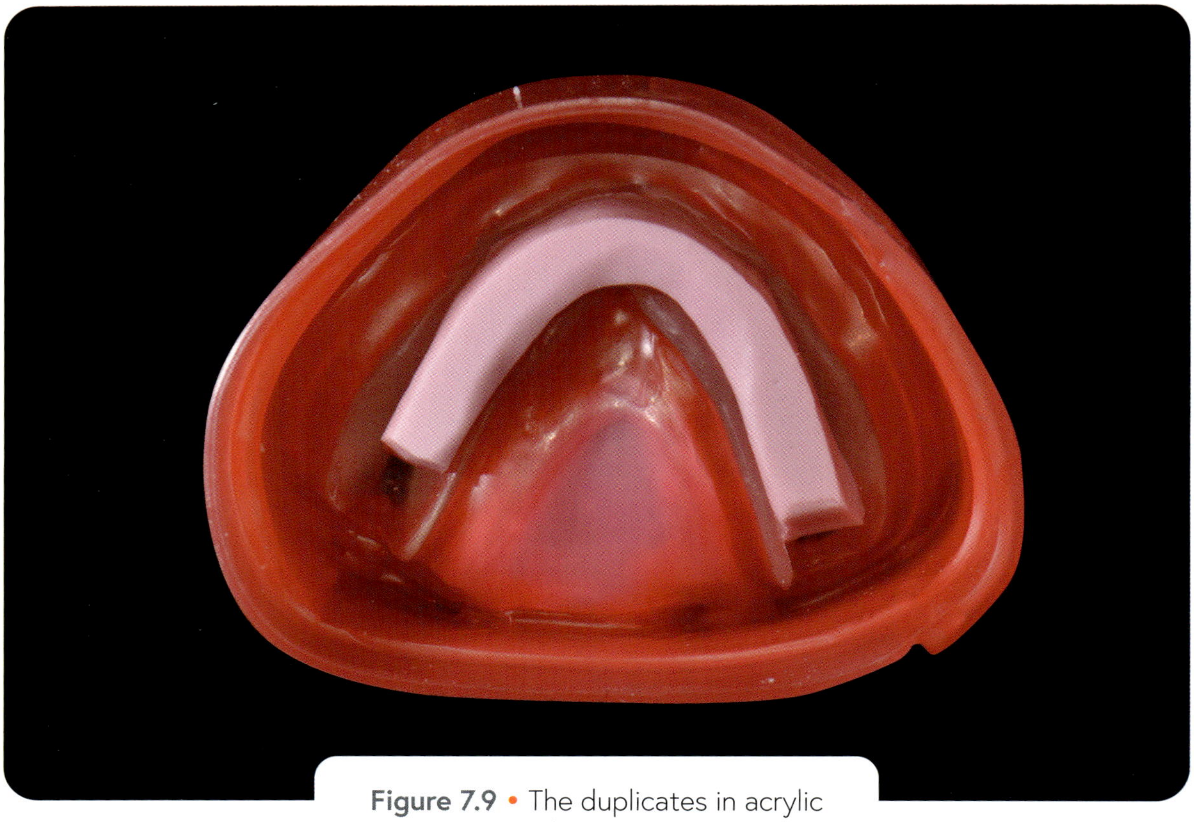

Figure 7.9 • The duplicates in acrylic resin are boxed with wax.

A silicone spacer is inserted on the impression surface of the lower duplicate, and then the level four plaster is poured **(Figures 7.10** and **7.11)**. This measure will make it possible for the model to be hollowed in the area where the implants are to be positioned according to the one-model technique [14] and, moreover, will allow the prosthesis duplicates of the model to be removed easily. The upper model will also be treated with the same method.

The models may be mounted in the articulator thanks to a previously recorded facebow. At this stage, it will therefore be possible to transfer the position of the maxilla into the space in a three-dimensionally correct manner.

Furthermore, thanks to the use of the duplicates, the intermaxillary relations between the edentulous arches can be easily reproduced **(Figure 7.12)**. When the duplicates are removed, the exact spatial reproduction that the patient has when the prostheses are in the maximum intercuspation relation will be obtained **(Figure 7.13)**.

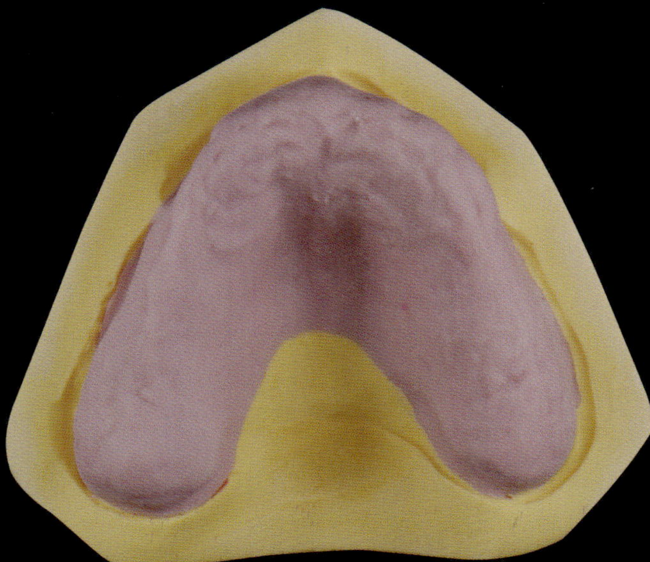

Figure 7.10 • Level four plaster is used to make the models.

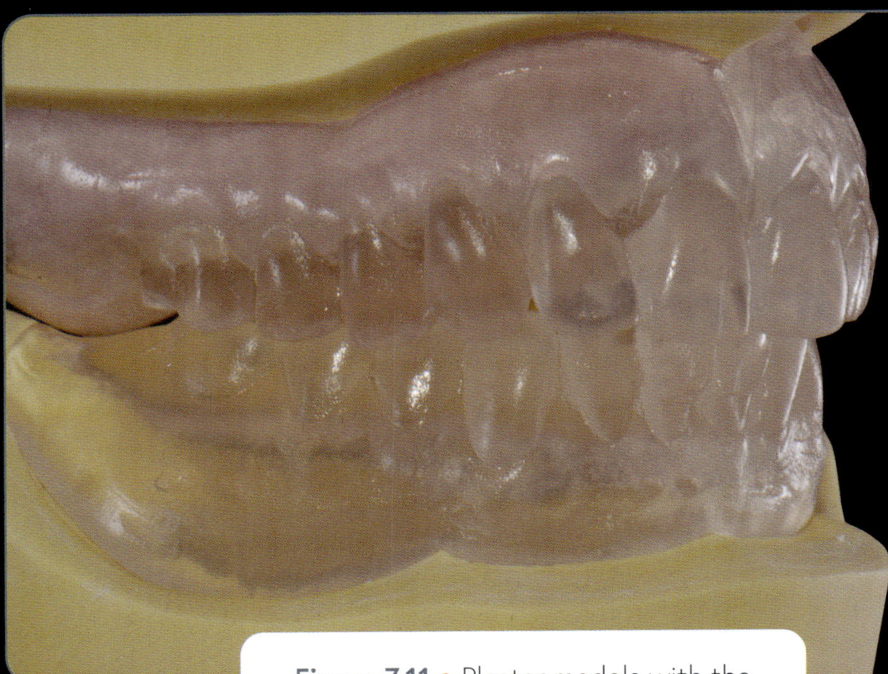

Figure 7.11 • Plaster models with the duplicates of the prosthesis in occlusion.

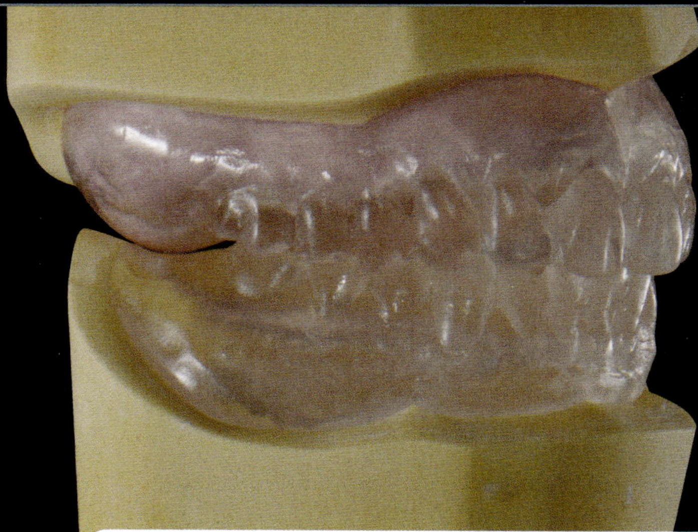

Figure 7.12 • The models are mounted in the articulator with the facial bow.

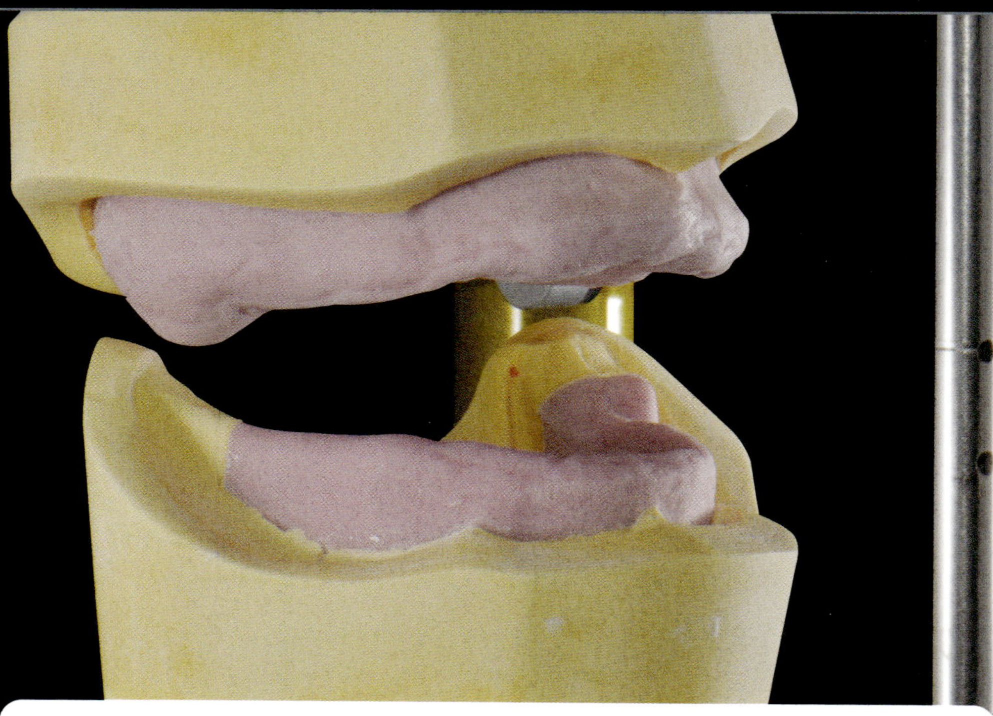

Figure 7.13 • After removing the duplicates, one may appreciate how the transfer of information relating to the vertical dimension and that relating to the sagittal intermaxillary relationships is extremely easy to perform.

Another resin replica of the prosthesis will be needed for diagnostic purposes. The individual acrylic teeth will be perforated and a groove will be carved in the centre of the ridge: both the channels obtained at the level of the artificial teeth and the centre-crestal sulcus will be filled with resin containing barium **(Figure 7.14)**. This is a radiopaque material that can be seen during the radiological examination with the aim of obtaining information regarding the available bone volumes for implant therapy in relation to the ideal prosthetic design.

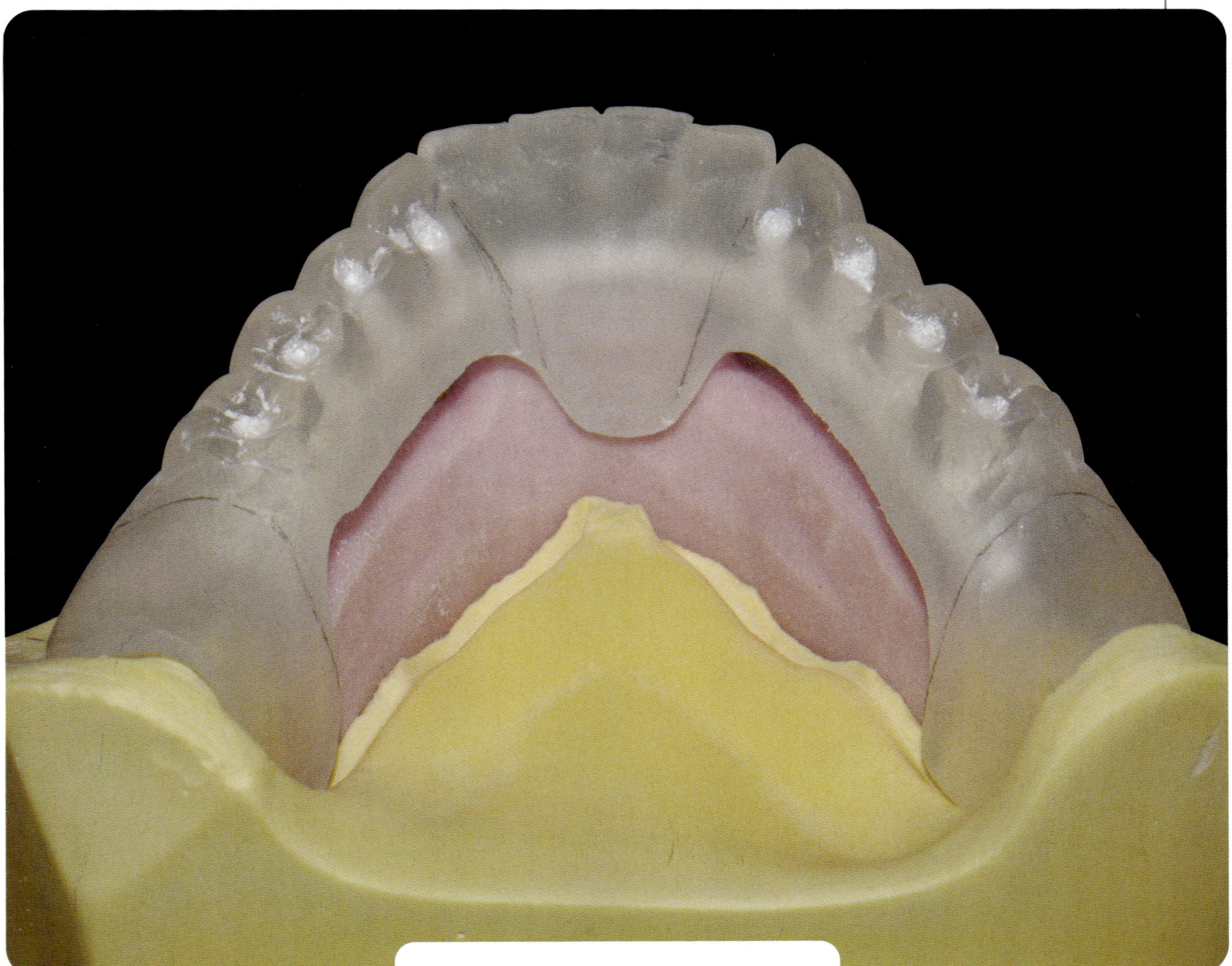

Figure 7.14 • Radiographic stent.

The patient will need to perform a three-dimensional cone beam radiograph (CBCT) wearing the barium X-ray template and the duplicate upper prosthesis, with mouth closed **(Figure 7.15)**. The DICOM files obtained will be loaded into an implant navigation software coDiagnostiX (Dental Wings, Montreal Canada) to evaluate:

- the mandible anatomy **(Figure 7.16)**;
- the thickness of the soft tissues **(Figure 7.17)**;
- the height and angle of the posts to be used to bring the prosthetic connection to the surface and make a screw retained hybrid prosthesis **(Figure 7.18)**;
- the ideal implant position to achieve a closed prosthetic polygon **(Figure 7.19)**;
- the ideal length and morphology of the implants to be used (see Figure 7.19).

Based on the prosthetic indications, the radiological template was modified to provide the surgeon with information on the ideal implant position in relation to the prosthetic design.

In the clinical case presented in this chapter, the surgical template had three stabilisation elements at the level of the lower ridge (concerned by the implant-prosthetic

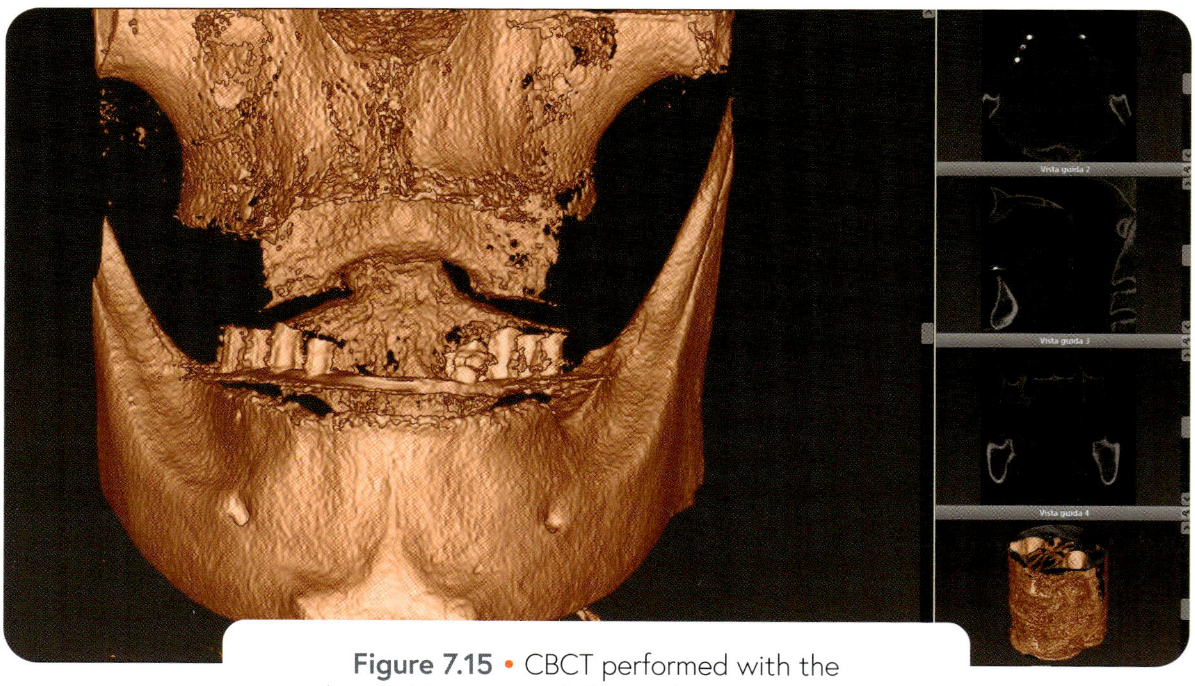

Figure 7.15 • CBCT performed with the radiographic stent and the duplicate of the upper prosthesis in occlusion.

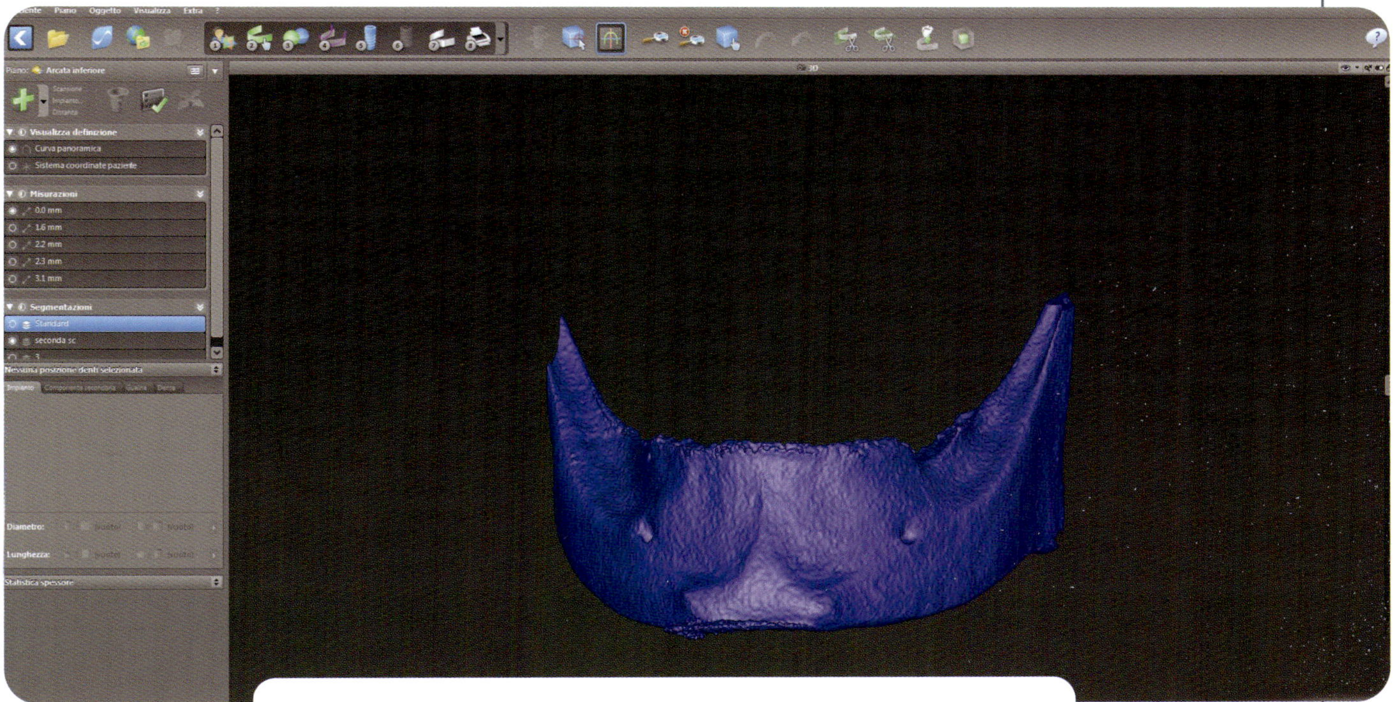

Figure 7.16 • Three-dimensional reconstruction of the mandible through DICOM file of the CBCT.

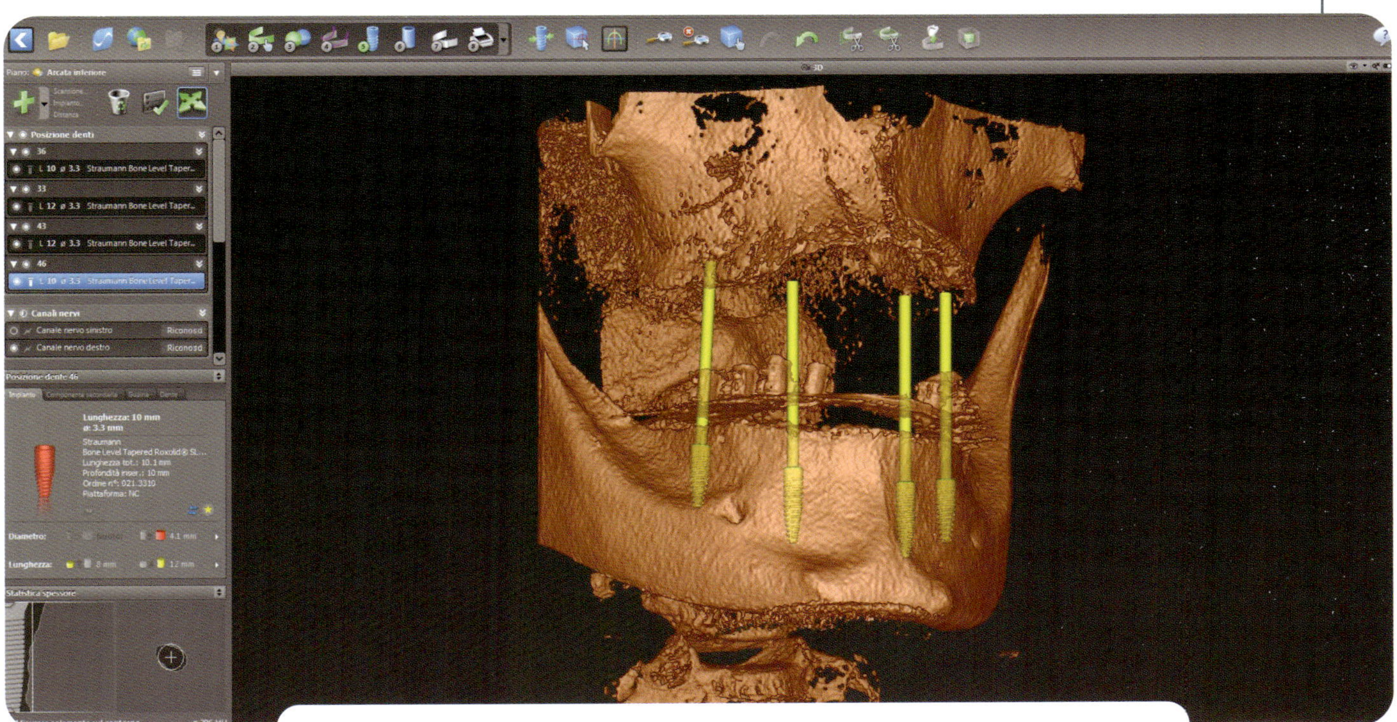

Figure 7.17 • Evaluation of the ideal position of the implants in relation to the thickness of the crest and that of soft tissues.

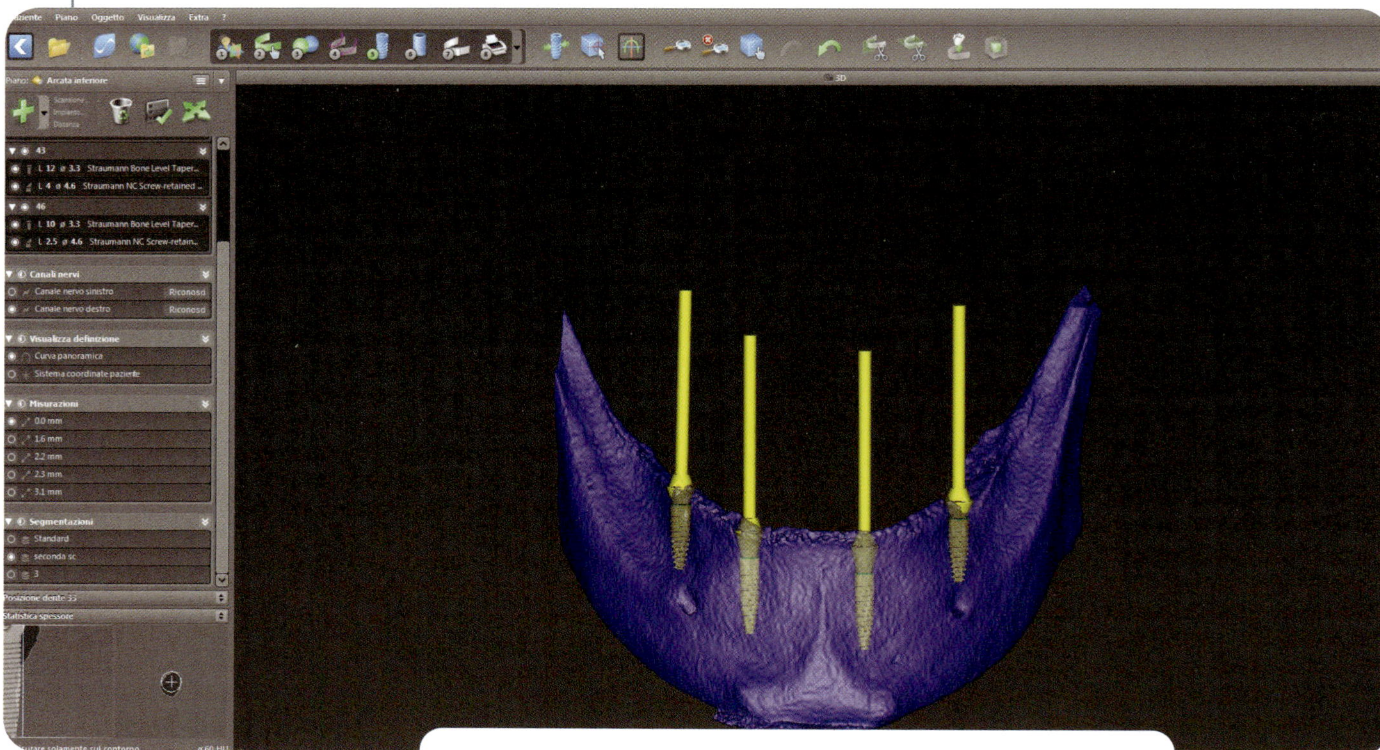

Figure 7.18 • Evaluation of the height of the abutments to be used to make a screw-on prosthesis.

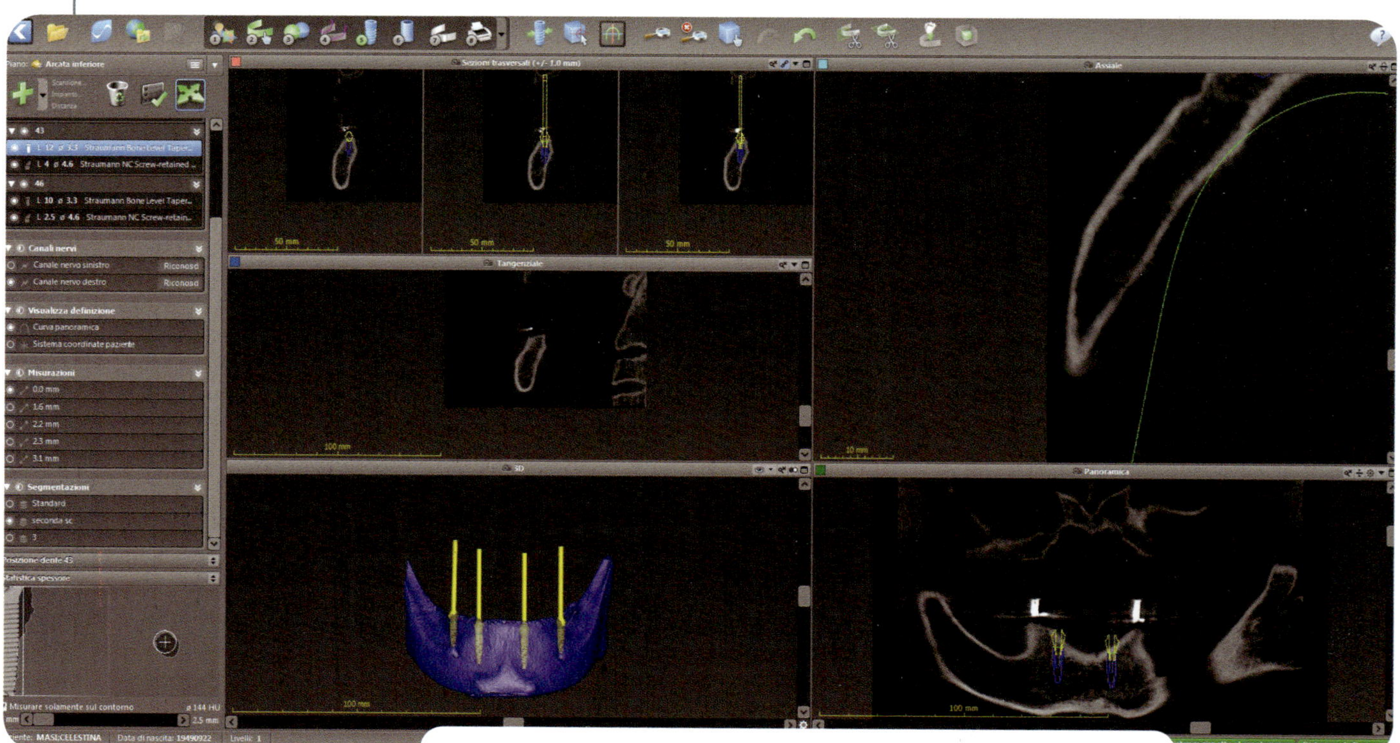

Figure 7.19 • Evaluation of the consistency of the implant design in the various sections.

therapy), two at the level of the trigone and the third one in the parasymphyseal area. Three other stabilisation points were designed on the occlusal table (two located in the molar area and the third one in the anterior area of the incisors) (**Figure 7.20**).

The registration plates (fenestrated in the lateral areas in order not to interfere with the procedures for registering the position of the implants) can thus be centred by making use of the patient's usual occlusion (**Figure 7.21**).

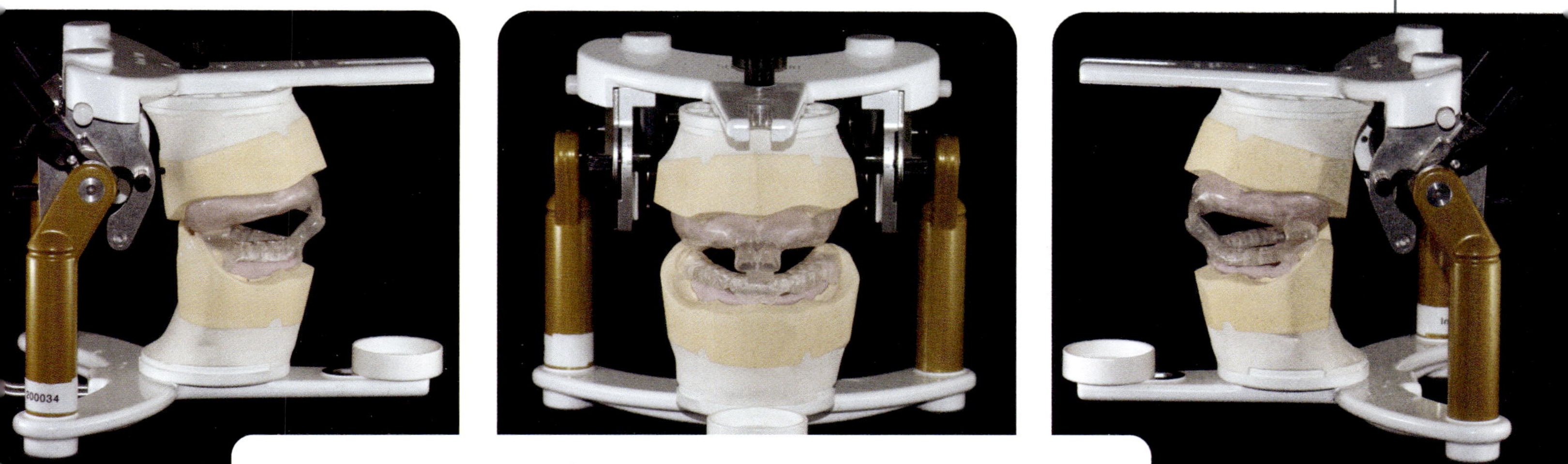

Figure 7.20 • Plates for carrying out the surgical phase and for registering the position of the implants mounted in the articulator.

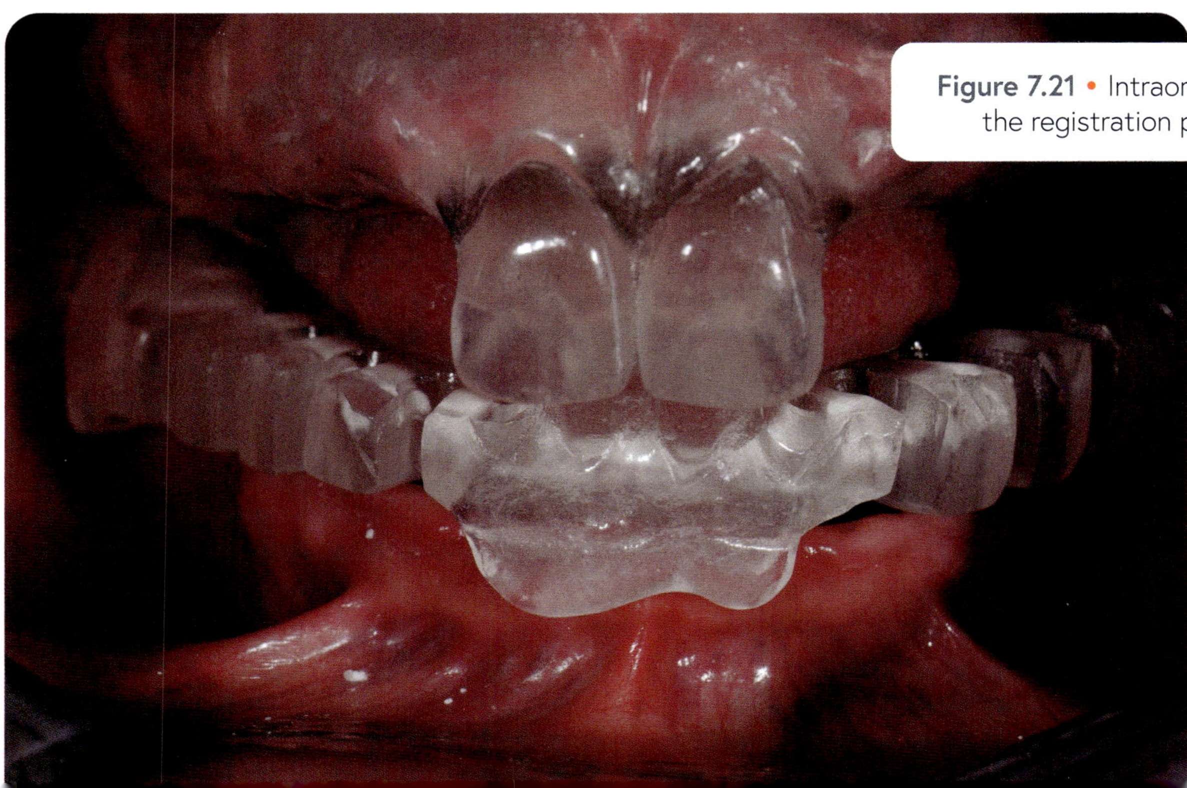

Figure 7.21 • Intraoral view of the registration plates.

On the day of the surgery, the consistency between the planned design and the patient's intraoral situation was ascertained (**Figures 7.22** and **7.23**).

After placing four implants (BLT, Straumann, Basel) the screw retained prosthetic posts were positioned (SRA Abutment, Straumann, Basel) required to bring the prosthetic connection to the surface and to make the screw-on prosthesis. They were tightened at 35 N using a torque wrench.

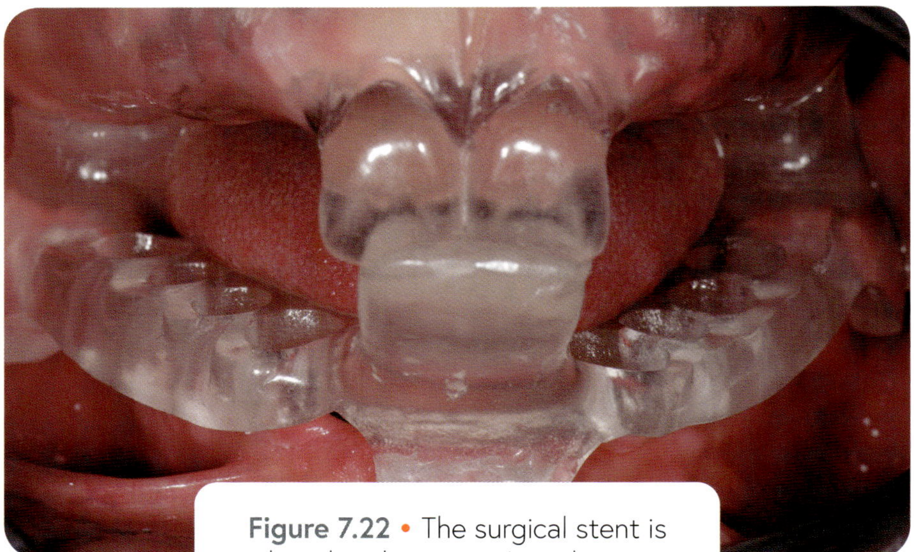

Figure 7.22 • The surgical stent is placed in the patient's oral cavity.

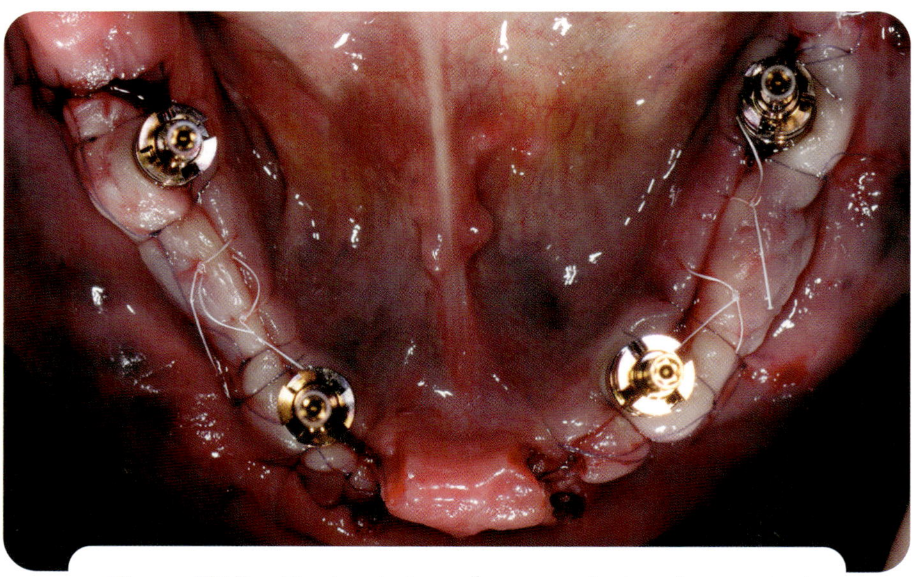

Figure 7.23 • Occlusal view after completing the surgical phase and positioning the abutments for screw-on prosthesis.

The impression transfers were screwed onto the posts and any interference between them and the transfer template were ruled out. One also ensured there was no interference between transfer and upper plate when in occlusion **(Figure 7.24)**.

A small amount of acrylic resin was applied (Pattern Resin, GC America) to attach the transfers to the bases made before **(Figure 7.25)**.

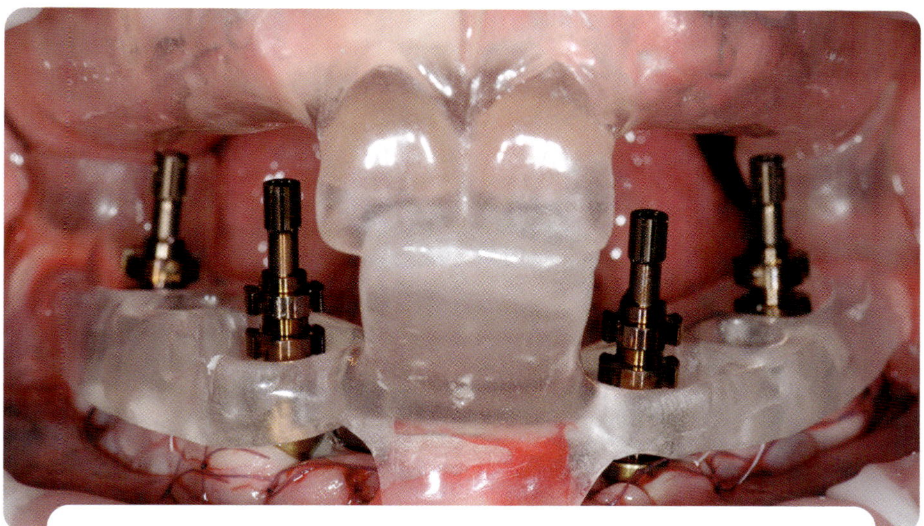

Figure 7.24 • Checking for interference between transfer plate and the mounted transfers from the SRA Abutments.

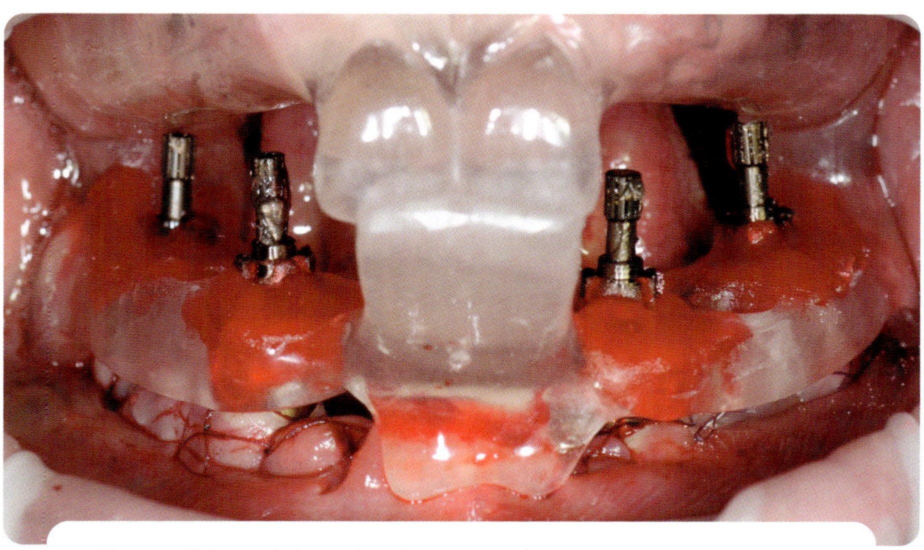

Figure 7.25 • A low shrinkage acrylic resin is used to attach the transfers to the transfer plate.

To make the control jig, SRA (Screw Retained Abutment) Abutments were fitted, titanium posts for screw retained prostheses, which were subsequently joined together with an orthodontic wire.

The posts were first joined together with a very rigid light-curing fluid composite (Bredent, Italy) then with Pattern Resin GC Italia (**Figure 7.26**).

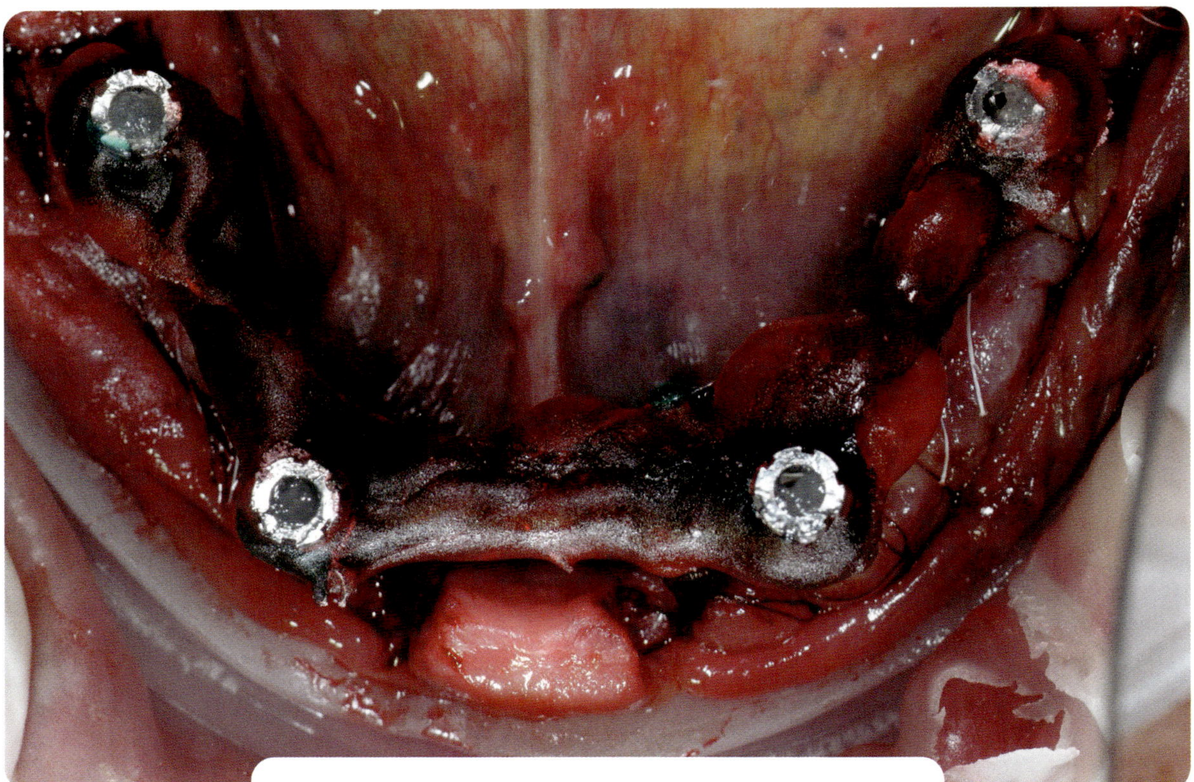

Figure 7.26 • Making the control index.

The control jig is required to validate the previous step. In the procedures to attach the transfers to the plate, errors may occur (lack of stability of an impression coping with respect to the plate, interference of the plate with the impression transfers), which might affect the making of the immediate loading prosthesis. The control jig is screwed onto the implant analogues and must be placed precisely and passively on them. If there is discrepancy in the position of one of the analogues, the control jig is essential to reposition it correctly in the master model after coring it.

The patient has completed the first stage of the treatment and has been discharged after placing four PEEK healing abutments on the implants **(Figure 7.27)**.

The implant analogues have been connected to the transfers **(Figure 7.28)**. The bases therefore allowed the prosthetic template-transfer-analogues complex to be repositioned on the carved master models already mounted in the articulator. The level four plaster has been cast into the model **(Figures 7.29** and **7.30)**; once hardened, the

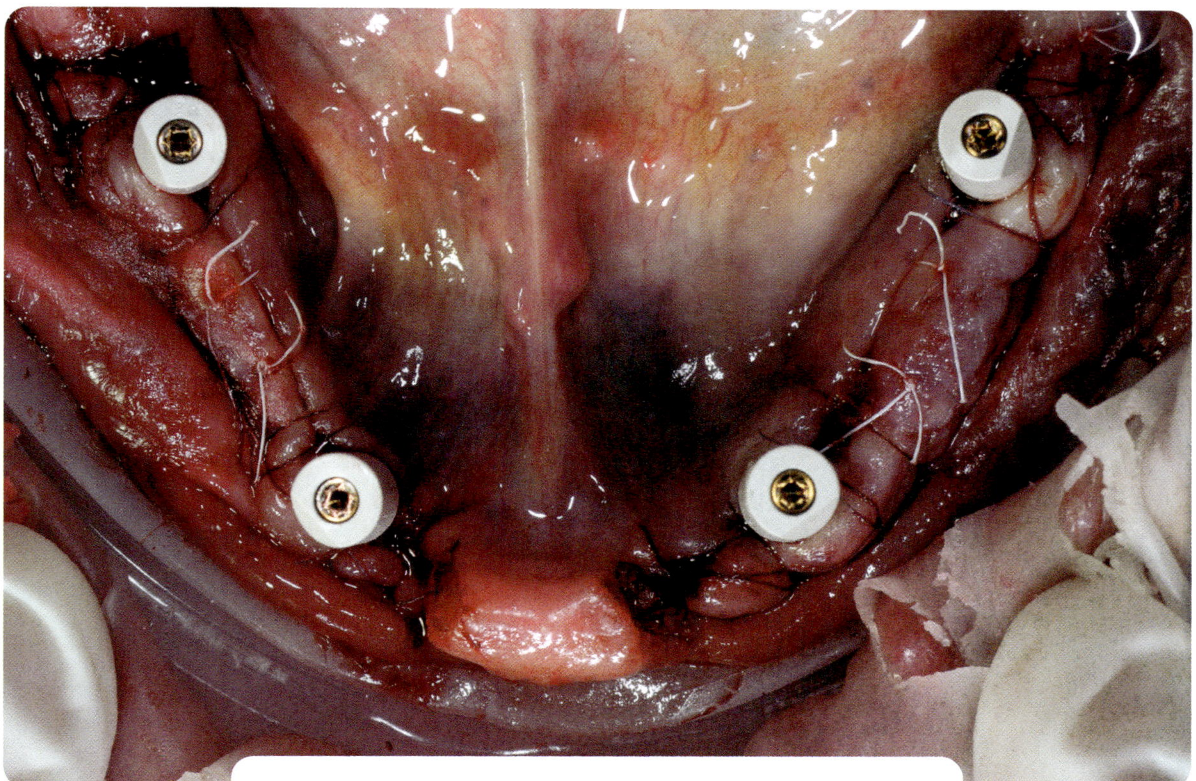

Figure 7.27 • The healing posts are inserted and the first appointment is thus completed.

The pattern resin LS (GC) is a material that has a wide range of applications in the office and in the laboratory. It consists of a powder (polymethyl methacrylate benzoyl peroxide) and a liquid (methyl methacrylate 2-hydroxyethyl methacrylate). The thixotropicity of the resin ensures optimal fluidity and excellent workability. The main advantages are: minimal shrinkage and easy finishing for perfect fit; high hardness and resistance; high stability even with thin layers.

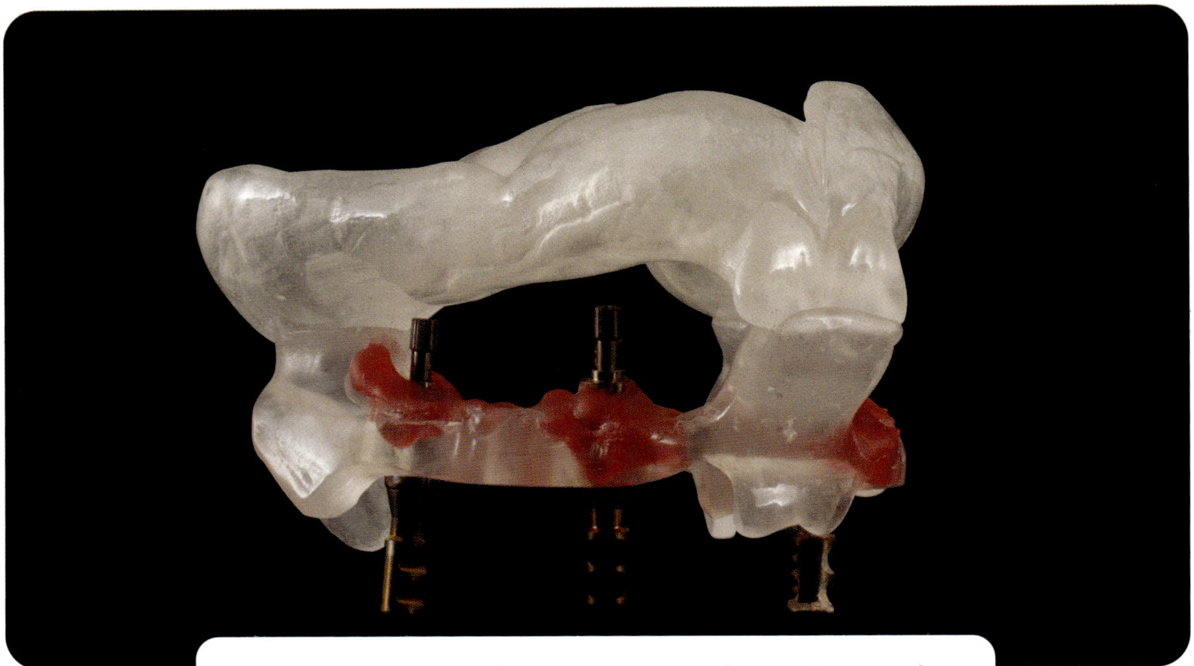

Figure 7.28 • The analogues are screwed onto the transfers.

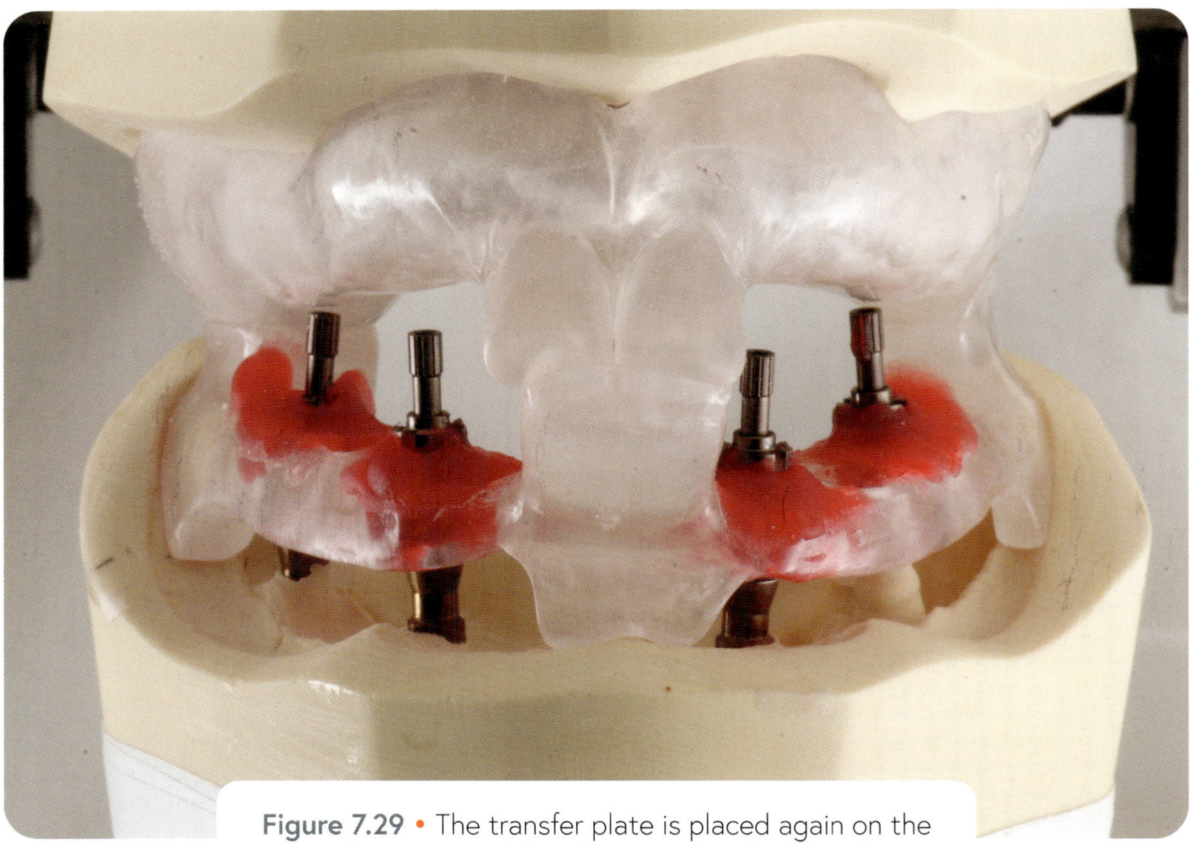

Figure 7.29 • The transfer plate is placed again on the carved master model and mounted in the articulator.

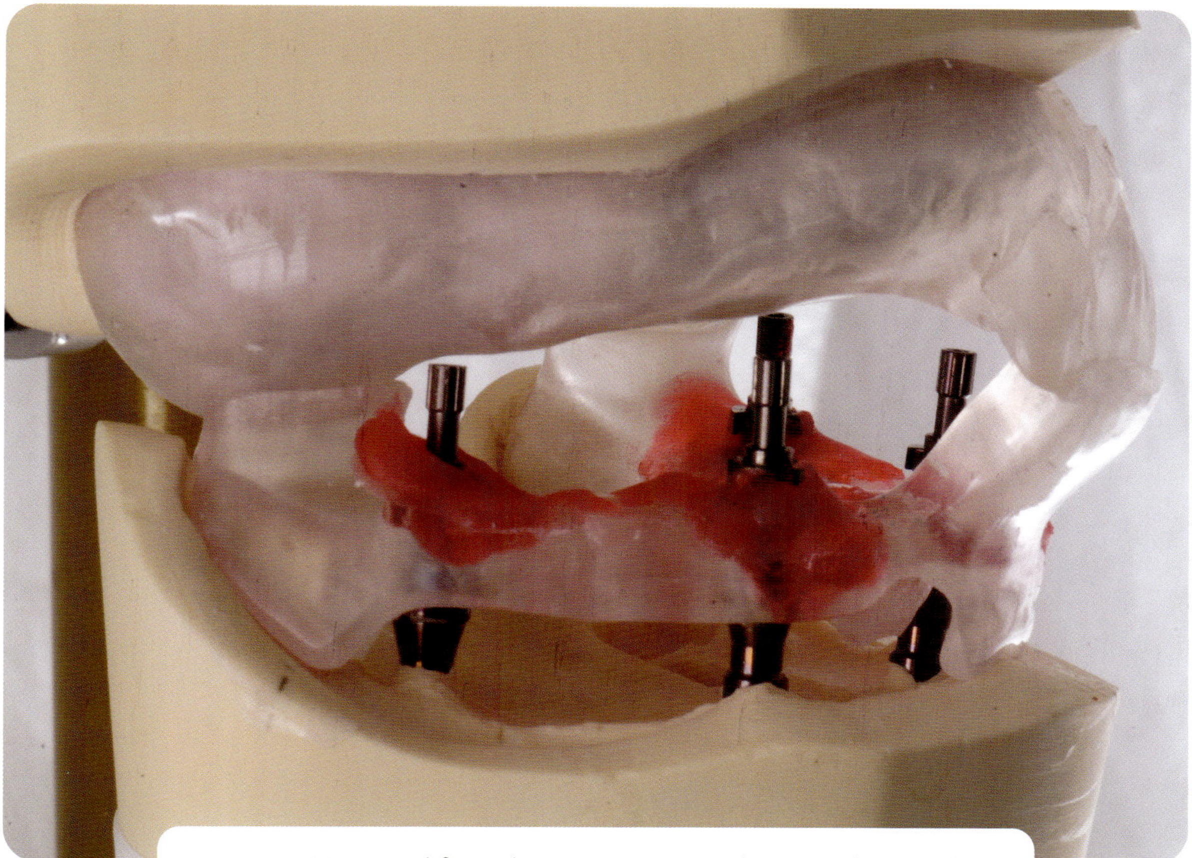
Figure 7.30 • Level four plaster is cast into the carved part which will encase and lock the analogues.

plate has been unscrewed and the analogues have thus remained encased in the model, providing the dental technician with the precise implant position.

The control jig has allowed the correctness of the implant position on the model to be verified (**Figure 7.31**). In addition, the soft tissues have been reproduced thanks to a silicone index (**Figure 7.32**).

At this point, it has been possible to make and deliver the hybrid prosthesis anchored on implants in the space of a few hours after performing the surgical procedures.

The space available for final rehabilitation is then evaluated using a silicone index obtained from the duplicates of the prosthesis mounted in the articulator (**Figure 7.33**).

Titanium posts have been used for prosthetic finalisation (**Figure 7.34**). These have been resized by evaluating the overall dimension of the final prosthesis.

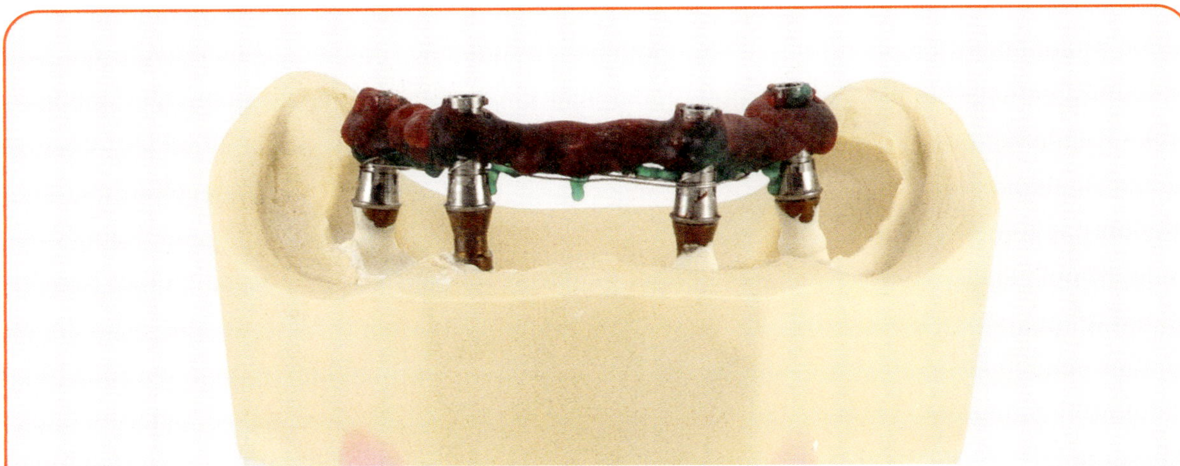

Figure 7.31 • The control index is used to check the proper registration of the implant position.

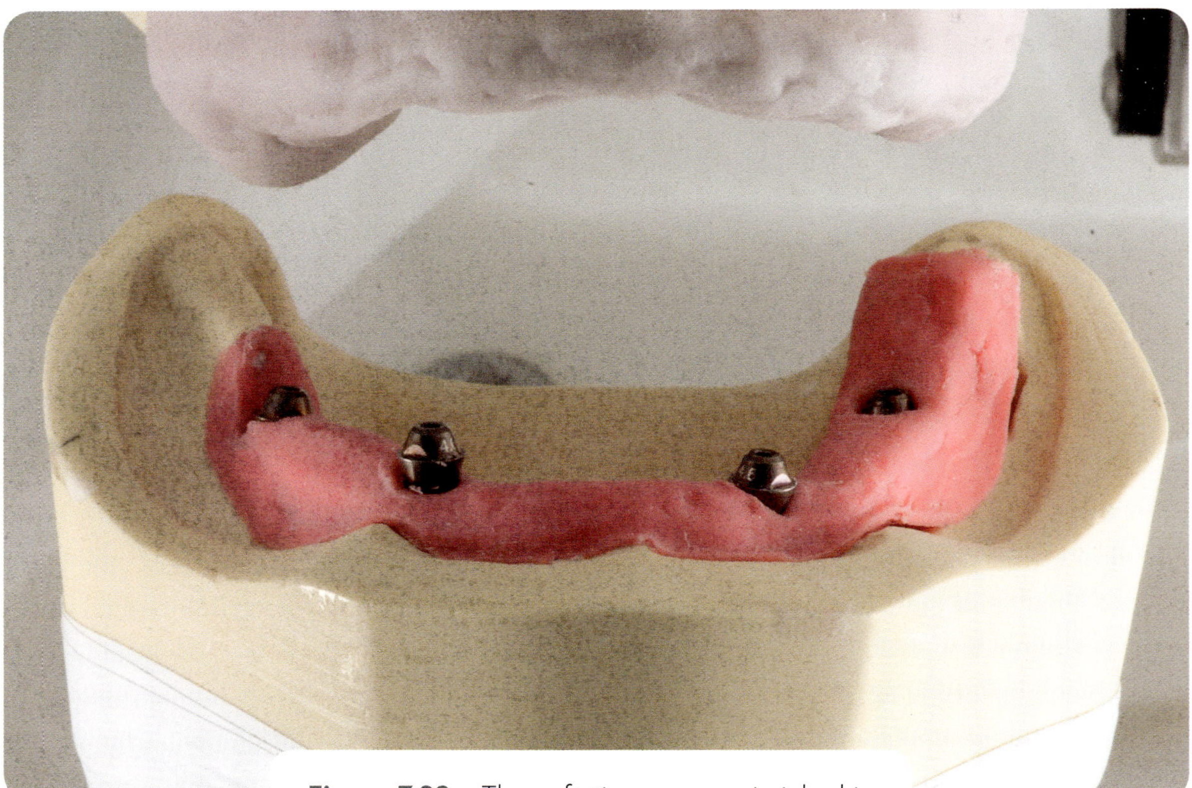

Figure 7.32 • The soft tissues are mimicked in silicone material.

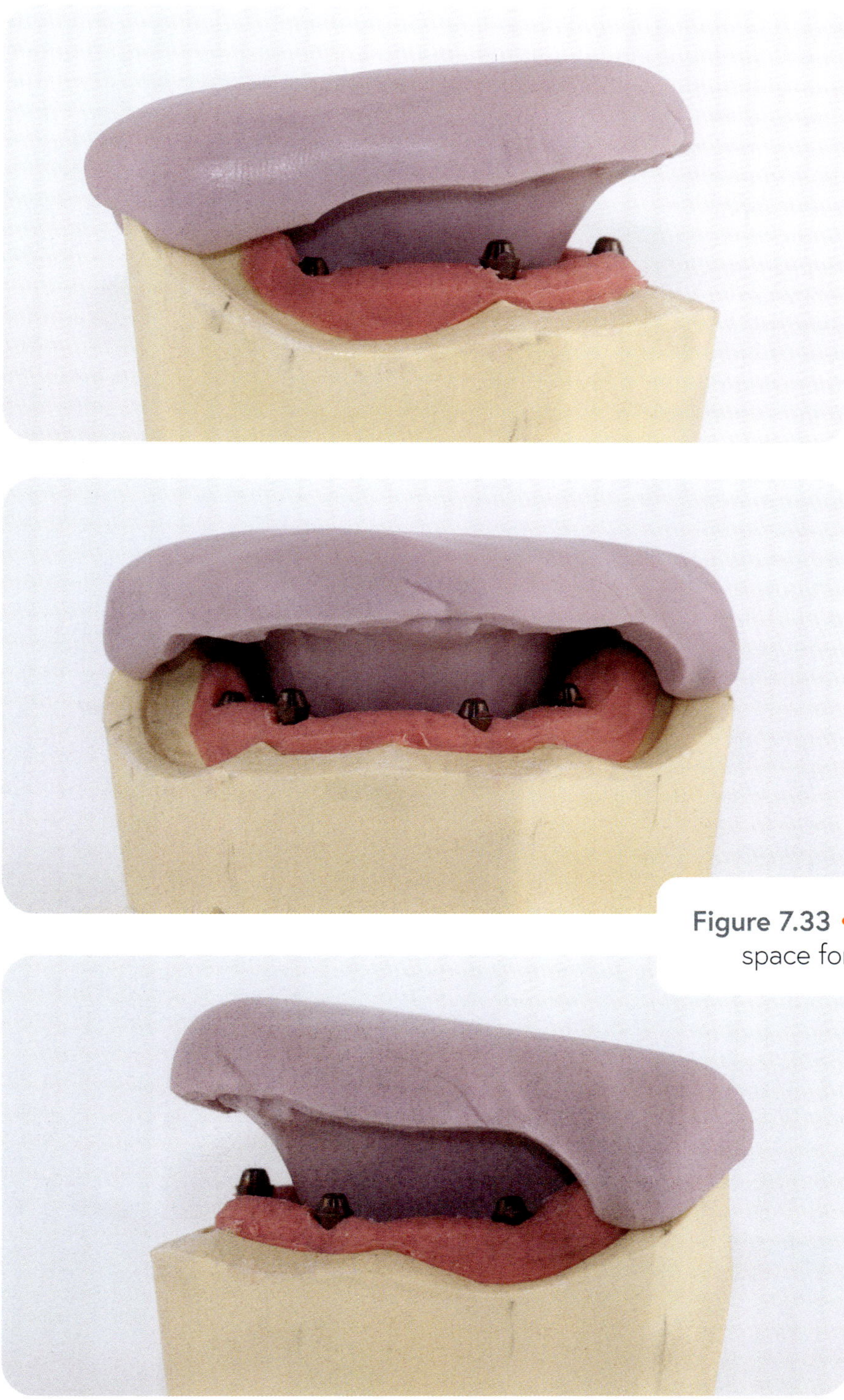

Figure 7.33 • Evaluation of the available space for the final rehabilitation.

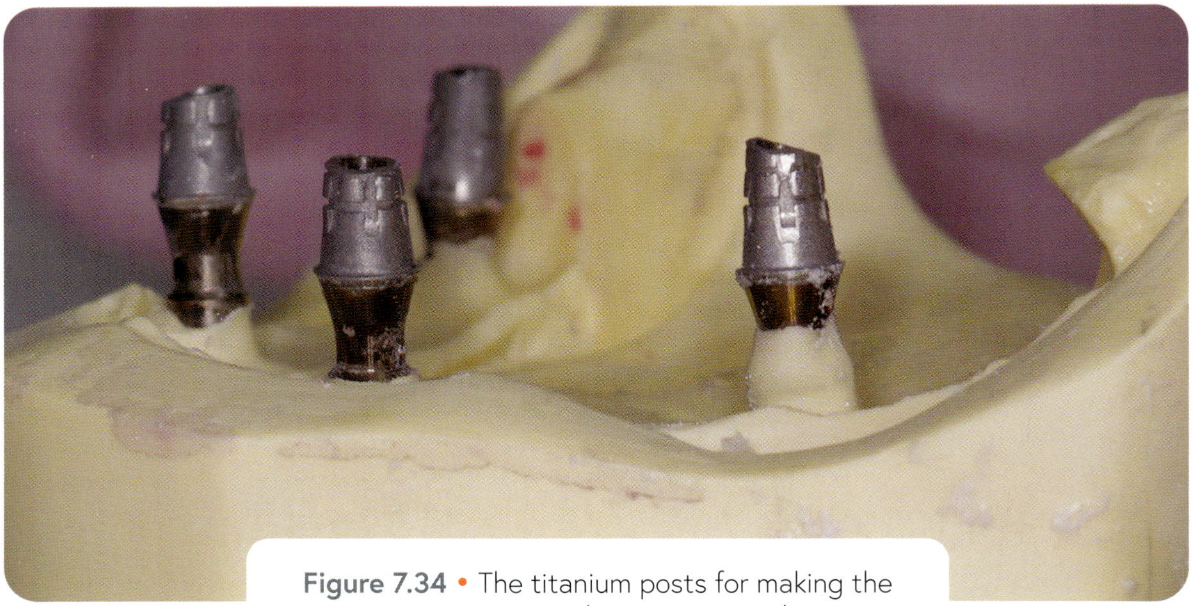

Figure 7.34 • The titanium posts for making the screw-on prosthesis are ground.

A fibre structure has been milled **(Figure 7.35)** in order to attach the implants to each other. The structure has been cemented to the abutments with anaerobic cement (Panavia^{TM} SA Cement, Kuraray Noritake, Hattersheim Germany) **(Figures 7.36** and **7.37)**.

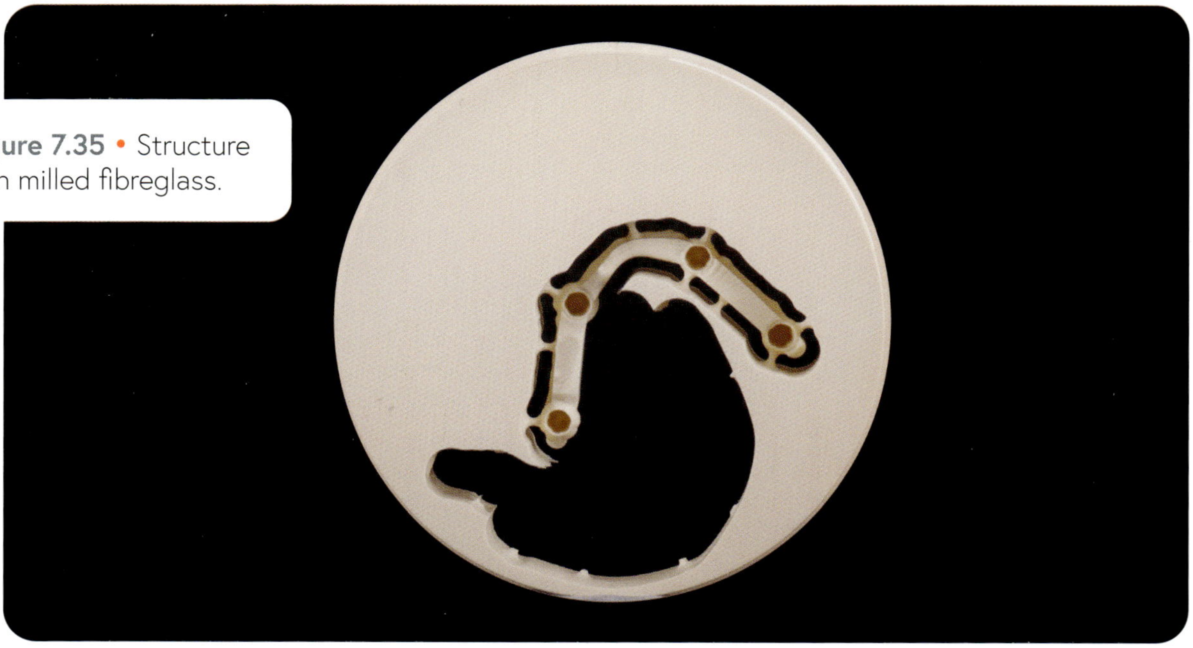

Figure 7.35 • Structure in milled fibreglass.

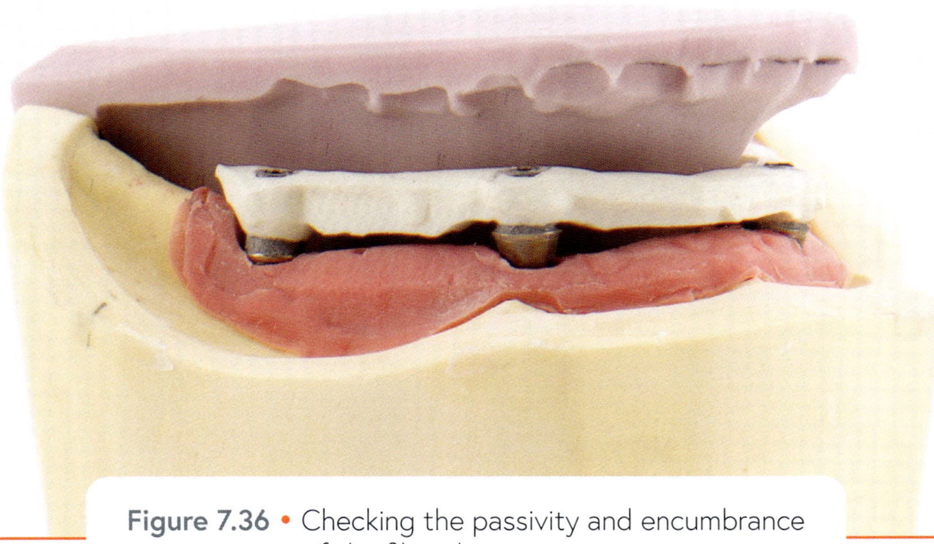

Figure 7.36 • Checking the passivity and encumbrance of the fibreglass structure.

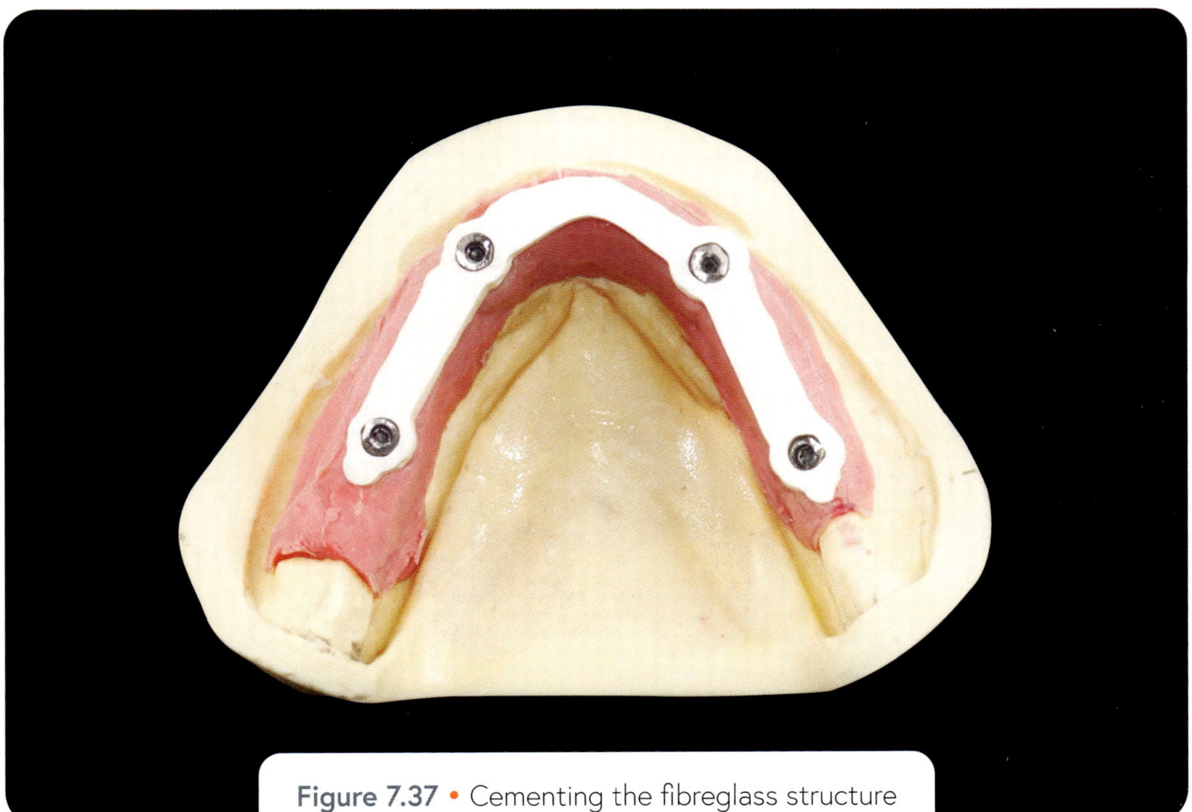

Figure 7.37 • Cementing the fibreglass structure onto the titanium posts.

The patient's lower prosthesis is carved **(Figure 7.38)** and repositioned on the model to evaluate the relations with the reinforcing structure and to check its passive fit.

The structure and the prostheses have been attached using resin for removable prostheses; the extension of the prostheses has then been reduced by removing part of the flange in order to ensure good hygiene of the rehabilitation **(Figure 7.39)**.

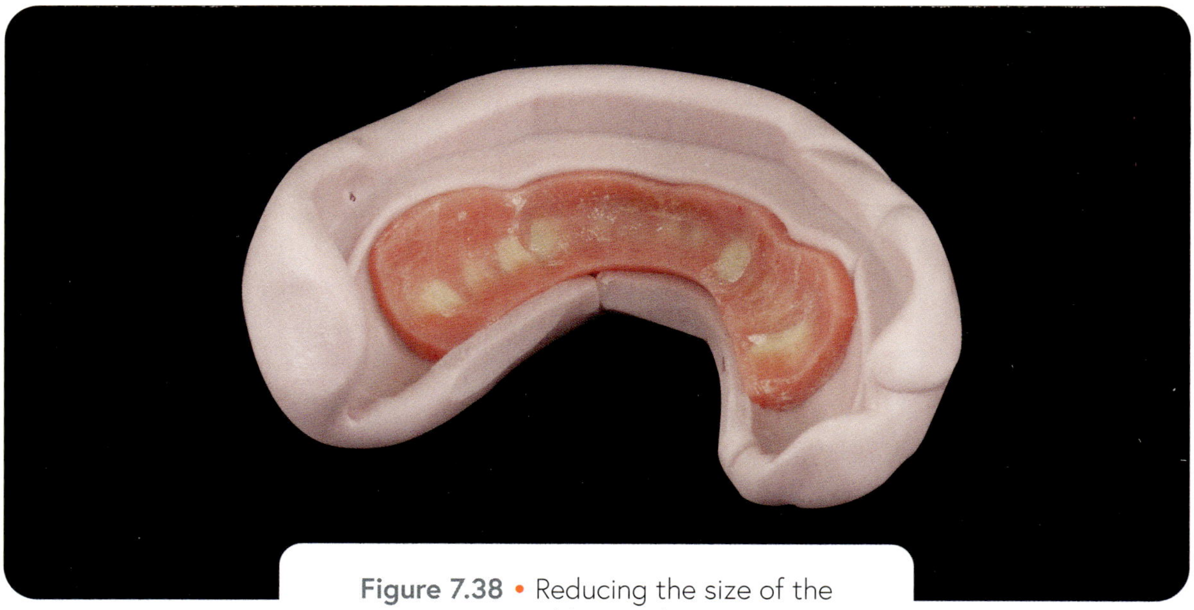

Figure 7.38 • Reducing the size of the removable prosthesis.

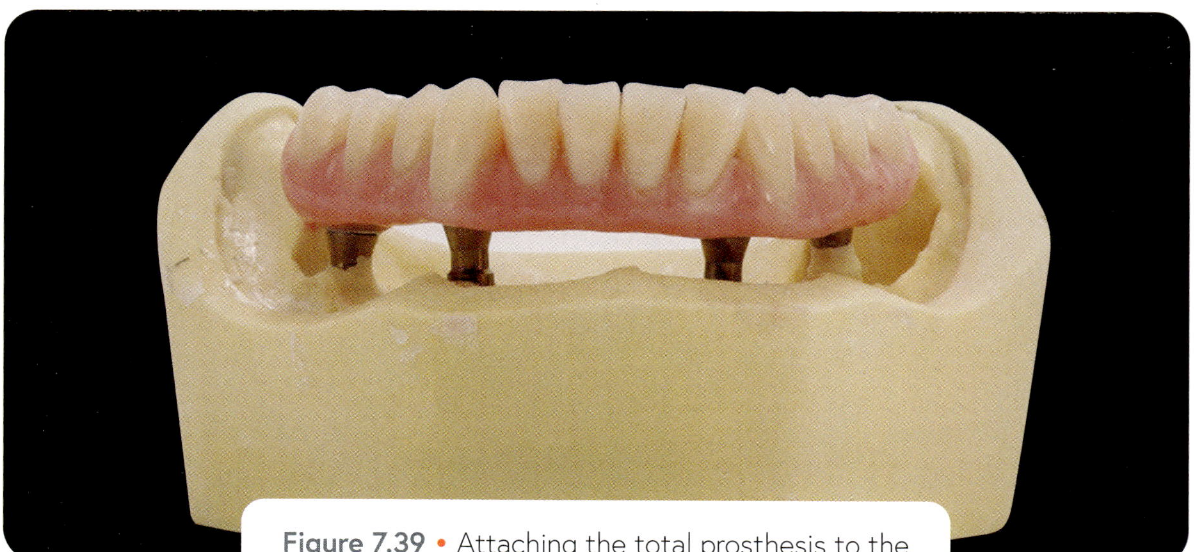

Figure 7.39 • Attaching the total prosthesis to the fibreglass bar.

The occlusal contacts are checked in the articulator **(Figure 7.40)**. Finally, the prostheses are polished.

Ultimately, at the end of this procedure, the removable mandibular prosthesis has been turned into a fixed screw-retained prosthesis.

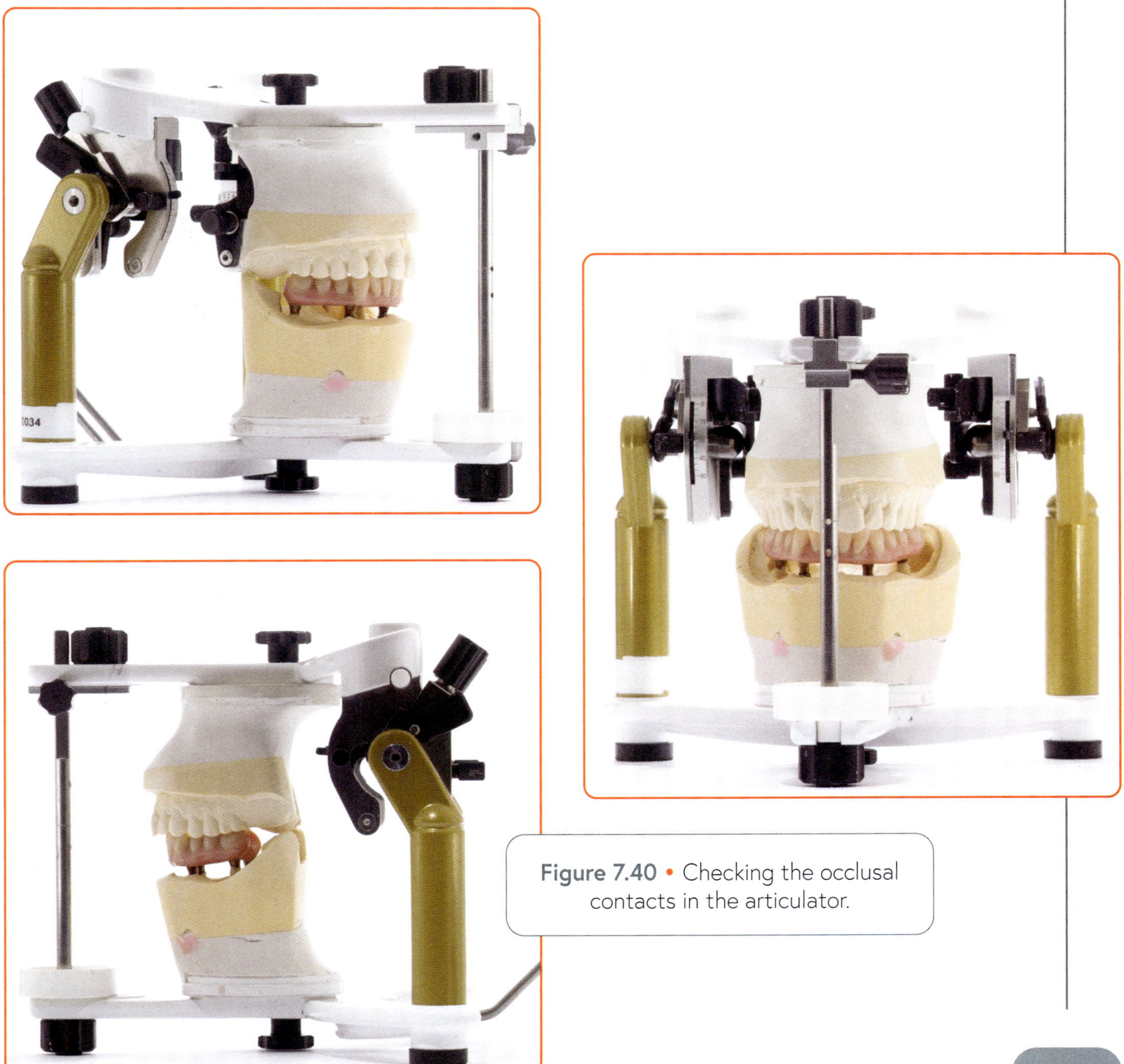

Figure 7.40 • Checking the occlusal contacts in the articulator.

The use of a rigid structure cemented to the abutments enabled rigid splinting of the implants to achieve passive adaptation, thus avoiding micro-movements that might interfere with the osseointegration of the implants [15-17]. The use of a milled structure cemented to the abutments has enabled rapid finalisation of the case, with the delivery of the prosthesis within 24 hours after placing the implants. A few hours later, the definitive prostheses have been delivered to the patient, and the screws have been tightened at 15 N/mm **(Figures 7.41-7.43)**.

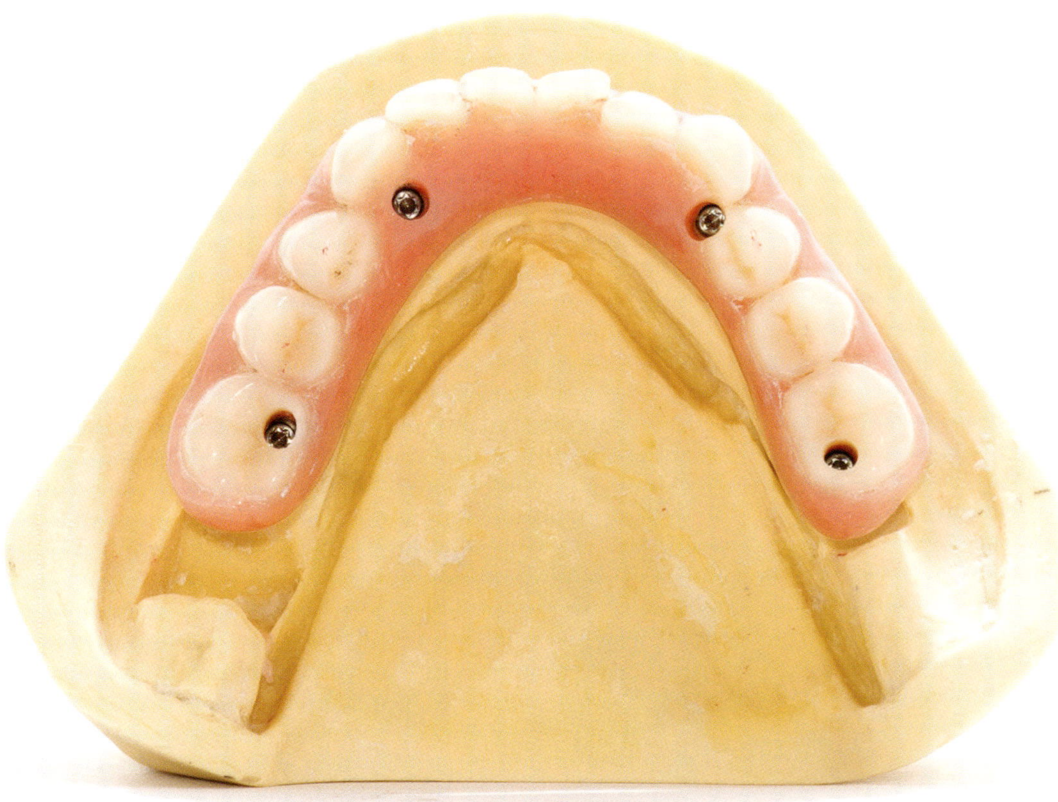

Figure 7.41 • Occlusal view of the hybrid prosthesis after polishing.

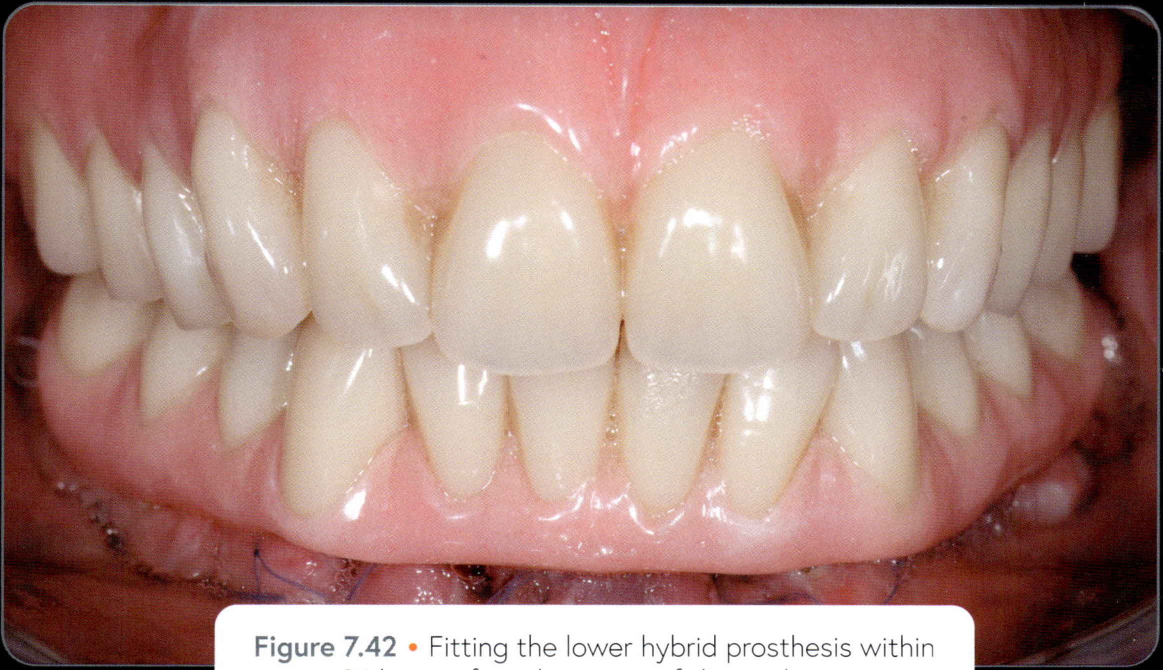

Figure 7.42 • Fitting the lower hybrid prosthesis within 24 hours after placement of the implants.

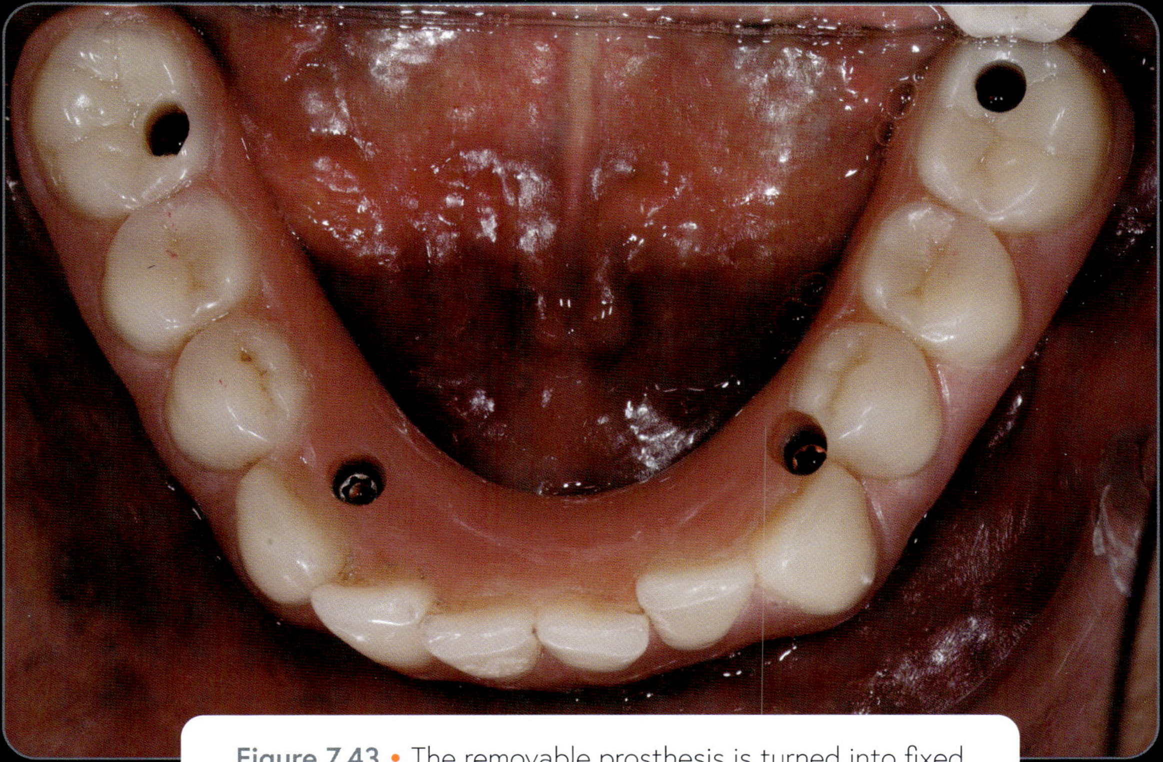

Figure 7.43 • The removable prosthesis is turned into fixed prosthesis. The fixing screws have been tightened at 15 N/mm.

The precision of the coupling between implants and posts for SRA screw-retained prostheses and titanium abutments was radiographically verified **(Figure 7.44)**.

The care taken in the information transfer procedures made it possible to avoid significant occlusal modifications at the time of delivery, as well as the maintenance of the esthetic and functional conditions that had already been widely tested for several weeks in the patient's mouth.

The sutures were removed after 8 days. The patient was monitored monthly after the surgery for a first period of 4 months.

Subsequently, the patient was entered in a maintenance session programme, with visits with the hygienist every 4 months and with a dental check-up once a year. At the 1-year follow-up visit, a good esthetic and functional result, and an excellent health condition of the soft tissues were evident **(Figures 7.45-7.47)**.

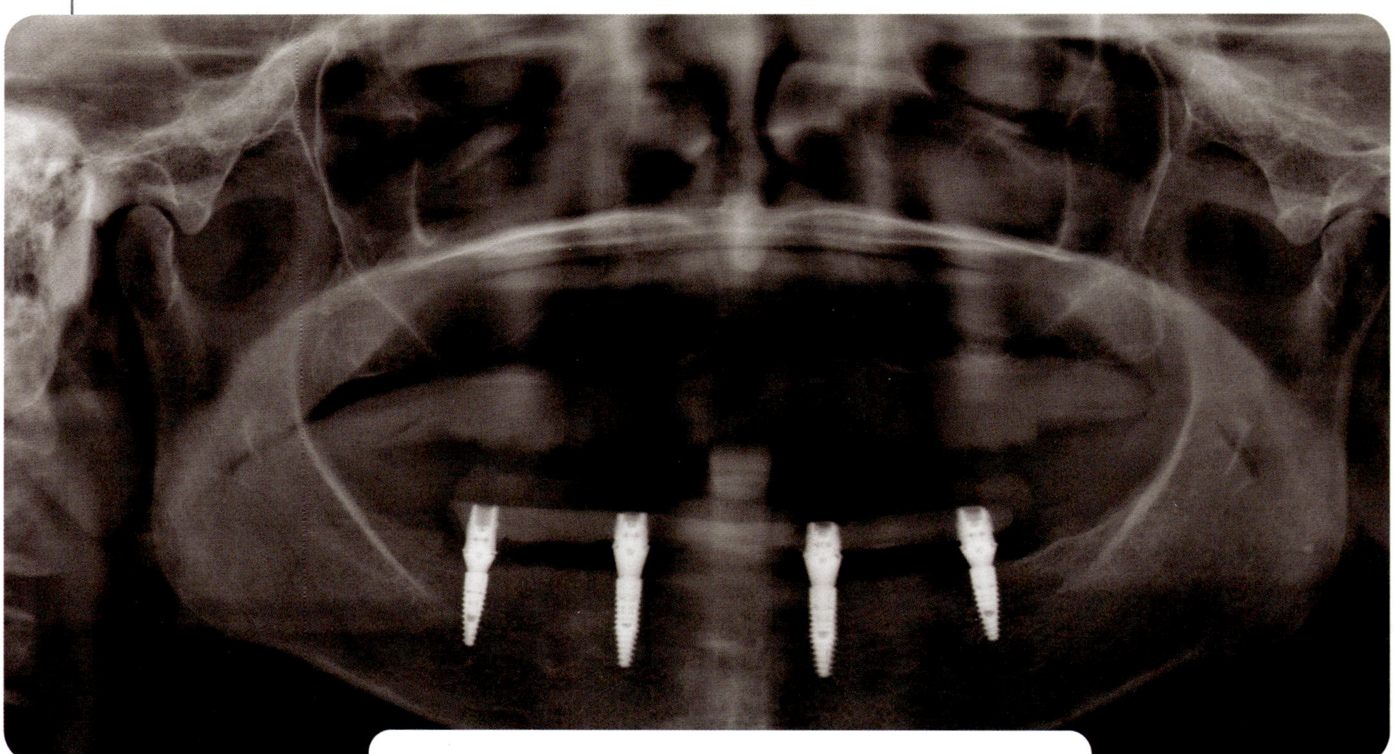

Figure 7.44 • Orthopantomography performed on the day of delivery of the rehabilitation.

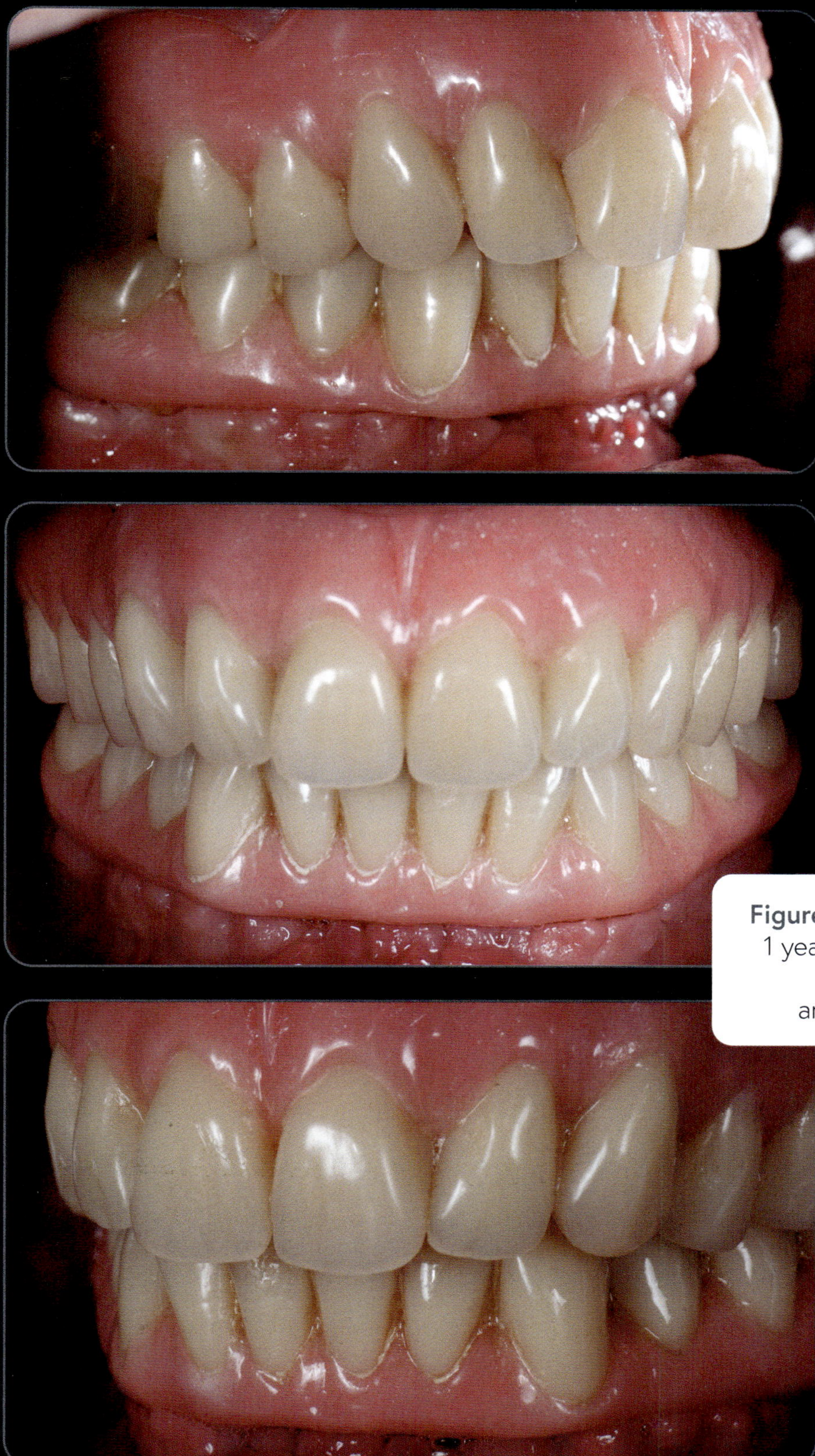

Figure 7.45 • Follow-up after 1 year. One may appreciate a good esthetic and functional result.

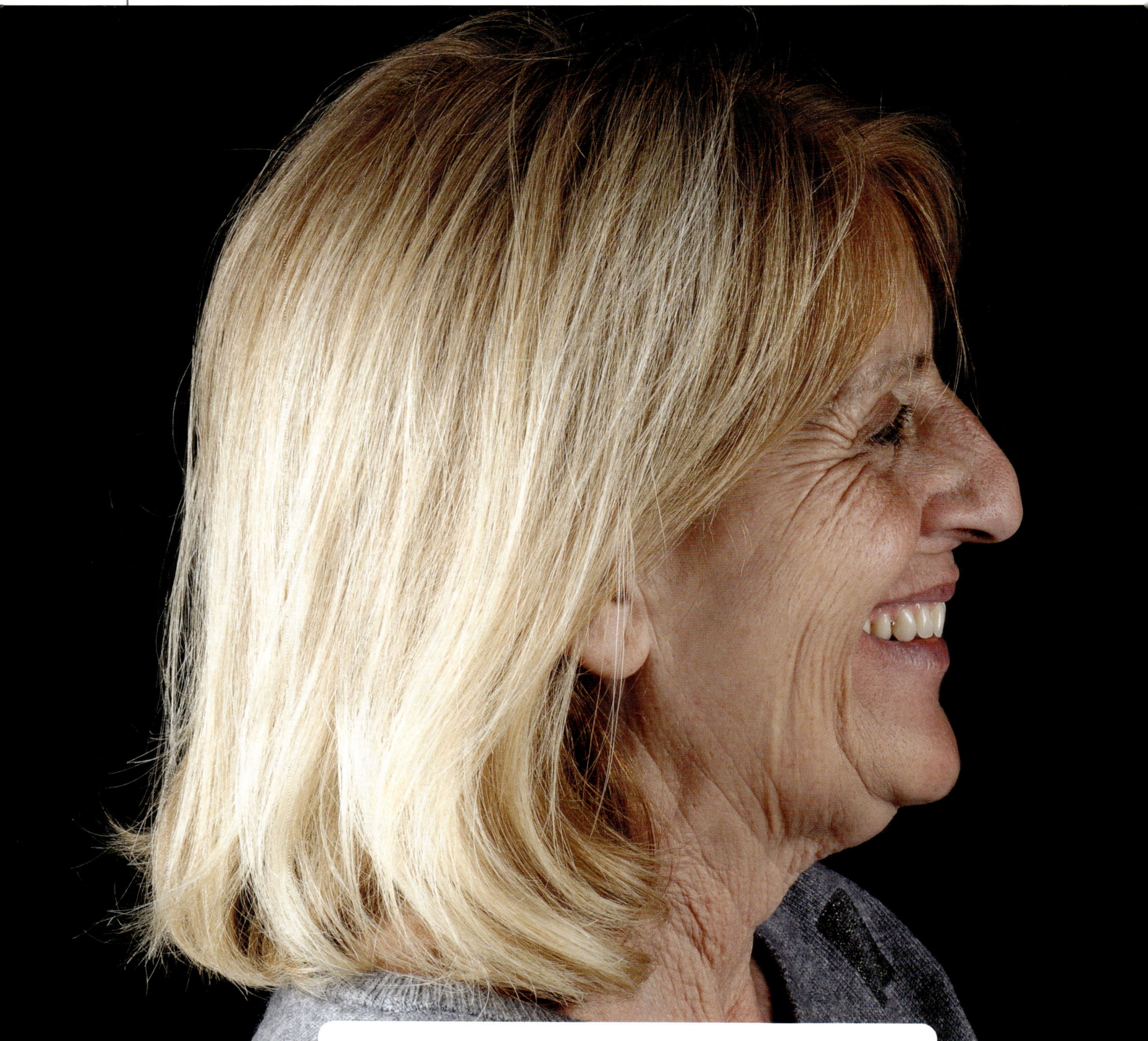

Figure 7.46 • Esthetic and functional rehabilitation of the patient after treatment with the B.A.R.I. Technique. Side view.

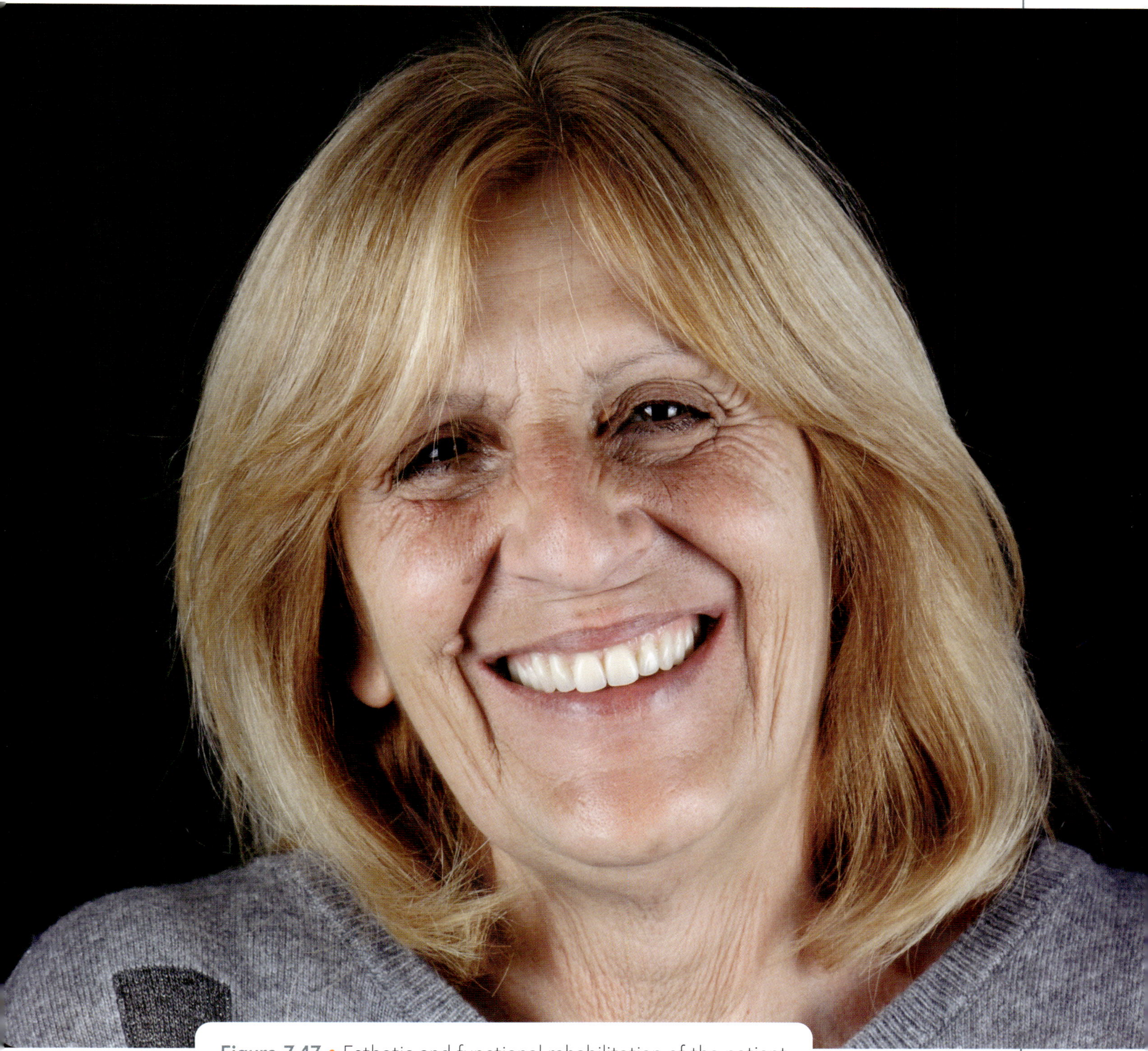

Figure 7.47 • Esthetic and functional rehabilitation of the patient after treatment with B.A.R.I. Technique. Front view.

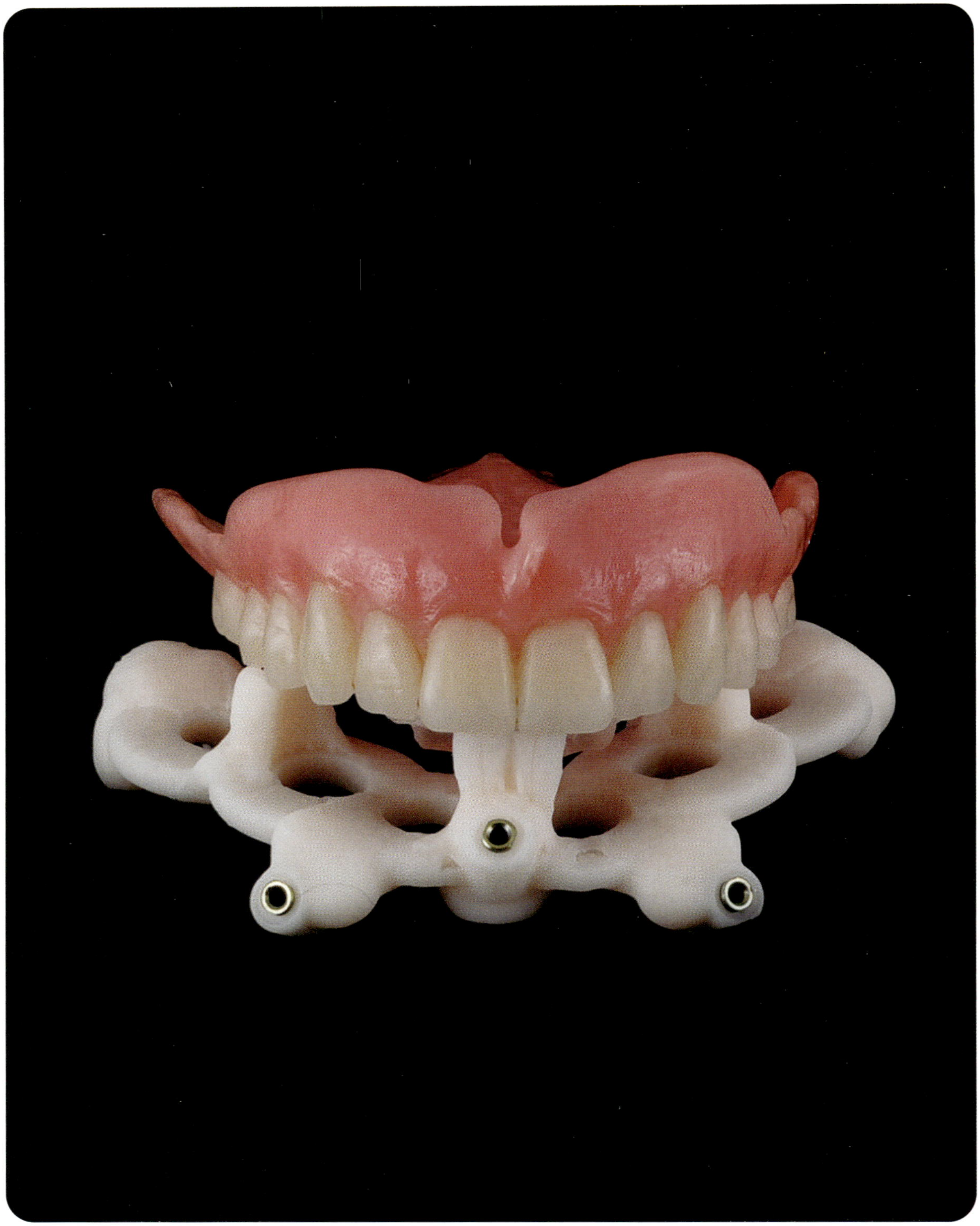

Digital flow

Immediate loading was proposed and used to rehabilitate the edentulous mandibular arches [18]. By definition, loading of the implants can be considered immediate when a fixed restoration, in occlusal function, is delivered within 48 hours after implant insertion [19,20]. Immediate loading in the mandible is a well documented and scientifically validated approach for both overdentures and fixed prostheses; less scientific evidence is available for immediate loading in the maxilla [3]. In the last twenty years, intense research activity, in the field both of the surface and design of implants and of prosthetic materials and procedures, has led to a change in the immediate loading protocols in order to reduce treatment time frames and achieve immediacy in the delivery of implant-supported restorations [21-25].

The treatment of patients with total edentulism or terminal dentition might be especially complex because these patients often have alterations in the cranio-mandibular relation, especially if they wear old prostheses that are by now inadequate with worn artificial acrylic resin teeth or when they have undergone migration of periodontally compromised teeth, with loss of vertical dimension [26]. In these cases, the physiological mandibular position must be established before treating the edentulous arches with immediate loading procedures and the use of temporary removable prostheses for a few weeks may be extremely useful [27].

A comprehensive approach to these complex rehabilitations has been proposed, with a particular focus on the diagnostic stage, performed with removable prostheses and based on the clinical and laboratory procedures used to record and store the occlusal information found in the diagnostic stage [28]. In recent years, digital technology has entered the dental profession and many procedures have been deeply renewed. The development of intraoral scanners, 3D printers and CAD/CAM machines (Computer Aided Design/Computer Aided Manufacturing) with superior performance, as well as the introduction of perfected materials, are shifting the paradigm towards a digital workflow [29-31].

One of the main advantages of removable prostheses is the possibility of easily modifying them several times until achieving a satisfactory esthetic and functional result. They can be used to test new intermaxillary and occlusal relations and must subsequently be replicated with a different and more durable material as definitive prostheses.

Clinical stage 1

The patient treated in the clinical case presented in this chapter received the maxillary and mandibular prosthesis according to the CAD/CAM protocol **(Figures 7.48-7.50)** [32,33] (see Chapter 5).

18 months after the rehabilitation with removable prostheses, the patient felt ready for a more efficient mandibular restoration. The first step, at this point, was to carefully check the previously fabricated prostheses from an esthetic and functional point of view. Two alternatives were proposed and illustrated to the patient: an overdenture and a hybrid prosthesis (a fixed total prosthesis with implant support) with a different

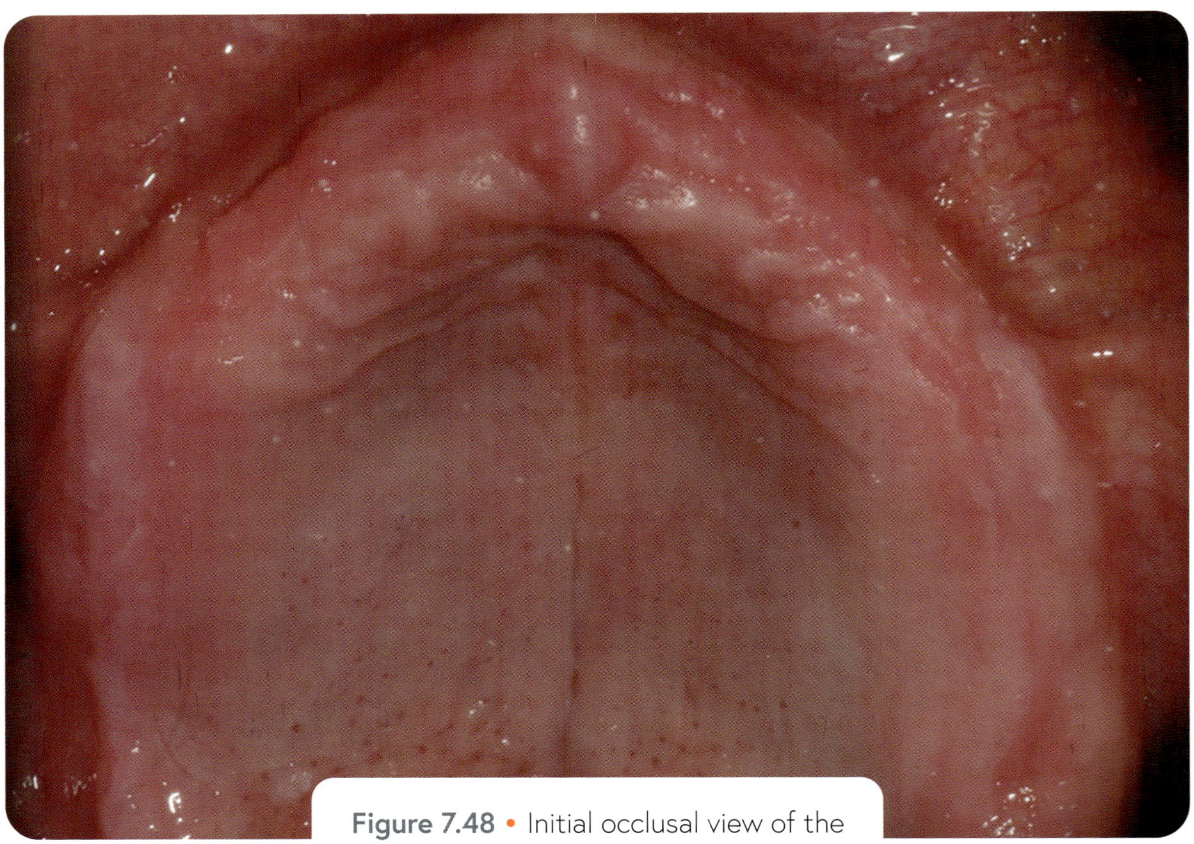

Figure 7.48 • Initial occlusal view of the patient's edentulous arches.

number of implants. The patient's choice fell on the hybrid prosthesis supported by six mandibular implants.

Guided surgery was planned for the patient as it has been shown to be an accurate method to reduce the likelihood of damaging anatomical structures and to simplify the prosthetic treatment [34-36]. Intra- and extraoral photographs of the patient were taken with and without the prostheses. Since the previous prosthetic design was already available, the maxillary and mandibular prostheses were easily duplicated with a 3D printer (Rapid Shape P20, Rapid Shape GmbH, Heimshein, Germany).

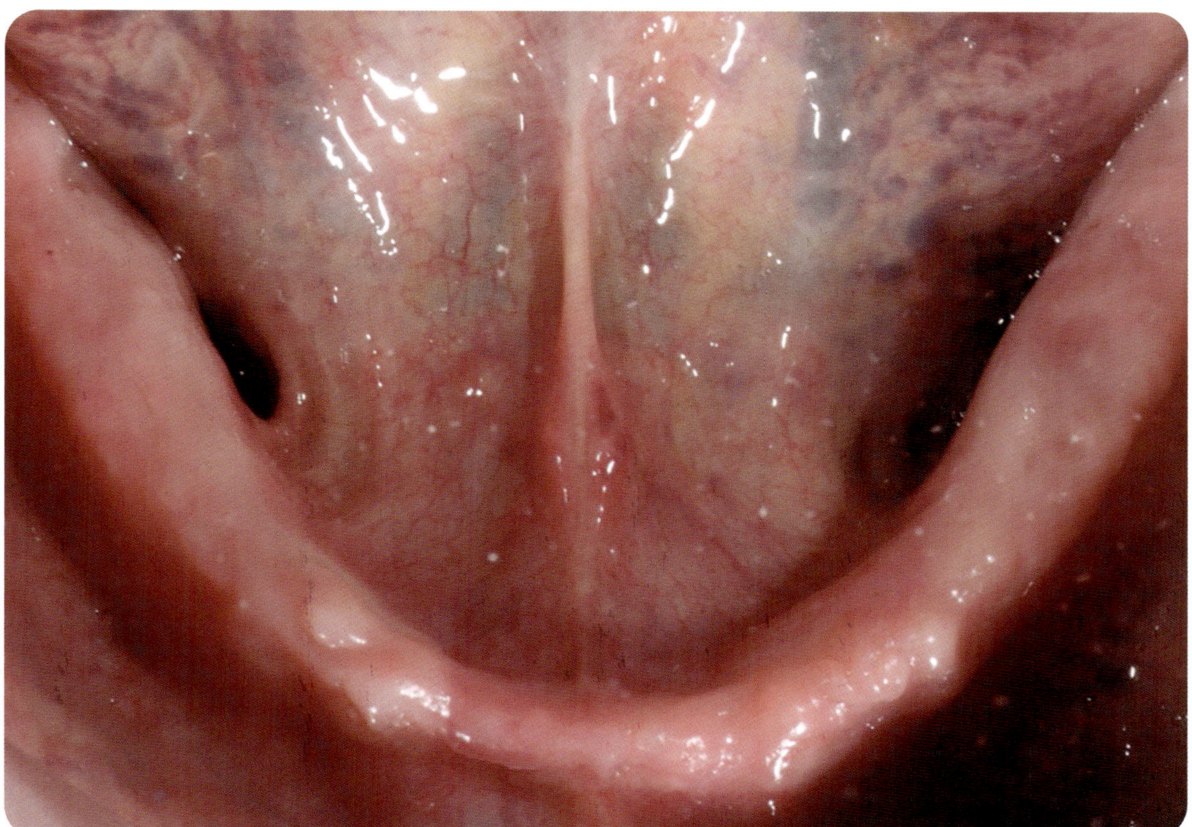

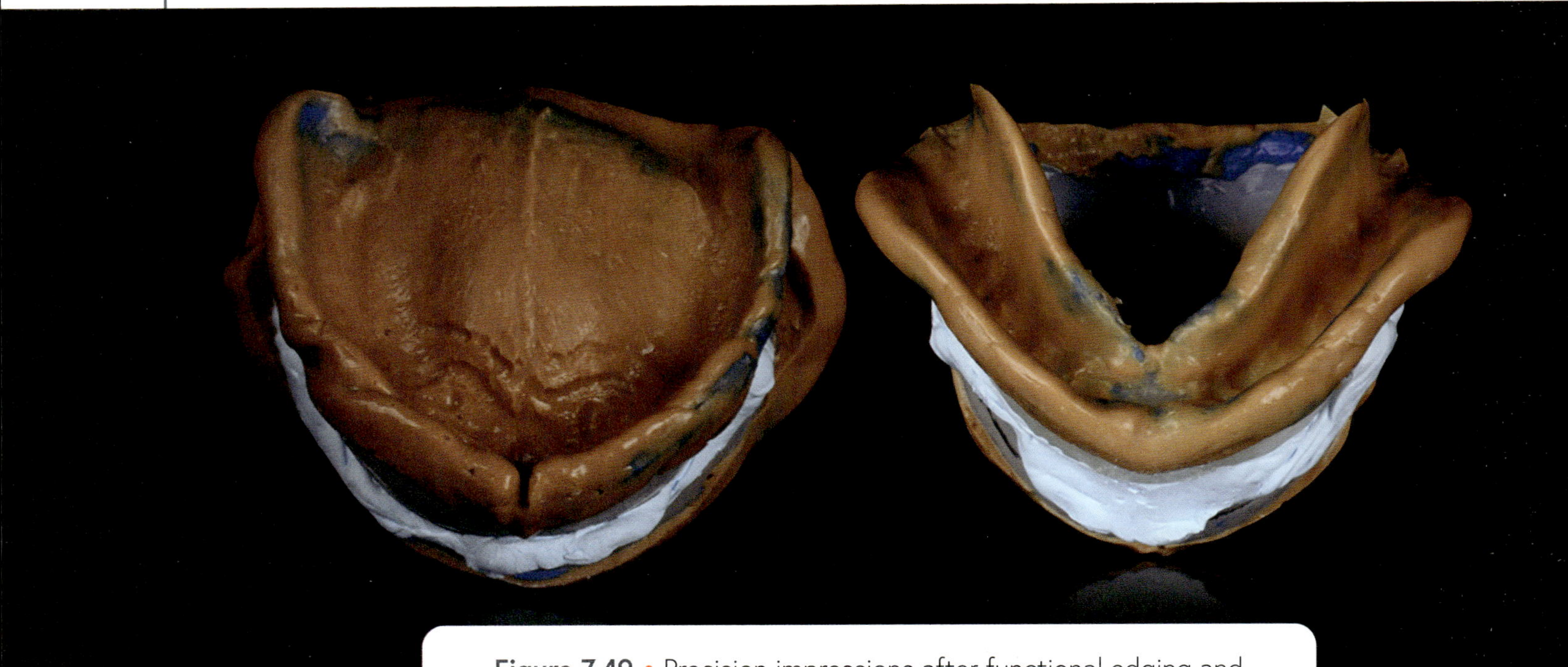

Figure 7.49 • Precision impressions after functional edging and registration of the vertical dimension and intermaxillary relationships.

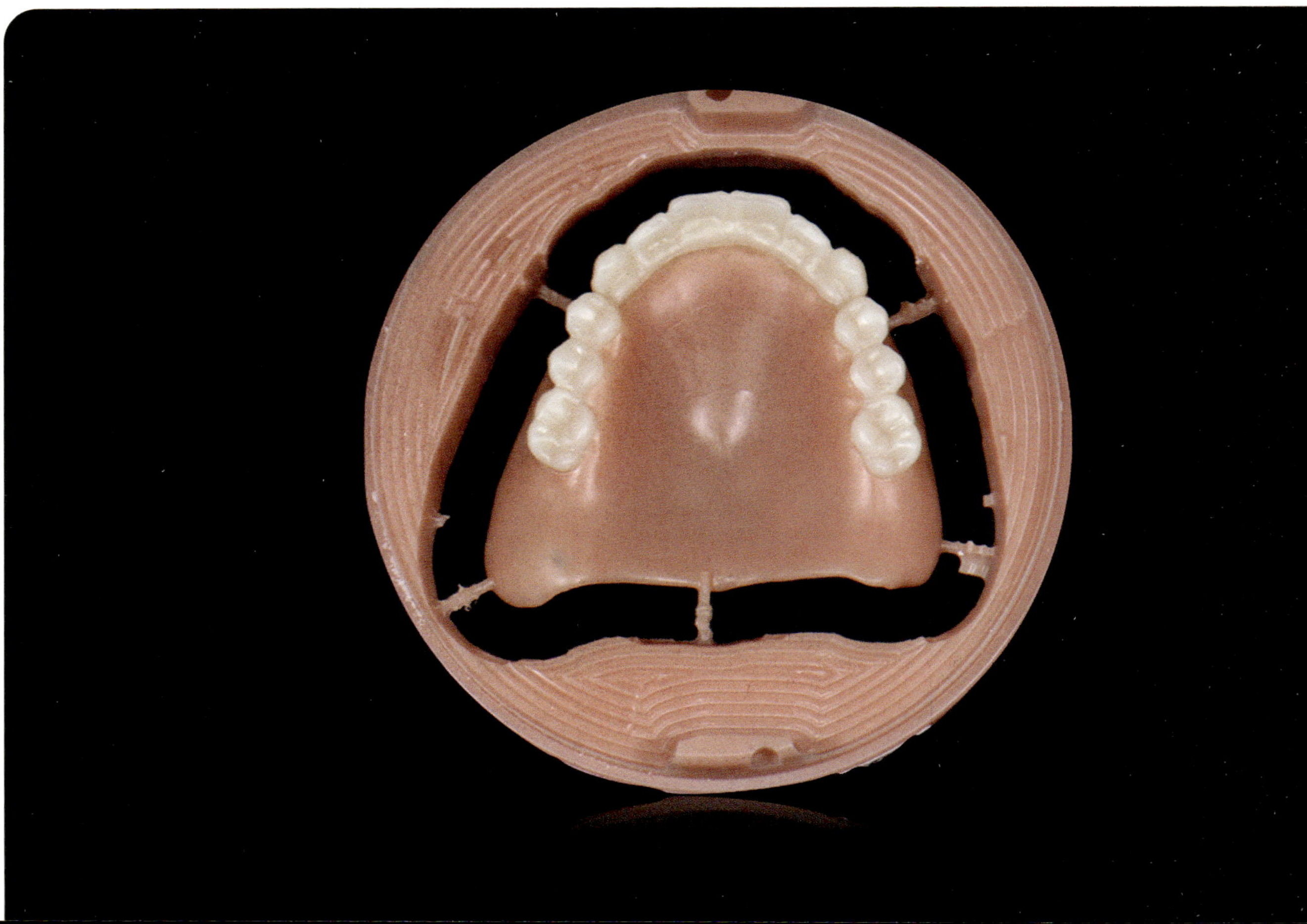

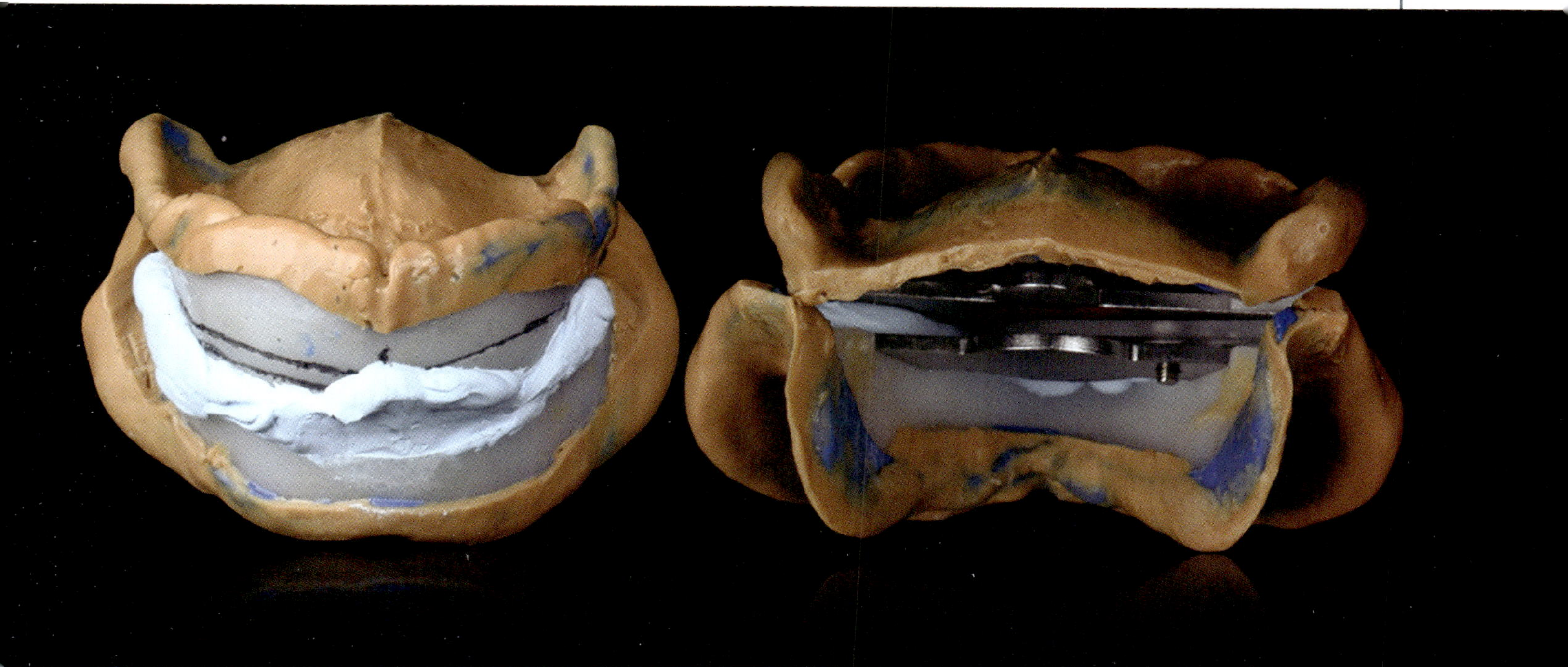

Figure 7.50 • Total prostheses finalised with CAD/CAM digital flow.

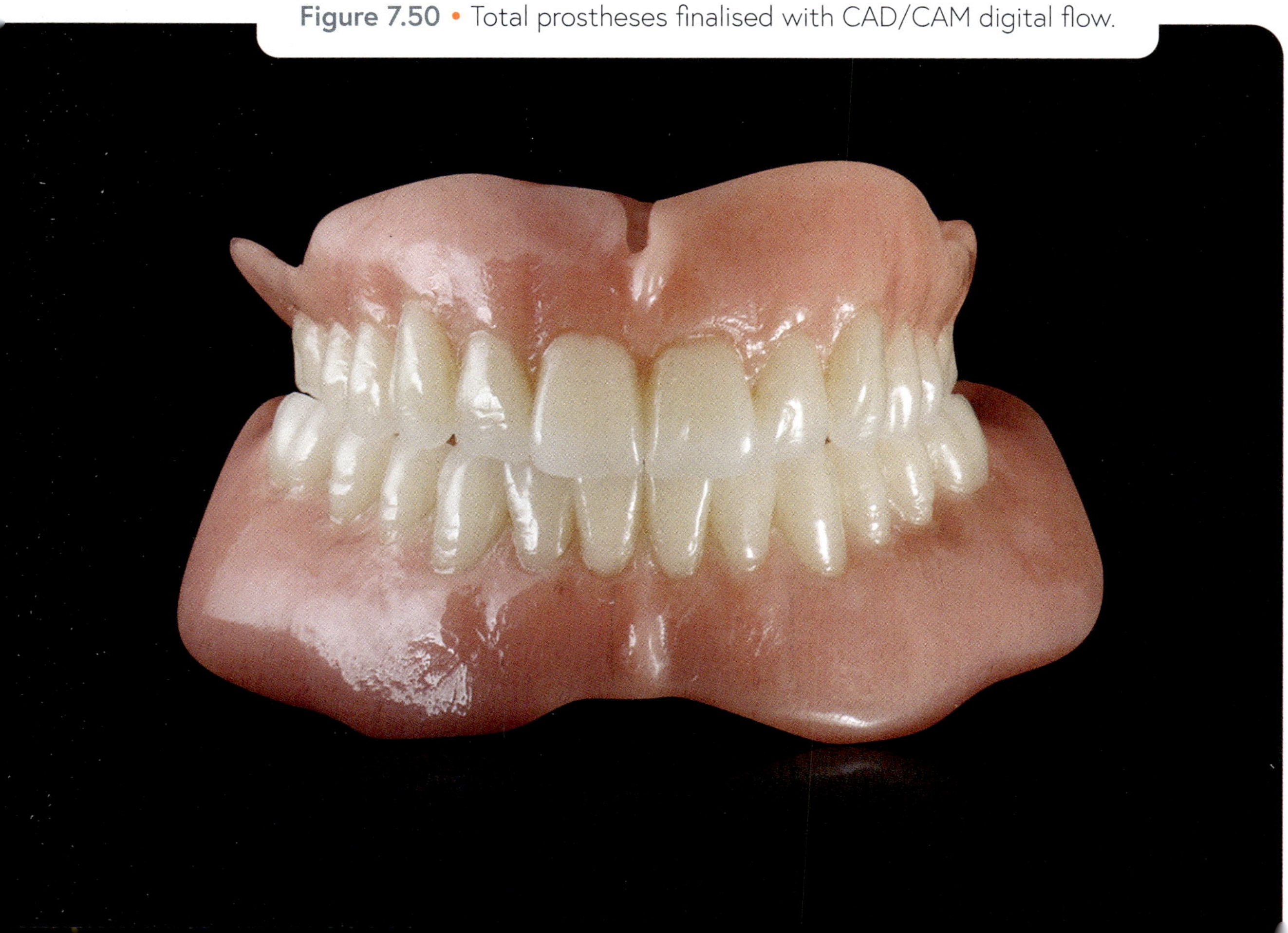

The resin used for the duplicate was radiolucent (SHERAprint-model plus UV sand, Shera, Lemforde, Germany), while a radiopaque resin (ACRY C&B colour RX, Rutinum Group, Badia Polesine, Italy) was used to add ten reference points on the duplicate of the total prosthesis, in order to create a radiographic stent which was then scanned with a laboratory CAD scanner (Scanner d710, Wieland Dental, Pforzheim, Germany), from which the STL files were obtained **(Figures 7.51** and **7.52)**.

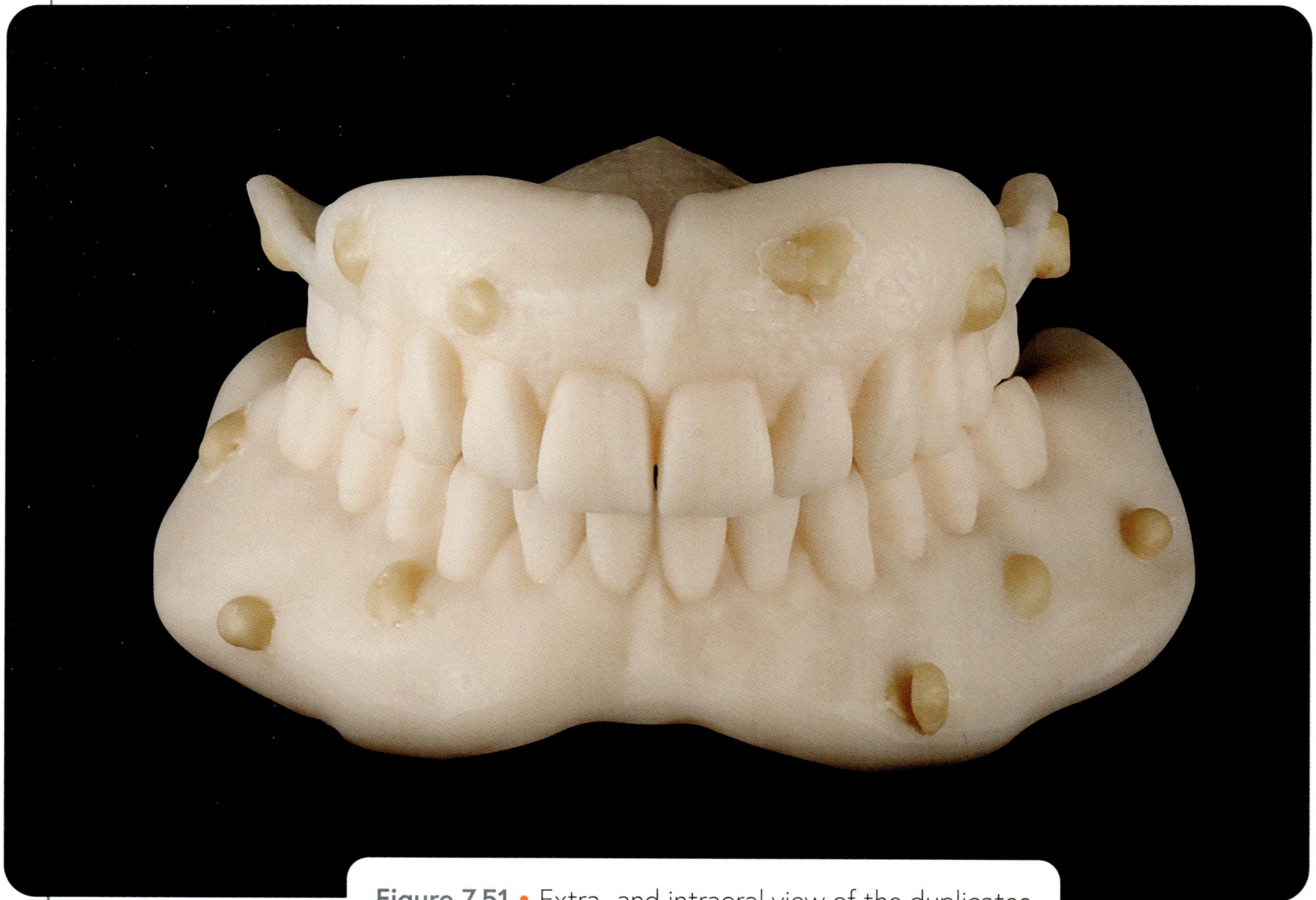

Figure 7.51 • Extra- and intraoral view of the duplicates of the total prostheses with radio-opaque landmarks.

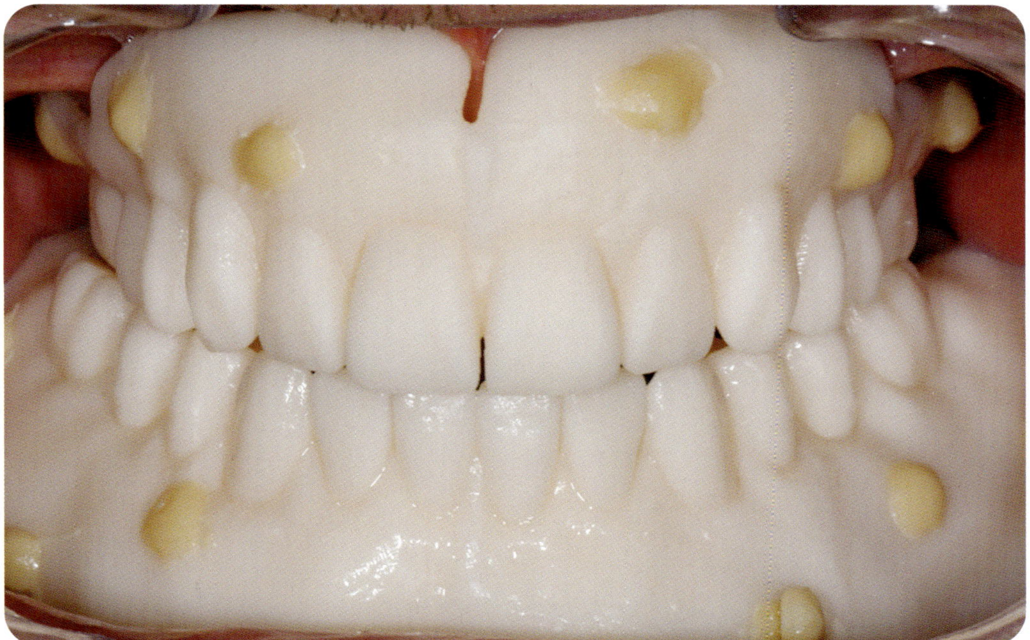

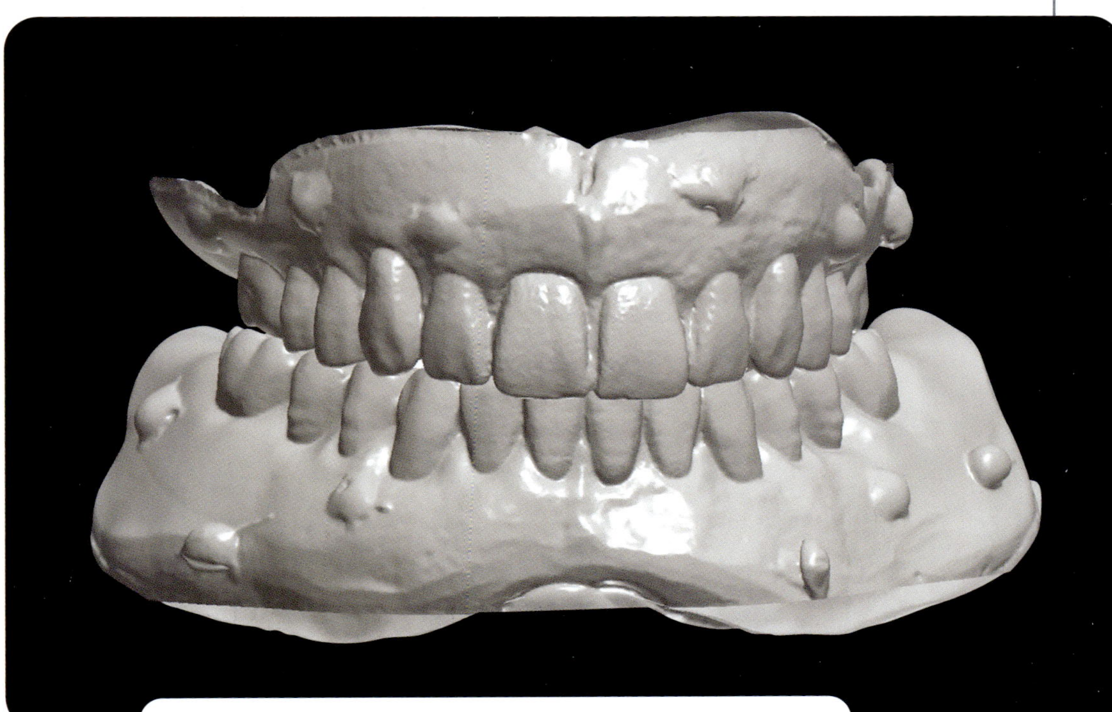

Figure 7.52 • Scan of the duplicate prostheses.

A CBCT was taken with the radiographic stent in position and the DICOM files were obtained. The STL and DICOM files were paired by superposing the reference points using an appropriate software (coDiagnostiX 9.12, Dental Wings, Montreal, Canada) [37] **(Figure 7.53)**.

The position of the implants was planned virtually on the coDiagnostix software. Special attention was paid to inserting the implants in the proper prosthetic position in relation to the patient's prosthesis. Furthermore, the intermediate abutments were selected during digital planning. The ferrules for guided surgery were chosen and positioned and a mucous membrane supported surgical stent was designed, paying particular attention to maintaining three occlusion points with the antagonist prosthesis. Three fixing pins were envisaged, in order to stabilise the stent during surgical procedures. The radiological stent was created according to the Layer Plastic Deposition (LPD) printing technology and it was tried on before starting the surgical procedure. The patient was asked to bite on the reference points placed on the stent in order to keep it in the proper position: the guide featured stability and fit [38] **(Figure 7.54)**.

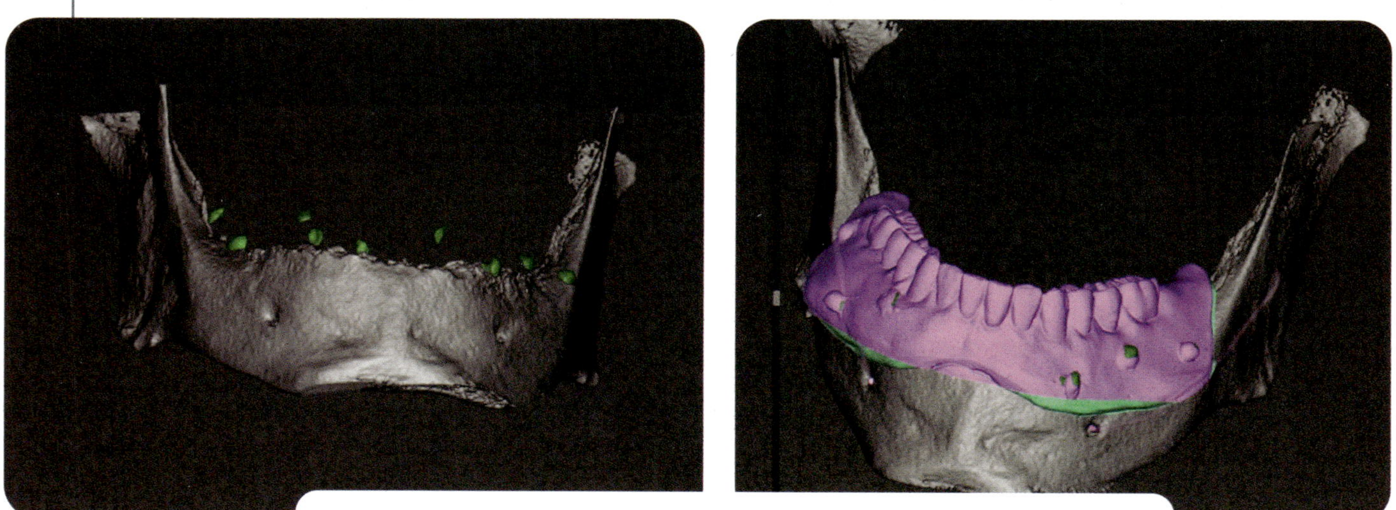

Figure 7.53 • Reconstruction of the mandible from DICOM file and its coupling with the STL files of the scan of the duplicate prosthesis thanks to radio-opaque landmarks.

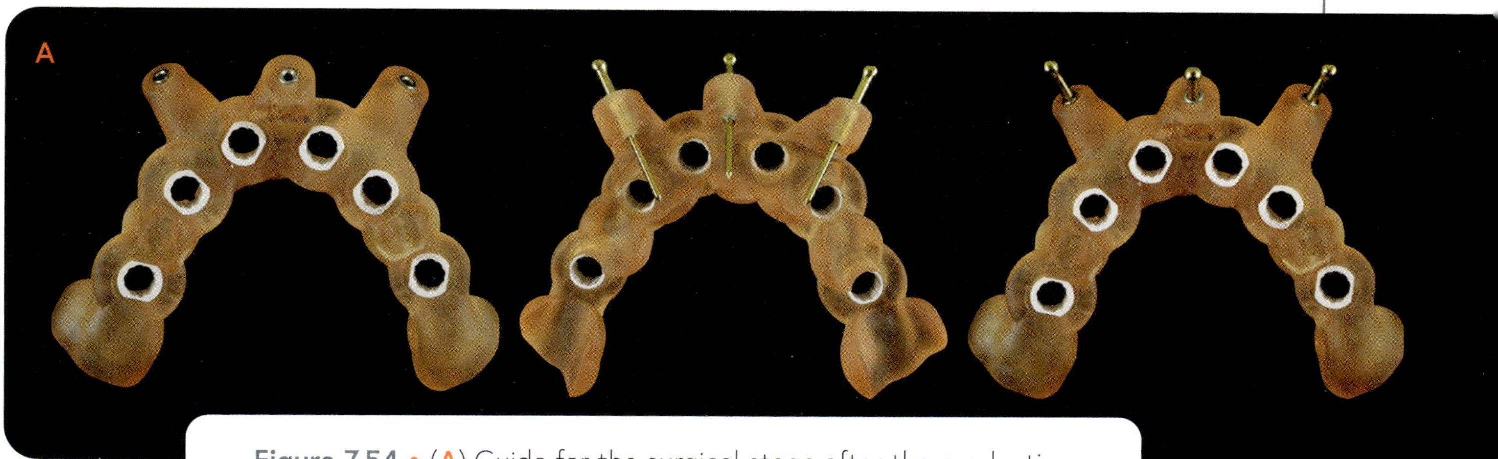

Figure 7.54 • (**A**) Guide for the surgical stage after the production process. (**B**) Intraoral view of the surgical guide in occlusion to the total prosthesis and before inserting the stabilisation pins.

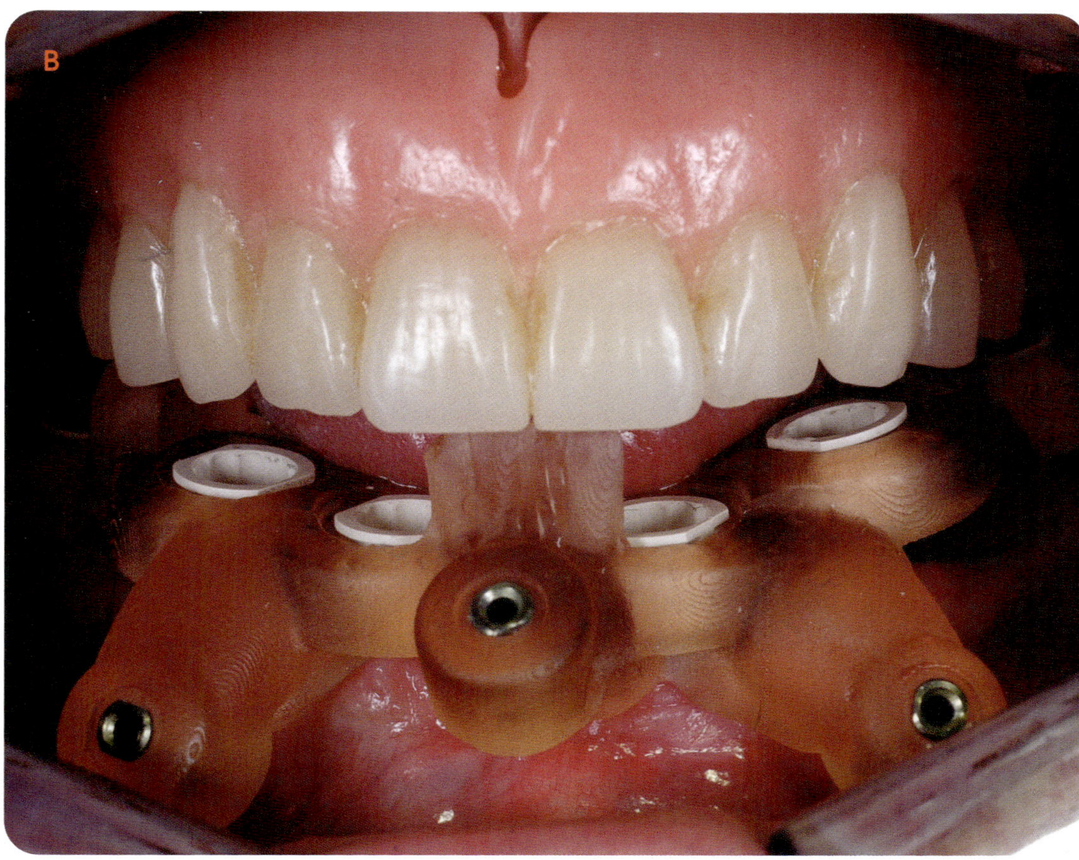

The surgery was carried out under local anesthesia. At this stage, the three pins (Anchor pin, Institut Straumann AG, Basel, Switzerland) were inserted in order to stabilise the surgical stent on the patient's mandible. The patient's arches were kept in occlusion during placement of the pins and, once inserted, the upper prosthesis was removed.

Microflaps were made with micro scalpels to displace the keratinised tissue, which had been thinned, as is often the case in edentulous lower jaws.

Six implants were inserted with a macro-design specifically designed for immediate loading and with a surface that promotes osseointegration (SLActive BLX implants, Institut Straumann AG) following the guided surgery protocol **(Figure 7.55)**. The surgical

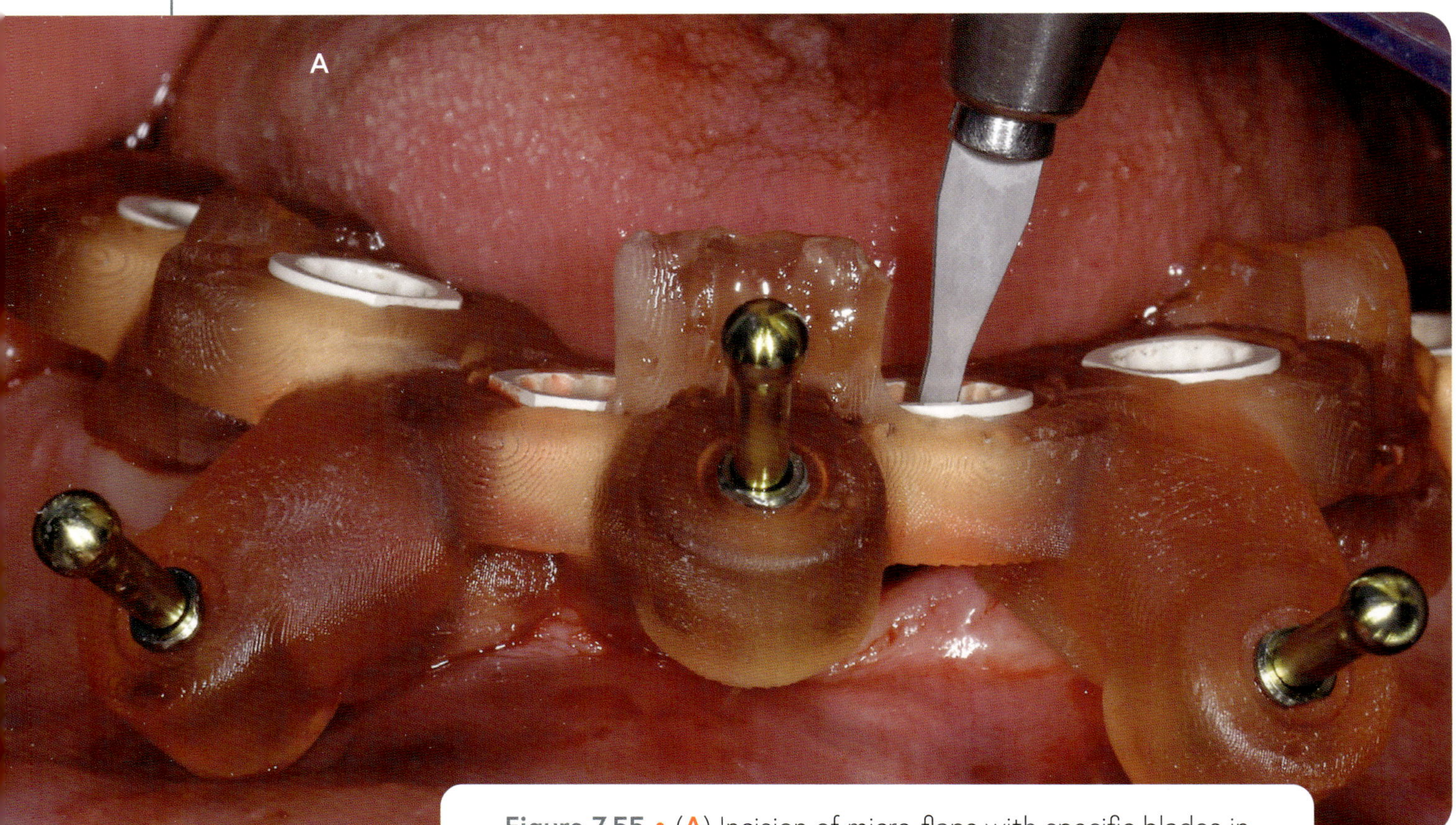

Figure 7.55 • (**A**) Incision of micro-flaps with specific blades in order to preserve the keratinised tissue. (**B**) Occlusal view of the lower arch upon completion of the surgical therapy.

guide was then removed and the intermediate abutments (SRA Abutment, Institut Straumann AG) were connected to the implants **(Figure 7.56)**.

The position of the scanbodies on the arches is registered through an intraoral scanner and reproduced on a virtual model.

The spatial position of the implants is then reconstructed thanks to the known dimensions of the scanbodies. As this was an edentulous case, it was necessary to manage some problems: few studies support the use of intraoral scanners for taking the impression on multiple implants aimed at making extended restorations supported by implants such as full-arch.

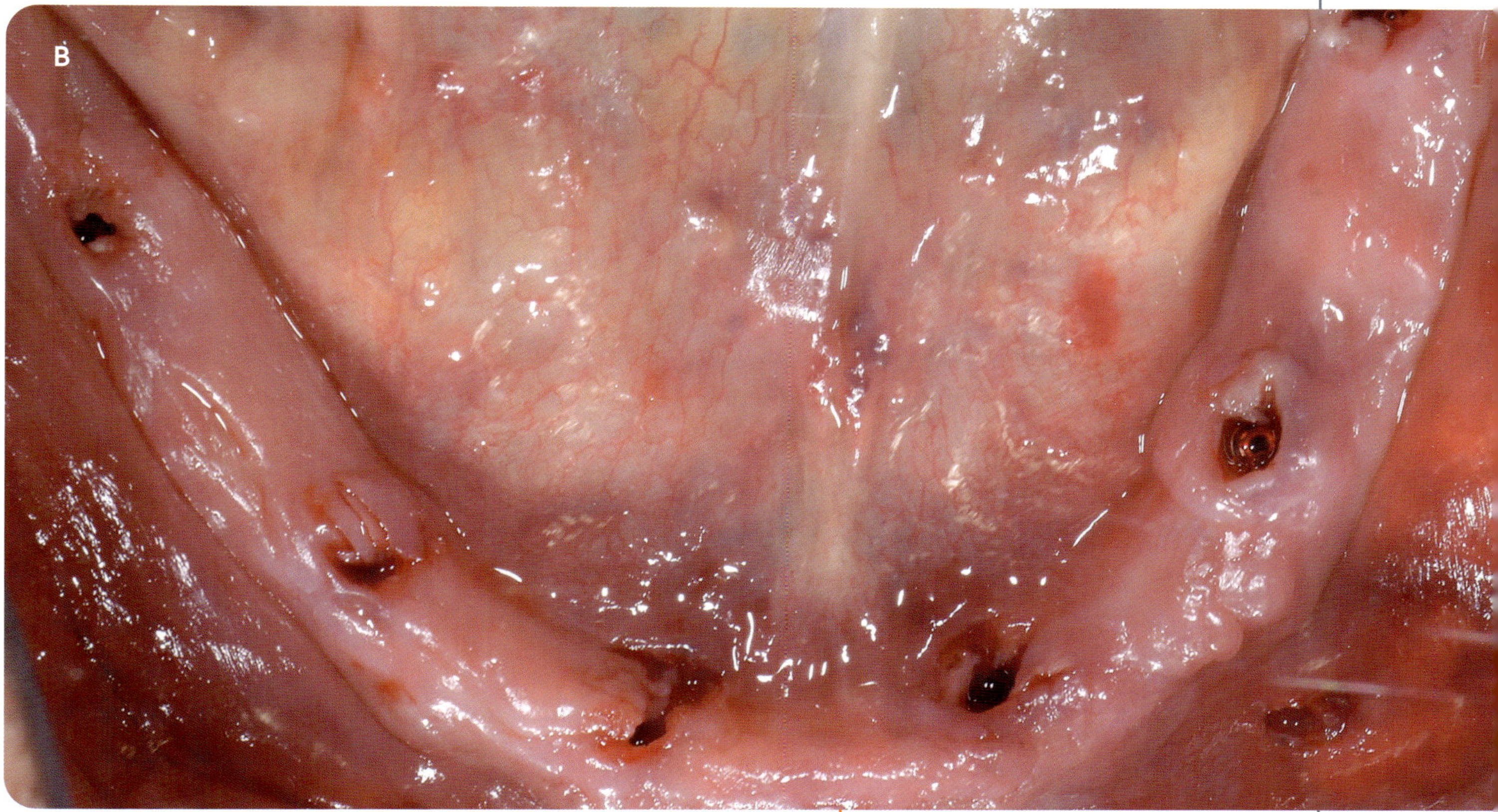

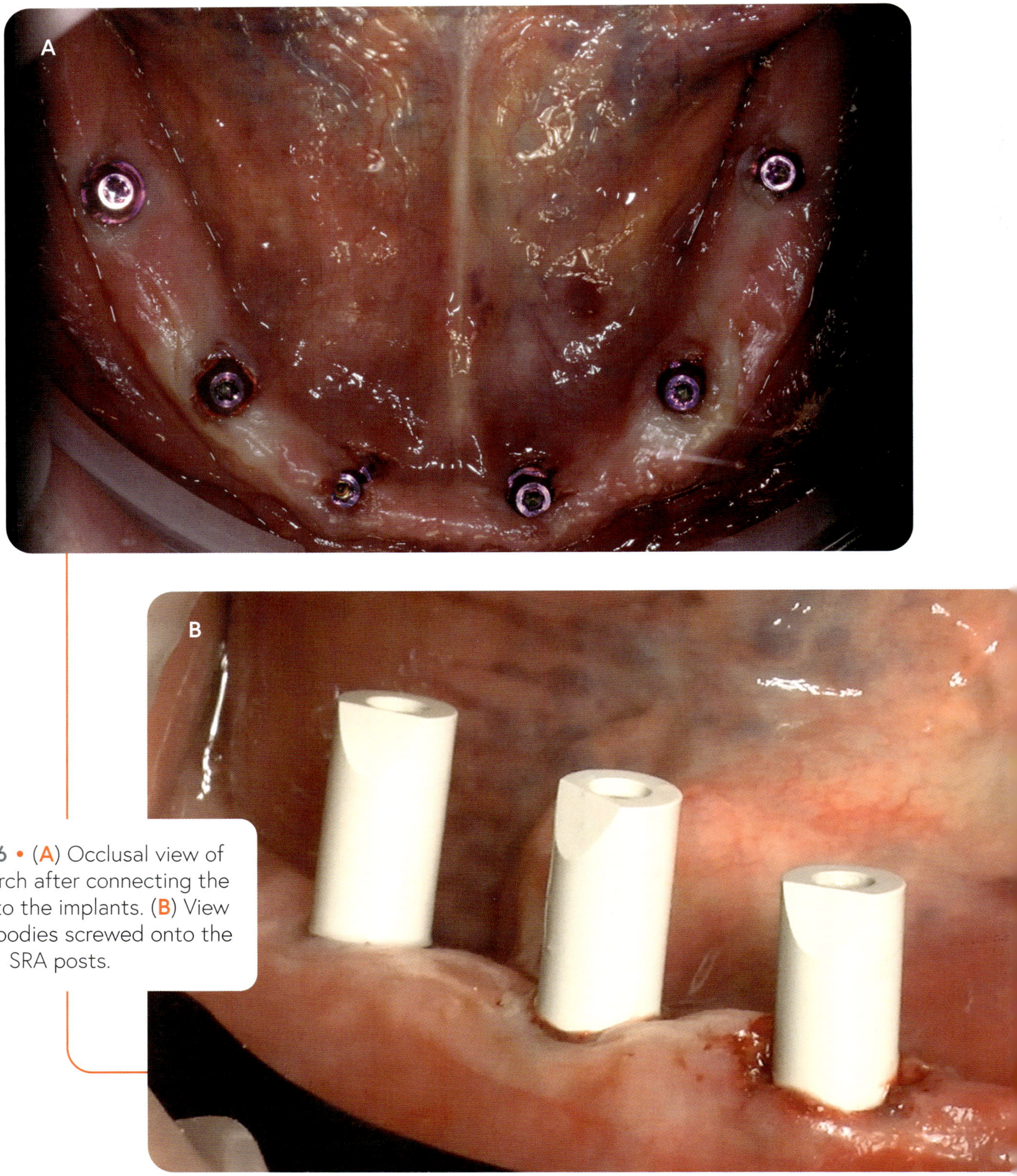

Figure 7.56 • (**A**) Occlusal view of the lower arch after connecting the SRA posts to the implants. (**B**) View of the scanbodies screwed onto the SRA posts.

This limitation is caused by the capture method of intraoral scanners and by the difficulty in reconstructing large surfaces [39]. Furthermore, it is particularly difficult to achieve accurate digital scans of the arch in which there are large homogeneous areas, such as the spaces between implants in edentulous arches. These difficulties are due to the absence of anatomical unevenness in the area to be scanned [40]. For this reason, an auxiliary device has been made with a dual function: to create the necessary unevenness in the scan area and register the intermaxillary relation. This special resin prosthetic stent was designed and 3D printed (SHERAprint-model plus UV sand, SHERA) from the digital design of the surgical guide with mucous support, especially for the area of the lower incisors and trigones. Furthermore, it featured the same three occlusal stops and the same sheaths for the pins as the surgical stent. Compared to the surgical guide, the prosthetic stent had six scanbody holes that were larger than the ferrule holes and were thinner in the scanbody regions. The increase in the space between the stent and the scan bodies allowed the intraoral scanner to recognise the scan bodies with the stent in place (**Figures 7.57** and **7.58**).

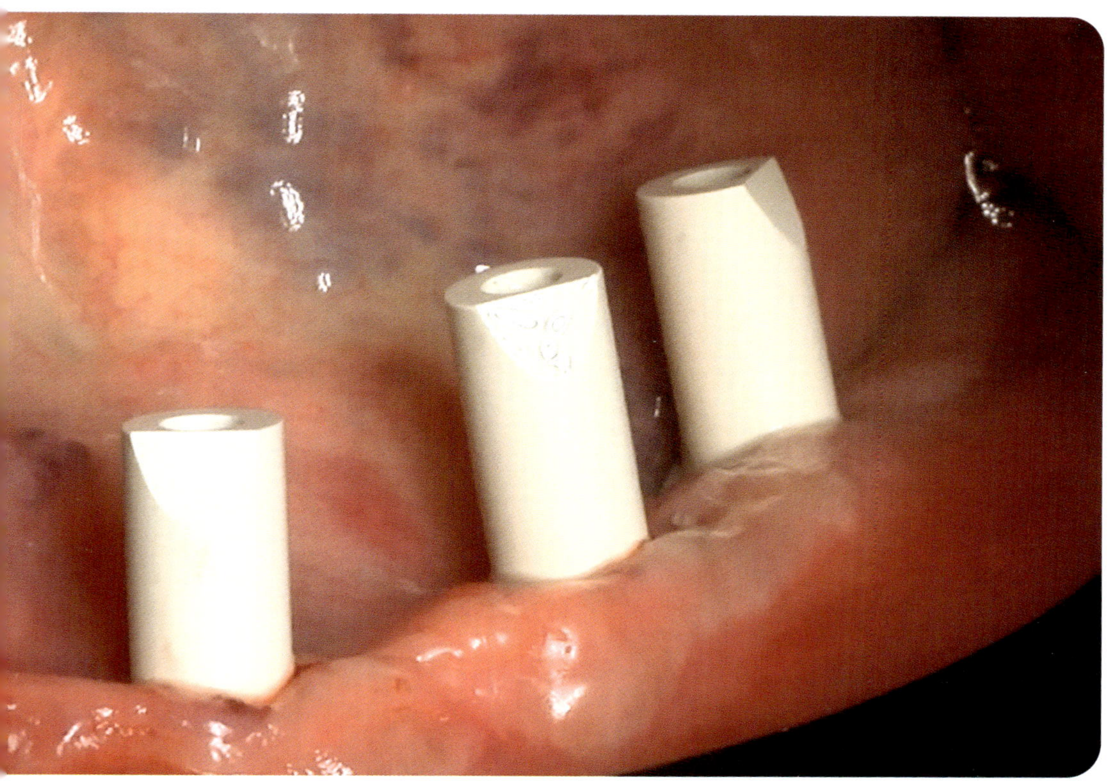

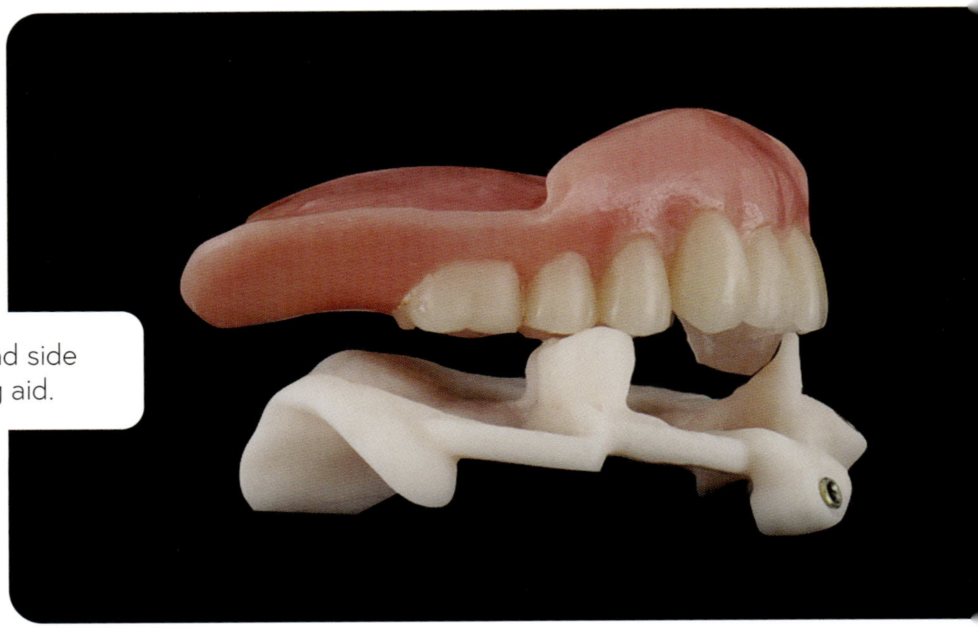

Figure 7.57 • Front and side view of the scanning aid.

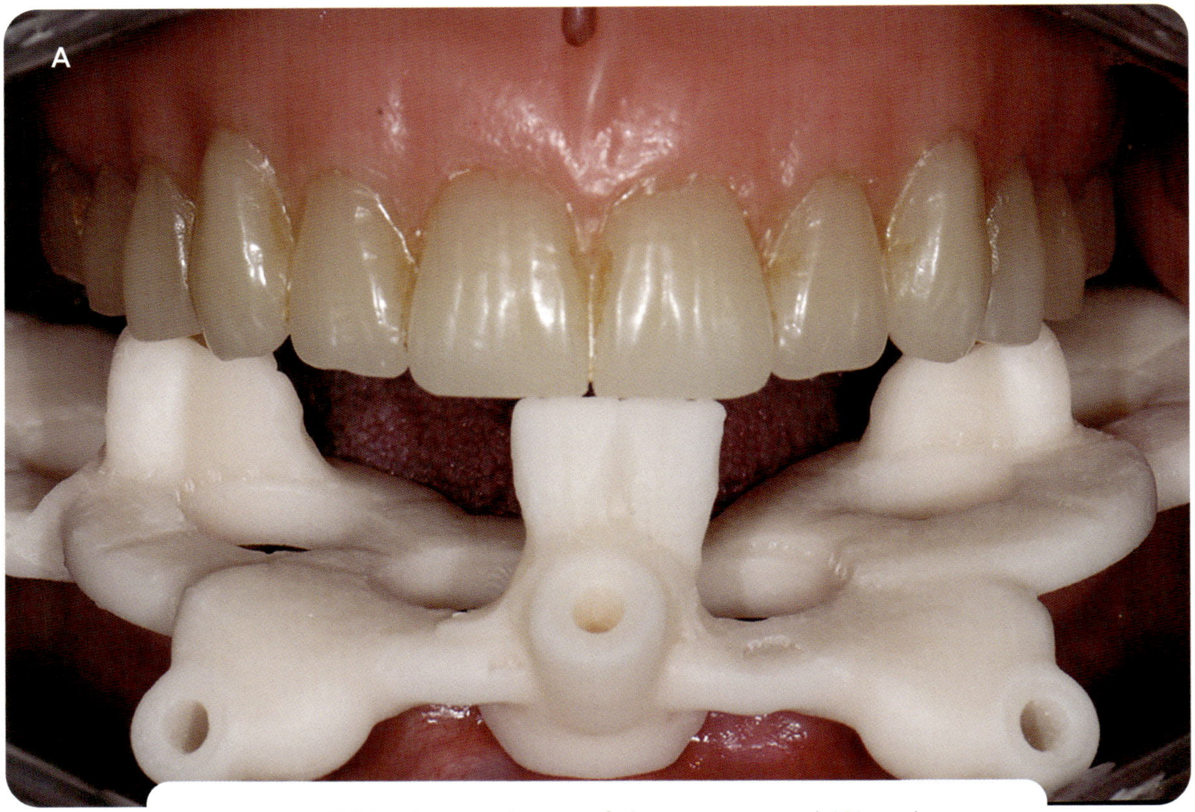

Figure 7.58 • Intraoral view of the scanning aid (A) and its occlusal view after stabilisation with the fixing pins (B).

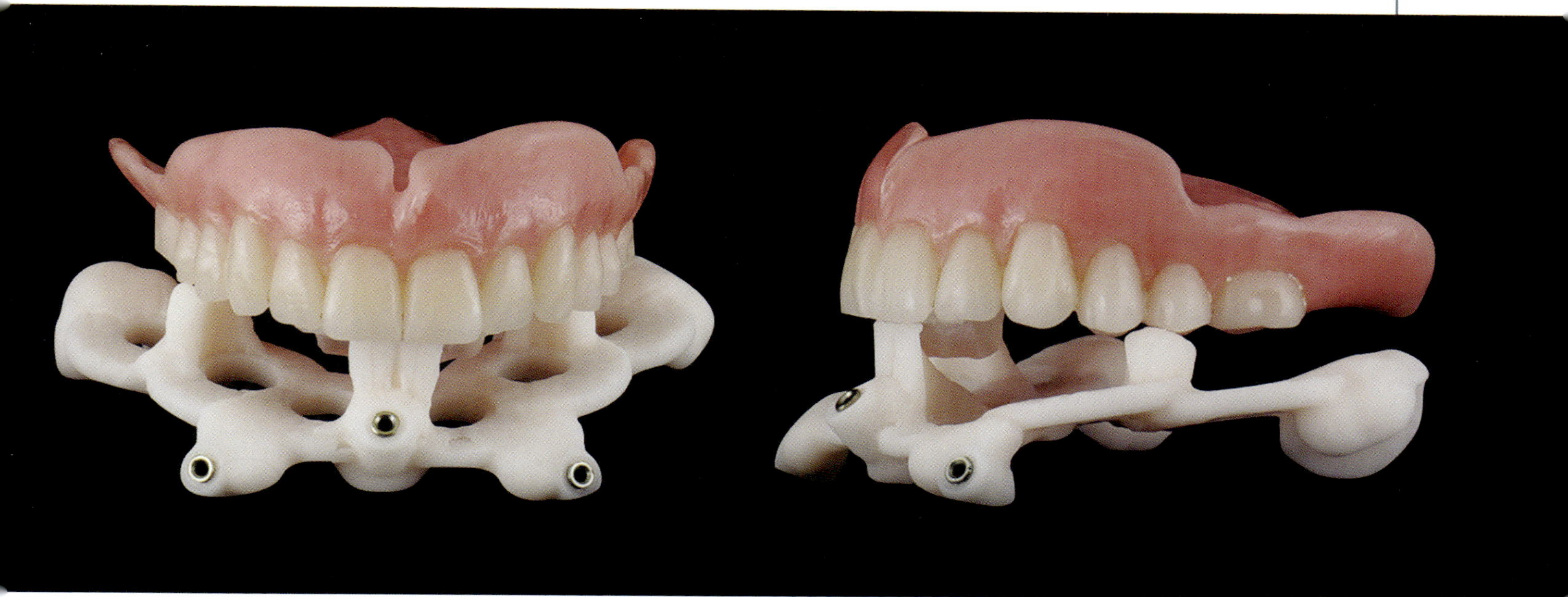

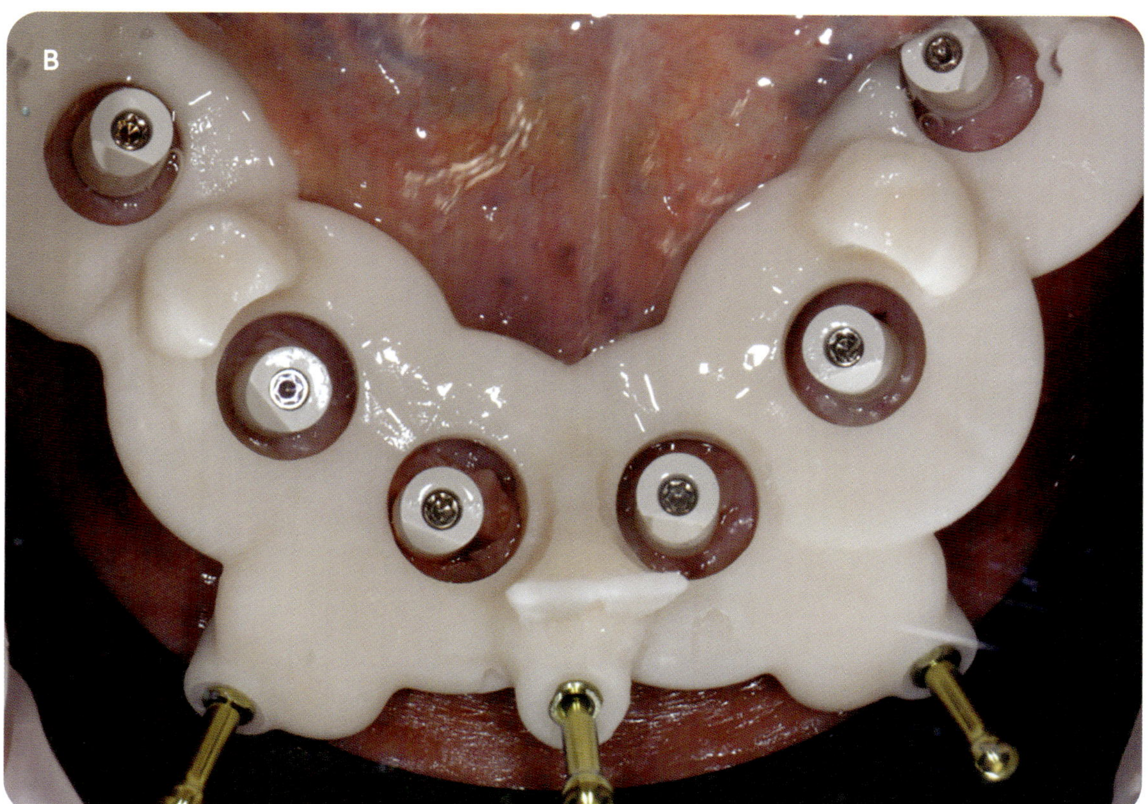
B

The scan of the maxillary prosthesis was easily taken outside the mouth. A digital impression was taken with an intraoral scanner (True Definition Scanner, 3M, Minneapolis USA) with the registration stent in place and, thanks to the occlusal reference points, it was possible to register the bite also on the left and right side **(Figures 7.59-7.62)**. The registered occlusal relation was exactly the same as the one the patient had with the two prostheses (an aspect that was very comfortable for him, as assessed in the treatment planning stage).

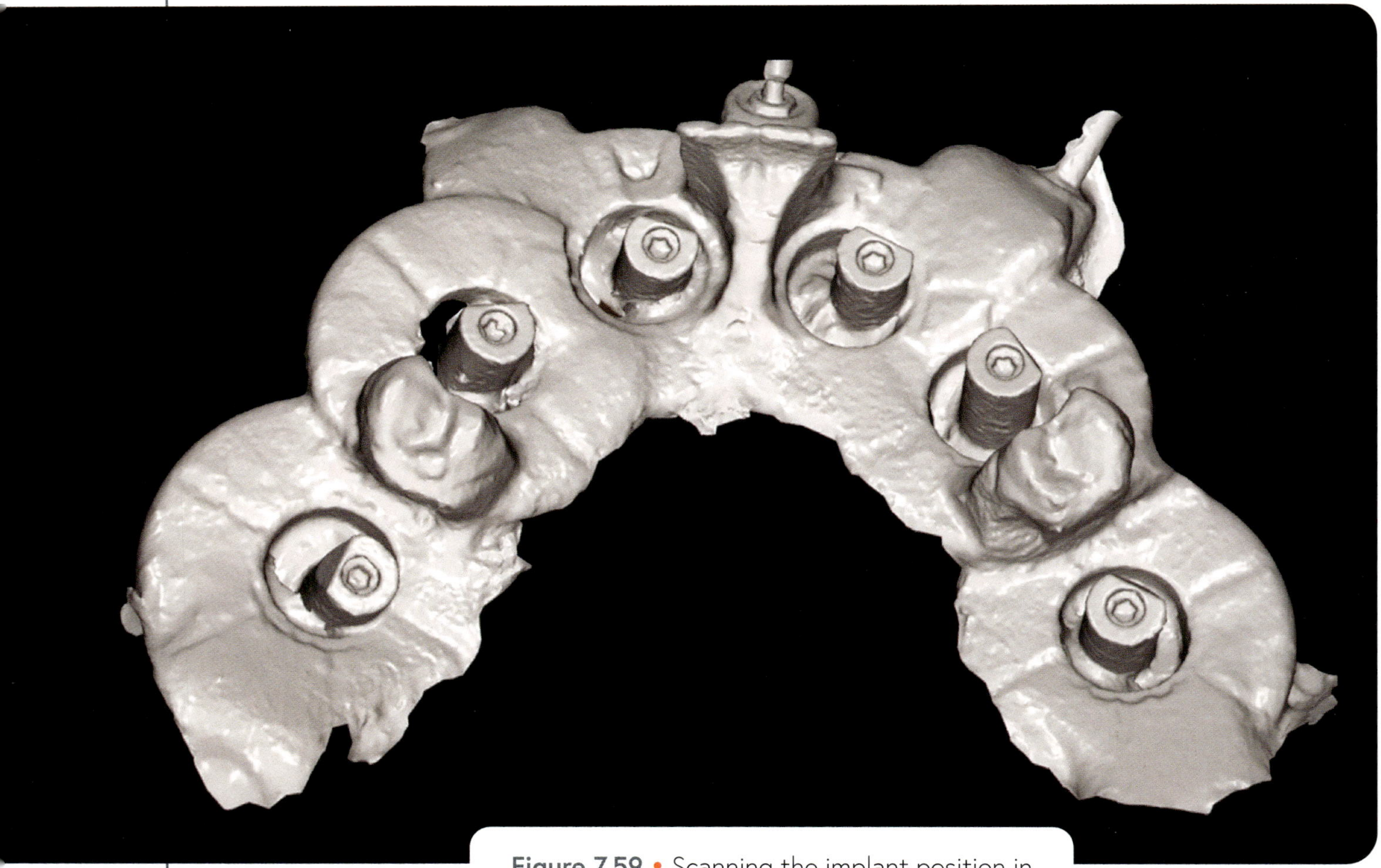

Figure 7.59 • Scanning the implant position in relation to the prosthetic stent.

At this stage of the treatment, the following STL files were available: one for the maxillary prosthesis, one for the mandibular implants plus the stent and two STL files for occlusion.

Since the soft tissues were missing in the lower impression with implants and stents, these were obtained virtually by superimposing the scan of the lower prosthesis and of the prosthetic stent.

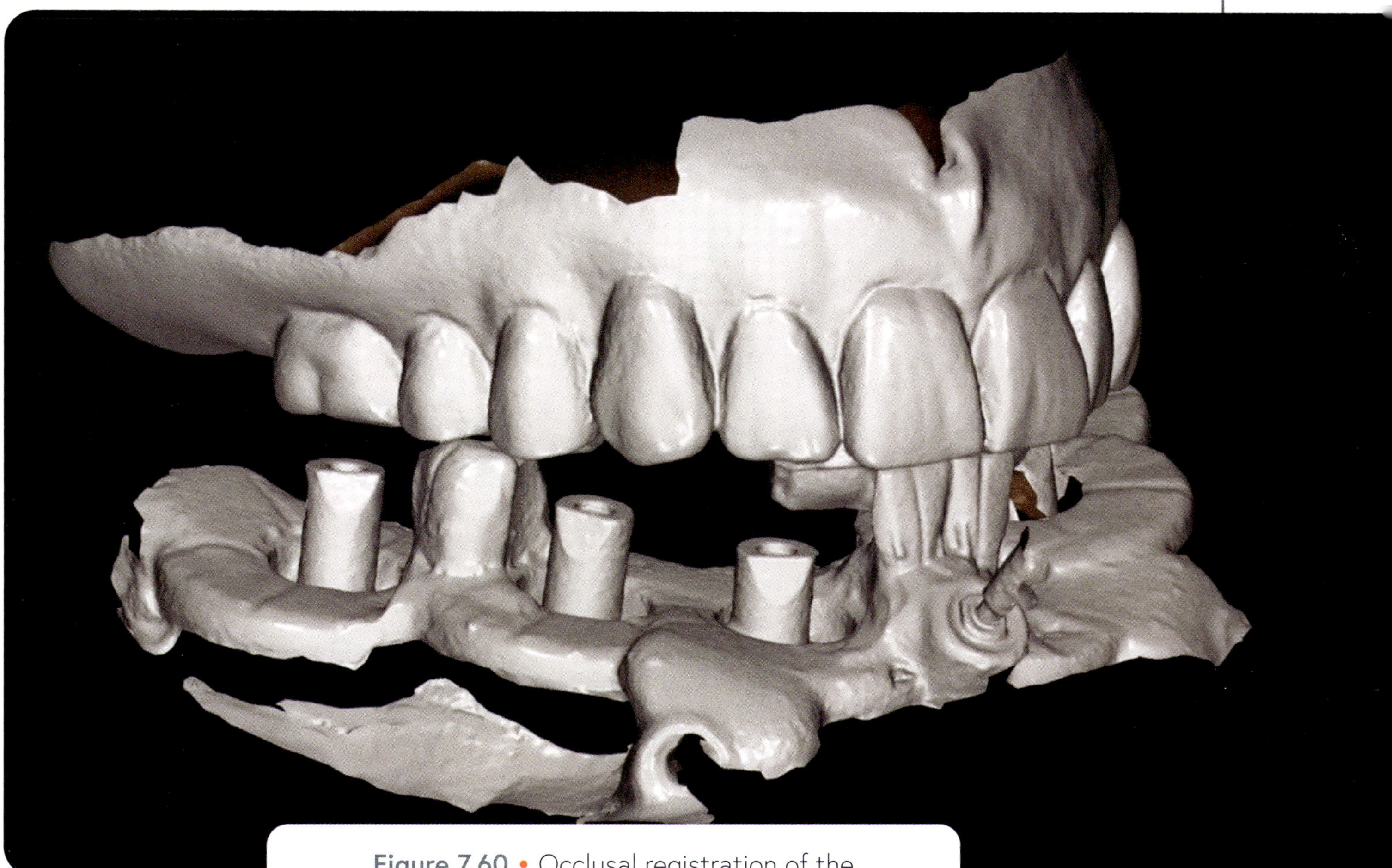

Figure 7.60 • Occlusal registration of the intermaxillary relationships between upper prosthesis and prosthetic stent.

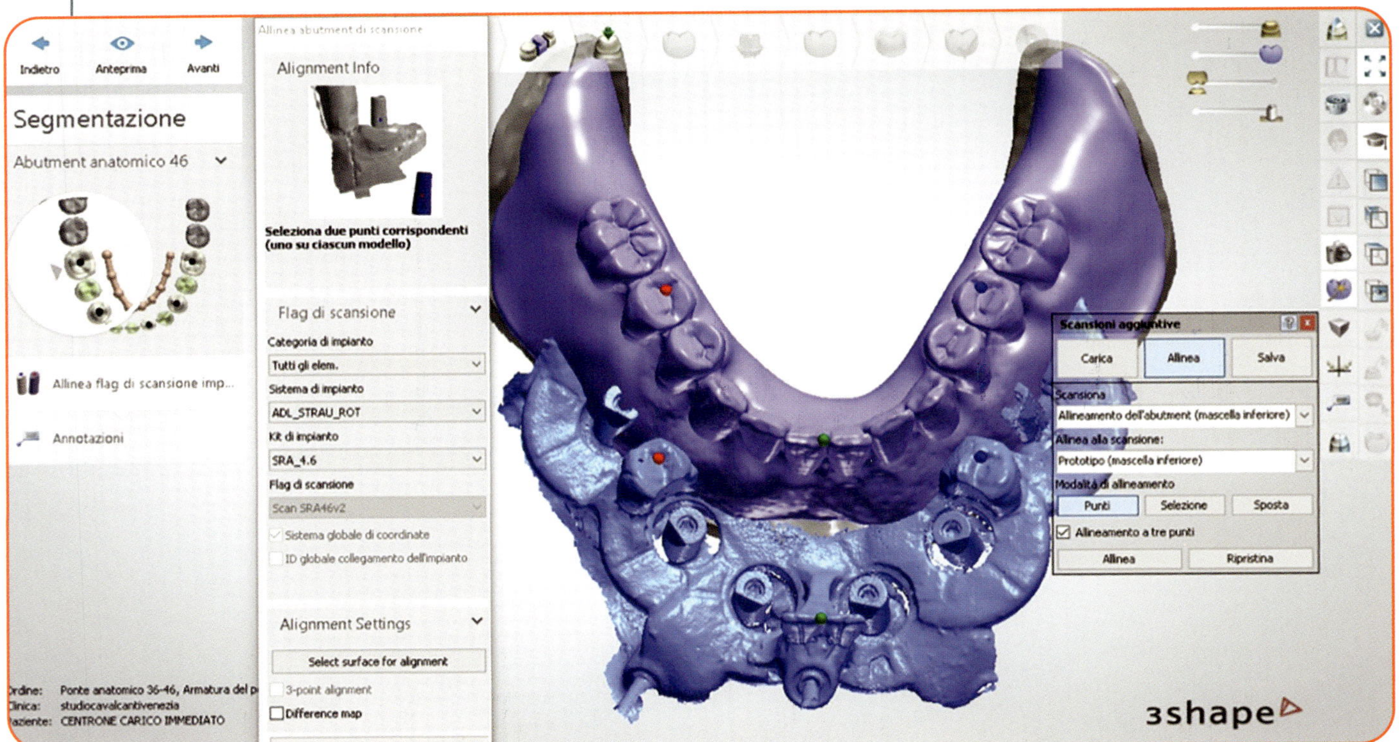

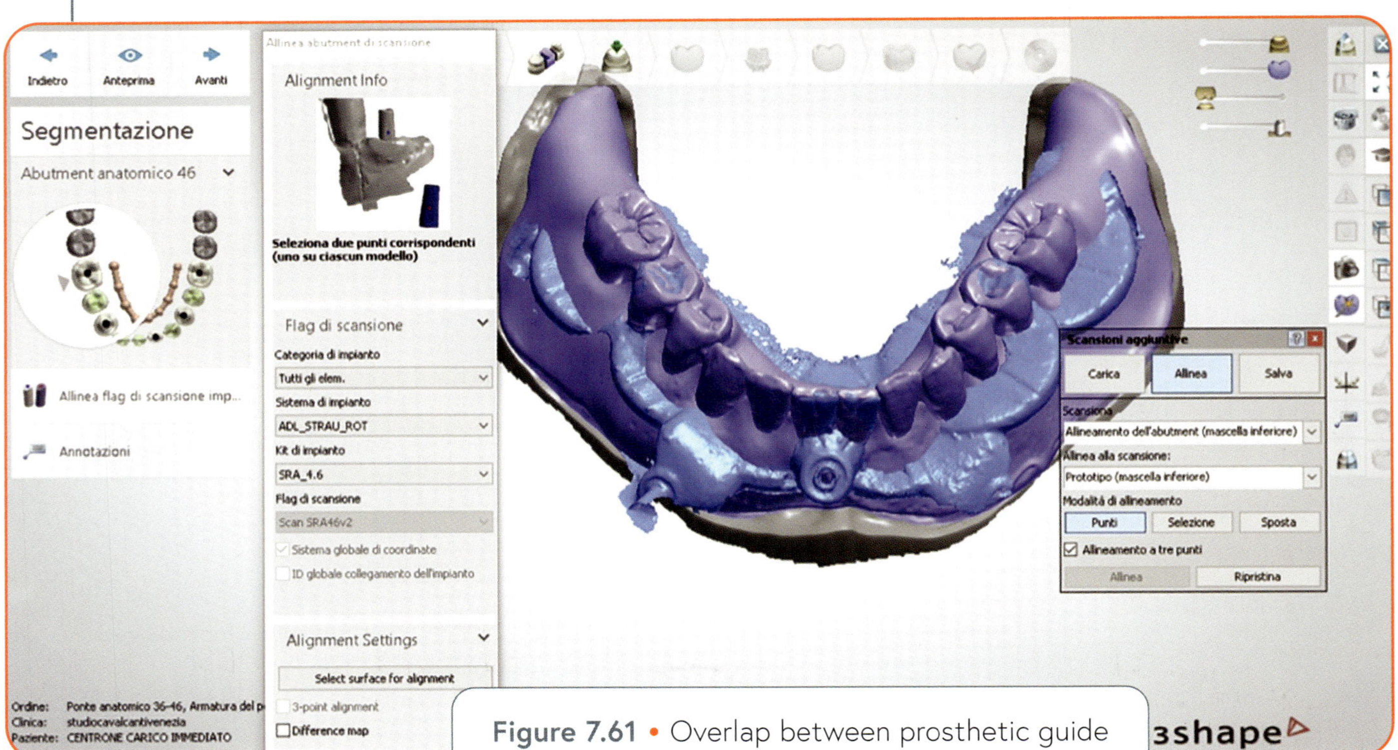

Figure 7.61 • Overlap between prosthetic guide and scan of the total lower prosthesis.

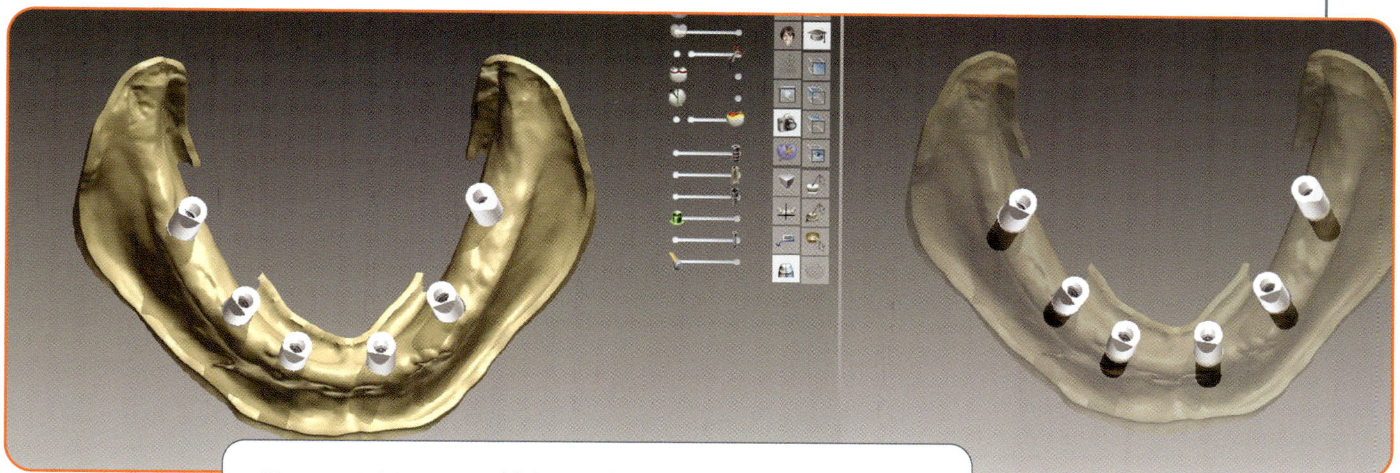

Figure 7.62 • Mandible model with registration of the scan bodies placed at the level of the SRA posts.

All previously registered information regarding the intermaxillary relations may be used for the implant-supported rehabilitation. The rehabilitation stage with the removable prostheses was carried out with care and with great effort to find the proper inter-arch relations. These data should be stored and, thanks to this technique, no information was lost. In this stage all the necessary information was in digital format: the scan of the mandibular arch with the implants and the stent in place, the scan of the opposite maxillary prosthesis, the file of the previous mandibular prosthesis and the bite registration with the intermaxillary relation taken with the prosthetic stent. All these files might be superposed thanks to consistent reference points.

It was possible to design a hybrid prosthesis using the Variobase titanium copy libraries (Institut Straumann AG), combined with the SRA abutments. The hybrid prosthesis was 3D printed (resin NEXTDENT C&B, Nextdent B.V., Soesterberg, Netherlands) and tried on 3D printed models (SHERAPRINT Model Plus UV GREY Resin, SHERA). It was then stained (Optiglaze, GC Europe, Leuven, Belgium) and finished, then the Variobase copings (Institut Straumann AG) were cemented using the digital models as reference **(Figure 7.63)**.

After polishing, the prosthesis made was delivered to the patient a few hours after the procedure. In this session, the fixing screws were tightened at 15 N/mm **(Figures 7.64-7.67)**.

The attention paid in the information transfer procedures made it possible to avoid significant occlusal modifications at the time of delivery, and the maintenance of the es-

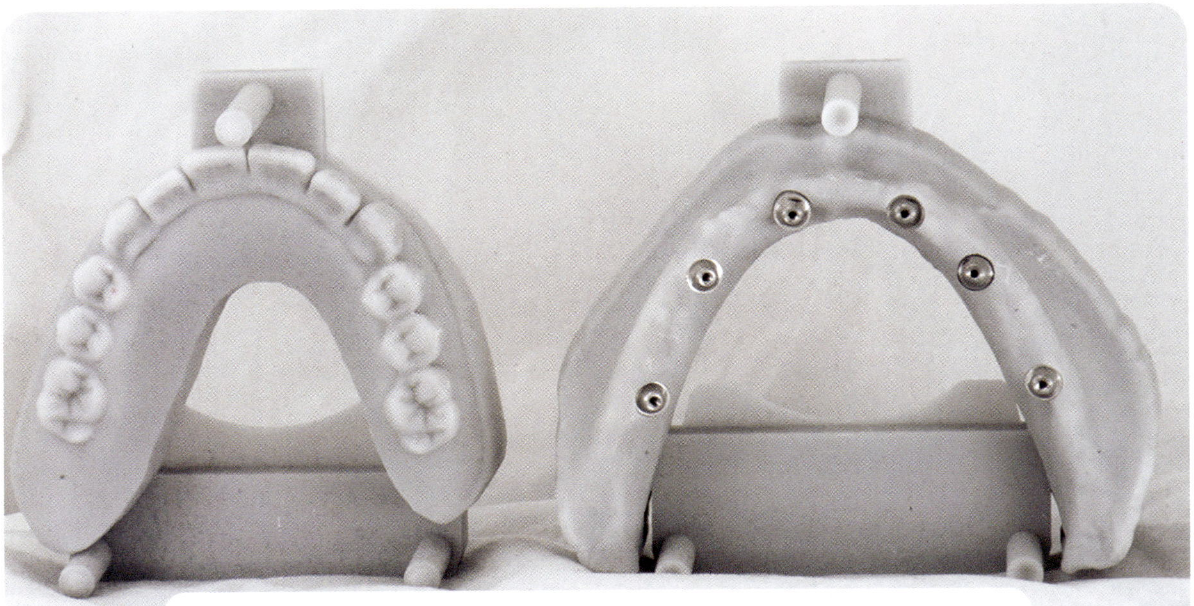

Figure 7.63 • Upper and lower models stereolithographed in occlusion at the vertical dimension previously registered.

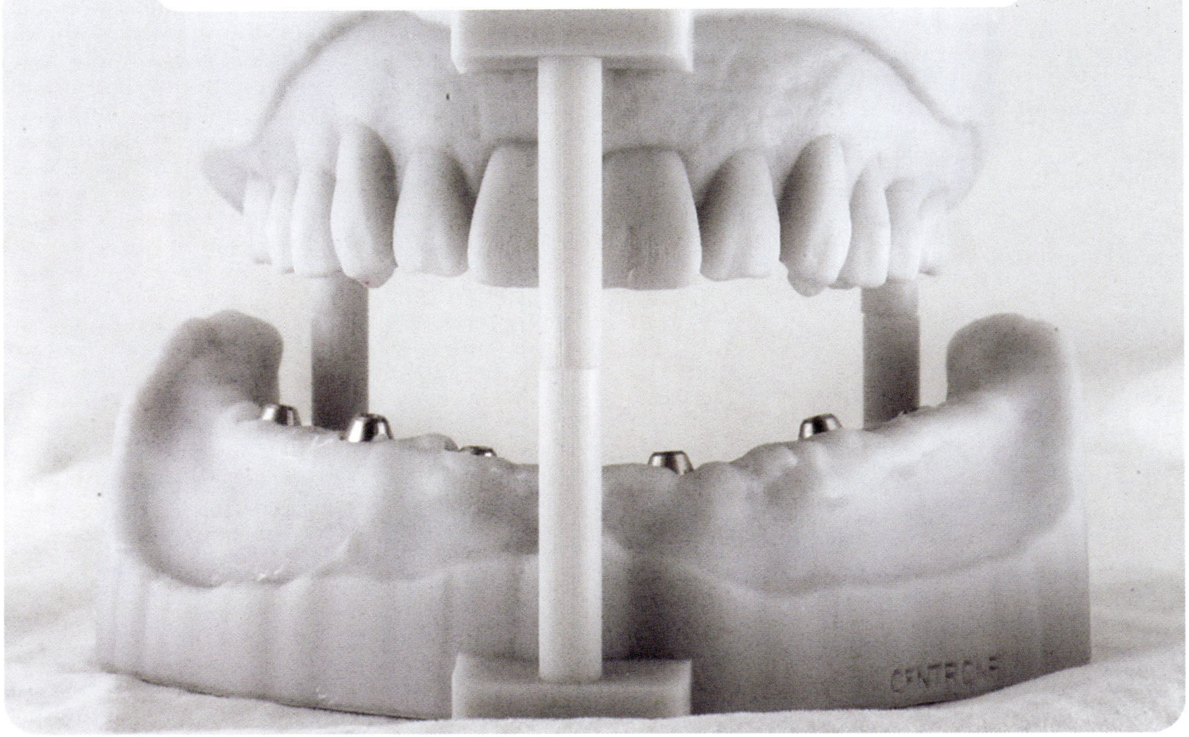

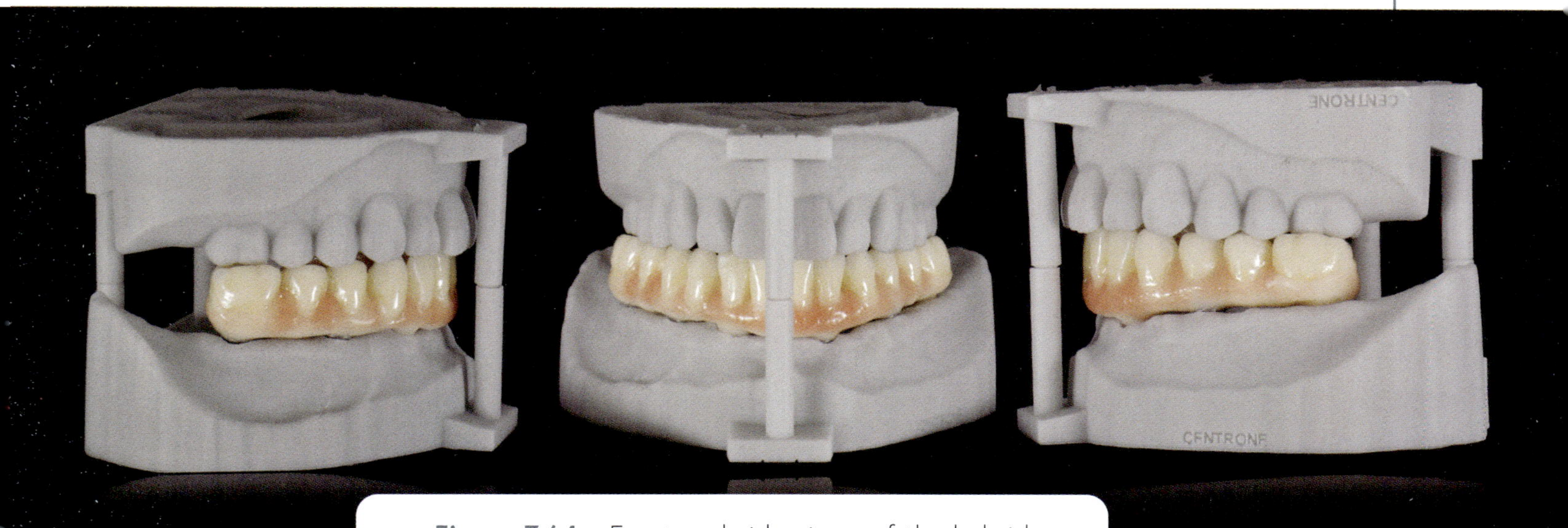

Figure 7.64 • Front and side views of the hybrid prosthesis made with 3D printing technology.

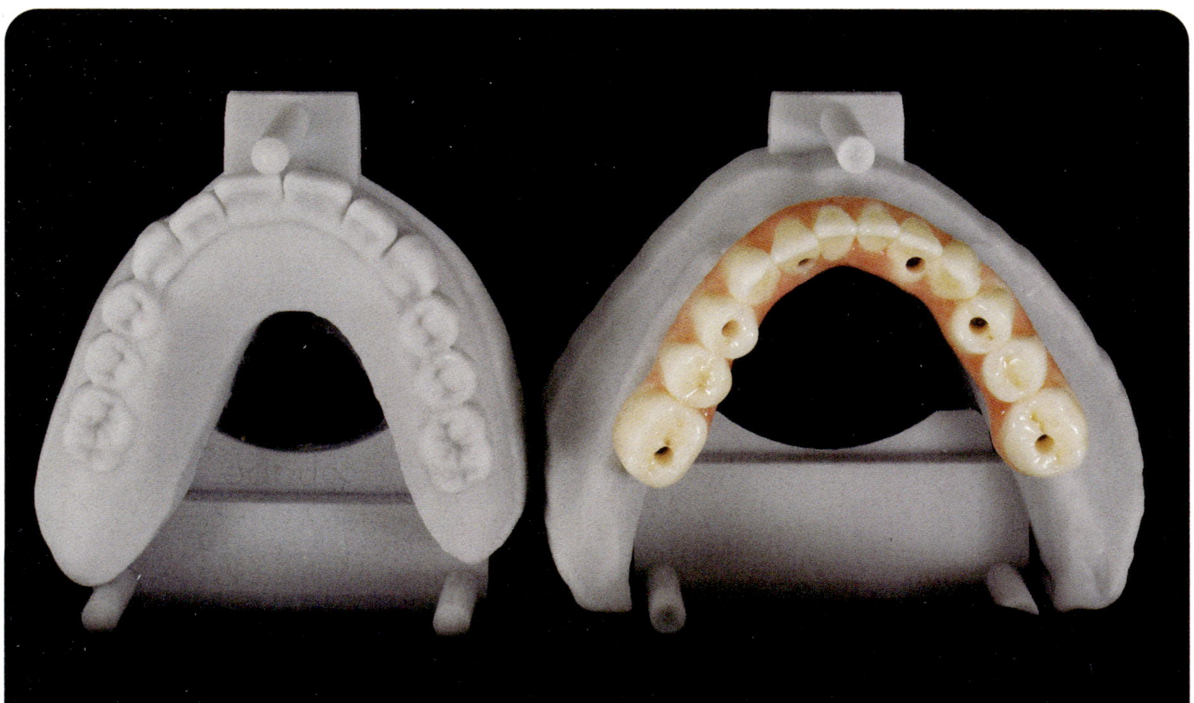

Figure 7.65 • Occlusal view of the hybrid prosthesis.

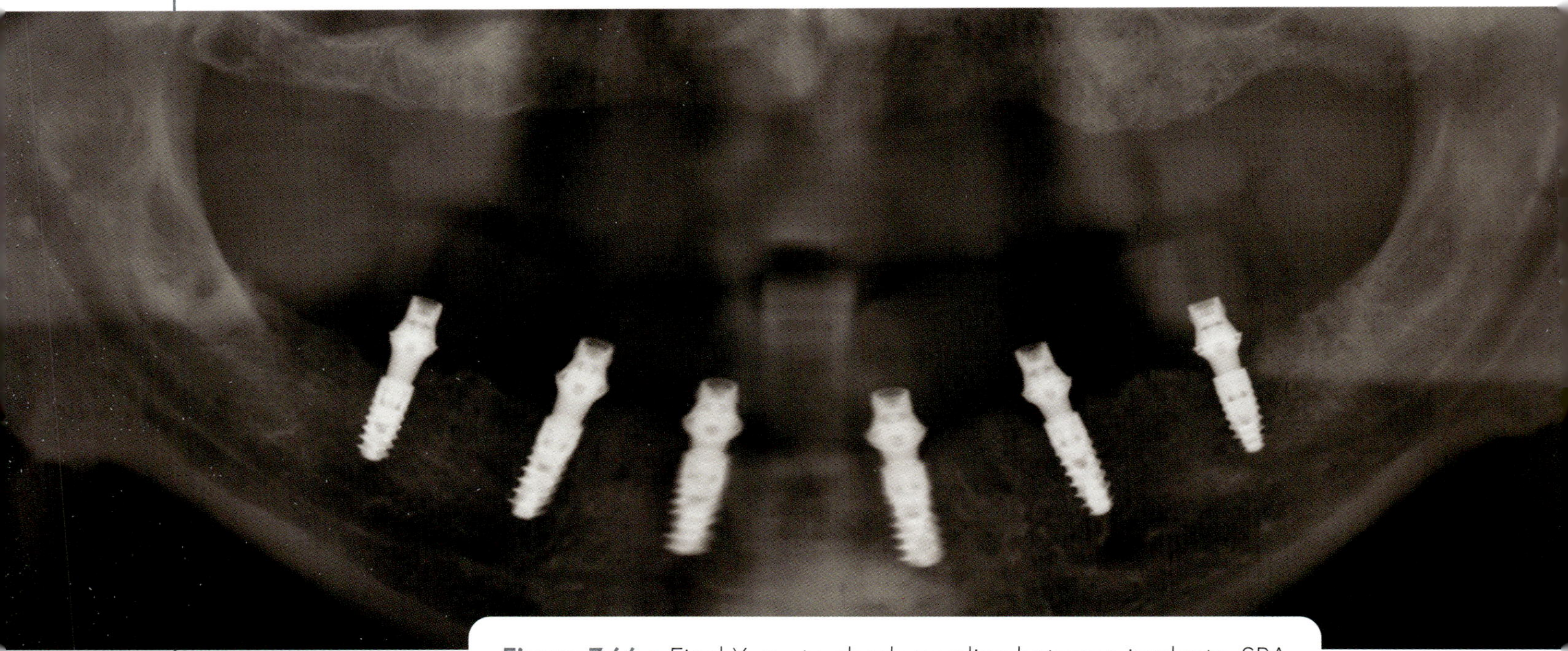

Figure 7.66 • Final X-ray to check coupling between implants, SRA posts and posts of the hybrid prosthesis.

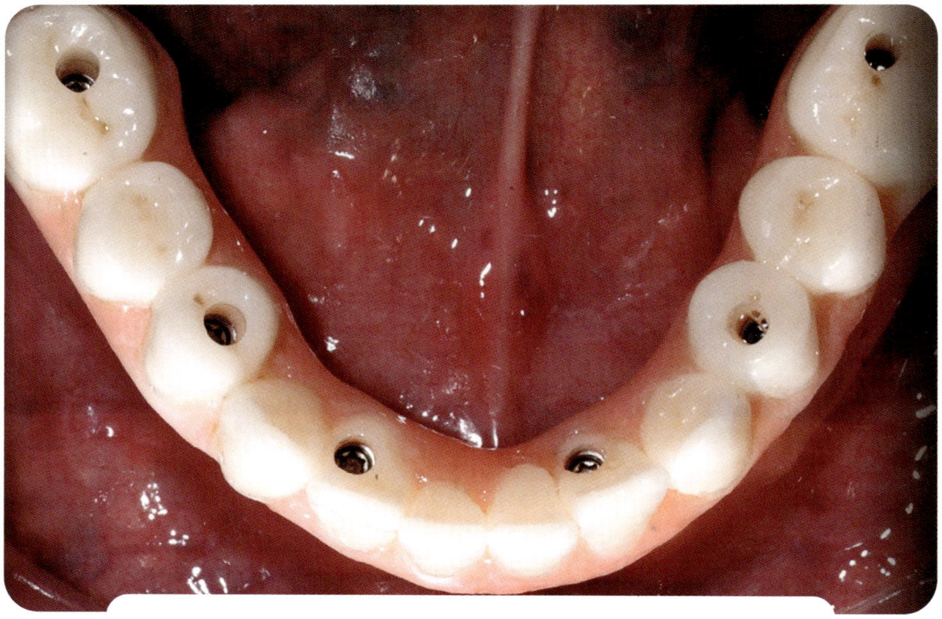

Figure 7.67 • Hybrid prosthesis seated on SRA posts after tightening the connection screws.

thetic and functional conditions already widely tested for several weeks in the patient's mouth. The provisional diagnostic stage with the removable prostheses was carried out with care and with great effort to find the proper intermaxillary relations. All previously registered information on the inter-arch relations was not lost and may be used for the implant-supported rehabilitation.

The delivery of the implant-supported hybrid prosthesis was carried out smoothly and with minimal occlusal adjustments, indicating that the technique enabled precise transfer of the prosthetic information. The patient was assigned to a maintenance programme with regular visits for professional oral hygiene and checks three times a year. The two-year follow-up showed a stable situation **(Figure 7.68)**.

The prosthetic stent used in this clinical case has a dual function. Firstly, the stent was useful for performing an accurate intraoral scan, as it is well documented that edentulous arches are critical clinical situations for intraoral scanning. The use of an auxiliary stent to increase the accuracy of intraoral scans has been described in the literature [41,42].

The device also enabled predictable registration of the intermaxillary relations.

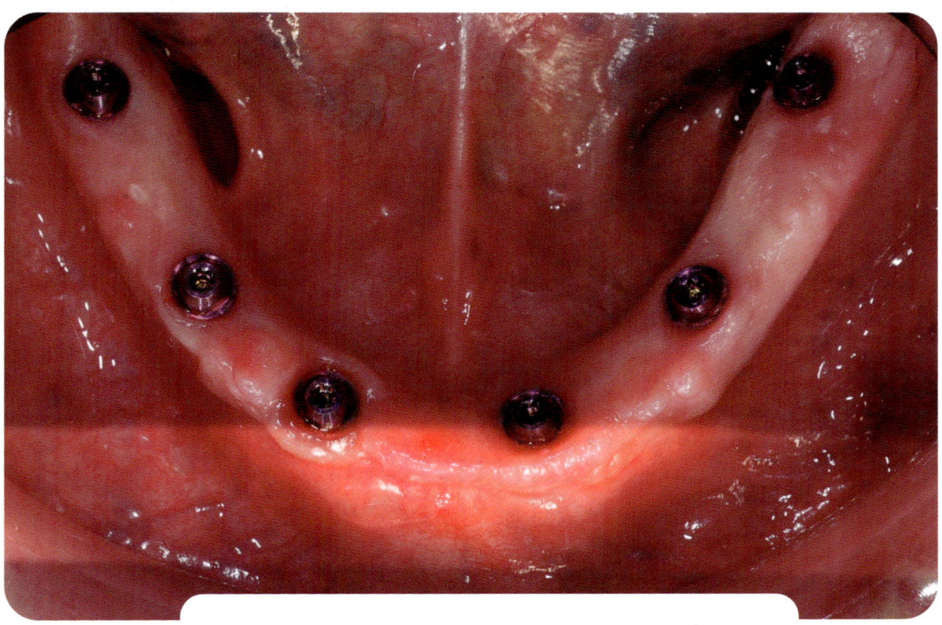

Figure 7.68 • Follow-up two years after fitting the lower fixed prosthesis.

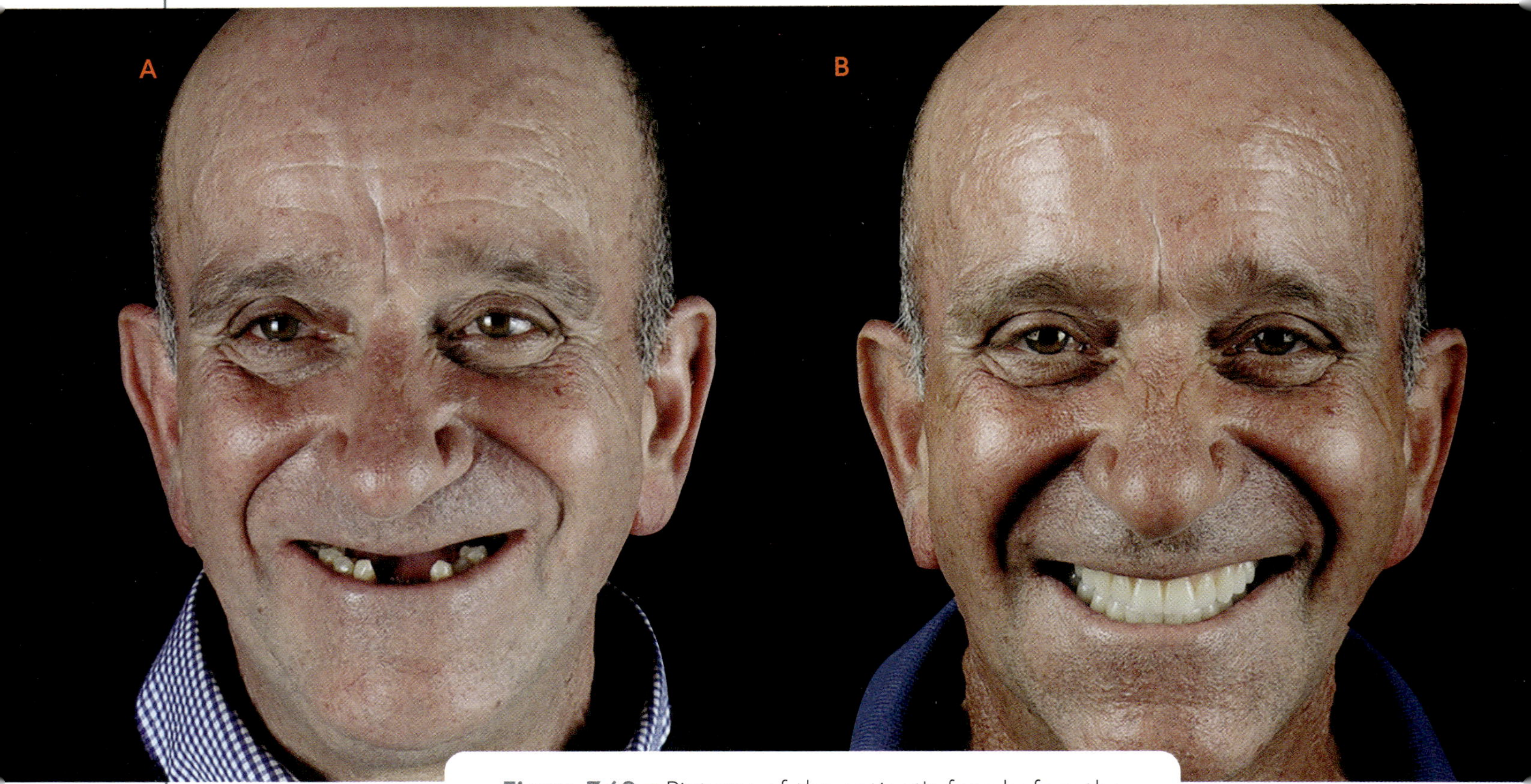

Figure 7.69 • Pictures of the patient's face before the treatment (**A**), after rehabilitation with full dentures made with CAD/CAM work flows (**B**) and after inserting the hybrid prosthesis in the lower arch (**C**).

In complex rehabilitations of already fully edentulous patients, the diagnostic phase is essential and must be carried out with a removable prosthesis. The subsequent steps, regardless of the analogue or digital workflows used, will be simple, reliable and predictable. New technologies and new materials can certainly aid in transferring the information obtained from the provisional prosthesis into the definitive one with implant anchoring.

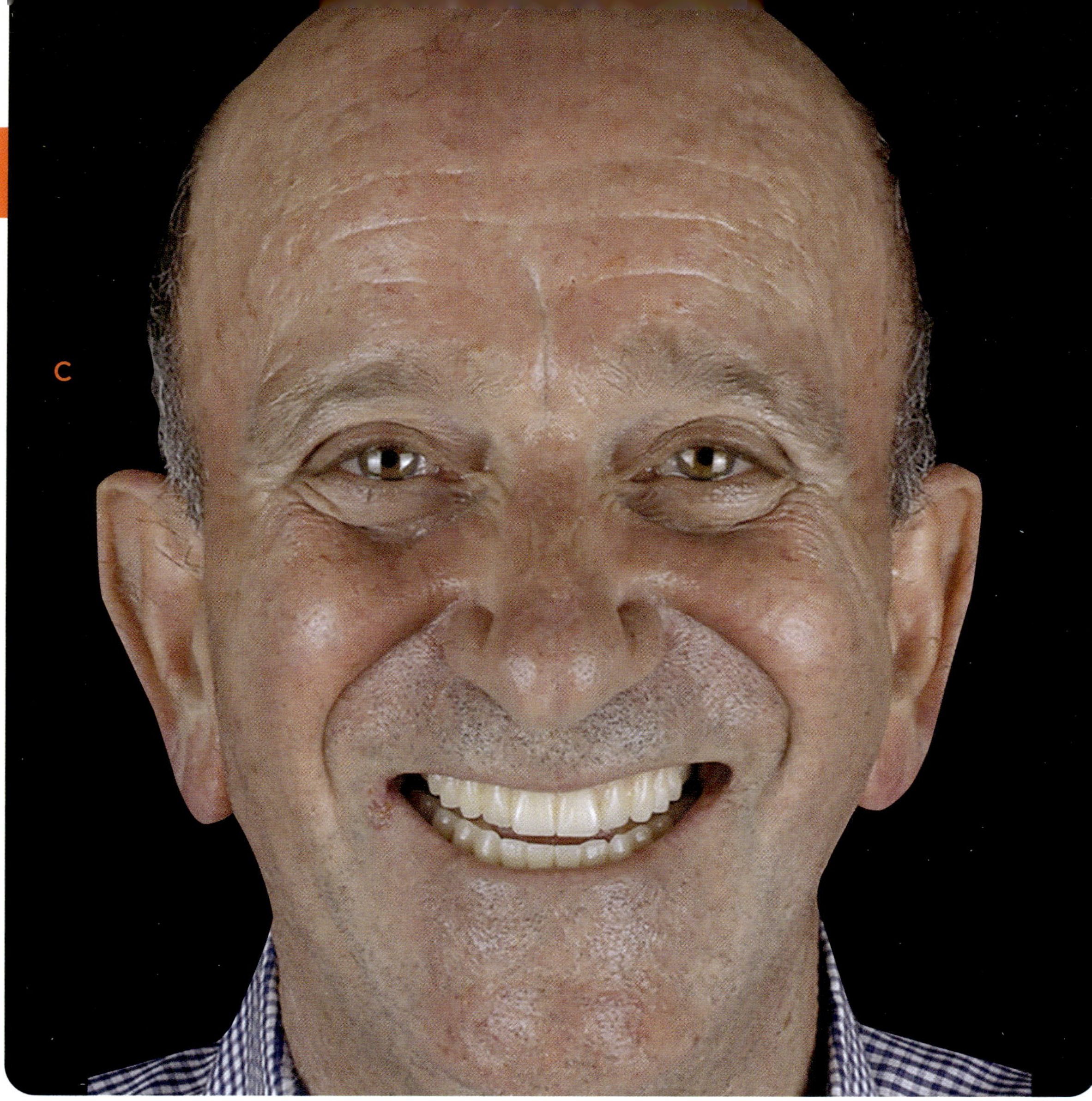

C

Final remarks

One of the difficulties in the prosthetic routine is to move from a satisfactory temporary restoration to an equally accurate final restoration. The B.A.R.I. Technique with an analogue workflow has therefore been described and proposed [28]. A protocol has also been proposed to digitally transfer prosthetic information (vertical dimension, centric relation, frontal and lateral guide and esthetics) in cases treated with fixed temporary prostheses [44]. The recording of intermaxillary relations has also been described for the fabrication of a 3D printed bite for patients with TMJ disorders [45].

Intraoral scans of edentulous arches can be challenging, mainly for two reasons: for intraoral scanners it is difficult to scan large edentulous areas and it is highly complex to record the correct relation between the arches.

Using a prosthetic stent makes it possible to solve both problems in an accurate and predictable manner.

References

1. Cochran DL, Morton D, Weber HP. Consensus statements and recommended clinical procedures regarding loading protocols for endosseous dental implants. *Int J Oral Maxillofac Implants*. 2004;(19, Suppl):109-13.
2. Gallucci GO, Morton D, Weber HP. Loading protocols for dental implants in edentulous patients. *Int J Oral Maxillofac Implants*. 2009;(24, suppl):132-46.
3. Chiapasco M, Gatti C, Rossi E et al. Implant-retained mandibular overdentures with immediate loading. A retrospective multicenter study on 226 consecutive cases. *Clin Oral Implants Res*. 1997;8(1):48-57.
4. Turkyilmaz I, Sennerby L, McGlumphy EA, Tözüm TF. Biomechanical aspects of primary implant stability: A human cadaver study. *Clin Implant Dent Relat Res*. 2009;11(2):113-9.
5. Wolfinger GJ, Balshi TJ, Rangert B. Immediate functional loading of Brånemark system implants in edentulous mandibles: clinical report of the results of developmental and simplified protocols. *Int J Oral Maxillofac Implants*. 2003;18(2):250-7.
6. Cooper LF, Rahman A, Moriarty J et al. Immediate mandibular rehabilitation with endosseous implants: simultaneous extraction, implant placement, and loading. *Int J Oral Maxillofac Implants*. 2002;17(4):517-25.
7. Gallucci GO, Bernard JP, Bertosa M, Belser UC. Immediate loading with fixed screw-retained provisional restorations in edentulous jaws: the pickup technique. *Int J Oral Maxillofac Implants*. 2004;19(4):524-33.
8. Maló P, Rangert B, Nobre M. "All-on-four" immediate-function concept with brånemark system® implants for completely edentulous mandibles: A retrospective clinical study. *Clin Implant Dent Relat Res*. 2003;5(Suppl. 1):2-9.
9. Cordaro L, Torsello F. Soft tissue conditioning by immediate restoration of immediately placed implants in full-arch rehabilitation: the double provisional technique. *Eur J Esthet Dent*. 2006;1(3):216-29.
10. Kozawa T, Igarashi Y, Yamashita S. Posterior occlusal support and bite force influence on the mandibular position. *Eur J Prosthodont Restor Dent*. 2003;11(1):33-40.
11. Cura C, Saraçoğlu A, Oztürk B. Prosthetic rehabilitation of extremely worn dentition: case reports. *Quintessence Int (Berl)*. 2002;33(3):225-30.
12. Millet C, Jeannin C, Vincent B, Malquarti G. Report on the determination of occlusal vertical dimension and centric relation using swallowing in edentulous patients. *J Oral Rehabil*. 2003;30(11):1118-22.
13. Coelho Goiato M, Garcia AR, Micheline dos Santos D. Electromyographic evaluation of masseter and anterior temporalis muscles in resting position and during maximum tooth clenching of edentulous patients before and after new complete dentures. *Acta odontológica Latinoam*. 2007;20(2):67-72.
14. Biscaro L, Becattelli A, Poggio PM et al. The one-model technique: a new method for immediate loading with fixed prostheses in edentulous or potentially edentulous jaws. *Int J Periodontics Restor Dent*. 2009;29(3):307-13.
15. Brunski JB. Avoid pitfalls of overloading and micromotion of intraosseous implants. *Dent Implantol Update*. 1993;4(10):77-81.
16. Szmukler-Moncler S, Salama H, Reingewirtz Y, Dubruille JH. Timing of loading and effect of micromotion on bone-dental implant interface: Review of experimental literature. J Biomed Mater Res. 1998;43:192-203.
17. Torsello F, Mirisola di Torresanto V, Cordaro L, Ercoli C. Evaluation of the marginal precision of one-piece complete arch titanium frameworks fabricated using five different methods for implant-supported restorations. *Clin Oral Implants Res*. 2008;19:772-9.
18. Chiapasco M, Gatti C, Rossi E et al. Implant-retained mandibular overdentures with immediate loading. A retrospective multicenter study on 226 consecutive cases. *Clin Oral Implant Res*. 1997;8:48-57.
19. Cochran DL, Morton D, Weber HP. Consensus statements and recommended clinical procedures regarding loading protocols for endosseous dental implants. *Int J Oral Maxillofac Implant*. 2004;19:109-13.
20. Gallucci GO, Morton D, Weber HP. Loading protocols for dental implants in edentulous patients. *Int J Oral Maxillofac Implant*. 2009;24:132-46.
21. Cooper LF, Rahman A, Moriarty J et al. Immediate mandibular rehabilitation with endosseous implants: Simultaneous extraction, implant place-

ment, and loading. *Int J Oral Maxillofac Implant*. 2002:17:517-25.
22. Wolfinger GJ, Balshi TJ, Rangert B. Immediate functional loading of Branemark system implants in edentulous mandibles: Clinical report of the results of developmental and simplified protocols. *Int J Oral Maxillofac Implant*. 2003;18:250-7.
23. Gallucci GO, Bernard JP, Bertossa M, Belser UC. Immediate loading with fixed screw retained provvisional restorations in edentulous jaws: The pickup technique. Int J Oral Maxillofac Implant 2004;19:524-33.
24. Maló P, Rangert B, Nobre M. "All-on-Four" immediate-function concept with Brånemark System implants for completely edentulous mandibles: A retrospective clinical study. *Clin Implant Dent Relat Res*. 2003;5(Suppl. 1):2-9.
25. Cordaro L, Torsello F. Soft tissues conditioning by immediate restoration of immediately placed implants in full-arch rehabilitation: The double provisional technique. *Eur J Esthet Dent*. 2006;1:216-29.
26. Kozawa T, Igarashi Y, Yamashita S. Posterior occlusal support and bite force influence on the mandibular position. *Eur J Prosthodont Restor Dent*. 2003;11:33-40.
27. Venezia P, Torsello F. Orientation of digital casts according to facial lines. *J Prosthet Dent*. 2018;120, 964-5.
28. Venezia P, Lacasella P, Cordaro L et al. The BARI technique: A new approach to immediate loading. *Int J Esthet Dent*. 2015;10:428-43.
29. Albdour EA, Shaheen E, Vranckx M et al. A novel in vivo method to evaluate trueness of digital impressions. *BMC Oral Health*. 2018;18:117.
30. Mangano F, Mangano C, Margiani B, Admakin O. Combining intraoral and face scans for the design and fabrication of computer-assisted design/ computer-assisted manufacturing (CAD/CAM) polyether-ether-ketone (PEEK) implant-supported bars for maxillary overdentures. *Scanning 2019*. 2019;4274715.
31. Jacobs R, Salmon B, Codari M et al. Cone beam computed tomography in implant dentistry: Recommendations for clinical use. *BMC Oral Health*. 2018;18:87.
32. Bonnet G, Batisse C, Bessadet M et al. A new digital denture procedure: A first practitioners appraisal. *BMC Oral Health*. 2017;17:155.
33. Unkovskiy A, Wahl E, Zander AT et al. Intraoral scanning to fabricate complete dentures with functional borders: A proof-of-concept case report. *BMC Oral Health*. 2019;19:46.
34. Tahmaseb A, Wu V, Wismeijer D et al. The accuracy of static computer-aided implant surgery: A systematic review and meta-analysis. *Clin. Oral Implant. Res.* 2018;29 (Suppl. 16):416-35.
35. Raico Gallardo YN, da Silva-Olivio IRT, Mukai E et al. Accuracy comparison of guided surgery for dental implants according to the tissue of support: A systematic review and meta-analysis. *Clin Oral Implant Res*. 2017;28:602-12.
36. Spielau T, Hauschild U, Katsoulis J. Computer-assisted, template-guided immediate implant placement and loading in the mandible: A case report. *BMC Oral Health*. 2019;19:55.
37. Colombo M, Mangano C, Mijiritsky E et al. Clinical applications and effectiveness of guided implant surgery: A critical review based on randomized controlled trials. *BMC Oral Health*. 2017;17:150.
38. Kühl S, Payer M, Zitzmann NU et al. Printed template for guided implantation. *Clin Implant Dent Relat Res*. 2015;17:e177-e182.
39. Mangano F, Hauschild U, Veronesi G et al. Trueness and precision of 5 intraoral scanners in the impressions of single and multiple implants: A comparative in vitro study. *BMC Oral Health*. 2019;19:101.
40. Osnes CA, Wu JH, Venezia P et al. Full arch precision of six intraoral scanners in vitro. *J Prosthodont Res*. 2020 Jan;64(1):6-11.
41. Brunsvold MA. Pathologic tooth migration. *J Periodontol*. 2005;6:859-66.
42. Iturrate M, Minguez R, Pradies G, Solaberrieta E. Obtaining reliable intraoral digital scans for an implant supported complete-arch prosthesis: A dental technique. *J Prosthet Dent*. 2019, 121, 237-41.
43. Iturrate M, Eguiraun H, Etxaniz O, Solaberrieta E. Accuracy analysis of complete-arch digital scans in edentulous arches when using an auxiliary geometric device. *J Prosthet Dent*. 2019;121: 447-54.
44. Venezia P, Torsello F, D'Amato S, Cavalcanti R. Digital cross-mounting: A new opportunity in prosthetic dentistry. *Quintessence Int*. 2017;48:701-9.
45. Venezia P, Lo Muzio L, De Furia C, Torsello F. Digital manufacturing of occlusal splint: From intraoral scanning to 3D printing. *J Osseointegr*. 2019;11(4):535-39.